Color Atlas of Hematology

An Illustrated Field Guide Based on Proficiency Testing

Atlas Subcommittee
of the
Hematology and Clinical Microscopy
Resource Committee

Eric F. Glassy, MD
Chairman and Editor

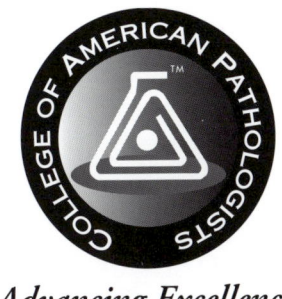

Advancing Excellence

College of American Pathologists
Northfield, Illinois

© 1998 College of American Pathologists (CAP). All rights reserved. None of the contents of this publication may be reproduced, stored in a retrieval system, or transmitted in any form or by any means (electronic, mechanical, photocopying, recording, or otherwise) without prior written permission from the publisher.

The inclusion of a product name or service in a CAP publication should not be construed as an endorsement of such product or service, nor is failure to include the name of a product or service to be construed as disapproval.

Library of Congress Catalog Card Number: 98-71043
ISBN: 0-930304-66-7

Printed in U.S.A.

Extra copies available from:
College of American Pathologists
325 Waukegan Road
Northfield, Illinois 60093-2750
800-323-4040

20004/00

Color Atlas of Hematology

An Illustrated Field Guide Based on Proficiency Testing

College of American Pathologists
Hematology and Clinical Microscopy
Resource Committee

Editor
Eric F. Glassy, MD

Atlas Subcommittee Members
Steven J. Agosti, MD
P. Joanne Cornbleet, MD, PhD
Katherine Galagan, MD
Amy S. Gewirtz, MD
Eric F. Glassy, MD
Robert Novak, MD
Catherine Spier, MD

Illustrations, Design and Layout
Eric F. Glassy, MD

Contents

Preface viii
Acknowledgements ix
Proficiency Testing in Hematology: An Overview 2

Granulocytic (Myeloid) Cells

Introduction 5
Myeloblast 6
   *A Closer Look At…*Acute Nonlymphocytic
      Leukemia 8
Promyelocyte 10
Myeloblast/Promyelocyte with Auer Rod(s) 12
   *A Closer Look At…*Auer Bodies 14
Myelocyte, Neutrophilic 16
   *A Closer Look At…*Post–Mitotic Myeloid
      Precursors 18
Metamyelocyte, Neutrophilic 20
Band, Neutrophilic 22
Segmented Neutrophil 24
   *A Closer Look At…*Is it a Band or Segmented
      Neutrophil? 26
Basophil 28
Eosinophil (any stage) 30
   *A Closer Look At…*Eosinophilia 32
Monocytes, Immature 34
Monocyte 36
   *A Closer Look At…*Life Cycle of Monocytes 38
Toxic Granulation and/or Multiple Toxic Vacuoles ... 40
Döhle Body with/without Toxic Granulation 42
   *A Closer Look At…*Acquired Neutrophil
      Abnormalities 44
   *A Closer Look At…*May-Hegglin Anomaly 46
Metamyelocyte, Giant (Bone Marrow) 48
Band Neutrophil, Giant (Bone Marrow) 50
Hypersegmented Neutrophil 52
Neutrophil with Dysplastic Nucleus/Agranular
   Cytoplasm 54
   *A Closer Look At…*Myelodysplastic Syndromes ... 56
Pelger–Huët Anomaly 58

Erythrocytic Cells and Inclusions

Introduction 61
Erythrocyte (Normocytic, Normochromic) 62
Acanthocyte 64
   *A Closer Look At…*How Acanthocytes Form 66
Bite Cell 68
   *A Closer Look At…*Bite Cell Formation and
      Morphology 70
Blister Cell (Pre-Keratocyte) 72
   *A Closer Look At…*Vacuolated Non-Nucleated
      Red Blood Cells 74
Echinocyte 76
   *A Closer Look At…*Spiculated Red Cells 78
Fragmented Cell (Schistocyte, Helmet Cell,
   Keratocyte) 80
   *A Closer Look At…*Microangiopathic Anemias ... 82
   *A Closer Look At…*Diagnostic Morphology
      in MAHA and Heinz Body Anemia 84
Macrocyte (Oval or Round) 86
Microcyte (with Central Pallor) 88
Ovalocyte (Elliptocyte) 90
   *A Closer Look At…*Hereditary Elliptocytosis 92
Polychromatophilic Red Cell (Non-Nucleated) 94
Sickle Cell 96
   *A Closer Look At…*Sickle Cell Anemia 98
Spherocyte 100
   *A Closer Look At…*Red Cell Membrane Loss
      and Spherocytosis 102
Stomatocyte 104
Target Cell 106
   *A Closer Look At…*How Target Cells Form 108
Teardrop Cell 110
   *A Closer Look At…*How Teardrop Cells Form ... 112
Reticulocyte (Supravital Stain) 114
Basophilic Stippling (Coarse) 116
   *A Closer Look At…*How Basophilic Stippling
      Forms 118
   *A Closer Look At…*Red Cell Inclusions 120
Heinz Body 124
   *A Closer Look At…*How Heinz Bodies Form ... 126
Hemoglobin C Crystal 128
Hemoglobin H Inclusions (Supravital Stain) 130
   *A Closer Look At…*Different Types of
      Precipitated Hemoglobin 132
Howell-Jolly Body (Wright-Giemsa stain) 134
Howell-Jolly Body (Iron Stain) 136
   *A Closer Look At…*Howell-Jolly Body Formation ... 138
Pappenheimer Bodies (Wright-Giemsa Stain) 140
Pappenheimer Bodies (Iron Stain) 142
   *A Closer Look At…*How Pappenheimer Bodies
      Form 144
Red Cell Agglutinates 146
Rouleaux 148
   *A Closer Look At…*Sticky Red Blood Cells 150

Nucleated Red Cells

Introduction 153
Pronormoblast (Bone Marrow) 154
  A Closer Look At...Red Cell Maturation and
    Cell Division 156
  A Closer Look At...Morphologic Keys to
    Identifying Early Normoblasts 158
Basophilic Normoblast (Bone Marrow) 160
Polychromatophilic Normoblast (Bone Marrow) ... 162
Orthochromic Normoblast (Bone Marrow) 164
Nucleated Red Cell, Megaloblastic
  (Bone Marrow) 166
  A Closer Look At...Megaloblastic Morphology 168
Nucleated Red Cell, Normal or Abnormal
  (Blood) 170
Nucleated Red Cell, Dysplastic (Bone Marrow) 172
  A Closer Look At...Megaloblastic vs.
    Megaloblastoid Erythroid Maturation 174
Sideroblast (Iron Stain) 176
  A Closer Look At...Sideroblasts and
    Siderocytes 178
Sideroblast, Ringed (Iron Stain) 180
  A Closer Look At...Hemoglobin Formation
    and Iron Utilization 182
  A Closer Look At...Formation of Ringed
    Sideroblasts 184

Megakaryocytic Cells and Thrombocytes

Introduction 187
Megakaryocyte or Precursor, Normal 188
  A Closer Look At...Megakaryocyte Maturation 190
Megakaryocyte or Precursor, Abnormal 192
  A Closer Look At...Dysplastic Megakaryocytes 194
Megakaryocyte Nucleus 196
Platelet, Normal 198
  A Closer Look At...Platelet Formation 200
Platelet, Giant 202
Platelet, Hypogranular 204
Platelet Satellitism 206
  A Closer Look At...Platelet Satellitism 208

Lymphocytic and Plasmacytic Cells

Introduction 211
Hairy Cell 212
  A Closer Look At...Hairy Cell Leukemia 214
Lymphoblast 216
Lymphocyte, Mature 218
  A Closer Look At...Normal vs.
    Reactive Lymphocytes 220
Lymphocyte, Reactive 222
  A Closer Look At...Reactive vs. Neoplastic
    Lymphocytes 226
Lymphoma Cell 228
  A Closer Look At...Normal Lymphocyte
    Maturation and Malignant Transformation 230
  A Closer Look At...B Cell Neoplasms 232
  A Closer Look At...T Cell and Putative NK Cell
    Neoplasms 236
Plasma Cell, Mature 238
  A Closer Look At...Plasma Cell Maturation 240
Plasma Cell, Immature or Abnormal
  (Myeloma Cell) 242
Plasma Cell or Precursor with Inclusion Body 244
Prolymphocyte 246
  A Closer Look At...Prolymphocytes 248
Sézary Cell 250

Microorganisms

Introduction 253
Babesia 254
  A Closer Look At...Babesiosis vs. Malaria 256
Bacteria (Cocci or Rod), Extracellular 258
Bacteria (Spirochete) 260
Fungi, Extracellular 262
Leukocyte (Blood) with Phagocytized Bacteria 264
Leukocyte (Blood) with Phagocytized Fungi 266
Macrophage with *Histoplasma*, *Leishmania*, or
  Toxoplasma 268
Macrophage with Phagocytized Mycobacteria 270
Malaria (Intracellular and Extracellular) 272
  A Closer Look At...Species Differences Among
    Malarial Parasites 274
Microfilaria 276
  A Closer Look At...Species Differences Among
    Microfilariae 278
Protozoan (Non-Malarial) 280
  A Closer Look At...African Trypanosomiasis 282

Artifacts
Introduction 285
Basket Cell or Smudge Cell 286
Neutrophil Necrobiosis 288
   *A Closer Look At...*Cell Death 290
Erythrocyte with Overlapping Platelet 292
Stain Precipitate 294

Miscellaneous Cells
Introduction 297
Blast Cell 298
   *A Closer Look At...*Antigen Markers in Blastic
      Cells 300
Alder's Anomaly Inclusion 302
Chédiak-Higashi Anomaly Inclusion 304
   *A Closer Look At...*Cytoplasmic Inclusions in
      Neutrophils 306
Endothelial Cell 308
Epithelial Cell 310
Lipocyte 312
   *A Closer Look At...*Bone Marrow
      Microenvironment 314
Macrophage (Histiocyte) 316
Macrophage with Phagocytized Red Cell
   (Erythrophagocytosis) 318
   *A Closer Look At...*Cytoplasmic Inclusions in Bone
      Marrow Cells 320
Gaucher Cell and Pseudo-Gaucher Cell 322
Histocyte, Sea Blue 324
Niemann-Pick Cell, Foamy Macrophage 326
Mast Cell 328
   *A Closer Look At...*Mast Cells vs. Basophils 330
Metastatic Tumor Cell 332
Mitotic Figure 334
Osteoblast 336
   *A Closer Look At...*Osteoblast vs. Plasma Cell 338
Osteoclast 340

Appendix A
Selected References 342

Appendix B
Hematology Master List (1997-1998)
   (with Proficiency Testing Codes) 344

Appendix C
How to Review Proficiency Testing
   Photomicrographs 346

Appendix D
CAP Hematology Proficiency Testing Challenges
   Listed by Master List Identification 347

Appendix E
CAP Hematology Proficiency Testing Challenges
   Listed by Year 356

Index 366

A Closer Look At... Discussions (Alphabetical Listing)

Acquired Neutrophil Abnormalities	44
Acute Nonlymphocytic Leukemia	8
African Trypanosomiasis	282
Antigen Markers in Blastic Cells	300
Auer Bodies	14
B Cell Neoplasms	232
Babesiosis vs. Malaria	256
Bite Cell Formation and Morphology	70
Bone Marrow Microenvironment	314
Cell Death	290
Cytoplasmic Inclusions in Bone Marrow Cells	320
Cytoplasmic Inclusions in Neutrophils	306
Diagnostic Morphology in MAHA and Heinz Body Anemia	84
Different Types of Precipitated Hemoglobin	132
Dysplastic Megakaryocytes	194
Eosinophilia	32
Formation of Ringed Sideroblasts	184
Hairy Cell Leukemia	214
Hemoglobin Formation and Iron Utilization	182
Hereditary Elliptocytosis	92
How Acanthocytes Form	66
How Basophilic Stippling Forms	118
How Heinz Bodies Form	126
How Howell-Jolly Bodies Form	138
How Pappenheimer Bodies Form	144
How Target Cells Form	108
How Teardrop Cells Form	112
Is it a Band or Segmented Neutrophil?	26
Life Cycle of Monocytes	38
Mast Cells vs. Basophils	330
May-Hegglin Anomaly	46
Megakaryocyte Maturation	190
Megaloblastic Morphology	168
Megaloblastic vs. Megaloblastoid Erythroid Maturation	174
Microangiopathic Anemias	82
Morphologic Keys to Identifying Early Normoblasts	158
Myelodysplastic Syndromes	56
Normal Lymphocyte Maturation and Malignant Transformation	230
Normal vs. Reactive Lymphocytes	220
Osteoblast vs. Plasma Cell	338
Plasma Cell Maturation	240
Platelet Formation	200
Platelet Satellitism	208
Post–Mitotic Myeloid Precursors	18
Prolymphocytes	248
Reactive vs. Neoplastic Lymphocytes	226
Red Cell Inclusions	120
Red Cell Maturation and Cell Division	156
Red Cell Membrane Loss and Spherocytosis	102
Sickle Cell Anemia	98
Sideroblasts and Siderocytes	178
Species Differences Among Malarial Parasites	274
Species Differences Among Microfilariae	278
Spiculated Red Cells	78
Sticky Red Blood Cells	150
T Cell and Putative NK Cell Neoplasms	236
Vacuolated Non-Nucleated Red Blood Cells	74

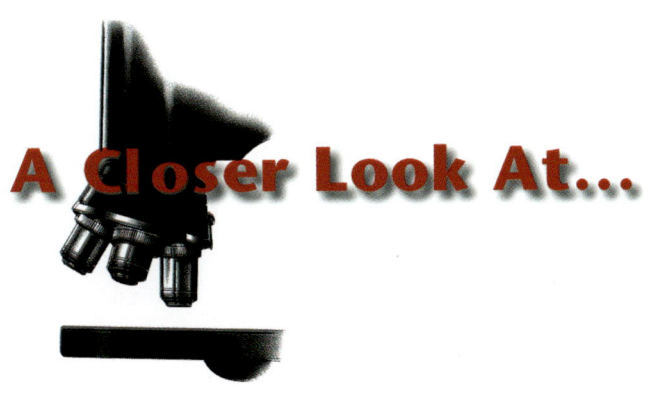

Preface

Proficiency testing (PT) is a core product of the College of American Pathologists (CAP). The photomicrographs in the hematology surveys provide a unique resource of referee and participant consensus cell identifications. This Atlas culls the best examples from our archives and lists the critical keys to successful morphologic identification.

We call it a *field guide* because it is an in-the-trenches, real-world look at cell identification—the important morphologic clues, the key features of differentiation, the look-alikes and the associated disease states. As laboratorians, we rely on microscopes instead of binoculars to identify our quarry. But it's still a jungle out there in CLIA-land. A good guidebook will focus your thinking and sharpen your diagnostic acumen. The world may not need another hematology atlas, but a field guide is another niche altogether. Consider it a signpost in the regulatory wilderness.

The Atlas is not meant to be comprehensive. We cover only the cells in the current Master List (the CAP cell identification choices in PT challenges). But the depth is sufficient to form a foundation on which to build a clear vision of hematologic morphology.

Each cell identification is divided into four parts. A **Vital statistics** section creates a checklist of important attributes, potential mimics, and associated conditions or disease states. **Glossary text** fleshes out this fact sheet. **Color illustrations** highlight the key differential points of identification. **Photomicrographs** on the facing pages are examples of actual proficiency testing challenges, listing referee and participant data in percentage format. The illustration on the bottom of the next page describes the photo layout.

Although individual cell identification is the centerpiece, we are particularly proud of the *A Closer Look At...* sections that highlight clinical information, pathophysiology, or identification details that cannot be covered in a pure "glossary" approach. In many ways, these sections are the most valuable because they hopefully expand the morphologic constructs to bring reality to the image and depth to the sketch, helping you move from a collection of images toward a deeper understanding of their meaning. They allow you to go beyond merely "passing PT" by reinterpreting the simple glossary definitions in light of expanded information. Consensus cell identification provides a nexus to a broader and deeper view of morphology. The Atlas then becomes a book that anyone involved in hematology can value, not just those that have grades and regulatory guidelines on their minds.

The design of the Atlas owes much to two hematology texts. The first was a Christmas present given to me by my father, Frank Glassy. He is a fellow pathologist with a love for family and hematology. *Blood Smears Reinterpreted*, by Marcel Bessis is a thin, unpretentious book that does not attempt to cover all the shifting sands that make up hematology. It is meant, in the author's words, "...to make dead blood cells come alive." But in addition to the diagnostic pearls, I was intrigued by the design of the book—it was a pleasure to read as well as view.

As a hematology fellow, I worked with Dr. Nora Sun at Harbor UCLA Medical Center on another influential tome, *Hematology, An Atlas and Diagnostic Guide*. The case study format and photographic layout that supports her excellent text also influenced the design of this Atlas. It was here that I was first exposed to the art and science of medical illustration. Besides sharing photographic duties with Dr. Sun, I did most of the drawings and charts without benefit of computer. In retrospect they look pretty crude; all were created by hand using rub-on letters, tape, razor blades, gray screens and technical pens.

As leader of the Atlas subcommittee, my goal was to create a consistent, visually appealing work that built on the styles of the other two books. I wanted it to be awash with color, like an illuminated manuscript that added visual impact to a dramatic story line. It took us four years to finish and represents a lot of weeknights, weekends, and holidays staring at a color monitor. It started life on an Apple Macintosh IIFX and ended up on a PowerPC 8500. I did the layout in PageMaker (versions 4 through 6.5) and all the illustrations in FreeHand (versions 4 through 8). The photomicrographs were scanned in Kodak PhotoCD format and color corrected in Adobe Photoshop. I have learned that printing is not an exact science. Some colors, particularly those that make up Wright-Giemsa stained cells, just don't translate well from glass slide to photographic film to printer's ink. Limitations of the medium aside, the final product is unique. Our committee hopes this Atlas provides insight, stimulation, enlightenment and, if you work in a laboratory, successful PT identifications. Utimately, we trust it will make better morphologists of us all.

Eric F. Glassy, MD

Acknowledgements

This book represents a four year gestation by the Atlas Subcommittee of the Hematology and Clinical Microscopy Resource Committee (HCMRC). We would like to acknowledge the many individuals who contributed to the final product; volunteer efforts such as the Atlas go far beyond the seven primary authors.

In the end, all the members, past and present of the HCMRC who contributed photomicrographs and case discussions share in the finished project. But we would be remiss in not listing several key individuals. Bong Hyun, MD, created the first detailed glossary of cell types that forms the basis of the atlas. The initial concept was born under the leadership of Albert (Rab) Rabinovitch, MD, chairman of the HCMRC from 1991 through 1993. Initial concepts, ideas, and case materials were contributed by Meryl Haber, MD, and Jerome Nosanchuk, MD.

Current members of the HCMRC made many valuable suggestions. Virgil Fairbanks, MD, reviewed the sections on hemoglobin H and Heinz bodies. LoAnne Peterson, MD edited the section on normal and activated lymphocytes. James Hoyer, MD added additional commentary.

We thank the past and current CAP staff who pulled all the photomicrographs and proficiency testing (PT) data, especially Stacy Junge, Mary Paton, and Jill Kachin. Jill in particular deserves credit for last minute data input. Joe Schramm heads the CAP publications department; he did the proof reading and helped ramrod the project through all the last minute glitches.

Nora Sun, MD, Frank Glassy, MD, and James Baker, MD added key suggestions.

Patrick Ward, MD, deserves special mention. It is hard to imagine a more entertaining and knowledgeable force in hematology. As an advisor to the HCMRC, he has provided photographic expertise over the last few years. With the Atlas project, Dr. Ward—as quick with a quip as he is with cell identification—spent countless hours with the illustrator, Eric F. Glassy, MD, agonizing over colors and singular details of morphology. He is a resource of incredible depth and an unparalleled morphologist. We all owe him a debt of gratitude. As an aside, his innumerable skills even extend to the fine art of finessing the craps table; he taught one of our wives that gambling sometimes does pay!

Volunteer projects such as the Atlas take time away from work and home. Each of us would also like to thank family and colleagues for their support and understanding.

Finally, we would like to thank the participants of the CAP proficiency testing program. This book is unique because it is based on the input of many thousands of laboratories. Thank you for subscribing to the "gold standard" in hematology PT. Any success we generate is to the participants' credit.

The Atlas Subcommittee of the HCMRC

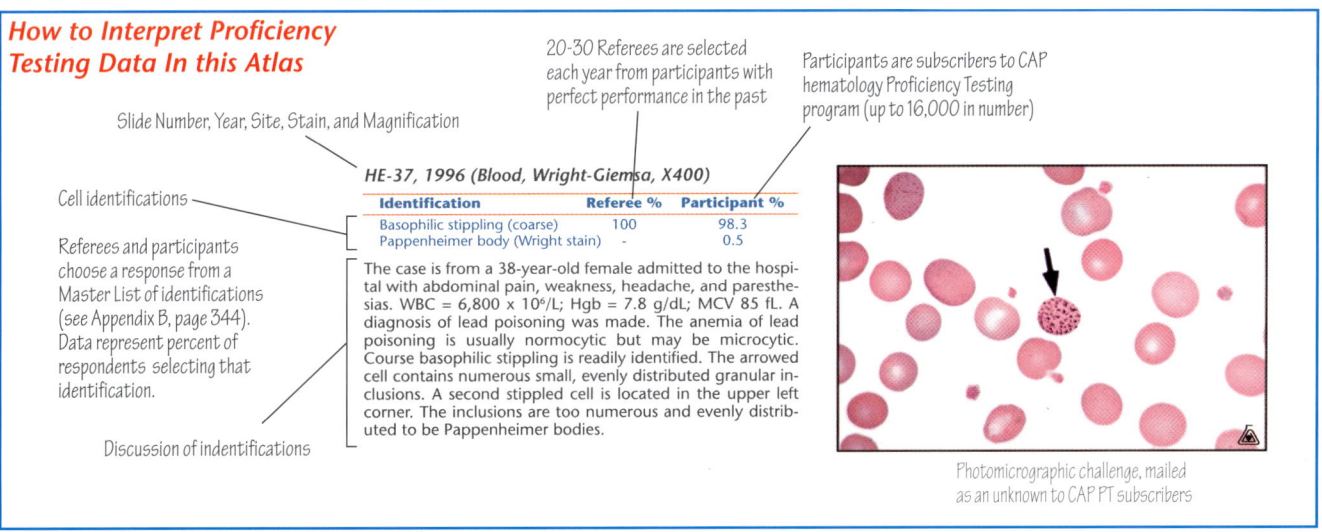

College of American Pathologists
Color Atlas of Hematology
An Illustrated Field Guide Based on Proficiency Testing

Section Lead Authors

Proficiency Testing in Hematology: An Overview
P. Joanne Cornbleet, MD, PhD

Granulocytic (Myeloid) Cells
Robert Novak, MD

Erythrocytic Cells and Inclusions
Catherine Spier, MD
Eric F. Glassy, MD

Nucleated Red Cells
Amy S. Gewirtz, MD

Megakaryocytic Cells and Thrombocytes
Eric F. Glassy, MD

Lymphocytic and Plasmacytic Cells
Steven J. Agosti, MD

Microorganisms
Katherine Galagan, MD

Artifacts
Eric F. Glassy, MD

Miscellaneous Cells
P. Joanne Cornbleet, MD, PhD

Proficiency Testing in Hematology: An Overview

The College of American Pathologists (CAP) was founded in 1947. One of its first tasks was to introduce a national proficiency testing program, which began in 1949. Initially 515 laboratories participated, and 10 chemistry constituents were offered. Hematology analytes first were offered in 1963, expanding to a menu that included both glass blood films for leukocyte differential and blood cell identification transparencies in 1970. Surveys in 1988 added material for a flow-through leukocyte differential with three cell subgroups. By 1991 the College produced the only hematology survey offering an automated differential with 5 cell types. Today, in 1998, 16,000 laboratories subscribe to the various hematology survey modules offered by the College.

In 1979, distribution of glass slides was discontinued, and only photomicrograph transparencies were used. The number of subscribers had increased to such a great number that the production of glass slides from a single blood sample was no longer feasible. Photomicrograph transparencies have advantages and disadvantages as compared to actual blood films for cell identification proficiency testing. While blood smears simulate the medium actually used in the laboratory for identifying blood cells, morphology and staining properties may deteriorate during production and shipping, and staining differences between laboratories may lead to misinterpretation. Furthermore, grading is difficult, since an aggregate number of each cell subtype is reported, influenced not only by differences between laboratories in cell classification, but by large variation attributed to the random distribution of cells on the blood smear (Rümke statistics). While the use of photomicrographs for cell identification has the disadvantage of displaying a limited field of the blood film, all participants identify the identical cell, which enables comparison of morphologic practice between individuals and laboratories. In addition, an educational discussion can be provided, highlighting the attributes that should lead to correct classification.

Production of the hematology proficiency testing surveys is under the purview of the Hematology and Clinical Microscopy Resource Committee (HCMRC). For cell identification proficiency testing, photomicrographs are taken by individual HCMRC members, then reviewed by the entire committee; only the most interesting cases and best cell examples are chosen. These are submitted to a group of 20-30 referees, chosen from laboratories participating in the cell identification survey with perfect performance. Referee results are reviewed by the HCMRC, with assignment of "good" and "acceptable" answers. In most cases, only photomicrographs that achieve referee consensus in identification are used for graded cell identification. In the past, 80 percent of referees selecting "good" or "acceptable" answers was considered consensus to qualify photomicrographs for evaluation, but rules adopted in response to CLIA '88 regulations now require 90 percent consensus for grading cell identification challenges.

Although cell identification proficiency testing serves a regulatory function, the HCMRC believes that this activity offers an opportunity for education and improvement in morphologic skills. A Glossary of Terms for Hematology was first written in 1980 to standardize identification of blood and bone marrow cells and provide survey participants with precise descriptions of the various cell types. Interesting or unusual cases are presented, even though participants may be asked to identify common cell types on these photomicrographs for graded challenges. Inclusion of pathologic material provides an opportunity for HCMRC members to write educational critiques in the participant summaries, discussing disease pathophysiology as well as morphologic features. In 1991, five ungraded photomicrograph challenges were added to the comprehensive hematology surveys, enabling the use of more difficult cell types, including bone marrow cells. Thus, the entire spectrum of hematologic findings—benign, reactive or malignant cells, mature or precursor cells, infectious agents in blood or marrow, and artifacts—could be included and discussed in the survey.

The CAP collection of survey photomicrographs represents a unique resource, since many individuals and laboratories have expressed an opinion about the identity of various hematologic elements rather than just one author. Review of the referee and participant data can suggest which morphologic variants illustrate unambiguous examples of the various cell types and which pose difficulty in classification.

The production of this atlas represents the culmination of four years of work of many HCMRC members. The Glossary of Terms for Hematology, provided to CAP proficiency testing subsribers, has been re-written to include vital information about each cell type or morphologic finding in a compact, uniform format. The best photomicrograph examples for each category have been selected, and a brief write-up highlights the most important features. Much of the credit belongs to Eric Glassy, MD, who designed the format, produced all of the illustrations, and performed the final atlas layout. We hope that this publication will further our goal of self-improvement in hematology cell morphology among CAP proficiency testing participants.

P. Joanne Cornbleet, MD, PhD
Advisor and former Chair
CAP Hematology and Clinical Microscopy
Resource Committee

Granulocytic (Myeloid) Cells

Introduction	5
Myeloblast	6
*A Closer Look At…*Acute Nonlymphocytic Leukemia	8
Promyelocyte	10
Myeloblast/Promyelocyte with Auer Rod(s)	12
*A Closer Look At…*Auer Bodies	14
Myelocyte, Neutrophilic	16
*A Closer Look At…*Post–Mitotic Myeloid Precursors	18
Metamyelocyte, Neutrophilic	20
Band, Neutrophilic	22
Segmented Neutrophil	24
*A Closer Look At…*Is it a Band or Segmented Neutrophil?	26
Basophil	28
Eosinophil (any stage)	30
*A Closer Look At…*Eosinophilia	32
Monocytes, Immature	34
Monocyte	36
*A Closer Look At…*Life Cycle of Monocytes	38
Toxic Granulation and/or Multiple Toxic Vacuoles	40
Döhle Body with/without Toxic Granulation	42
*A Closer Look At…*Acquired Neutrophil Abnormalities	44
*A Closer Look At…*May-Hegglin Anomaly	46
Metamyelocyte, Giant (Bone Marrow)	48
Band Neutrophil, Giant (Bone Marrow)	50
Hypersegmented Neutrophil	52
Neutrophil with Dysplastic Nucleus/Agranular Cytoplasm	54
*A Closer Look At…*Myelodysplastic Syndromes	56
Pelger–Huët Anomaly	58

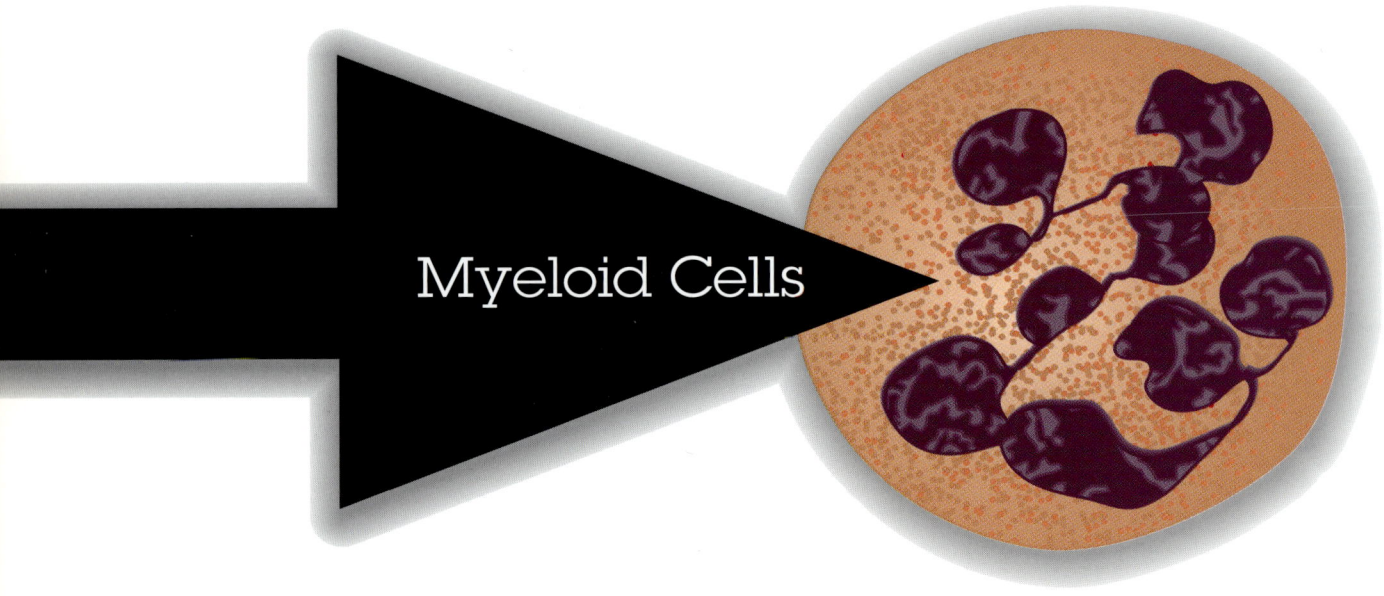

Myeloid Cells

Introduction

Pleuripotential hematopoietic stem cells in the bone marrow are influenced by cytokines to become first broadly committed precursor cells (colony forming unit—granulocyte/monocyte) and then unipotential precursor cells (colony forming unit—neutrophil, basophil or eosinophil). The granulocytes which result after division and maturation of these cells are among the most common white cells in the blood and have the important function of serving as the major line of defense against invading pathogens. Morphologically cells which show generalized granulocytic lineage and then specific granulocyte lineage can be identified cytologically in the bone marrow. The myeloblast and promyelocyte are cells that have cytochemical and immunophenotypic markers compatible with myeloid differentiation but the specific type of granulocyte that will result cannot be defined; their cytoplasm contains more and more primary granules, membrane-bound packets of enzymes which are common to all members of the myeloid series (hence the name granulocytes); their nuclei are round and contain open chromatin. After a series of divisions, the nucleus begins to flatten and indent and its chromatin clumps. The cytoplasm begins to contain secondary or specific granules, characteristic of only one of the types of granulocytes. This is the myelocyte stage; it is the first stage where the final type of granulocyte which will be produced can be designated and it is the last stage of the granulocyte precursors that can divide. After this stage there is progressive indentation of the nucleus (metamyelocyte and band stage) and ultimately segmentation (segmented stage) and accumulation of specific granules in the cytoplasm. Under normal circumstances this process from stem cell in the marrow to mature granulocyte in the blood takes 10 to 14 days. Alterations in DNA structure and function can lead to a failure of maturation and abnormal precursor proliferation which is manifest as an acute leukemia or a myelodysplastic state. Lack of factors essential to DNA replication can impair nuclear maturation and result in a granulocyte precursor which have distinct abnormalities in nuclear development. Infection and other toxic states can lead to increased cytokine stimulation which results in cytoplasmic abnormalities collectively referred to as toxic changes in the cytoplasm of these cells. The pages which follow will attempt to define this maturation process and illustrate how genetic and acquired abnormalities of myelopoiesis are manifest.

Myeloblast

SYNONYMS
none

VITAL STATISTICS
- size .... 15 to 20 μm
- N:C ratio .... 7:1 to 5:1
- cell shape .... round to oval
- nuclear shape .... round to oval
- chromatin .... finely reticular
- nucleoli .... distinct, 2 to 5
- cytoplasm .... scant, basophilic

KEY DIFFERENTIATING FEATURES
high N:C, finely reticular chromatin with nucleoli
basophilic cytoplasm without granules

OTHER FEATURES
Auer rods (needle–like granules, see pages 12 and 14) may be present; they are diagnostic of acute myelogenous leukemia

POTENTIAL LOOK–ALIKES
other blasts (monoblasts, lymphoblasts)
rarely atypical lymphocytes

ASSOCIATED DISEASE STATES AND CONDITIONS
acute myelogenous leukemia
acute myelomonocytic leukemia
erythroleukemia
myeloproliferative states
rarely severe leukemoid reactions

Myeloblasts are the most immature cells in the myeloid series. They are normally confined to the bone marrow where they constitute <3% of the nucleated cells. They are seen circulating in the blood in the acute non–lymphoid leukemias (see *A Closer Look At…* page 8), in chronic myeloproliferative and myelodysplastic states (see *A Closer Look At…* page 56) and rarely in leukemoid reactions. The normal myeloblast is a fairly large cell, 15 to 20 μm in diameter. In pathologic states such as leukemias, small micromyeloblasts (cells with the nuclear and cytoplasmic characteristics of blasts but the size of mature myeloid cells) may be seen. The nucleus has a finely reticulated chromatin and distinct nucleoli are present. The nucleus is usually round, but nuclear clefting or folding may rarely be seen, again mainly in pathologic states. The cytoplasm is basophilic and usually agranular. In leukemic states, cells with the nuclear characteristics of myeloblasts, may be seen with cytoplasm containing no granules (type I myeloblasts); with cytoplasm containing rare delicate granules and/or single Auer bodies (type II myeloblasts) or cytoplasm containing numerous azurophilic granules (type III myeloblasts).

Distinguishing one type of blast cell from another in a patient with a leukemic process is not always possible using Wright–Giemsa stains alone. In the absence of Auer bodies, characteristic cytoplasmic granules, cytochemical data (e.g. peroxidase activity or sudan black reactivity), or cell surface marker data (e.g. CD 13, 15, and 33) it is not possible to define the lineage of a given blast cell.

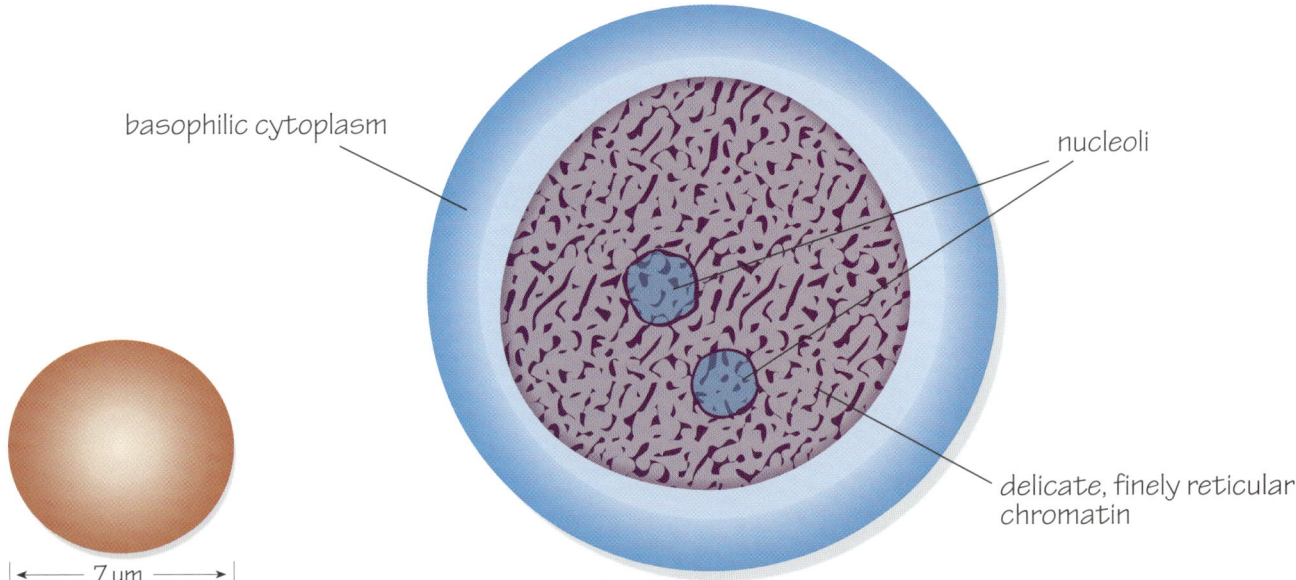

Myeloblast
- basophilic cytoplasm
- nucleoli
- delicate, finely reticular chromatin
- 7 μm — size of normal red blood cell

Granulocytic (Myeloid) Cells

HE-53, 1992 (Blood, Wright-Giemsa, X450)

Identification	Referee %	Participant %
Myeloblast	50	23
Blast cell	50	55
Lymphoblast		12

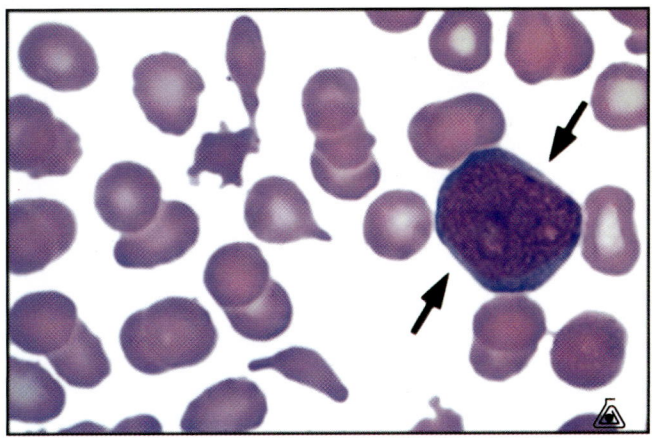

Between the arrows is a typical myeloblast. It does not contain an Auer body or show granules characteristic of a myeloid cell so it can only be identified in the context of the case. Thus, blast cell is certainly an acceptable identification; lymphoblast is not optimal but it cannot be ruled out. The cell has a modest amount of basophilic cytoplasm and a nucleus with finely granular chromatin in which is seen two distinct nucleoli. Red cells visible in the slide show morphologic abnormalities which include fragmentation and dacryocytes (teardrop cells).

H1-41, 1986 (Blood, Wright-Giemsa, X400)

Identification	Referee %	Participant %
Myeloblast	77	55
Blast cell	23	34

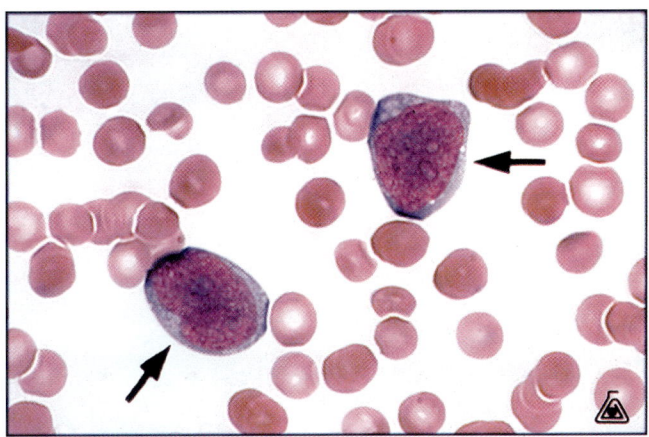

Each arrow points to a myeloblast. Once again, lacking specific findings, blast cell is also an acceptable answer. The myeloblast in the center of the field has scant basophilic cytoplasm with pale areas and vacuoles. The nucleus is round, has loose chromatin and contains three distinct nucleoli. The myeloblast in the lower portion of the field shows a nucleus which is clefted and has a less distinct nucleolus. Its cytoplasm is scant, basophilic, and lacks identifiable granules. The red cells in the field show some overlapping suggesting that this is not at the feathered edge of the blood smear.

H1-42, 1986 (Blood, Wright-Giemsa, X400)

Identification	Referee %	Participant %
Myeloblast	71	54
Blast cell	24	33

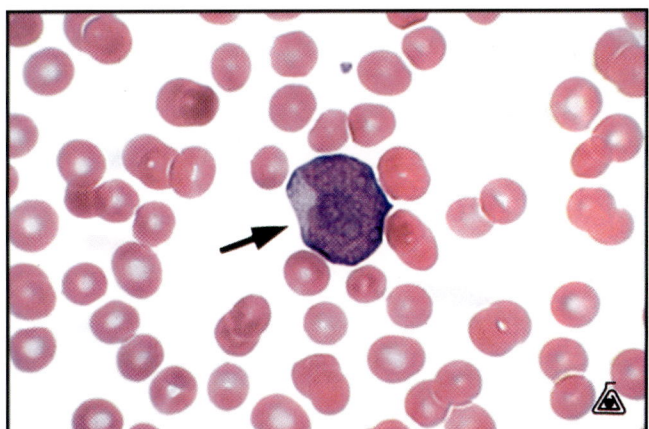

The illustrated white cell is clearly a blast cell. There is a high nuclear to cytoplasmic ratio, the nuclear chromatin is finely granular and there are distinct nucleoli. The nucleus is folded and no granules are seen in the cytoplasm. The cell in context is a myeloblast, but the answer blast cell is completely appropriate.

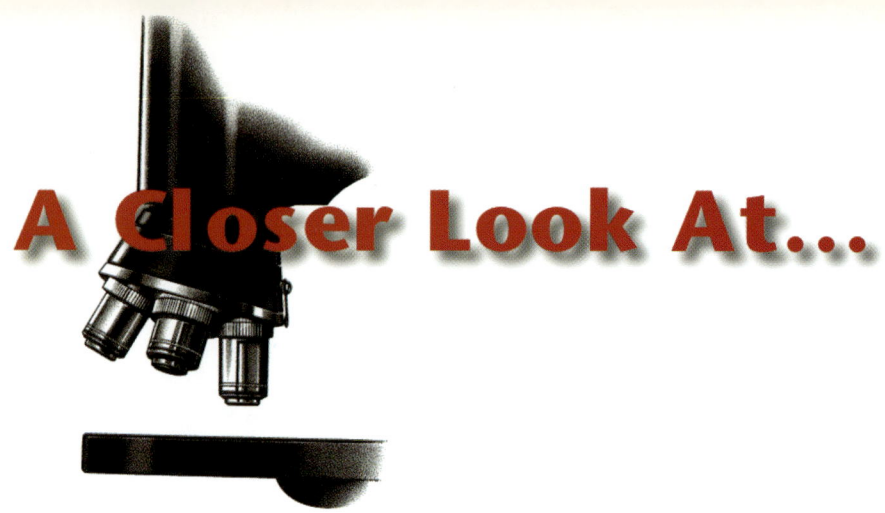

A Closer Look At...

Acute Nonlymphocytic Leukemia

Leukemias are malignancies that arise from uncontrolled clonal proliferation of hematopoietic cells. The acute nonlymphocytic leukemias (ANLL) arise from myeloid, monocytic, erythrocytic, and megakaryocytic precursors and account for 45% of acute leukemias, 80% of those seen in adults and 20% of those seen in children. The number and type of precursor cells in the marrow determine the type of ANLL according to the French–American–British (FAB) classification scheme. The nature of precursor cells is determined by their cytology, cytochemistry, and immunophenotype. It is beyond the scope of this atlas to provide a comprehensive discussion of ANLL. The table on the opposite page outlines the definition of blast cells and the nature of the blast cell populations in the FAB categories of acute leukemia.

French-American-British Classification of Acute Nonlymphocytic Leukemia

FAB Category	Bone Marrow Morphology	Cytochemistry Results	Immunophenotype Results
M0 Undifferentiated	Blasts with no morphologic differentiation	All stains are negative	Only CD 13 and 33 are positive
M1 Myeloblastic without differentiation	>90% blasts in marrow; <10% of blasts show maturation	>3% of blasts are MPO or SB positive	CD 13, 15, 33, 34, and DR positive
M2 Myeloblastic with differentiation	>30% but <90% blast cells; >30% of cells demonstrate myeloid differentiation; <20% are monoblasts	Many cells are MPO, SB, and CE positive	CD 13, 15, 33, 34, and DR positive
M3 Promyelocytic	>30% of leukemic cells are promyelocytes	Strong MPO, SB, and CE positivity	CD 13, 15, and 33 positive; DR is negative
M4 Myelomonocytic	>30% blasts; <80% myeloid blasts or precursors; >20% monoblasts or precursors	MPO and SB positive; Myeloid CE positive; Monocytic NSE positive	CD 11b, 13, 14, 15, 33, 36, and DR positive
M5 Monoblastic	>80% monoblasts and monocyte precursors	MPO, SB, NSE positive	CD 11b, 13, 14, 15, 33, 36, and DR positive
M6 Erythroleukemia	>50% of cells are nucleated red cell precursors with prominent dyserythropoiesis >30% non-erythroid cells are myeloblasts	Erythroid cells are PAS positive	Erythroid cells are CD71 and glycophorin A and C positive
M7 Megakaryocytic	>30% of cells are blasts; some show budding	Megakaryoblasts PAS and NSE positive	Megakaryoblasts are CD 41 and 61 positive

MPO= myeloperoxidase SB= sudan black CE= chloracetate esterase
NSE= nonspecific esterase CD= cluster designation DR= HLA DR antigen

Promyelocyte

SYNONYMS
  progranulocyte

VITAL STATISTICS
  size .... 12 to 24 μm
  N:C ratio .... 5:1 to 3:1
  cell shape .... round to oval
  nuclear shape .... round to oval
  chromatin .... finely reticular, slight clumping
  nucleoli .... distinct, 1 to 3
  cytoplasm .... blue, contains numerous azurophilic granules

KEY DIFFERENTIATING FEATURES
  high N:C, finely reticular chromatin with nucleoli, blue cytoplasm with azurophilic granules

OTHER FEATURES
  may contain collections of Auer rods in M3 ANLL

POTENTIAL LOOK-ALIKES
  type II or III myeloblasts
  rarely atypical lymphocytes

ASSOCIATED DISEASE STATES AND CONDITIONS
  acute myelogenous leukemia with maturation
  acute promyelocytic leukemia
  myeloproliferative disorders
  rarely severe leukemoid reactions

Promyelocytes are round to oval cells that are generally slightly larger the myeloblasts. A cell is considered to be a promyelocyte when it develops distinct primary granules in the cytoplasm. Promyelocytes still have a high N:C and their nuclei have fine chromatin and nucleoli like myeloblasts. They are normally confined to the marrow where they generally constitute <2% of the nucleated cells. The primary granules are coarse and azurophilic, and they may or may not overlie the nucleus. In pathologic states both hypergranular and microgranular forms of promyelocytes can be observed.

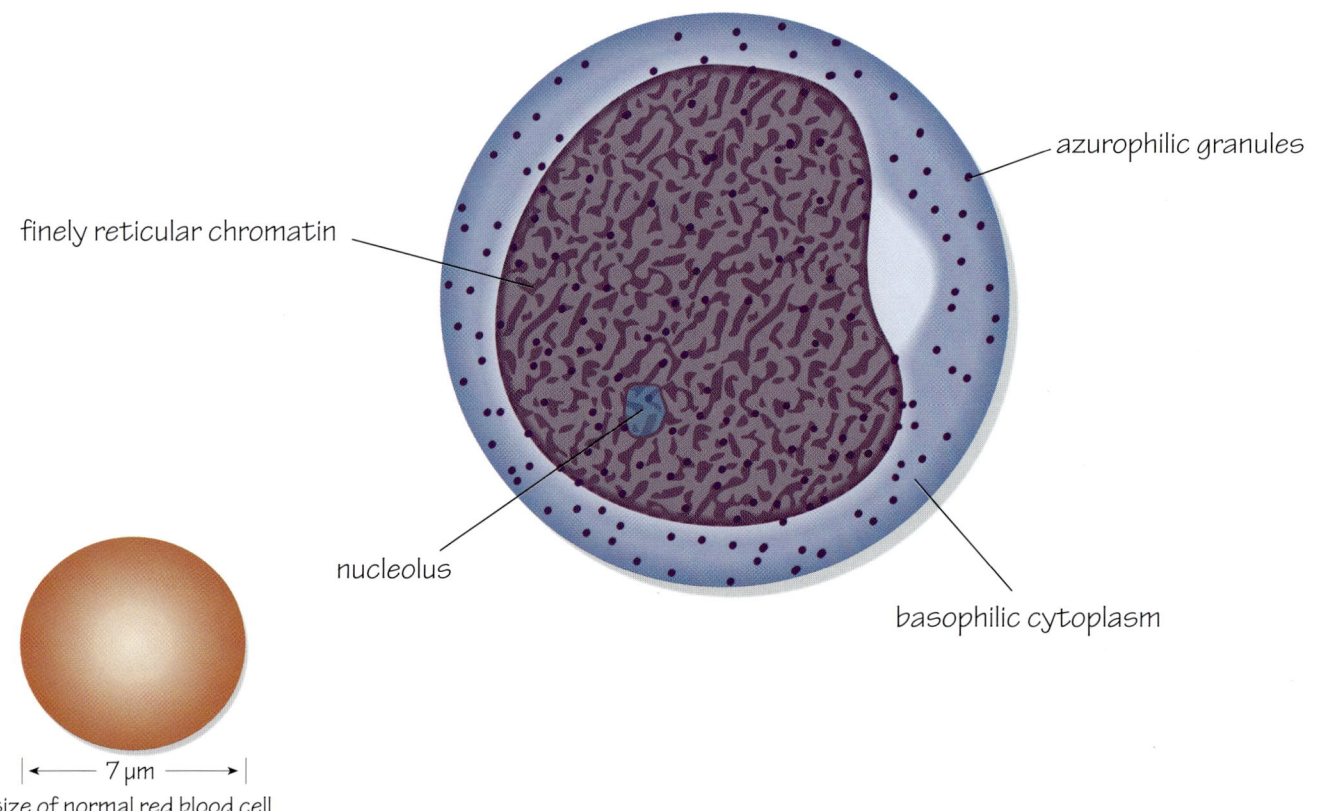

Promyelocyte
- finely reticular chromatin
- nucleolus
- azurophilic granules
- basophilic cytoplasm

|← 7 μm →|
size of normal red blood cell

Granulocytic (Myeloid) Cells

HE-08, 1995 (Blood, Wright-Giemsa, X400)

Identification	Referee %	Participant %
Promyelocyte	96.4	81.8
Myelocyte	-	13.2

The indicated cell is a promyelocyte. It is larger than a myeloblast and demonstrates cytoplasm containing numerous azurophilic primary granules. The nucleus is round and demonstrates distinct nucleoli. The combination of a blast–like nucleus and a cytoplasm showing differentiation due to the presence of primary granules is characteristic of this cell type.

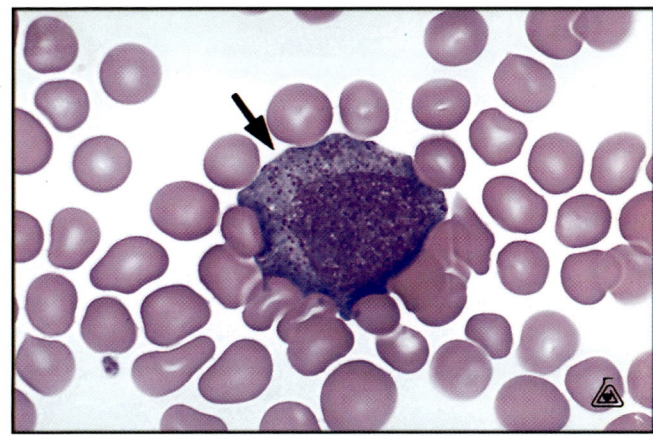

HE-30, 1996 (Bone Marrow, Wright-Giemsa, X400)

Identification	Referee %	Participant %
Promyelocyte	92.9	74.1
Myeloblast	3.6	6.2

The cell indicated by the arrow is a promyelocyte. It is a large cell with a high N:C ratio and the nuclear chromatin is loose with a definite nucleolus visible. The cytoplasm contains numerous azurophilic primary granules. The presence of a blast-like nucleus and primary granules define the promyelocyte. The cell is adjacent to other maturing myeloid elements.

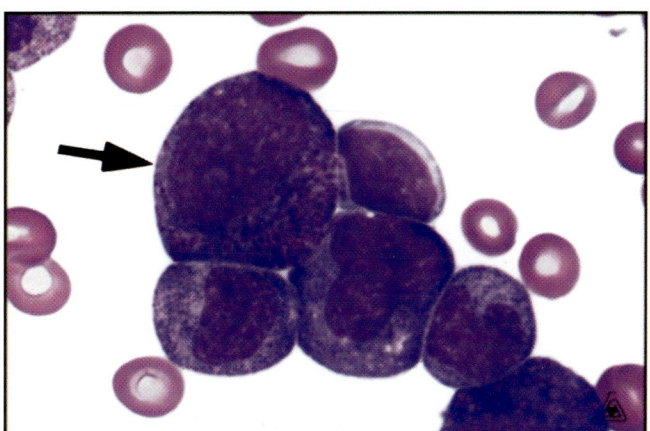

Granulocytic (Myeloid) Cells

Myeloblast/Promyelocyte with Auer Rod(s)

SYNONYMS
myeloblast with Auer body

VITAL STATISTICS
size .... 15 to 20 μm
N:C ratio .... 7:1 to 5:1
cell shape .... round to oval
nuclear shape .... round to oval
chromatin .... finely reticular
nucleoli .... distinct, 2 to 5
cytoplasm .... scant, basophilic; contains azophilic rod-like inclusion(s) measuring 0.2-0.5 μm in length; may be multiple; progranulocytes contain numerous azurophilic granules

KEY DIFFERENTIATING FEATURES
azurophilic rods measuring 0.2 to 0.5 μm in length; often overlap nucleus

OTHER FEATURES
may be multiple (faggot cells)

POTENTIAL LOOK-ALIKES
Chédiak-Higashi syndrome
inclusions in rare cases of chronic lymphocytic leukemia
toxic granulation

ASSOCIATED DISEASE STATES AND CONDITIONS
acute myelogenous leukemia
acute myelomonocytic leukemia
erythroleukemia

Approximately one-third of acute myelogenous leukemias are associated with red, round, or rod shaped cytoplasmic inclusions called Auer rods or Auer bodies. When present, they are found in only 1 to 10% of blast cells. Demonstration of one or several Auer rods in a blast is generally considered diagnostic of acute non-lymphocytic leukemia.

Auer bodies are seen mostly in immature granulocytes and rarely in immature monocytes. More mature cells may contain Auer rods as well, although very uncommonly.

Promyelocytes containing multiple Auer rods lumped together in a bundle is referred to as Sultan bodies or *faggot cell*. The word *faggot* is derived from the British term for a *cord of wood*.

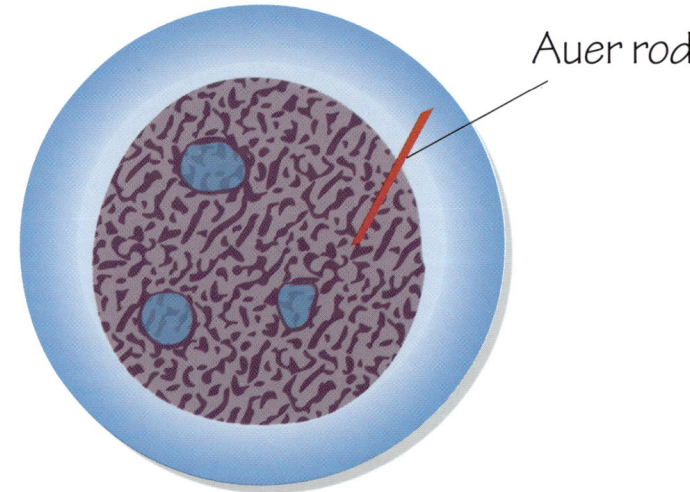

Myeloblast with Auer Rod

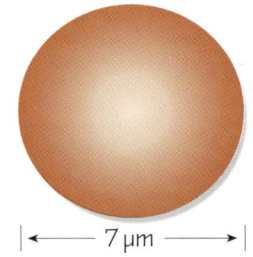

|← 7 μm →|
size of normal red blood cell

A-08, 1987 (Blood, Wright-Giemsa, X360)

Identification	Referee %	Participant %
Myeloblast with Auer rod	95	95

The three cells on the left side of the photograph have characteristics of blast cells. The middle cell, indicated by the arrow, contains a red, rod–like structure which is an example of an Auer rod. In the center of the photograph, the nucleated cell is a lymphocyte. On the right are two mature neutrophils.

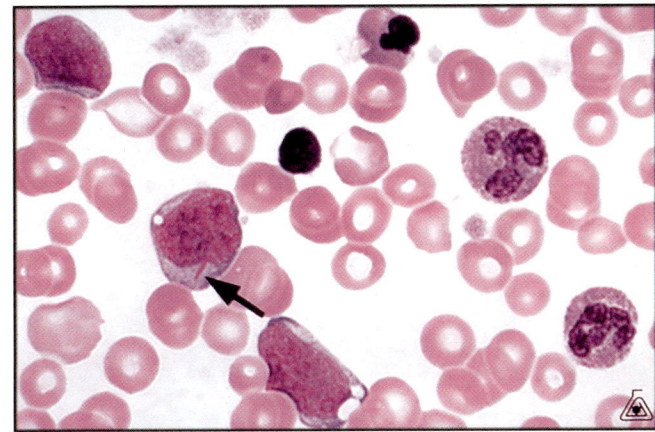

HE-06, 1995 (Blood, Wright-Giemsa, X400)

Identification	Referee %	Participant %
Myeloblast with Auer rod	89.3	91.4
Myeloblast	3.6	2.0

The cell indicated by the arrow is a myeloblast; the N:C ratio is high, the nucleus has a open chromatin pattern and contains multiple distinct nucleoli. Adjacent to the nucleus is a red rod–like structure, an Auer rod. There are no other specialized structures in the nucleus. Because of the presence of the Auer rod, a definite identification of myeloblast is appropriate.

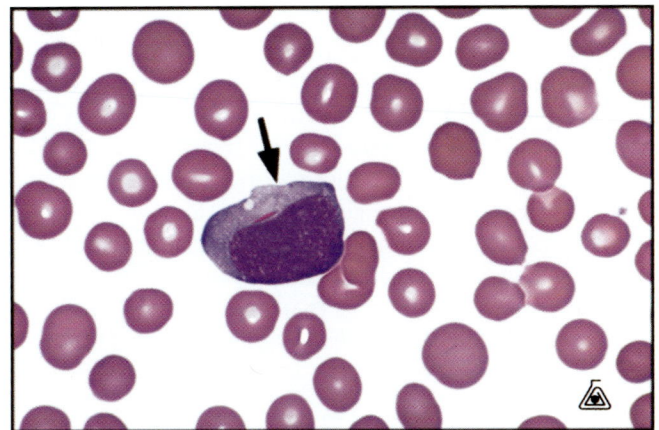

HE-29, 1996 (Blood, Wright-Giemsa, X400)

Identification	Referee %	Participant %
Myeloblast with Auer rod	92.3	86
Myeloblast	3.8	0.9

The cell indicated by the arrow is a blast cell (high N:C, immature nucleus with nucleolus) that contains in its cytoplasm large numbers of eosinophilic rods with the characteristics of Auer rods. Cells with multiple Auer rods are called faggot cells as the groups of rods resemble cords of wood. The cell was found in a patient with the microgranular varient of M3, AML, which explains the large number of abnormal cells in the blood. All three leukocytes in the field are blast cells.

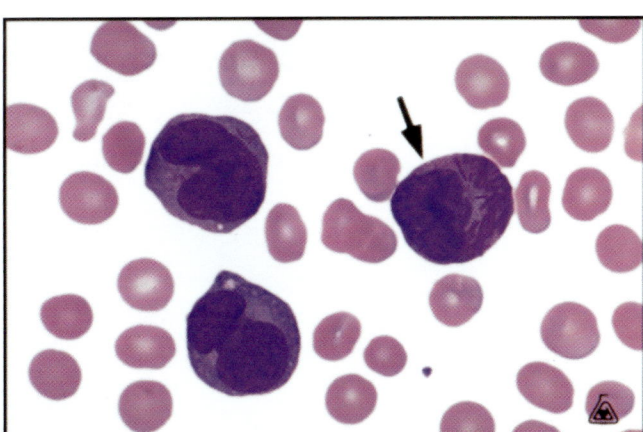

A Closer Look At...

Auer Bodies

Auer bodies are cytoplasmic inclusions representing an agglomeration of azurophilic (primary) granules. They are similar in staining properties and content to normal azurophilic granules but are abnormally large, measuring 0.2 to 5 µm in length. Auer bodies contain peroxidase, lysosomal enzymes, and large crystalline inclusions. Cells with multiple Auer bodies lumped together are called *faggot cells*.

The Chédiak–Higashi syndrome, a rare autosomal recessive condition characterized by albinism and increased susceptibility to infection, also mainfests an abnormality of azurophilic granules. Early in the promyelocytic stage, normal azurophilic granules form, but they then fuse to form megagranules. This abnormal fusion of lysosomes is manifest in other cells and tissues (see *Chédiak-Higashi Anomaly*, page 304).

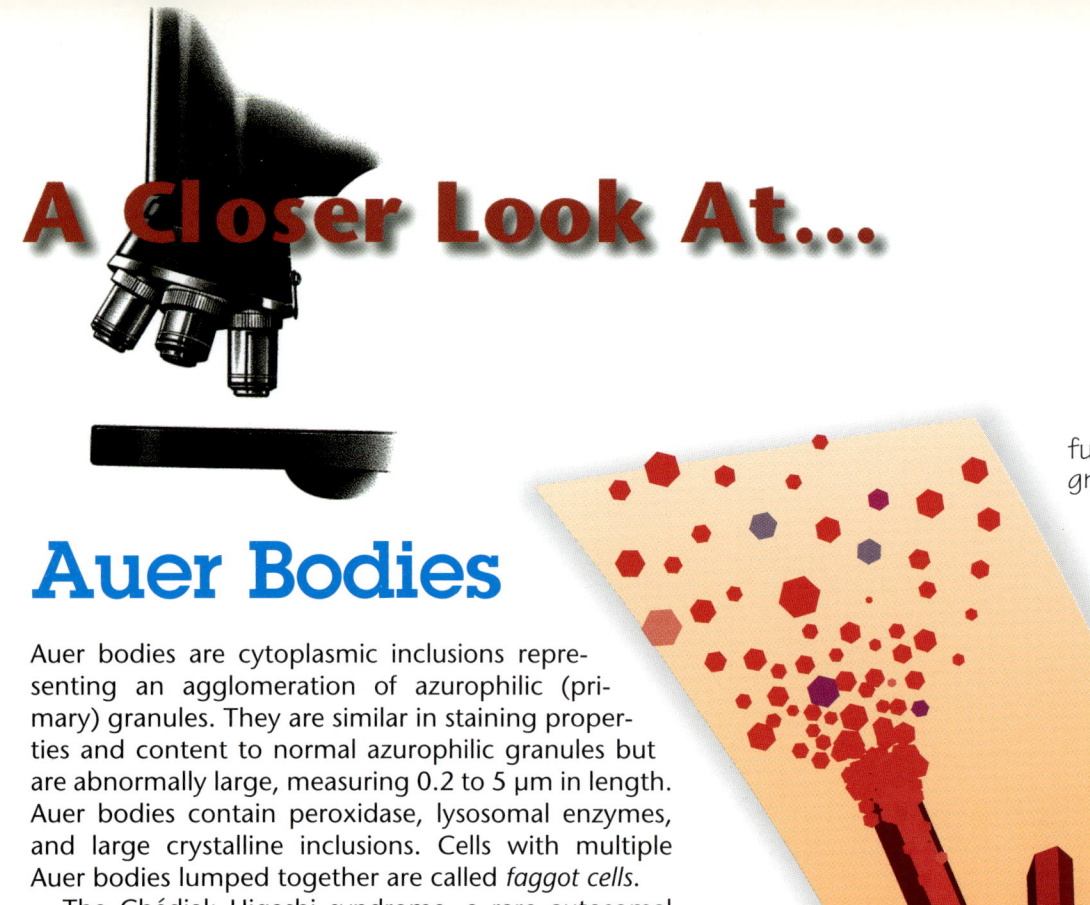

fusion of primary granules

rod-like bundles form

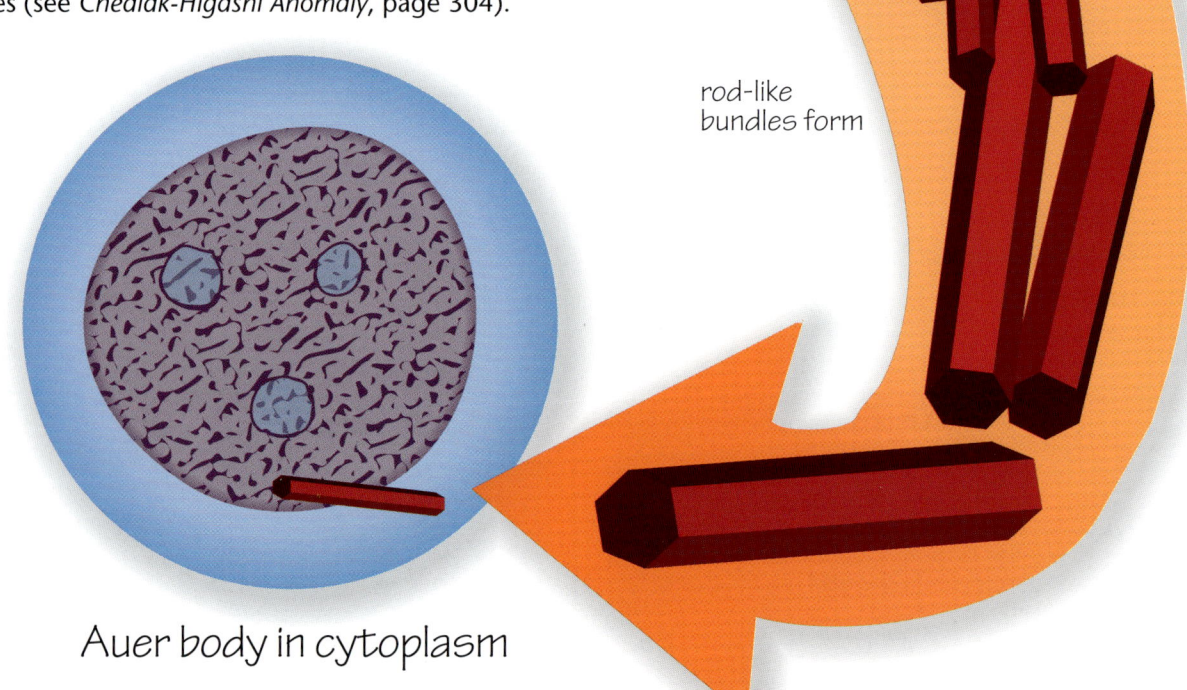

Auer body in cytoplasm

Finding Auer bodies is diagnostic of acute nonlymphocytic leukemia

Auer Body Facts

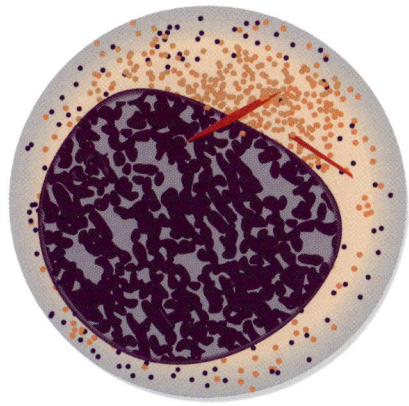
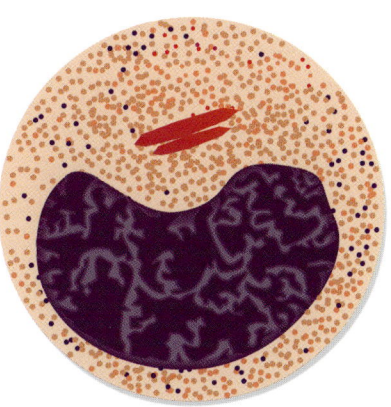

Auer bodies may occasionally be found in cells more mature than blasts, such as myelocytes and metamyelocytes. They are peroxidase and sudan black B positive.

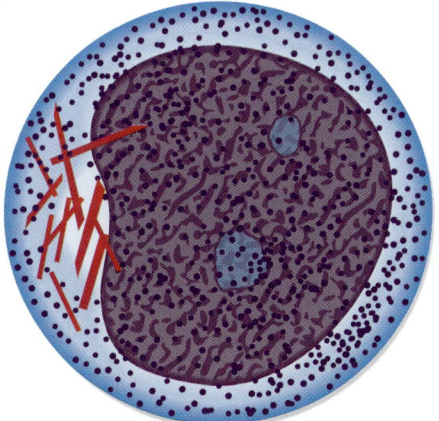

Cells with multiple Auer bodies are called Sultan bodies or "faggot cells." (Faggot comes from the British word meaning cord of wood). They are seen in acute promyelocytic leukemia.

Myelocyte, Neutrophilic

SYNONYMS
none

VITAL STATISTICS
- size .... 10 to 18 μm
- N:C ratio .... 2:1 to 1:1
- cell shape .... round to oval
- nuclear shape ..... oval, slightly indented or flattened
- chromatin .... variable amount of clumping
- nucleoli .... absent
- cytoplasm .... bluish–pink; contains both azurophilic (primary) and lilac (specific) granules

KEY DIFFERENTIATING FEATURES
absence of nucleoli and chromatin clumping
presence of both azurophilic and lilac granules

OTHER FEATURES
first morphologic stage where one can distinguish neutrophilic, eosinophilic, and basophilic precursors easily

POTENTIAL LOOK-ALIKES
monocytes
rarely atypical lymphocytes

ASSOCIATED DISEASE STATES AND CONDITIONS
myeloproliferative states, especially chronic myelogenous leukemia
acute myelocytic leukemia with maturation (M2)
leukemoid reactions

The transition from promyelocyte to myelocyte occurs with the end of production of azurophilic (primary) granules and the beginning of production of lilac (specific or secondary) granules. Myelocytes constitute approximately 10% of the nucleated cells in a normal marrow. The nucleus is somewhat eccentric, lacks a nucleolus, and begins to demonstrate chromatin clumping. Sometimes a clear region or hof is seen adjacent to the nucleus corresponding to location of the Golgi apparatus. The cytoplasm is relatively more abundant than in earlier stages and is amphophilic. Both primary and specific granules are present with the specific granules coming to predominate as maturation progresses.

Neutrophilic Myelocyte

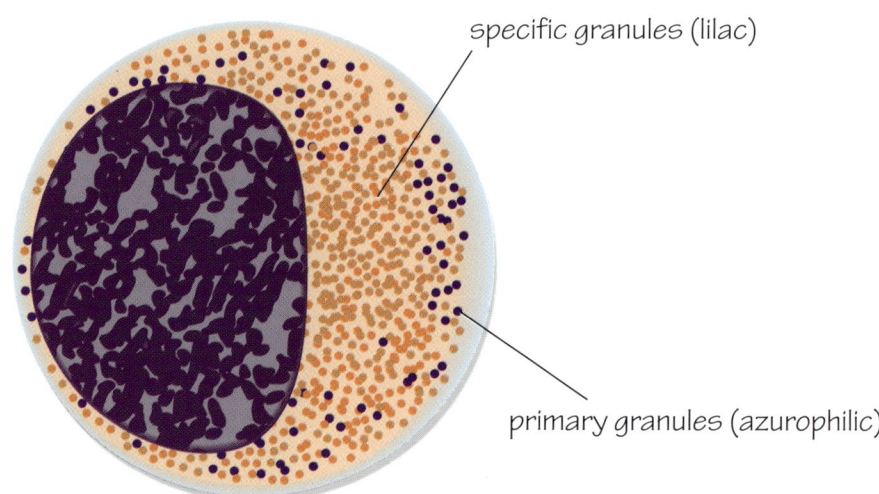

specific granules (lilac)

primary granules (azurophilic)

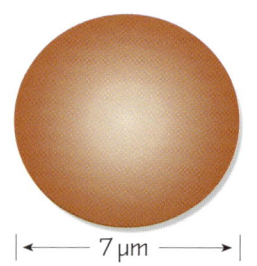

|← 7 μm →|

size of normal red blood cell

A-47, 1982 (Blood, Wright-Giemsa, X400)

Identification	Referee %	Participant %
Myelocyte	100	82.1

The arrowed cell is a myelocyte. The N:C is approximately 1:1 and the nucleus is somewhat flattened with clumping of the chromatin. Next to the nucleus there is a suggestion of a clear hof. The cytoplasm is pale and contains scattered coarse azurophilic granules and numerous fine lilac granules. Also present in the field presented are a neutrophil and a orthochromatic normoblast about to lose its nucleus.

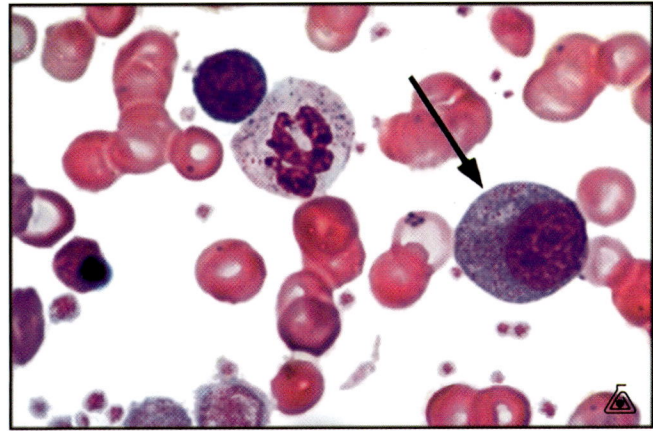

HE-58, 1991 (Blood, Wright-Giemsa, X400)

Identification	Referee %	Participant %
Myelocyte	90	73.9
Metamyelocyte	-	12.5

The cell indicated with an arrow is a myelocyte. It has an oval nucleus with some chromatin clumping. The nuclear indentation is not so great that the cell should be called a metamyelocyte. The cytoplasm has abundant azurophilic granules and a considerable number of lilac specific neutrophilic granules adjacent to nucleus, giving the cytoplasm a pale pink appearance.

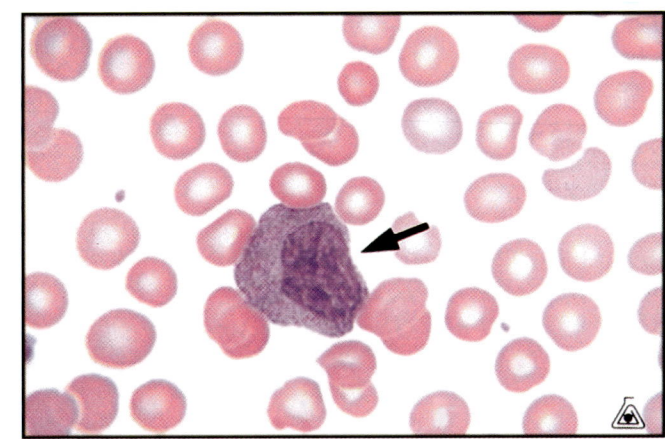

H1-21, 1988 (Bone Marrow, Wright-Giemsa, X330)

Identification	Referee %	Participant %
Myelocyte	58.8	58.5
Metamyelocyte	29.4	33.1

The cells indicated by the arrows are from a cellular area of bone marrow. All the cells show oval to somewhat indented nuclei with clumped chromatin. All are of neutrophilic lineage as their cytoplasm contains specific granules. The cells indicated were presented as myelocytes but the nuclei are such that a significant number of both referees and participants felt that they were more mature. To make consistent distinctions between two stages in what is essentially a continuous process always presents somewhat of a problem. All of the white cells indicated are myelocytes or more mature myeloid elements.

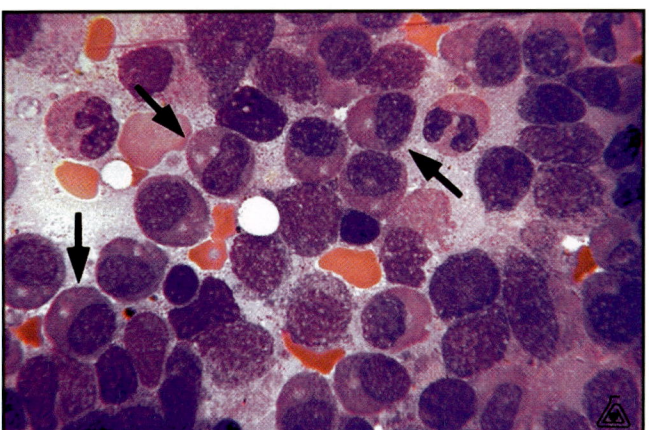

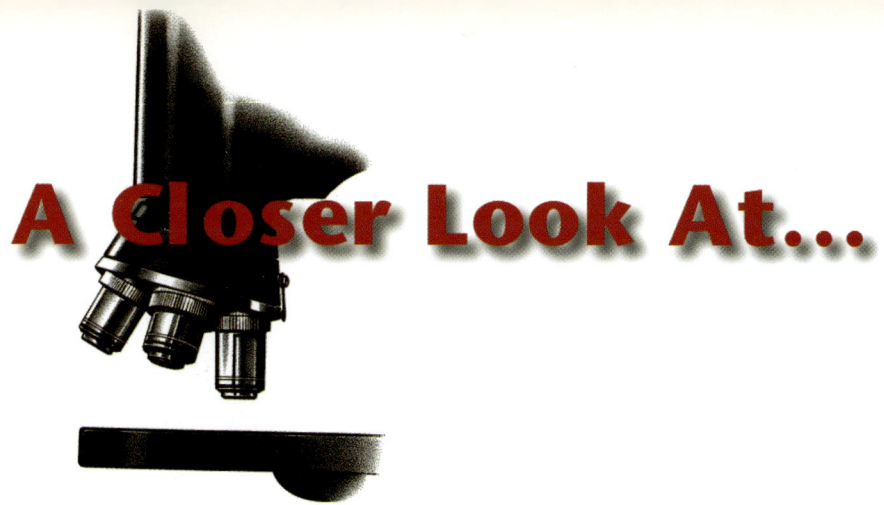

A Closer Look At...

Post-Mitotic Myeloid Precursors

All of the post–mitotic myeloid precursors (metamyelocytes, bands and segmented neutrophils) have a similar type of cytoplasm; their stage is determined by the degree of nuclear indentation and the presence or absence of nuclear segmentation. The metamyelocyte is indented to less than one half the theoretical round nucleus, while the band is indented to more than one half the theoretical round nucleus. The segmented form shows lobes connected only by a thin filament. The figure on the next page summarizes these stages.

The post-mitotic myeloid precursors constitute the maturation and storage pool of myeloid cells in the marrow. This pool contains the majority of myeloid cells in the marrow and the average cell spends approximately 10 days in this pool. The maturation portion of the process consists of the nuclear changes described above and the accumulation of specific granules in the cytoplasm. The pool is considered a storage pool because the neutrophils and band forms are readily mobilized into the blood in stressful situations, resulting in the so-called "left shift" phenomenon. Cytokines cannot induce cells in this group to divide but they do apparently activate these cells resulting in "toxic changes" in their appearance and in increased functional activity which can be demonstrated in in vitro studies (See Toxic Granulation, page 40 and A Closer Look At…Acquired Neutrophil Abnormalities, page 44). The severe neutropenia that occurs in overwhelming sepsis is due to an absolute depletion in the storage pool. The smaller relative size of the maturation and storage pool in neonates appears to predispose them to exhaustion of this pool in sepsis and accounts in part for the high mortality they experience when bacteria invade their blood stream.

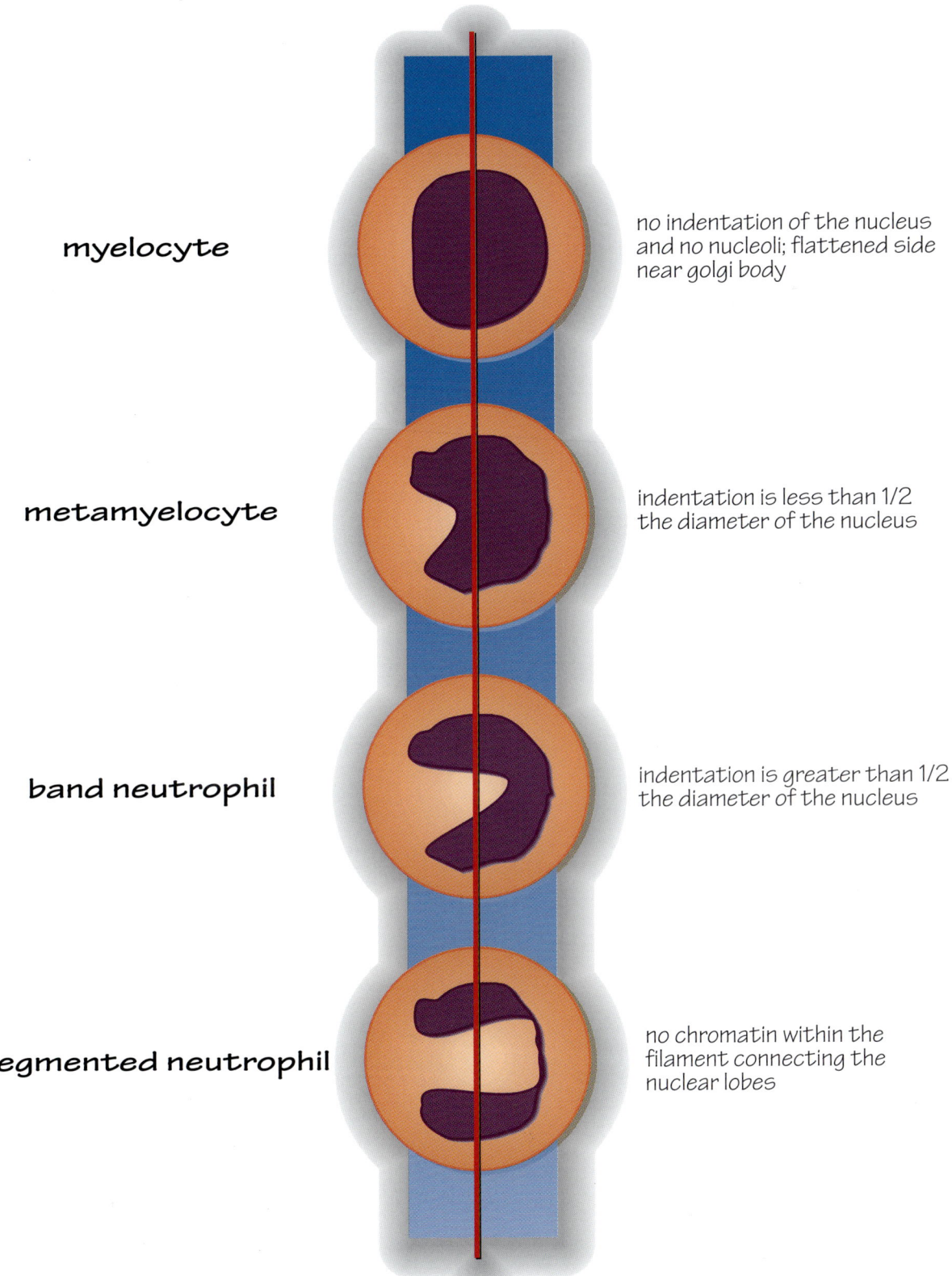

Metamyelocyte, Neutrophilic

SYNONYMS
  juvenile

VITAL STATISTICS
  size .... 10 to 18 µm
  N:C ratio .... 1.5:1 to 1:1
  cell shape .... round to oval
  nuclear shape .... indented, kidney shaped
  chromatin .... clumped with distinct regions
  nucleoli .... none
  cytoplasm .... pink, plentiful; contains many specific granules, rare azurophilic granules

KEY DIFFERENTIATING FEATURES
  neutrophil cytoplasm with indented nucleus
  indentation less than one half of theoretical round nucleus

OTHER FEATURES
  giant forms (one and one half times normal) may be seen in megaloblastic states (see page 48)

POTENTIAL LOOK-ALIKES
  monocytes
  rarely atypical lymphocytes

ASSOCIATED DISEASE STATES AND CONDITIONS
  acute myelocytic leukemia with maturation (FAB M2)
  myeloproliferative disease, especially chronic myelogenous leukemia
  neutrophil left-shift in stress and infection
  leukemoid reactions

Metamyelocytes are the first of the post-mitotic myeloid precursors. They are slightly smaller than myelocytes and constitute 15–20% of the nucleated cells in a normal bone marrow. Their nuclear chromatin is clumped and the nucleus is indented to less than half the diameter of the potential round nucleus (i.e., the indentation is less than half of the distance to the farthest nuclear margin). The cytoplasm is abundant and contains rare azurophilic (primary) granules and many fine lilac (specific) granules.

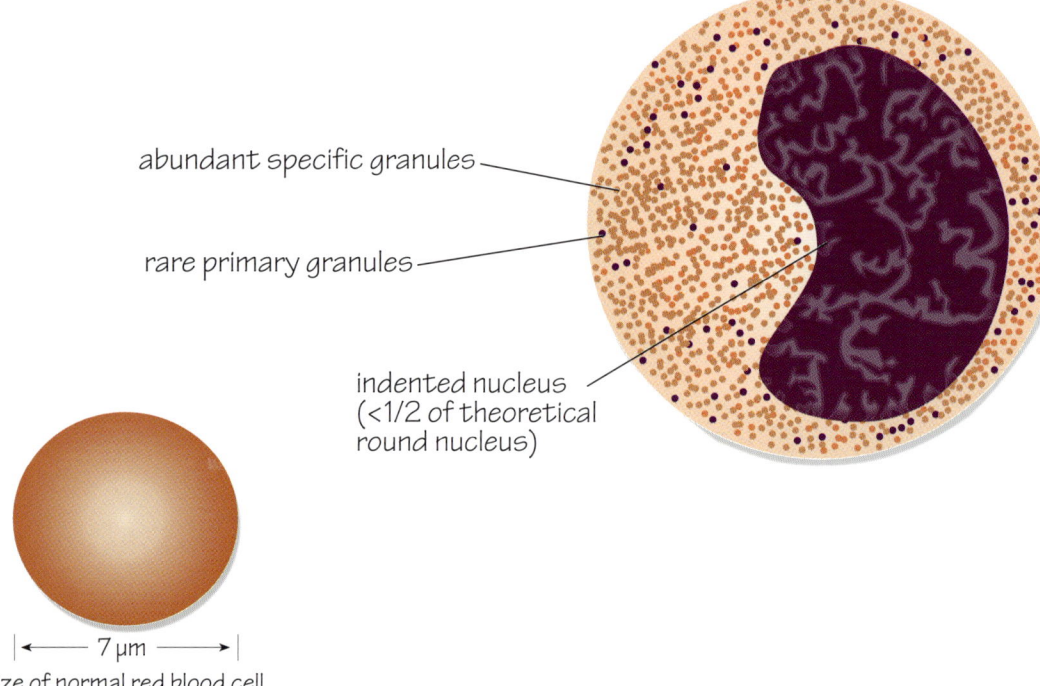

Neutrophilic Metamyelocyte

- abundant specific granules
- rare primary granules
- indented nucleus (<1/2 of theoretical round nucleus)

|← 7 µm →|
size of normal red blood cell

Granulocytic (Myeloid) Cells

H-38, 1981 (Blood, Wright-Giemsa, X330)

Identification	Referee %	Participant %
Metamyelocyte	100	73.8
Monocyte or precursor	-	19.6

The arrowed cell is a metamyelocyte. The nucleus is kidney shaped with a modest indentation. The cytoplasm is pink and contains neutrophilic granules, identifying this cell as a member of the myeloid, not the monocytic series. There is a segmented neutrophil below the arrowed cell; note how similar the cytoplasm appears. There is a clump of platelets in the upper right hand corner. The red cells present show some variation in size and shape.

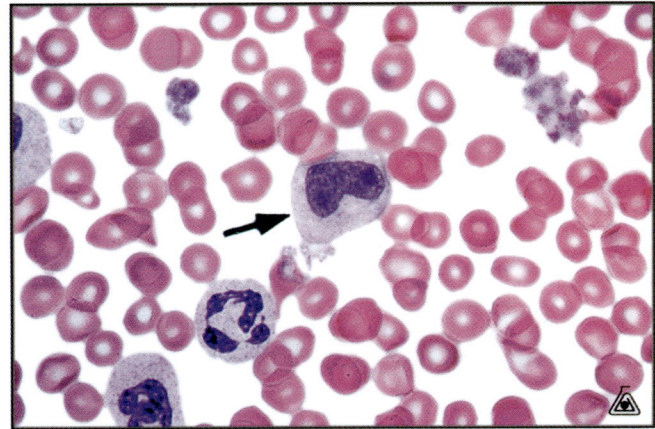

XH-06, 1990 (Blood, Wright-Giemsa X400)

Identification	Referee %	Participant %
Metamyelocyte	100	84.7
Band neutrophil	-	11

The central cell, indicated with an arrow, is a metamyelocyte. It has a granular cytoplasm and a kidney shaped nucleus. There are two small vacuoles in the cytoplasm, an indication of activation or degeneration. To the left of the cell is a cell with similar cytoplasm but with a nucleus with much greater indentation, giving the nucleus a "C" shape. This is a band neutrophil in contrast to the cell indicated with an arrow.

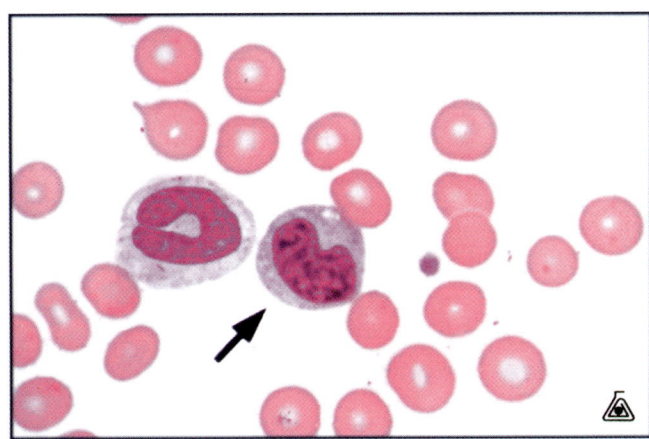

H1-6, 1985 (Blood, Wright-Giemsa, X450)

Identification	Referee %	Participant %
Metamyelocyte	100	93.8

The cell indicated with an arrow is a metamyelocyte. It has coarser granulation than the previously illustrated metamyelocytes. The nucleus is indented and kidney shaped. Two platelets are immediately adjacent to the cell at 12 o'clock and at 3 o'clock. The other nucleated cell in the field has a nonsegmented, band–like nucleus and eosinophilic granules. There are some red cells in the field that appear crenated or burred.

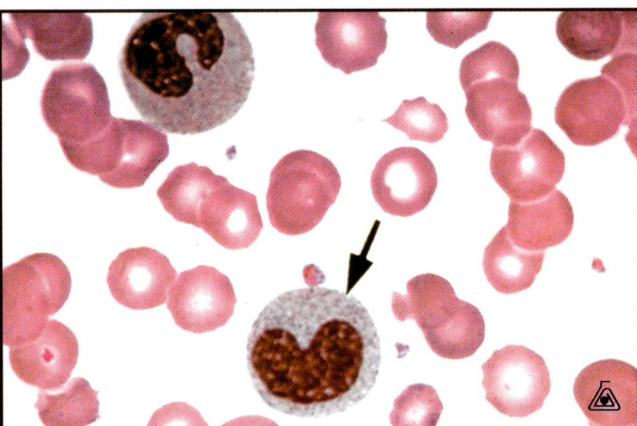

Granulocytic (Myeloid) Cells

Band, Neutrophilic

SYNONYMS
stab

VITAL STATISTICS
- size .... 10 to 18 μm
- N:C ratio .... 1:1.5 to 1:2
- cell shape .... round to oval
- nuclear shape .... S, C, U, or lobated, visible chromatin in isthmus
- chromatin .... coarse, clumpy
- nucleoli .... none
- cytoplasm .... pink, plentiful, mainly specific granules, rare primary (azurophilic) granules

KEY DIFFERENTIATING FEATURES
neutrophil cytoplasm with nucleus that is deeply indented (more than half of theoretical round nucleus) in all areas chromatin is present between edges of nuclear membrane

OTHER FEATURES
enlarged forms may be seen in megaloblastic states (see page 50)

POTENTIAL LOOK-ALIKES
monocytes
segmented neutrophils with folded nuclei

ASSOCIATED DISEASE STATES AND CONDITIONS
normal constituent of peripheral blood
increased in:
  myeloproliferative disorders
  neutrophil left shift in stress and infection
  leukemoid reactions

Band neutrophils constitute 10-15% of the nucleated cells in the marrow and 5-10% of the nucleated cells in blood. Their nuclear chromatin is clumped and the nucleus is indented to more than half the distance from the farthest nuclear margin. The nucleus can assume many shapes; band-like, sausage-like, S, C, U, and lobated. It may be twisted or folded on itself. It never constricts to the point of a filament. The cytoplasm is similar to that of other post-mitotic neutrophils with the lilac (specific) granules predominating.

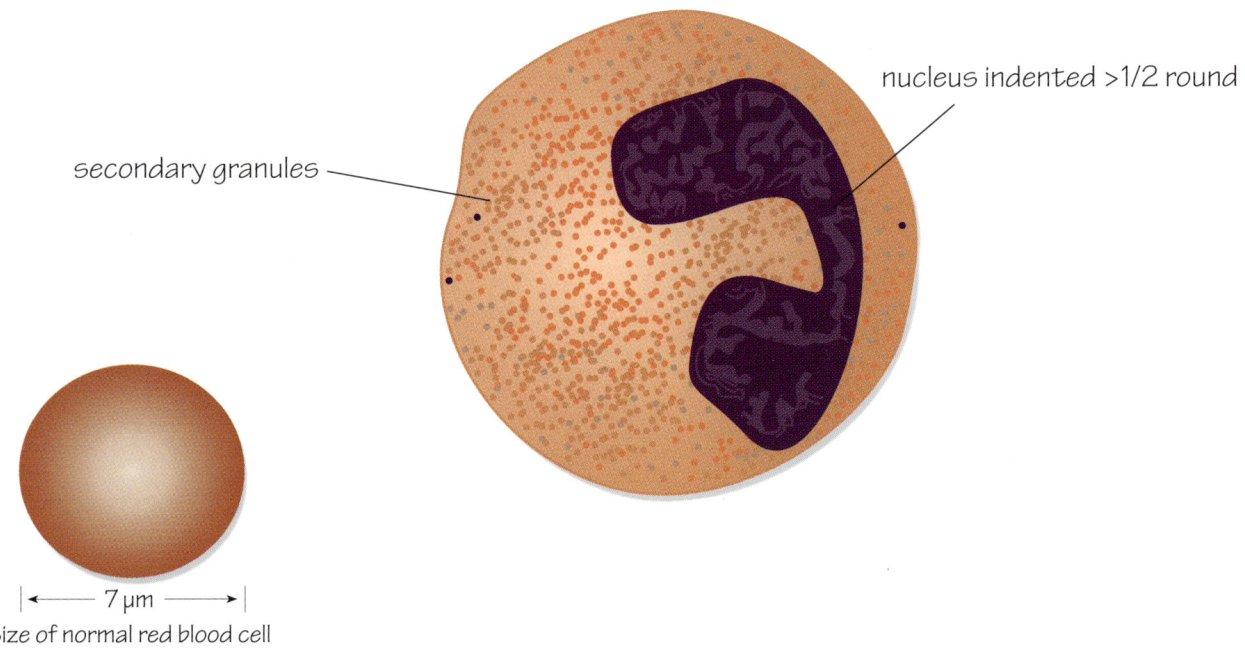

Band Neutrophil
- nucleus indented >1/2 round
- secondary granules
- 7 μm — size of normal red blood cell

Granulocytic (Myeloid) Cells

XL-06, 1987 (Blood, Wright-Giemsa, X400)

Identification	Referee %	Participant %
Band neutrophil	94.7	94.9
Segmented neutrophil	5.3	3.8

The cell indicated by the arrow is a band neutrophil. The cytoplasm contains many fine lilac granules characteristic of a neutrophil. The nucleus is deeply indented but is not constricted to the point that a filament that does not contain chromatin separates the nucleus into distinct lobes. Several red cells in the field are hypochromic.

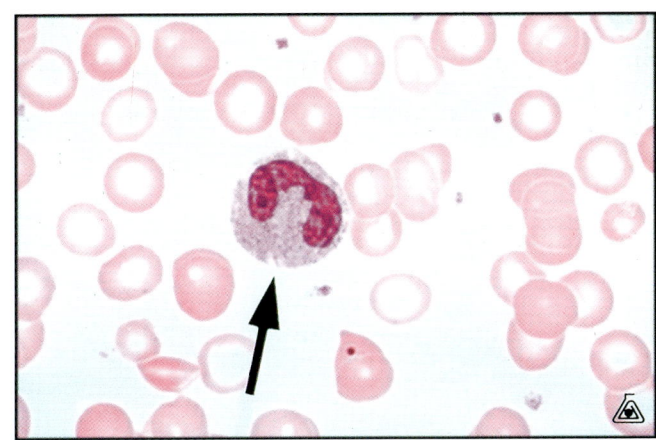

XL-72, 1987 (Blood, Wright-Giemsa, X400)

Identification	Referee %	Participant %
Band neutrophil	88.9	91.1
Segmented neutrophil	5.6	5.5

The cell indicated is a band neutrophil. The nucleus is U-shaped with no constrictions. The cytoplasm is filled with fine lilac granules. Several spherocytes are present among the red cells in the background.

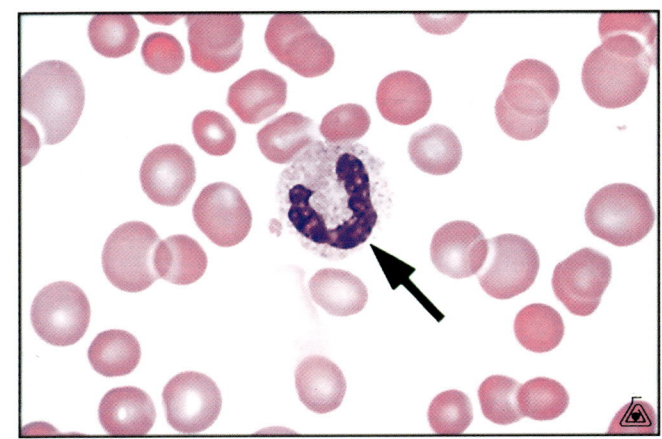

A-69, 1987 (Blood, Wright-Giemsa, X400)

Identification	Referee %	Participant %
Band neutrophil	100	97
Segmented neutrophil	-	2.3

The cell indicated is a band neutrophil. It has a U-shaped nucleus with no filaments or lobation. The cytoplasm contains many fine lilac granules. The surrounding cells are ovalocytes (elliptocytes). The patient has hereditary ovalocytosis.

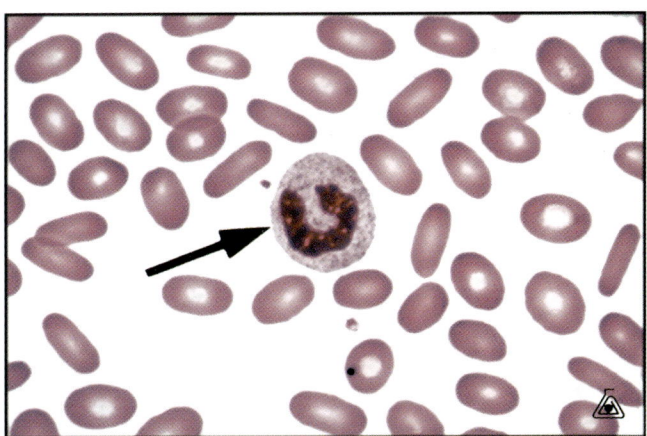

Granulocytic (Myeloid) Cells

Segmented Neutrophil

SYNONYMS
poly, PMN, seg

VITAL STATISTICS
- size .... 10 to 15 μm
- N:C ratio 1:3
- cell shape .... round to oval
- nuclear shape .... segmented, 2 to 5 lobes connected by filaments
- chromatin .... clumped
- nucleoli .... none
- cytoplasm .... pale pink with many specific (lilac) granules

KEY DIFFERENTIATING FEATURES
neutrophil cytoplasm with nucleus that is divided by thin filaments containing no internal chromatin into 2 to 5 lobes

OTHER FEATURES
forms with loss of nuclear–cytoplasm synchrony can be hypersegmented or agranular; these occur in megaloblastic and myelodysplastic states
activated forms show coarse (toxic) granulation and cytoplasmic vacuolization

POTENTIAL LOOK-ALIKES
monocytes

ASSOCIATED DISEASE STATES AND CONDITIONS
increased in infection, stress situations
leukemoid reactions

The segmented neutrophil is the most mature form of the myeloid series and the predominant white cell in the blood. It mimics its immediate precursors in size, shape, and the character of the cytoplasm. However, the nucleus is segmented or lobated (2-5 lobes normally), connected by thin filaments of chromatin. The filament appears as a solid thread-like dark line, so narrow that there is no visible chromatin between the two sides. The nuclear chromatin is clumped with no internal structure. N:C is 1:3, the lowest of the myeloid series. The cytoplasm is pale with lilac (specific) granules predominating.

Segmented Neutrophil

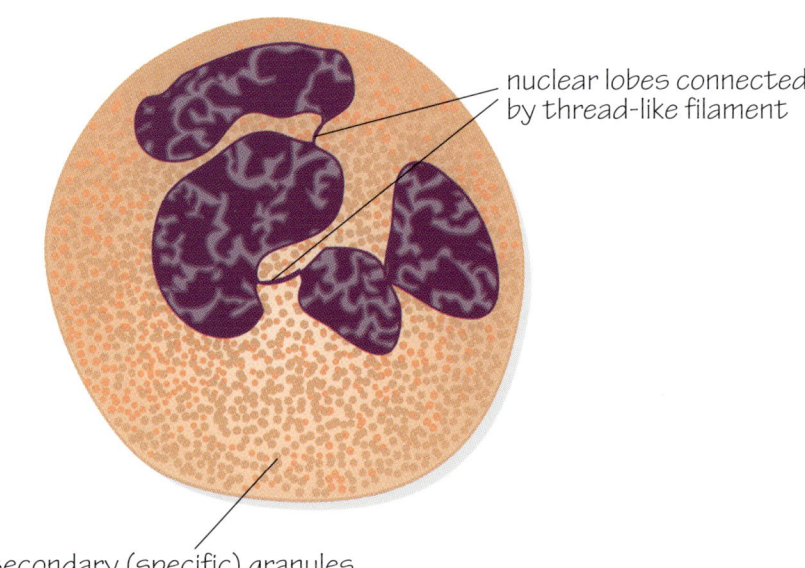

nuclear lobes connected by thread-like filament

secondary (specific) granules

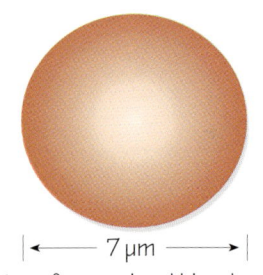

|← 7 μm →|

size of normal red blood cell

HE–38, 1992 (Blood, Wright-Giemsa, X440)

Identification	Referee %	Participant %
Segmented neutrophil	90	96
Band neutrophil	5.6	1.3

The cell between the two arrows is a segmented neutrophil. Its nucleus is divided into two lobes by a thin filament; there is no visible chromatin within the filament. The cytoplasm is a pale pink and contains many fine lilac granules. The red cells in the field show no distinctive abnormalities.

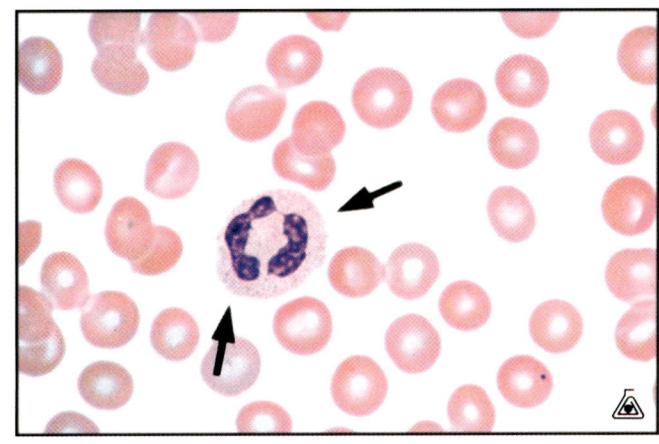

HE-7, 1996 (Blood, Wright-Giemsa, X400)

Identification	Referee %	Participant %
Segmented neutrophil	100	96.9
Hypersegmented neutrophil	-	1.3

The cell indicated by the arrow is a segmented neutrophil. It is divided into three distinct lobes by a thin filament of nuclear material; the nuclear cytoplasmic ratio is approximately 1:3. The cytoplasm is pale pink and contains fine lilac (secondary or specific) granules. The presence of a clearly segmented nucleus distinguishes the cell from other classes of leukocytes (monocytes and lymphocytes) and the nature of the granules distinguishes it from other blood granulocytes (eosinophils and basophils).

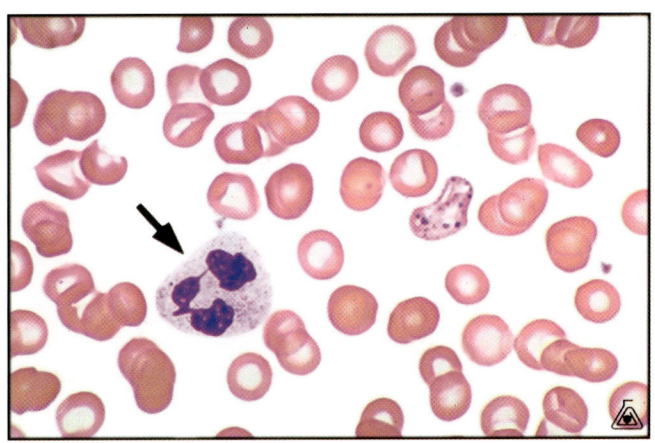

XH-17, 1995 (Blood, Wright-Giemsa, X400)

Identification	Referee %	Participant %
Segmented neutrophil	100	94.5

The cell is an example of a segmented neutrophil. The nucleus is divided into discrete lobes which are connected by thin filaments with no internal structure. The cytoplasm contains fine pink granules. A stomatocyte-like red cell is seen adjacent to this segmented neutrophil.

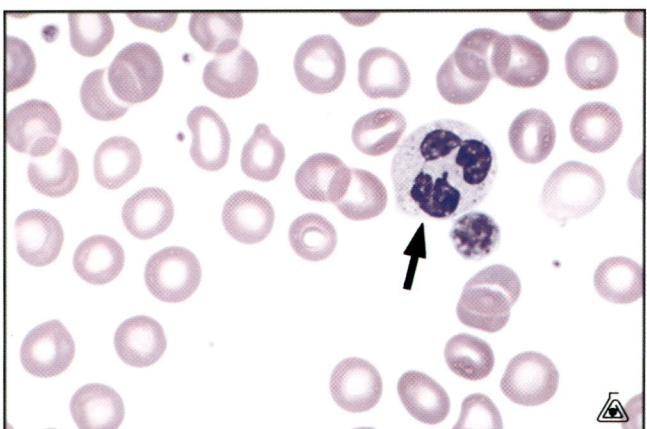

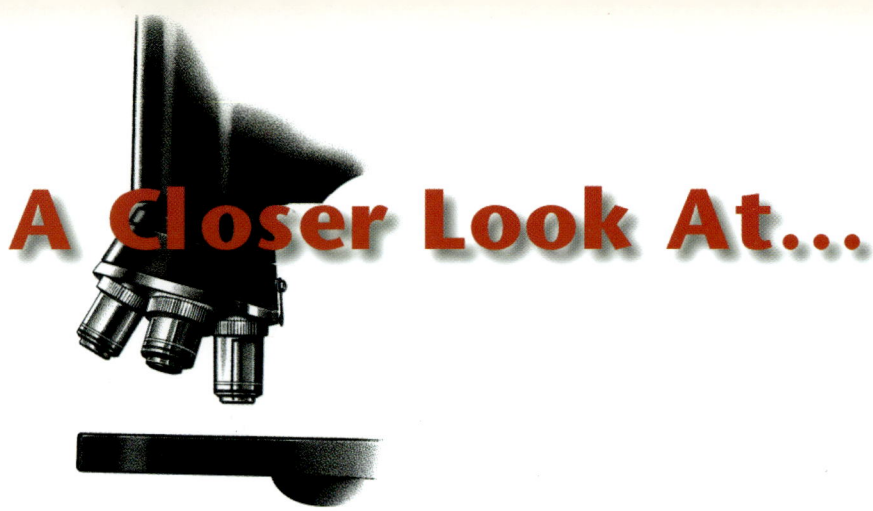

A Closer Look At...

Is it a Band or Segmented Neutrophil?

The classic band neutrophil with the S or C shaped nucleus or the classic segmented neutrophil with clearly evident filaments are no problem to distinguish. At times, however, the nucleus may be twisted or folded so that the connecting filaments are difficult, if not impossible, to visualize. In analyzing cells with touching or superimposed nuclear lobes, use the following considerations:

Assume a hidden filament is present and classify the cell as a segmented neutrophil if:
1. the margins of two adjacent lobes are completely separated
2. the width of either of the two adjacent lobes markedly narrows or converges toward the junction of the lobes, making it possible that a thin filament is hidden
3. the nucleus is so extensively folded that it cannot be determined if a filament is present.

Assume the cell is a folded band neutrophil if:
1. an elongated band crosses over itself without evidence of a constriction
2. only the distal tip of the nucleus is slightly bent back upon itself
3. the hidden area in the fold between two superimposed lobes is so small and the lobe width so plump, that it is unlikely a thin filament could form.

The diagram on the next page illustrates these rules.

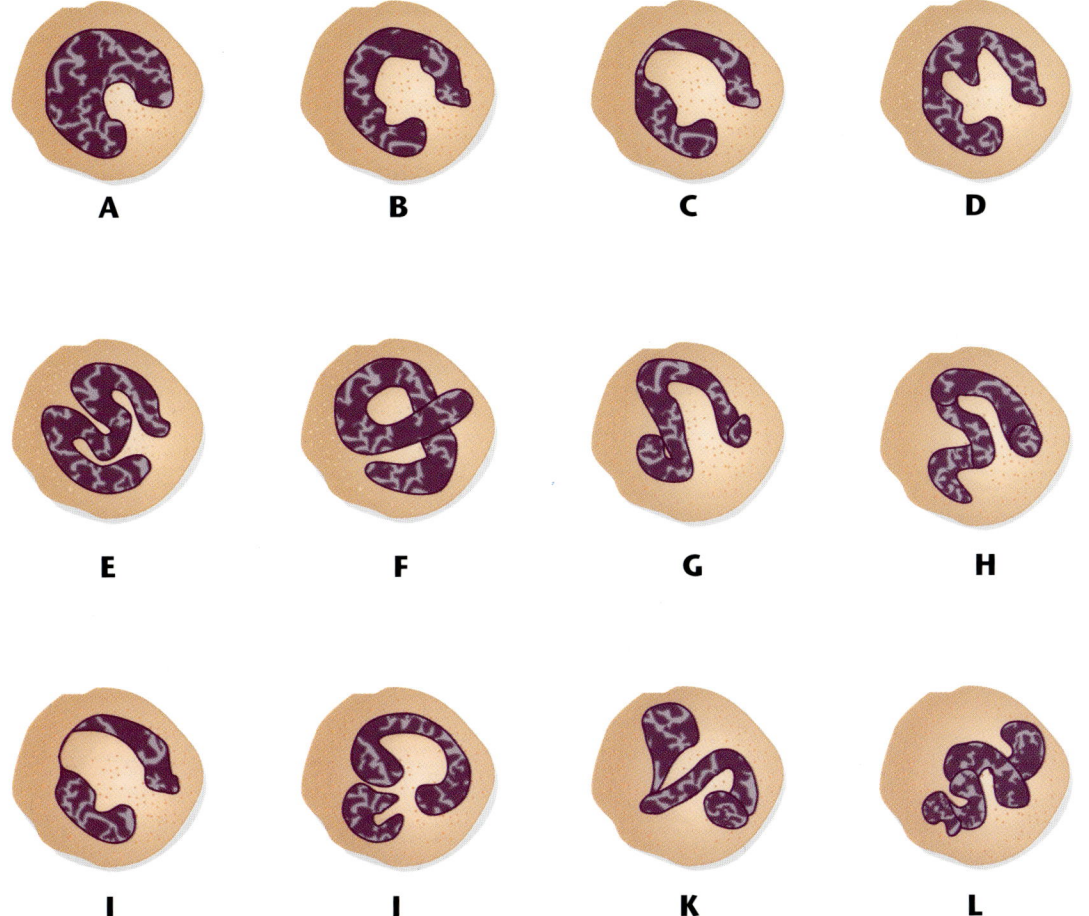

- A. **METAMYELOCYTE:** The nucleus is indented less than half the distance from the farthest nuclear margin.
- B. **BAND:** The nucleus is indented more than half the distance from the farthest nuclear margin.
- C. **BAND:** The nucleus has a constricted portion or isthmus connecting two lobes, but chromatin clearly is visible between the dark, parallel nuclear margins.
- D. **BAND:** A small extension or appendage of the nucleus is present, but the cell still is classified as a band because a filament is not visible.
- E. **BAND:** The nuclear contour is tortuous, but the no nuclear lobes or filaments are evident.
- F. **BAND:** The elongated band-shaped nucleus crosses over itself, but no lobes or filaments are visible.
- G. **BAND:** Only the distal tip of the nucleus is folded back upon itself.
- H. **BAND:** The hidden region between the lobes is small: it is unlikely that the nucleus could constrict down to a thin filament from the plump width of the adjoining lobes.
- I. **SEGMENTED NEUTROPHIL:** Complete constriction to a thin filament has occurred; no chromatin is visible between two margins.
- J. **SEGMENTED NEUTROPHIL:** Although no filament is visible, the margins of two adjacent lobes are completely separated.
- K. **SEGMENTED NEUTROPHIL:** The width of one of the lobes narrows as it approaches the border of another lobe, making it possible for a filament to be hidden behind the fold.
- L. **SEGMENTED NEUTROPHIL:** The nucleus is so extensively folded, it is impossible to determine whether a filament is present.

Granulocytic (Myeloid) Cells

Basophil

SYNONYMS
none

VITAL STATISTICS
size .... 10 to 15 µm
N:C ratio .... 1:2 to 1:3
cell shape .... round to oval
nuclear shape .... segmented, often obscured by granules
chromatin .... clumped
nucleoli .... none
cytoplasm .... coarse, dense granules

KEY DIFFERENTIATING FEATURES
appearance of mature myeloid cell with coarse, dense cytoplasmic granules that overlay the nucleus

OTHER FEATURES
mimics other mature myeloid cells in size and shape
shows alterations in megaloblastic and toxic states

POTENTIAL LOOK-ALIKES
rarely eosinophils and neutrophils with toxic granulation

ASSOCIATED DISEASE STATES AND CONDITIONS
myeloproliferative states
hypersensitivity reactions
myxedema
tuberculosis
diabetes
increased at onset of menses
increased number seen in blood smears collected in the afternoon and evening

Basophils, mature and immature are characterized by the presence of a small to moderate number of coarse, densely stained granules of different sizes and shapes. Basophilic granules are specific granules and are generally larger than neutrophilic granules and about the same size as eosinophilic granules. Most are roughly spherical but they may be irregular. The predominant color is blue–black, but some may stain purple to red. The granules are unevenly distributed and frequently overlay and obscure the nucleus. In cell size, shape, and nuclear morphology, the basophils mimic their neutrophil or eosinophil counterparts.

Basophil

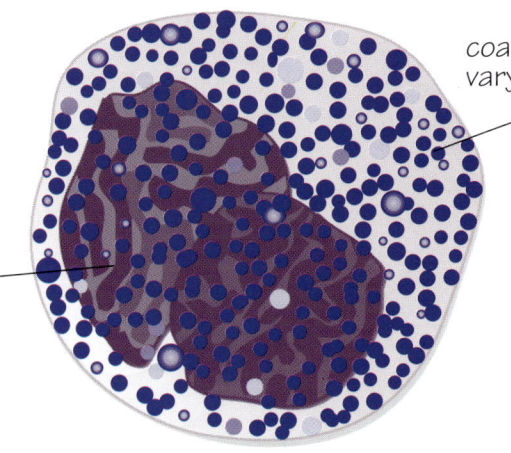

coarse, dense purple granules varying in size and shape

segmented nucleus, obscured by granules

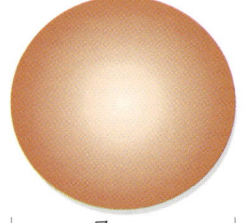

|← 7 µm →|
size of normal red blood cell

H-08, 1981 (Blood, Wright-Giemsa, X400)

Identification	Referee %	Participant %
Basophil	100	98.5

The cell indicated by the arrow and the cell opposite are basophils. A lobated nucleus is evident in both cells and the cytoplasm contains large dense granules which are over and partially obscure the nucleus. The nucleated cell in the center of the field is a lymphocyte.

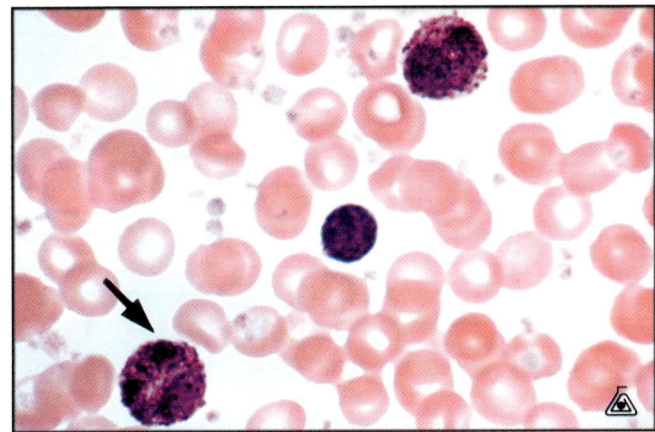

A-46, 1986 (Blood, Wright-Giemsa, X400)

Identification	Referee %	Participant %
Basophil	100	95.4

The cell indicated by the arrow is a basophil. The cytoplasm has a number of large coarse granules that range in color from dark purple to red purple. The red cells in the field are abnormal with a drepanocyte (sickle cell) and target cell adjacent to the basophil.

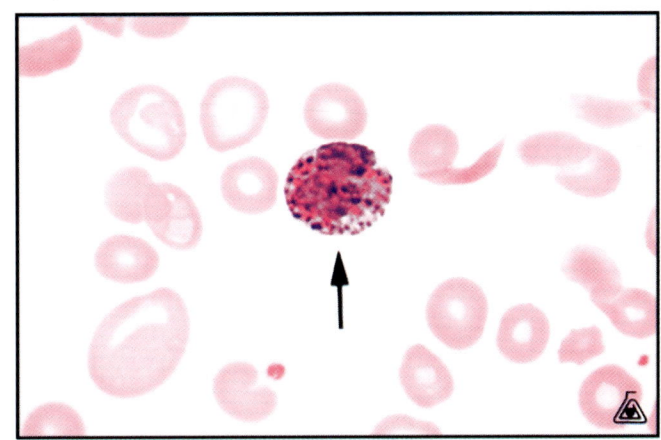

A-30, 1984 (Blood, Wright-Giemsa, X450)

Identification	Referee %	Participant %
Basophil	94.4	80.1

The cell indicated by the arrow has coarse, dense granules in its cytoplasm. Its nucleus, however, does not appear lobated or segmented. It is a basophil precursor, probably a basophilic myelocyte. Basophil granules are specific granules and become evident at the myelocyte stage. The nuclear maturation sequence in basophils is analogous to that in neutrophils.

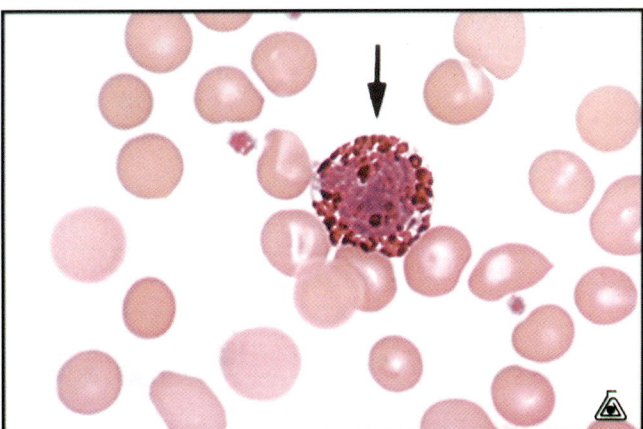

Eosinophil (any stage)

SYNONYMS
eo

VITAL STATISTICS

size	10 to 15 μm for mature forms; 10 to 18 μm for immature forms
N:C ratio	1:3 for mature forms and 1:2 to 2:1 for immature forms
cell shape	round to oval
nuclear shape	segmented with 2-3 lobes connected by a thin filament of chromatin; band, metamyelocyte, and myelocyte forms (generally found only in the bone marrow) have nuclear characteristics identical to the corresponding neutrophilic cells
chromatin	dense and compact in the segmented and band forms; less dense and finer in metamyelocyte and myelocyte forms
nucleoli	none
cytoplasm	filled by coarse, spherical, uniform orange-red refractile granules; may be partially degranulated; younger forms may contain a few dark purplish primary granules

KEY DIFFERENTIATING FEATURES
larger cells with nuclear characteristics identical to neutrophilic cells
abundant cytoplasm filled by large uniform, coarse, orange-red granules

POTENTIAL LOOK-ALIKES
neutrophil, with or without toxic granulation
basophil

ASSOCIATED DISEASE STATES AND CONDITIONS
normal constituent of peripheral blood
increased numbers seen in:
 drugs reactions
 invasive parasitic infections
 some chronic infections
 some carcinomas
 myeloproliferative disorders
 pernicious anemia
 Hodgkin's and non-Hodgkin's lymphomas
 collagen vascular disease
 various allergic and skin disorders
 sarcoidosis
 certain pulmonary diseases

Eosinophils are present in blood, bone marrow, and tissues. Their abundant cytoplasm is generally evenly filled by numerous, coarse, orange-red granules of uniform size. The granules rarely overlie the nucleus and exhibit a refractile appearance, due to their crystalline structure. Occasionally, eosinophils can become degranulated with only a few orange-red granules remaining visible within faint pink cytoplasm.

About 80% of mature segmented eosinophils have two round or ovoid nuclear lobes that are of equal size. The remainder of segmented eosinophils have three lobes and an occasional cell will have 4-5 lobes.

Immature eosinophils exhibit nuclear characteristics identical to the corresponding neutrophilic cell. These cells are rarely seen in the blood, but are found in bone marrow smears. Immature eosinophils may have fewer granules than more mature forms. The earliest recognizable eosinophilic form by light microscopy is the eosinophilic myelocyte. Eosinophilic myelocytes often contain a few dark purplish primary granules in addition to the orange-red secondary granules.

The characteristic bright color of eosinophilic granules makes these cells easily recognizable on well stained blood films. The granules may appear lighter or darker on photomicrographs due to problems with color rendition. Discoloration may give these granules a blue, brown, or even pink tint. Nonetheless, the uniform, coarse nature of eosinophilic granules is characteristic and differs from the smaller, finer granules of neutrophilic cells.

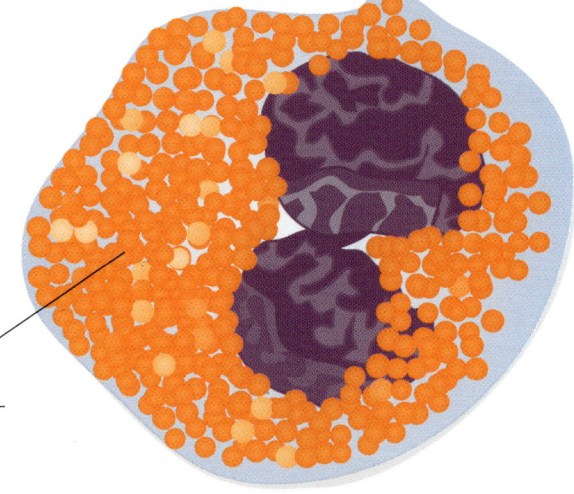

Eosinophil — bright orange-red refractile granules

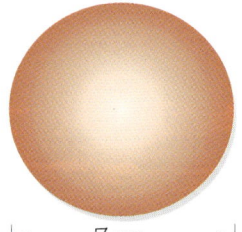

7 μm — size of normal red blood cell

H1-46, 1990 (Blood, Wright-Giemsa, X375)

Identification	Referee %	Participant %
Eosinophil	94.1	98.1

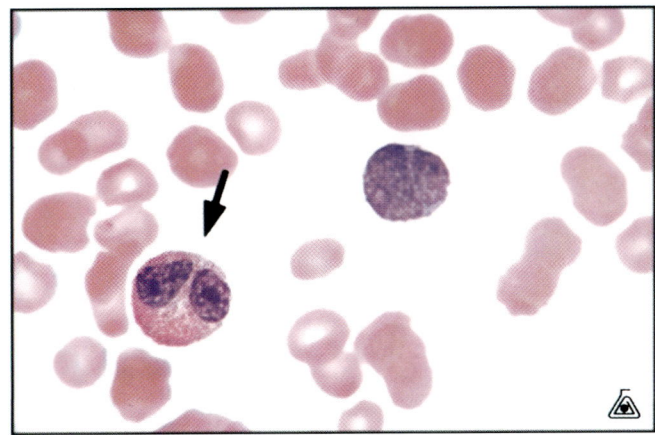

This blood film shows a mature eosinophil. No platelets are visible. The red blood cells exhibit artifacts from the thick area of the blood film. The arrowed cell has a bilobed nucleus separated by a barely visible thin filament. The chromatin is compact and dark with large clumps. No nucleoli are present. The abundant cytoplasm is filled by numerous, uniform, coarse, red-orange granules. The other leukocyte in the field is a lymphoma cell as recognized by its moderately fine chromatin, nuclear cleft, small nucleolus and scant cytoplasm. This case is from a 60-year-old man with circulating intermediate grade (small cleaved cell) lymphoma cells.

HE-22, 1991 (Blood, Wright-Giemsa, X350)

Identification	Referee %	Participant %
Eosinophil	100	99.1

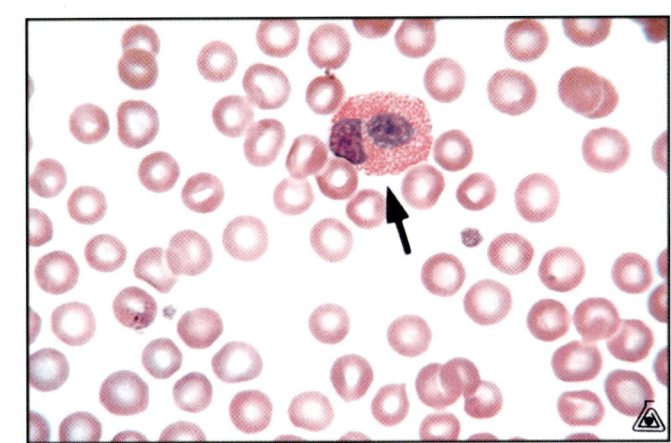

A mature eosinophil is illustrated in this blood film. Two normal platelets are seen. The red blood cells are normochromic and normocytic. The arrowed cell exhibits a bilobed nucleus separated by a barely visible thin filament. The chromatin is compact and dark. The cytoplasm contains uniform coarse, red-orange granules. This case is from a 24-year-old black female with sickle cell trait.

HE-36, 1992 (Blood, Wright-Giemsa, X375)

Identification	Referee %	Participant %
Eosinophil	100	98.8

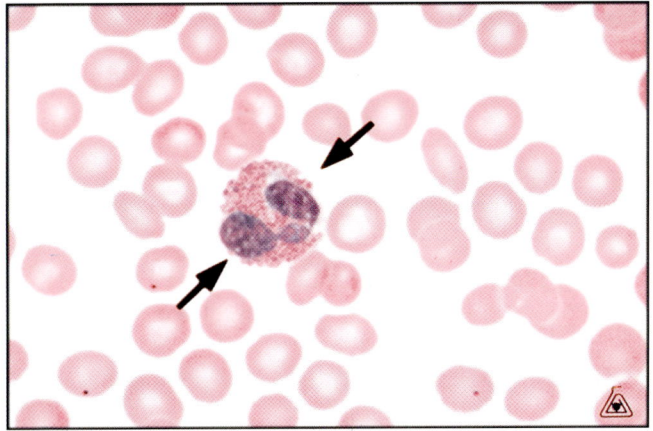

This blood film shows an eosinophil. No platelets are present. Red blood cells are normochromic and normocytic. Three red blood cells in the field contain Howell-Jolly bodies, which are slightly out of the plane of focus. A few ovalocytes are present. The arrowed cell contains a three lobed nucleus with the lobes connected by thin filaments. The chromatin is dark and compact without nucleoli. The cytoplasm is partially degranulated, but still contains numerous, coarse red-orange granules of uniform size. This case is from a 30-year-old woman with idiopathic thrombocytopenic purpura (ITP).

Granulocytic (Myeloid) Cells

A Closer Look At...

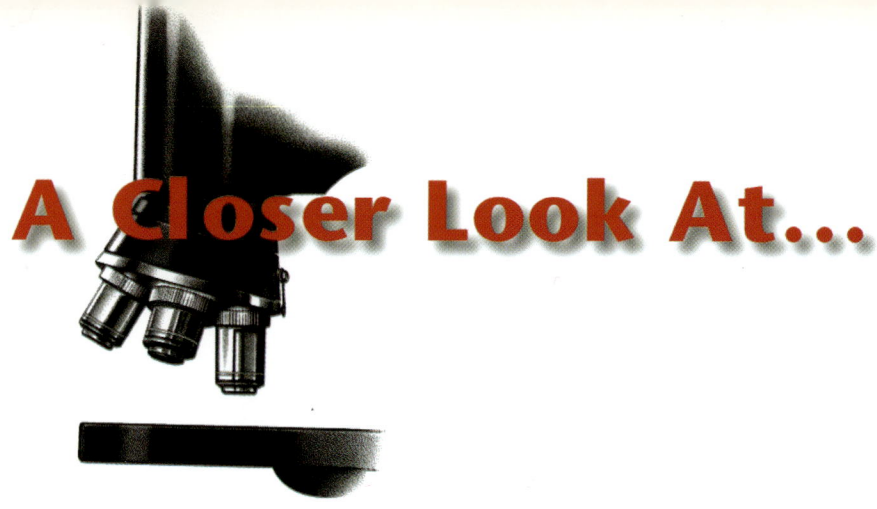

Eosinophilia

Eosinophils have receptors for IgE, histamine, the Fc portion of immunoglobulin, and complement. Their granules contain numerous enzymes including major basic protein, peroxidase, phospholipase D, catalase, acid phosphatase, and vitamin B_{12}-binding proteins. While eosinophils can phagocytize bacteria, their ability to kill bacteria is less than neutrophils. The primary function of eosinophils is in fighting protozoal, helminth, and other parasitic infections. They also participate in hypersensitivity (allergic) reactions and nonimmunologic inflammatory responses.

Eosinophilia in the blood and bone marrow can be found in a variety of disorders. Blood eosinophilia has been defined as an absolute eosinophil count greater than 0.6×10^9/L. The most common causes are drug reactions, allergies, and parasitic infections. Allergic conditions such as asthma, hay fever, and urticaria can all cause eosinophilia. Numerous drugs have been associated with eosinophilia and are probably the most common cause of this phenomenon in hospitalized patients. Parasitic infections due to organisms that are tissue invasive, such as trichinosis, filariasis, and visceral larva migrans (Toxocara), result in eosinophilia. In contrast, noninvasive parasitic infections due to organisms such as Giardia and Trichomonas do not cause eosinophilia.

A variety of chronic infections (Brucellosis, fungi, leprosy, tuberculosis, etc.), malignancies (carcinomas of the lung, stomach, ovaries, etc.), collagen vascular diseases, pulmonary diseases (hypersensitivity pneumonitis, Löffler's syndrome, etc.), sarcoidosis, and some types of dermatitis (pemphigus, bullous pemphigoid, dermatitis herpetiformis, etc.) are associated with eosinophilia. Increased numbers of eosinophils can be seen in any of the myeloproliferative disorders, which include chronic myelogenous leukemia (CML), essential thrombocythemia, polycythemia vera, and myelofibrosis with myeloid metaplasia. Eosinophilia is classically associated with Hodgkin's disease, but can also be found in non-Hodgkin's lymphomas, graft versus host disease, and pernicious anemia.

Occasional cases of marked eosinophilia without known cause are termed idiopathic hypereosinophilic syndrome. Some recently identified causes of reactive eosinophilia include eosinophilia-myalgia syndrome due to L-tryptophan ingestion and therapy with recombinant human interleukins.

A major constituent of the eosinophil is Charcot-Leyden protein, which is composed of lysophospholipase. Intense or prolonged eosinophilic inflammatory conditions can lead to the formation of Charcot-Leyden crystals. They are bipyramidal, hexagonal crystals found in tissues, fluids, and secretions. They are most commonly associated with asthma, parasitic infections, and the eosinophilic variant of acute myelomonocytic leukemia (M4Eo). In the latter leukemic condition, the crystals display a refractile glassy blue appearance and are several times longer than myeloblasts.

Formation of Charcot-Leyden Crystals

Causes of Eosinophilia

Allergies
  asthma, hayfever, urticaria
  drug allergies (gold, allopurinol, eosinophilia-myalgia syndrome)
Parasitic Infections
  ascariasis, filariasis, ancylostomiasis, trichinosis, toxocariasis
Skin Disorders
  psoriasis, eczema, dermatitis herpetiformis
Malignancies
  Hodgkin's and non-Hodgkin's lymphoma, carcinoma
Leukemia
  chronic myeloproliferative disorders, eosinophilic leukemia, eosinophilic variant of myelomonocytic leukemia
Miscellaneous Conditions
  immunodeficiency diseases, eosinophilic granuloma, erythema multiforme, polyarteritis nodosa, sarcoidosis, hypereosinophilic syndrome, post-irradiation, pulmonary eosinophilia, tropical eosinophilia, pernicious anemia, collagen vascular diseases, recombinant human interleukin therapy

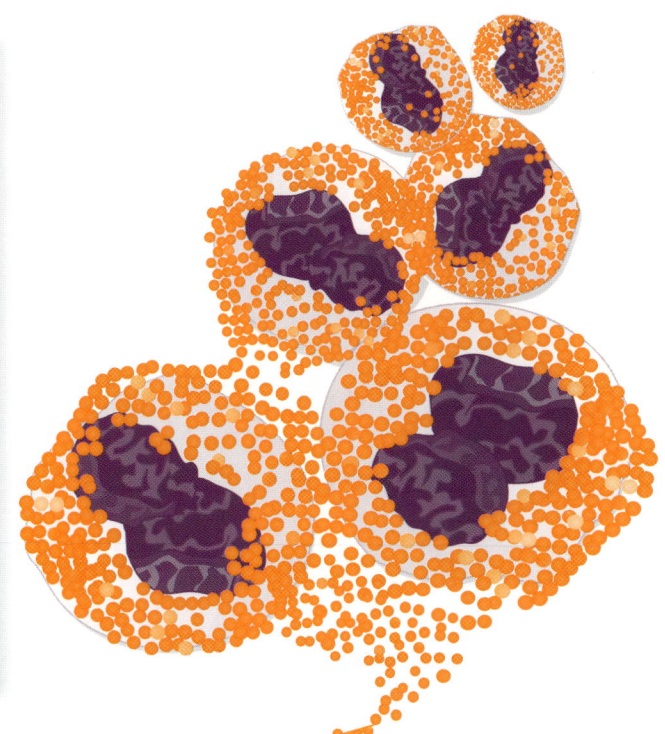

Massive infiltration of tissue or fluid by eosinophils often leads to disintegration of cells and formation of Charcot-Leyden crystals.

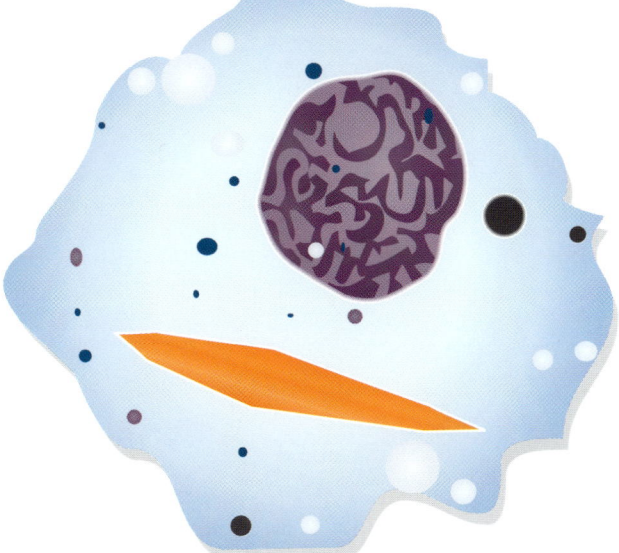

Some of the crystals may be phagocytized by macrophages.

Granulocytic (Myeloid) Cells

Monocytes, Immature

SYNONYMS
monoblast, promonocyte

VITAL STATISTICS
- size .... 15 to 25 µm
- N:C ratio .... 7:1 to 3:1
- cell shape .... round to oval
- nuclear shape .... round or indented
- chromatin .... reticular, lacy
- nucleoli .... 1 to 2 present
- cytoplasm .... gray to cloudy blue, few red granules

KEY DIFFERENTIATING FEATURES
high N:C, nucleoli, indented nucleus, gray cytoplasm

OTHER FEATURES
may appear as undefined "blast cell"
vacuoles may be seen in cytoplasm

POTENTIAL LOOK-ALIKES
other blasts (myeloblast, lymphoblast, megakaryoblast)
mature monocyte
macrophage
atypical lymphocyte (rarely)
lymphoma cell
carcinoma

ASSOCIATED DISEASE STATES AND CONDITIONS
acute monocytic leukemia
acute myelomonocytic leukemia
chronic myelomonocytic leukemia

Immature monocytes are not usually seen in any significant numbers except in malignancies involving the monocytic cell line. The morphologic characteristics of monoblasts are similar to other blast forms, although the cytoplasm is generally more abundant and the nucleus more folded than myeloblasts. Immature monocytes include a spectrum of cells whose morphology ranges from a blast cell to a monocyte having a somewhat enlarged nucleus with a small nucleolus.

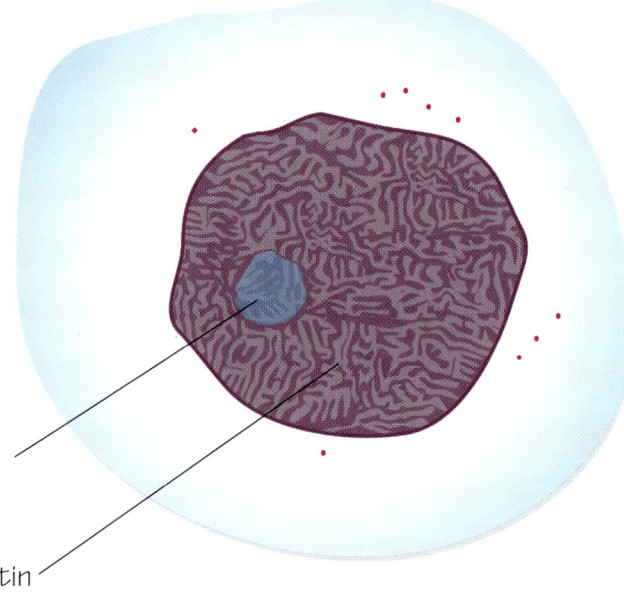

Monoblast
- prominent nucleolus
- lacy chromatin

Promonocyte
- few red granules
- coarse chromatin
- gray-blue cytoplasm
- nucleoli

|← 7 µm →|
size of normal red blood cell

Granulocytic (Myeloid) Cells

H-58, 1982 (Blood, Wright-Giemsa, X400)

Identification	Referee %	Participant %
Immature monocyte	66.7	59.7
Monoblast	28.2	17.5

The cell indicated by the arrow is an immature monocyte or monoblast. There is a high N:C ratio and the nucleus has lacy chromatin with nucleoli present. The nucleus is also indented. The cytoplasm is gray–blue and contains several vacuoles. The other nucleated cells in the field have similar nuclear and cytoplasmic characteristics and are also examples of immature monocytes.

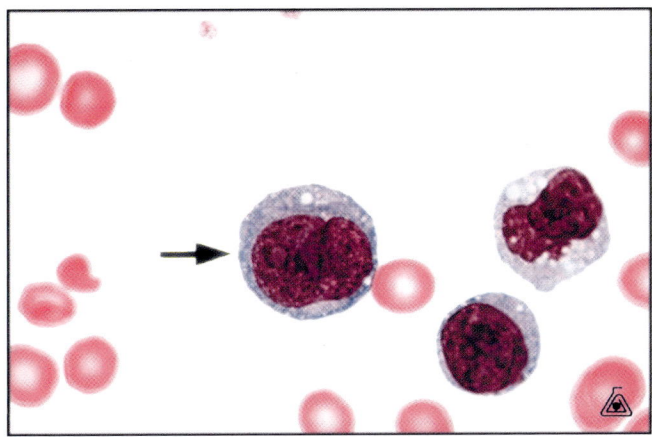

HE-28, 1994 (Blood, Wright-Giemsa, X400)

Identification	Referee %	Participant %
Monocyte	86.2	78.3
Immature monocyte	6.8	6.1

Two immature and dysplastic monocytes are seen. The nucleus is bean-shaped typical of a monocyte, but immature characteristics include blast-like, non-condensed chromatin and a high N:C ratio. The cytoplasm is also dysplastic; it is pale rather than the usual gray-blue. Because the cytoplasm is pale, these cells can be confused with giant bands or dysplastic neutrophils.

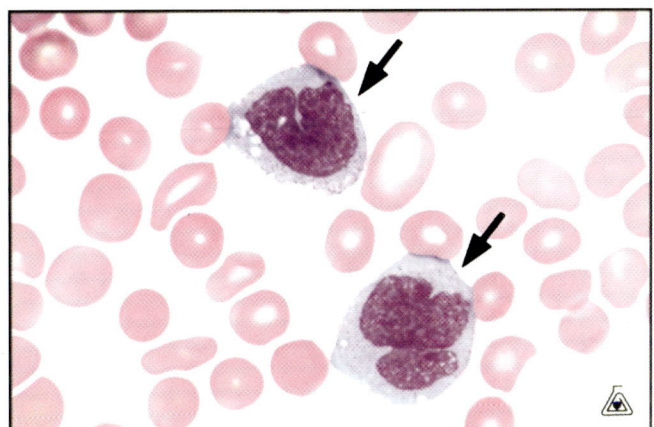

Monocyte

SYNONYMS
monos

VITAL STATISTICS
- size .... 12 to 20 μm
- N:C ratio .... 4:1 to 2:1
- cell shape .... round, may demonstrate pseudopods
- nuclear shape .... round to oval, indented
- chromatin .... slight clumping
- nucleoli .... none
- cytoplasm .... gray–blue, scattered vacuoles

KEY DIFFERENTIATING FEATURES
abundant gray blue cytoplasm often with vacuoles, indented nucleus

OTHER FEATURES
- sparse lilac granules
- may contain phagocytized material in cytoplasm

POTENTIAL LOOK–ALIKES
- atypical lymphocytes
- myelocytes, metamyelocytes
- band neutrophils
- immature monocytes

ASSOCIATED DISEASE STATES AND CONDITIONS
- normal constituent of peripheral blood
- increased in cases of:
  - chronic neutropenia
  - collagen vascular diseases
  - inflammatory bowel disease
  - sarcoid
  - chronic infections (CMV, syphilis and tuberculosis)
  - malignancy

Mature monocytes are slightly larger than neutrophils. The majority are round with smooth edges, but some may have pseudopod-like cytoplasm extensions. The nucleus is usually indented, often resembling a three-pointed hat, but can be folded or even band-like. The chromatin is somewhat clumped but usually less dense than the neutrophil or lymphocyte. There is no nucleolus. The cytoplasm is abundant and gray to gray-blue (ground–glass appearance) and may contain fine, evenly distributed pink azurophilic granules and/or vacuoles. Phagocytized material may be present in the cytoplasm.

Mature Monocytes

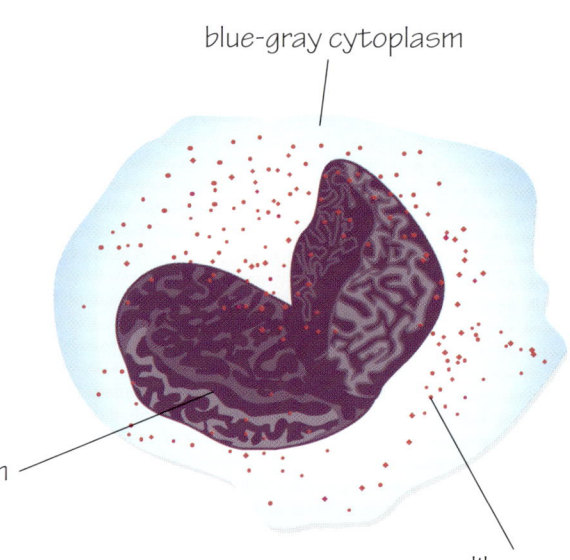

blue-gray cytoplasm

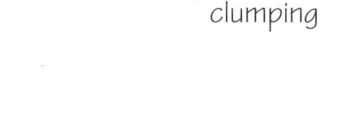

slight chromatin clumping

sparse lilac granules

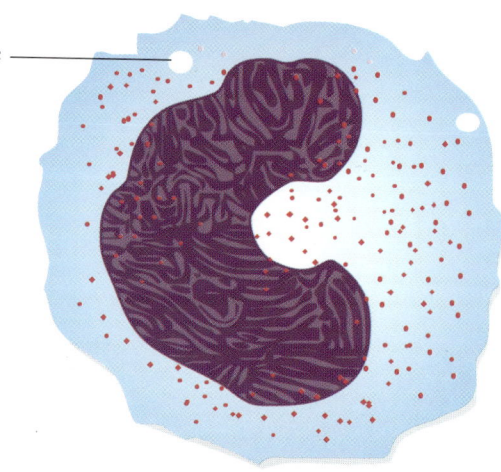

vacuole

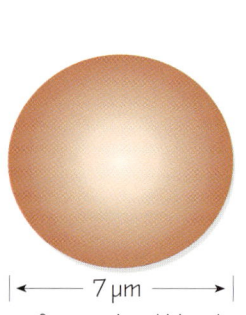

|← 7 μm →|

size of normal red blood cell

Granulocytic (Myeloid) Cells

HE-24, 1992 (Blood, Wright-Giemsa, X330)

Identification	Referee %	Participant %
Monocyte	85	82.7
Band neutrophil	15	6.7

The cell indicated by the arrow is a monocyte. It has an S-shaped nucleus with loose chromatin that is much less clumped than that which would be seen in a band neutrophil. The cytoplasm has a ground glass appearance with no evident granules. Surrounding the cell are normal platelets and red cells.

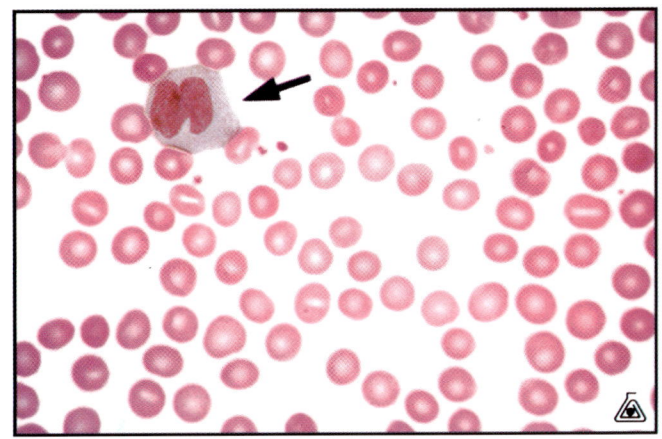

HE-4, 1992 (Blood, Wright-Giemsa, X450)

Identification	Referee %	Participant %
Monocyte	95	88.9
Immature monocyte	5	7.5

The cell indicated by the arrow is a monocyte. Its nucleus has the sponge–like chromatin and trilobate configuration often seen in monocytes. The cytoplasm has a grayish, ground glass appearance and numerous empty vacuoles are present. The other nucleated cell present is a segmented neutrophil, with its lobated nucleus and pink granular cytoplasm.

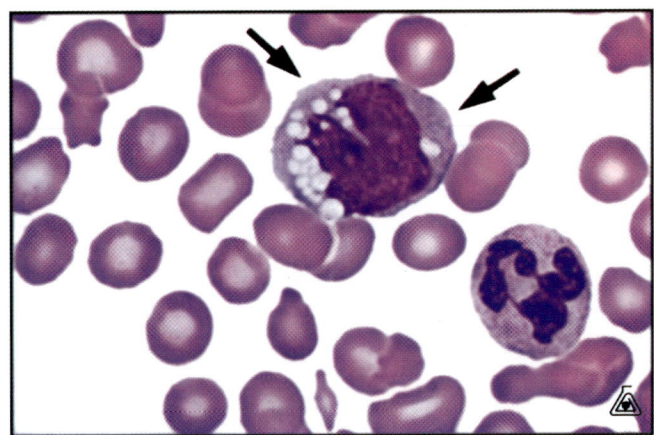

XH-10, 1994 (Blood, Wright-Giemsa stain, X400)

Identification	Referee %	Participant %
Monocyte	100	90
Atypical lymphocyte	-	6

The cell indicated by an arrow is a monocyte. It has an indented, somewhat lobulated nucleus with slightly clumped chromatin, clearly different from the adjacent band neutrophil. The cytoplasm has a gray-blue color and contains clear vacuoles. The adjacent band neutrophil can be used to contrast the tinctoral properties of the cytoplasm of the neutrophil (pale pink with readily apparent granules) and the monocyte (gray-blue with vacuoles). The nuclear characteristics and extent of cytoplasmic vacuolation distinguish this cell from an atypical lymphocyte.

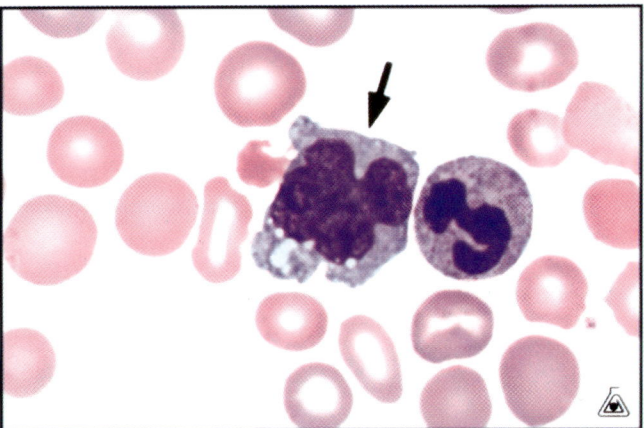

Granulocytic (Myeloid) Cells

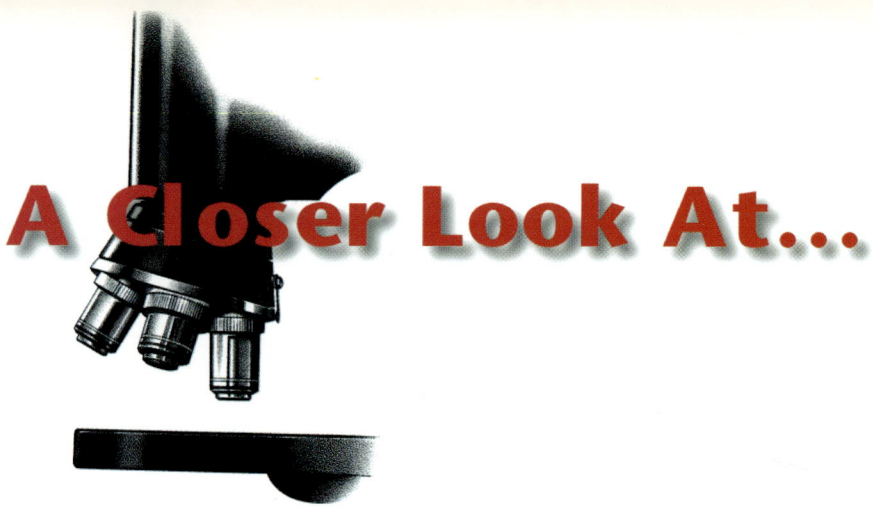

A Closer Look At...

Life Cycle of Monocytes

Monocytes share common stem cells with myeloid cells; the CFU-GM is the last cell type in the common lineage. The first committed monocyte precursor is the CFU-M. This cell gives rise to the monoblast, promonocyte, and monocyte. It is inferred that three to four cell divisions occur between the monoblast and monocyte and that once mature, monocytes exit the marrow fairly rapidly. The distinction between myeloblast and monoblast is difficult on a morphologic basis. It has been suggested that early monocyte precursors may be counted as myeloid precursors because no significant maturing monocyte population is usually recognized in normal bone marrow. The marrow promonocyte can best be defined using histochemical techniques, especially the nonspecific esterases. Promonocytes are large cells with an indented nucleus that may or may not demonstrate a discrete nucleolus. They have a moderate amount of gray-blue cytoplasm that may contain a few pink granules. Monocyte precursors are most readily recognized in pathologic states, specifically acute myelomonocytic leukemia (M4) and acute monoblastic leukemia (M5).

Once monocytes enter the blood they circulate for 12 to 24 hours and enter the tissue where they are transformed into macrophages without dividing. Tissue macrophages may survive a long period. Alveolar, splenic, and peritoneal macrophages, Kupffer cells of the liver, osteoclasts of the bone and microglial cells of the nervous system are all derived from bone marrow monocytes. Blood monocytosis is associated with infectious diseases (tuberculosis, leprosy, Salmonellosis, Brucellosis), collagen vascular diseases and hematologic diseases, as noted above.

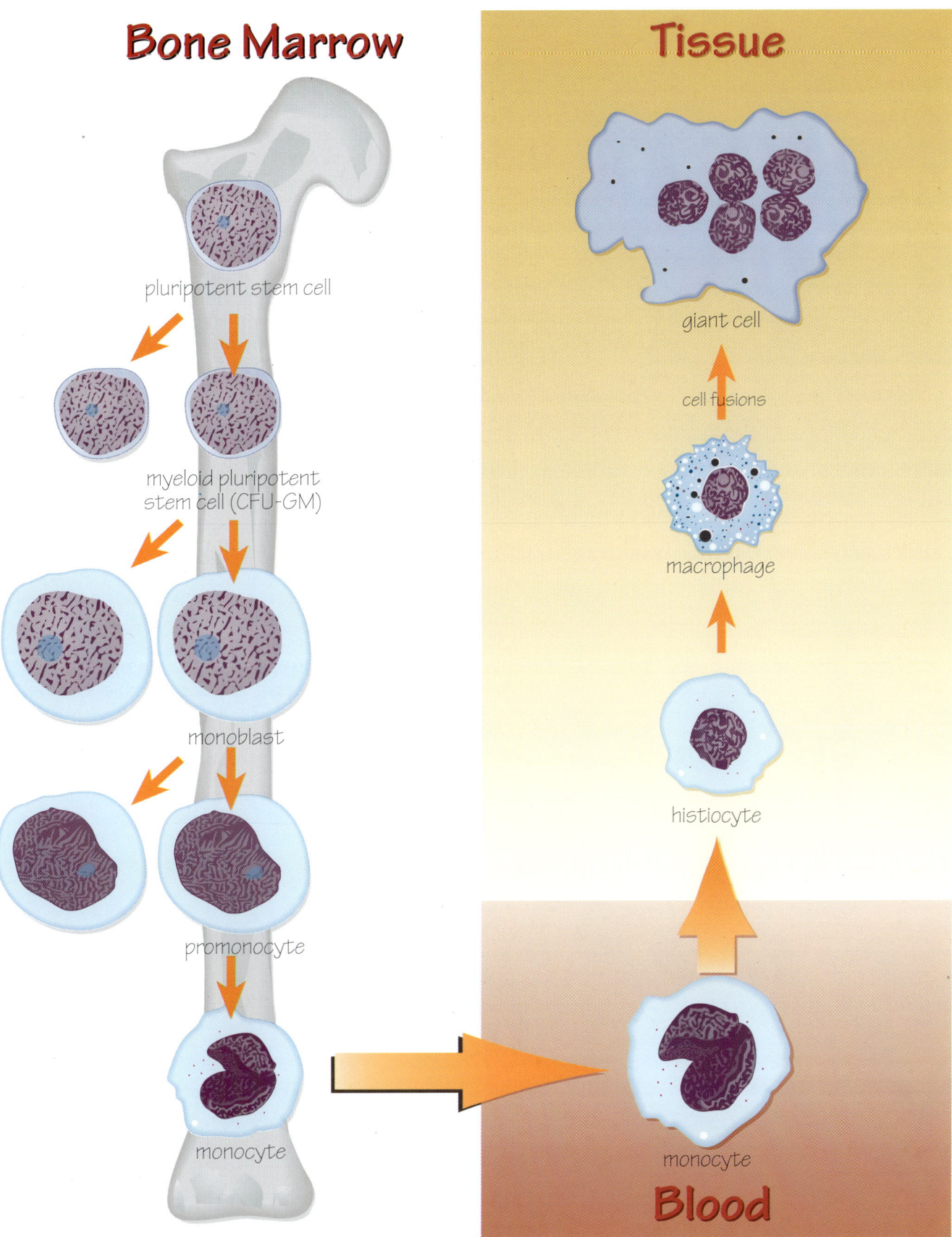

Granulocytic (Myeloid) Cells

Toxic Granulation and/or Multiple Toxic Vacuoles

SYNONYMS
activated neutrophils

VITAL STATISTICS
size	10-15 µm
N:C ratio	1:3
cell shape	round to oval
nuclear shape	segmented and band forms
chromatin	clumped
nucleoli	none
cytoplasm	large dark granules, multiple empty vacuoles, sometimes Döhle bodies

KEY DIFFERENTIATING FEATURES
dark granules
multiple vacuoles, often of varying size

OTHER FEATURES
vacuoles may contain ingested organsims
Döhle bodies may be present (if so, for proficiency testing purposes, use the Döhle body identification)

POTENTIAL LOOK-ALIKES
Alder's anomaly
monocytes
basophils
degenerating neutrophils

ASSOCIATED DISEASE STATES AND CONDITIONS
infection
trauma
burns
colony stimulating factor therapy

Toxic granulation is manifest by the presence of large purple or dark blue granules, resembling the primary granules of promyelocytes, metamyelocytes, bands, and segmented neutrophils. Histochemical stains and electron microscopy indicate that these granules are primary (azurophilic) granules. Even though about one third of the granules in a segmented neutrophil are azurophilic, they are difficult to recognize because they become progressively less basophilic as the cell matures. In neutrophil activation states, the primary granules retain their basophilia in mature neutrophils. They are also larger and more deeply staining than normal due to enhanced lysosomal enzyme production and packaging (see *A Closer Look At...page 44*).

Toxic granulation of neutrophils should not be confused with eosinophils. Toxic granules are smaller than eosinophilic granules, but larger than normal neutrophilic granules. Toxic granules are morphologically similar to the inclusions of Alder's anomaly (page 302).

Toxic vacuolization sometimes accompanies toxic granulation cells or may be found independently. Vacuoles are round clear spaces in the cytoplasm which represent the sites of digestion of phagocytized material. The presence of vacuoles may be clinically important because they occur in many cases of septicemia. When combined with a high neutrophil count and left shift, the sensitivity for the presence of sepsis is greater than 95%.

One or two small vacuoles may not be clinically significant; they may represent degenerative changes in blood stored in EDTA. Toxic vacuoles are larger and more numerous; they may coalesce into prominent groups that appear to disrupt the cytoplasm.

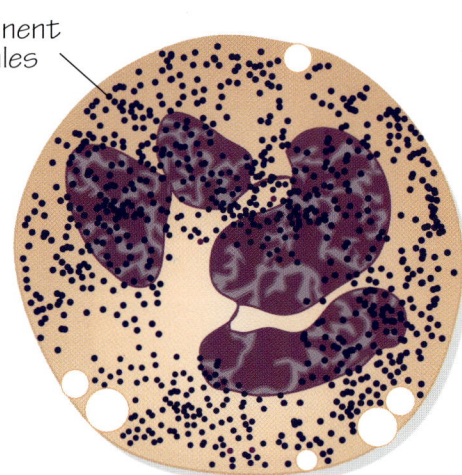

Toxic Segmented Neutrophils

A-68, 1985 (Blood, Wright-Giemsa, X400)

Identification	Referee %	Participant %
Neutrophil with toxic granulation	100	95.4

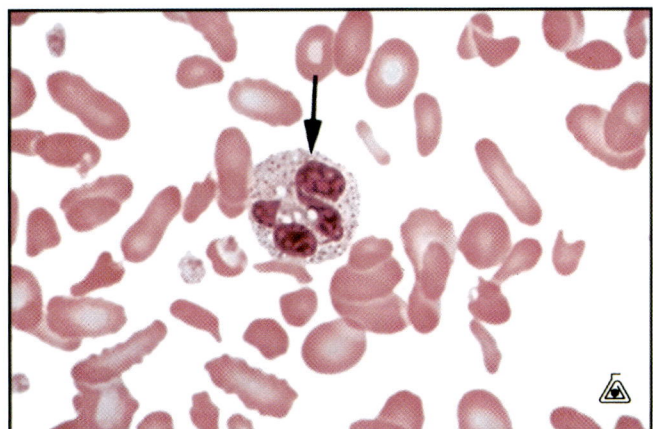

The arrowed cell in the center of the field is a segmented neutrophil which demonstrates both toxic granulation and toxic vacuolation. The nucleus is lobated and lobes are connected by a thin filament. The cytoplasmic granules are coarser and darker than normal. There are a number of empty, round vacuoles in the central portion of the cytoplasm. This is a case of hereditary elliptocytosis, status post splenectomy. Notice the abnormal red cell morphology. There are ovalocytes, crenated cells, and shistocytes (fragmented cells) present.

XH-11, 1997 (Blood, Wright-Giemsa, X400)

Identification	Referee %	Participant %
Neutrophil with toxic granulation	100	95.4

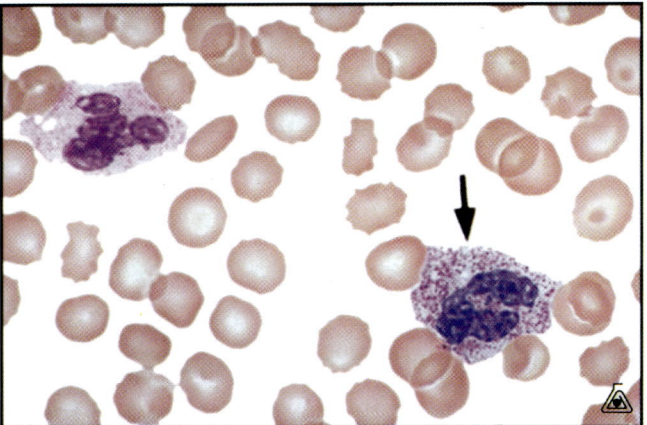

The arrowed cell is a segmented neutrophil which shows toxic granulation. The cytoplasm contains numerous course azurophilic granules. These are larger and darker than normal secondary neutrophilic granules. Another toxic change is the presence of cytoplasmic vacuoles. The clear spaces represent the sites of digestion of phagocytized material. The presence of vacuoles should always be noted because they are often associated with septicemia. Many of the background red cells are echinocytes. Platelets appear to be decreased in this field.

Döhle Body with/without Toxic Granulation

SYNONYMS
none

VITAL STATISTICS
- size .... 2-5 μm
- shape .... fusiform, rounded, oblong, crescent-shaped
- color .... blue; often more intensely staining in May-Hegglin anomaly
- location .... usually at periphery of cell in toxic conditons, randomly located in May-Hegglin anomaly

KEY DIFFERENTIATING FEATURES
blue fusiform or crescentic neutrophil cytoplasmic inclusion, most commonly located at the periphery of the cell

OTHER FEATURES
may be associated with vacuoles and toxic granulation in neutrophil activation states or with large platelets in May-Hegglin anomaly

POTENTIAL LOOK-ALIKES
inclusions in Chédiak-Higashi
phagocytized debris

ASSOCIATED DISEASE STATES AND CONDITIONS
May-Hegglin anomaly
Alder's anomaly
infection
trauma
burns
colony stimulating factor therapy
pregnancy

Döhle bodies appear as single or multiple blue to gray–blue inclusions of variable size and shape in the cytoplasm (often adjacent to the membrane) of neutrophils, bands, and metamyelocytes. These inclusions represent denatured aggregates of free ribosomes or stacks of rough endoplasmic reticulum. The inclusions often appear in association with other features of neutrophil activation: toxic granulation and vacuolization.

In May-Hegglin anomaly, Döhle bodies are found in almost all granulocytes and some monocytes. The inclusions are generally more basophilic and distinct than those seen in toxic or activated neutrophil conditions. The cytoplasm of May-Hegglin neutrophils does not show toxic changes unless there is concomitant infection. Giant platelets are always seen in this hereditary disorder. See *A Closer Look At...* page 46 for a more detailed discussion.

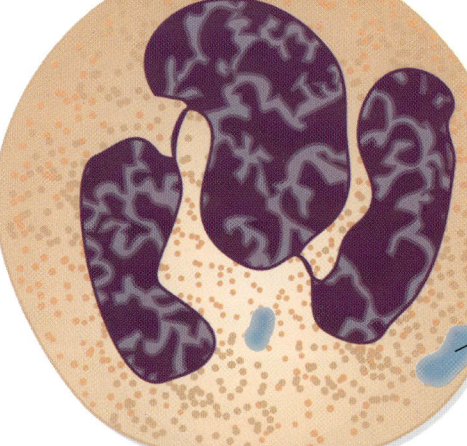

Toxic PMN — vacuoles, toxic granulation, Döhle body

PMN in May-Hegglin Anomaly

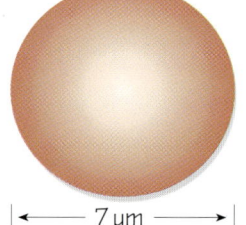

7 μm — size of normal red blood cell

Granulocytic (Myeloid) Cells

H-43, 1982 (Blood, Wright-Giemsa, X400)

Identification	Referee %	Participant %
Döhle body with or without toxic granulation	100	92.4

The central neutrophil has an arrow pointing to a bluish, rectangular inclusion adjacent to the cell membrane. This is a Döhle body. This segmented neutrophil also shows coarse, dark granules in its cytoplasm indicative of toxic granulation.

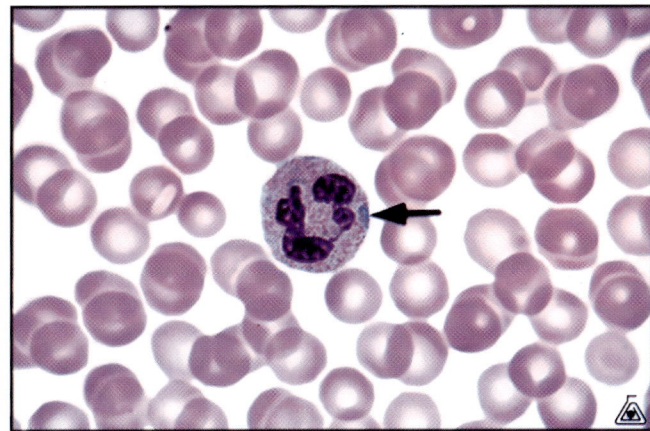

HE-51, 1996 (Blood, Wright-Giemsa, X400)

Identification	Referee %	Participant %
Döhle body with or without toxic granulation	91	95.3

This is a case of May-Hegglin anomaly. The arrowed cell is a segmented/band neutrophil containing a large blue inclusion near the cytoplasmic membrane. The cytoplasm is not toxic—there are no vacuoles and the granules are not prominent. Giant platelets are needed to confirm the diagnosis, but they are not visible in this field. See *A Closer Look At...* page 46 for a more detailed discussion of this disorder.

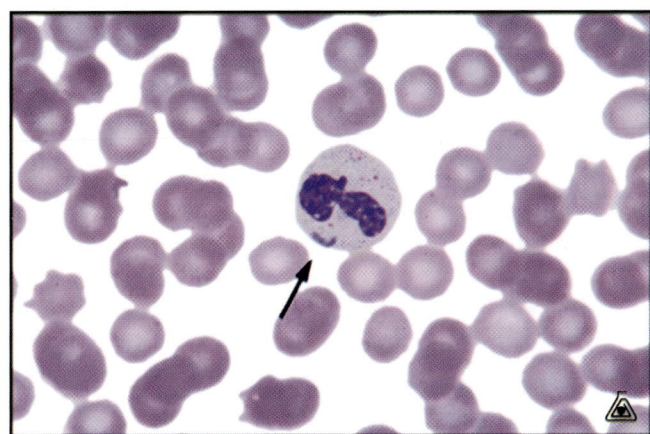

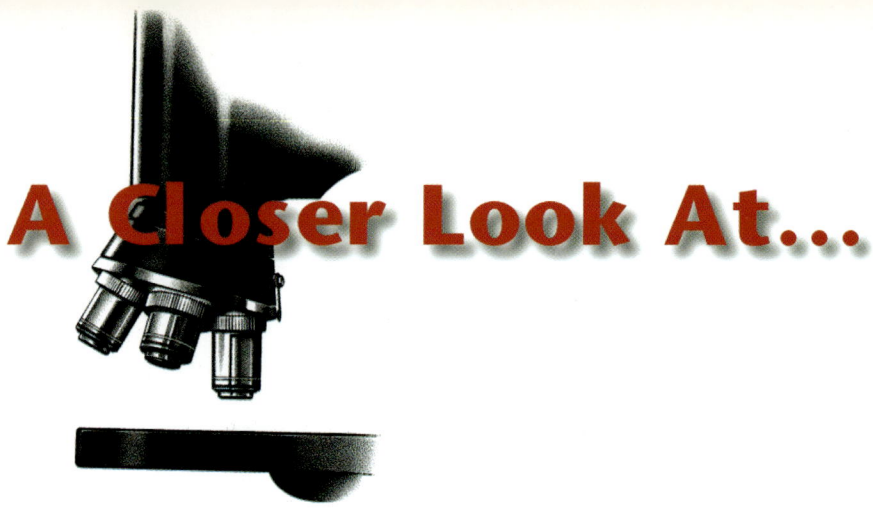
A Closer Look At...

Acquired Neutrophil Abnormalities

Two major acquired and reversible changes can be observed in granulocyte morphology: *megaloblastic myelopoiesis* (giant metamyelocytes, giant bands and hypersegmented neutrophils) and *cytokine induced activation* of granulocyte production.

Megaloblastic myelopoiesis results when there is a reduced rate of DNA synthesis but unaffected RNA synthesis and processing. Protein synthesis is therefore unaffected as well. This most commonly occurs when there is a deficiency of vitamin B_{12} or folic acid or when there is drug-induced suppression of DNA synthesis. A dyssynchrony in nuclear and cytoplasmic development is the result. In the myeloid lineage this creates enlarged precursors (giant metamyelocytes and bands) probably on the basis of missed cell divisions. The cytoplasm appears inappropriately mature—the nuclear chromatin of any given stage is less clumped than normal. Segmented neutrophils show increased lobation (by definition a hypersegmented neutrophil has six or more lobes) with the nuclear chromatin once again somewhat less dense than normal. Upon correction of the nutrient deficiency or discontinuation of the interfering agent, the morphology of the granulocytic cells returns to normal.

Toxic changes consist of toxic granulation, toxic vacuolation, and Döhle bodies. These changes result when cytokines (granulocyte colony stimulating factor for example) increase and induce shortened transit and activation of granulocytic elements. The toxic granules are larger and stain more darkly. Döhle bodies are remnants of rough endoplasmic reticulum that normally do not persist in the cytoplasm of normal granulocytes. Toxic vacuoles are clear spaces indicative of increased spontaneous phagocytic activity. Therapeutic administration of cytokines results in these "activation" changes and it is presumed that the toxic changes in granulocytes seen in severe infections, after trauma, and in significant burns are a result of bursts of cytokine release associated with these disease states.

How Toxic Changes Develop

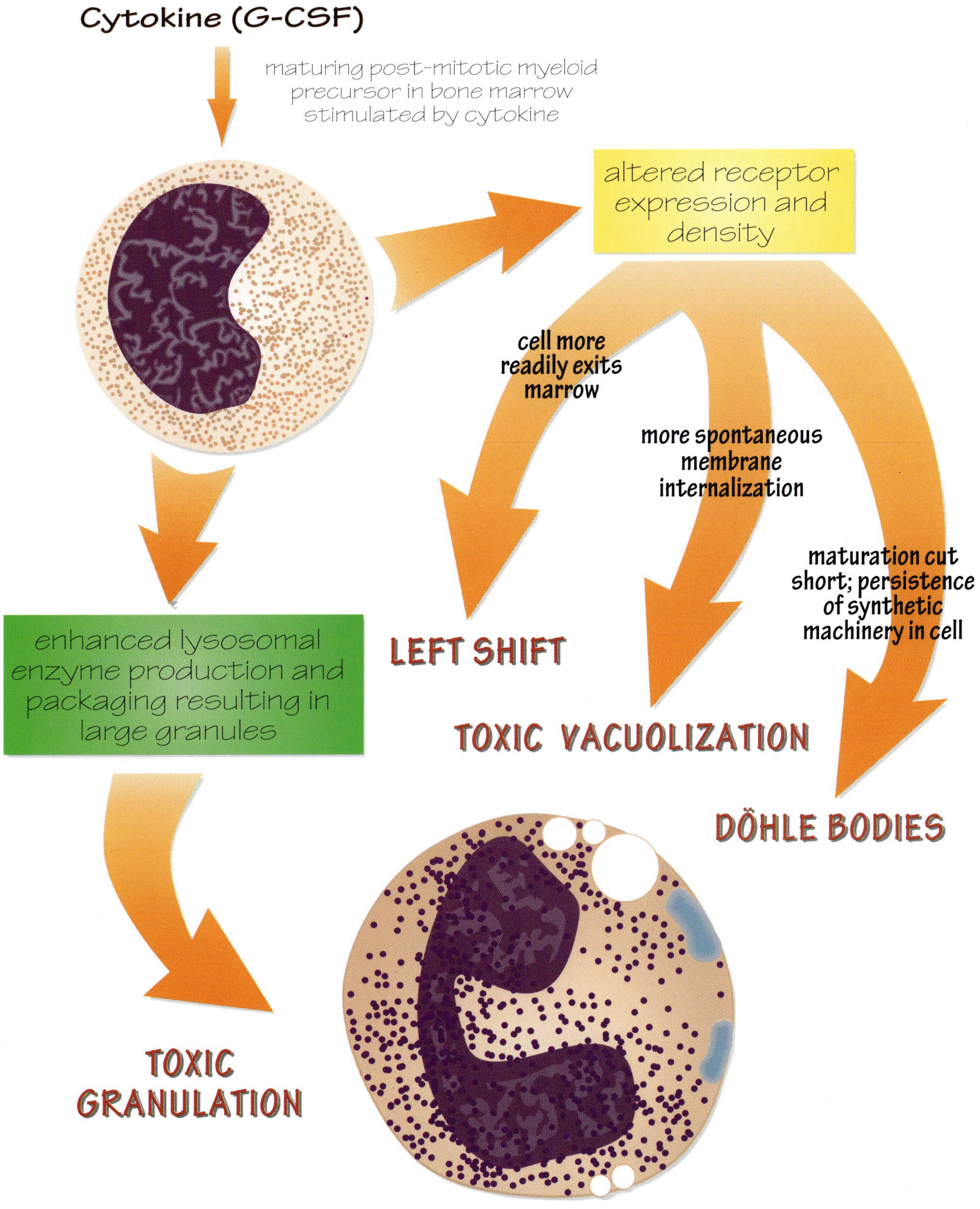

Cytokine (G-CSF)

maturing post-mitotic myeloid precursor in bone marrow stimulated by cytokine

altered receptor expression and density

cell more readily exits marrow

more spontaneous membrane internalization

maturation cut short; persistence of synthetic machinery in cell

enhanced lysosomal enzyme production and packaging resulting in large granules

LEFT SHIFT

TOXIC VACUOLIZATION

DÖHLE BODIES

TOXIC GRANULATION

Granulocytic (Myeloid) Cells

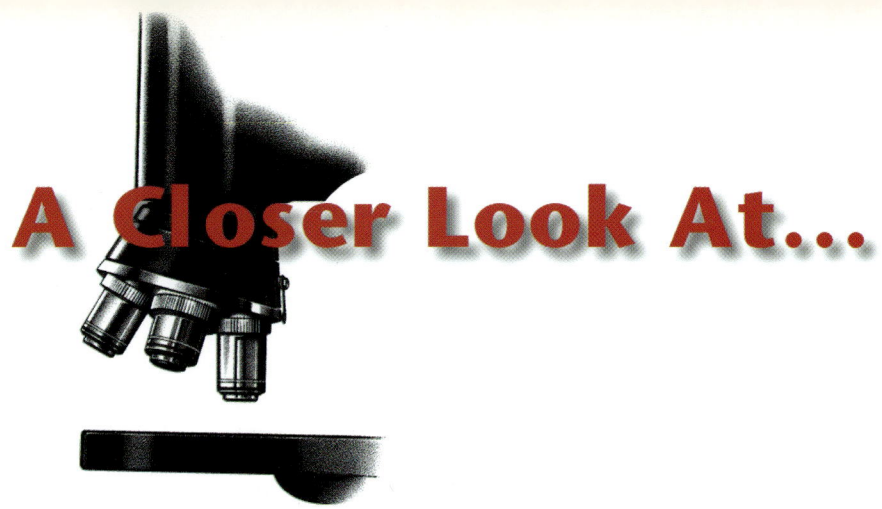

A Closer Look At...

May-Hegglin Anomaly

May-Hegglin anomaly is a rare autosomal dominant disorder characterized by prominent Döhle bodies in granulocytic cells, poorly granulated giant platelets, and variable thrombocytopenia that may cause purpura.

The mild bleeding problems seen in about 40% of cases are related to the degree of thrombocytopenia. Purpura may be prominent and lead to the incorrect diagnosis of thrombotic thrombocytopenic purpura. Although abnormally large, the platelets in May-Hegglin are functionally normal. Total platelet mass and platelet survival are also normal. The large platelet size and mild bleeding diathesis are probably due to premature megakaryocyte fragmentation. The platelets in May-Hegglin anomaly typically vary from 4 to 8 µm. Some may be much larger. They are often cigar-shaped or elliptical.

The key distinguishing morphologic feature of May-Hegglin anomaly is the presence of prominent Döhle bodies. Almost all neutrophils—and sometimes a few monocytes—are affected. Basophils and eosinophils may also contain the inclusions.

The Döhle bodies in May-Hegglin anomaly often display features that distinguish them from their counterparts found in infections, as shown in the table below. In most instances, they are larger (2-5 µm in size), more round, more sharply defined, and more intensely blue staining. But some examples of May-Hegglin anomaly demonstrate Döhle bodies indistinguishable from those of infection. By the same token, some infections display very prominent inclusions. In either case, the bodies are oblong, crescentic or spindle-shaped and are composed of RNA. By electron microscopy, the RNA is structurally different compared to other Döhle bodies. The inclusions in May-Hegglin anomaly are not peripherally placed but are distributed randomly within the granulocyte; they are often found between the lobes of the cell nucleus. Toxic granulation and cytoplasmic vacuoles are not present unless there is concomitant infection. The finding of large, well-stained inclusions in non-toxic neutrophils plus presence of giant platelets is pathognomonic of the May-Hegglin abnormality.

	Döhle Bodies in Toxic States	Döhle Bodies in May-Hegglin Anomaly
Morphology	1-2 µm in diameter; light blue or blue-gray; fusiform, spindle or crescent shape; fuzzy edges	2-5 µm in diameter; light blue; round, oval or crescent shape; sharply defined edges
Location	usually peripheral	random distribution, sometimes between nuclear lobes
Composition	RNA; aggregates of ribosomes or stacks of rough endoplasmic reticulum	RNA; similar to toxic states but ultrastructurally the RNA is altered
Cells Involved	neutrophils only	all mature granulocytes, monocytes, and lymphocytes
Clinical Associations	transient manifestation of neutrophil activation; most commonly seen in severe infection and burns; numerous other causes	autosomal dominant trait; associated leukopenia and thrombocytopenia with giant platelets; mild bleeding problems in 40% of patients

May-Hegglin Anomaly

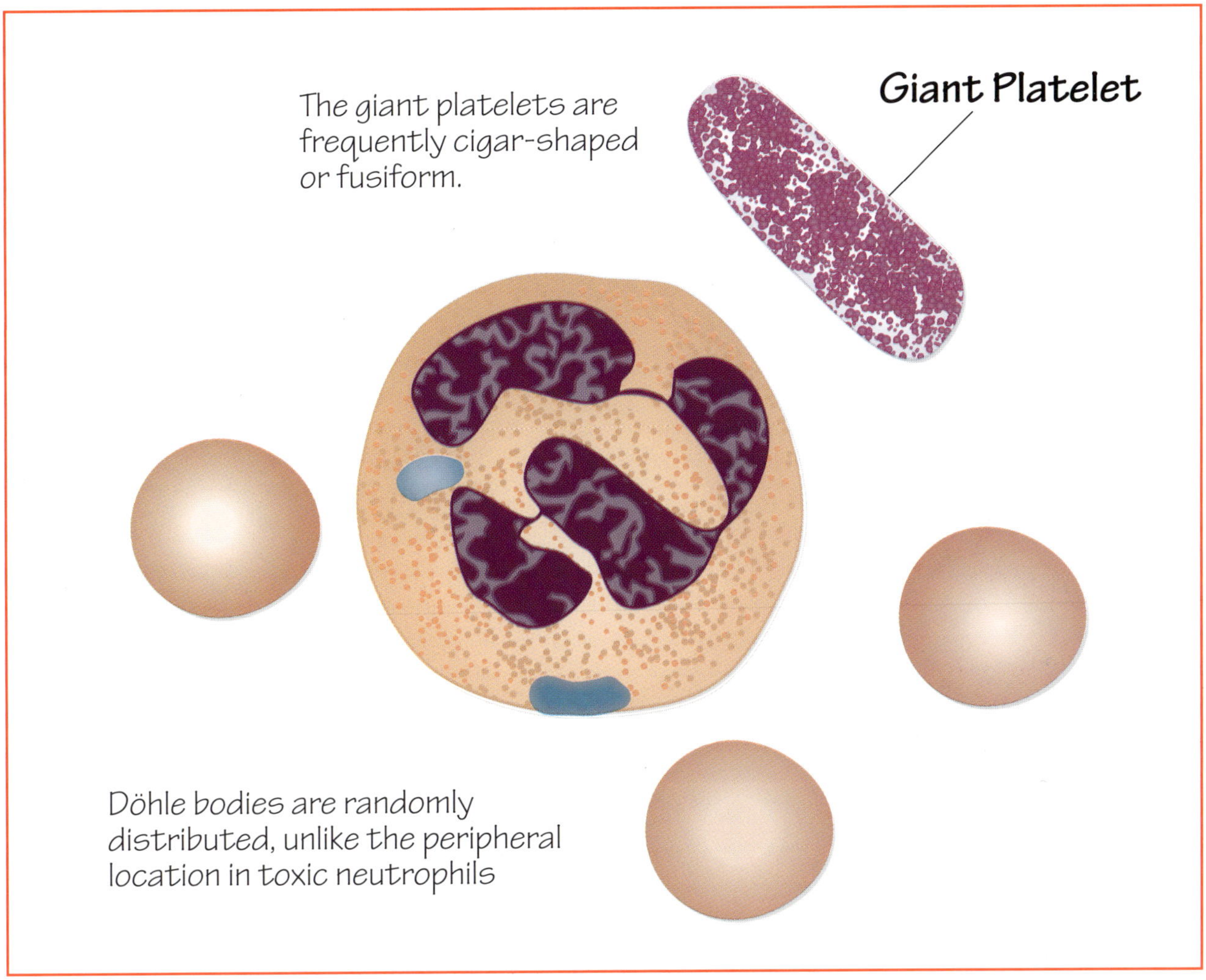

The giant platelets are frequently cigar-shaped or fusiform.

Giant Platelet

Döhle bodies are randomly distributed, unlike the peripheral location in toxic neutrophils

Döhle bodies can also be found in monocytes, basophils, and eosinophils.

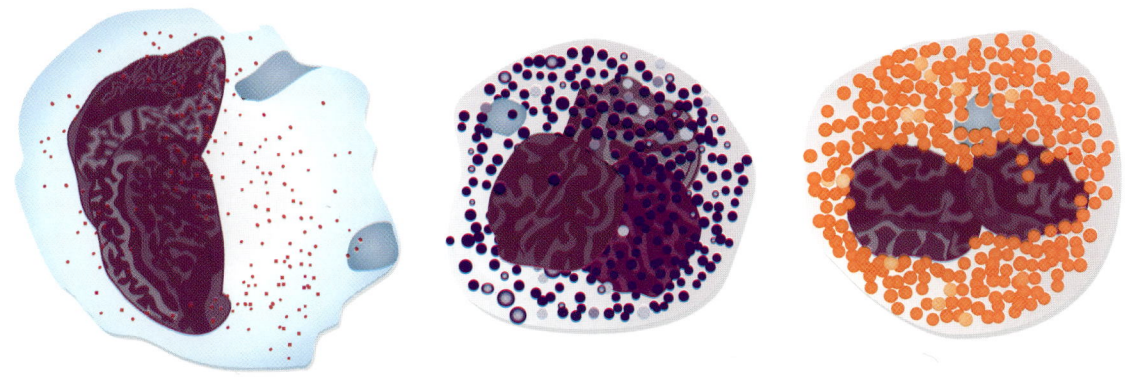

Granulocytic (Myeloid) Cells

Metamyelocyte, Giant (Bone Marrow)

SYNONYMS
giant meta

VITAL STATISTICS
size .... 15 to 25 μm
N:C ratio 1.5:1
cell shape .... round to oval
nuclear shape .... indented, kidney shaped
chromatin .... loosely clumped, less condensed than normal metamyelocyte
nucleoli .... none
cytoplasm .... pale pink with many lilac granules

KEY DIFFERENTIATING FEATURES
increased size and decreased clumping of nuclear chromatin

OTHER FEATURES
loss of nuclear-cytoplasmic synchrony
accompanying red blood cell changes (megaloblastic, oval macrocytes)

POTENTIAL LOOK-ALIKES
dysplastic myeloid precursors
giant band
normal metamyelocyte
normal band

ASSOCIATED DISEASE STATES AND CONDITIONS
vitamin B_{12} deficiency
folate deficiency
anti-metabolite therapy
alcoholism

Larger than normal (1.5 times the normal size or greater) metamyelocytes with decreased chromatin clumping are seen in the marrow of patients where synthesis of DNA is compromised or abnormal. Such states include deficiency of cofactors for nucleotide synthesis such as vitamin B_{12} and folate deficiency and cases where the patient is receiving a nucleotide analog (such as 6-mercaptopurine) or a cofactor blocking agent (such as methotrexate). The finding in the bone marrow of giant metamyelocytes and giant bands is possibly the most dependable single indication of a megaloblastic process.

Some of the cells may be quite dramatically enlarged—3 or more times normal size—as depicted in the illustration on the right. The nucleus is sometimes irregular in shape, reflecting the over abundance of DNA material in a cell that has not divided in concert with cytoplasmic maturation. The nuclear chromatin is more open and resembles the almost "salami-like" changes seen in megaloblastic normoblasts.

Giant Neutrophilic Metamyelocyte

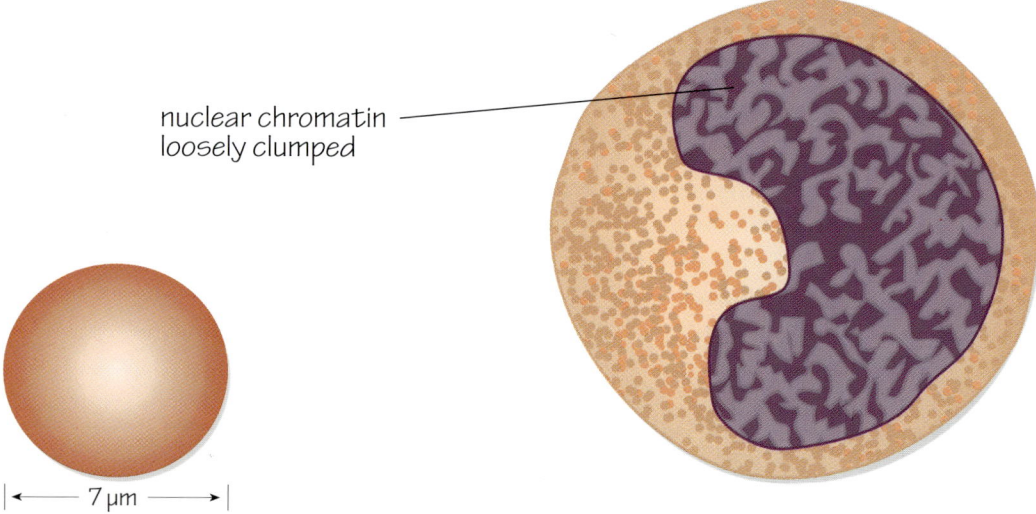

nuclear chromatin loosely clumped

|← 7 μm →|
size of normal red blood cell

Granulocytic (Myeloid) Cells

HE-43, 1996 (Bone Marrow, Wright-Giemsa, X400)

Identification	Referee %	Participant %
Metamyelocyte, giant	78.6	71.0
Band, giant	14.3	13.7

The cell indicated by the arrow is quite large (compare it to the adjacent segment neutrophil) and has a kidney shaped nucleus (indented less than one-half of the diameter of the nucleus). The degree of nuclear chromatin clumping is less than expected for a myeloid precursor of this stage. The cytoplasm contains neutrophilic granules. The findings are characteristic of a metamyelocyte which is clearly abnormally large. The finding of giant metamyelocyte and band forms is characteristic of megaloblastic hematopoiesis.

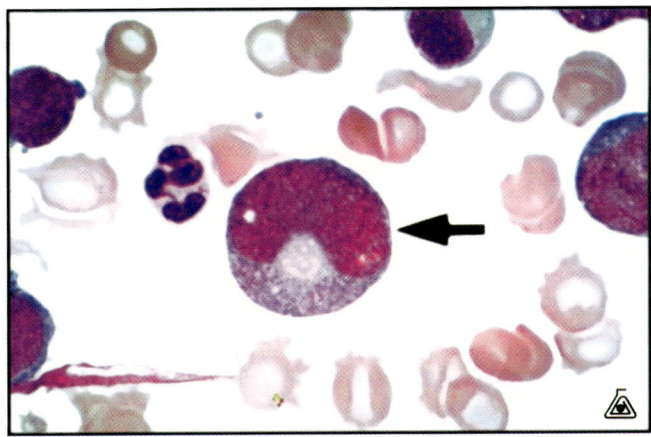

Comparison of Normal and Giant Neutrophilic Metamyelocytes

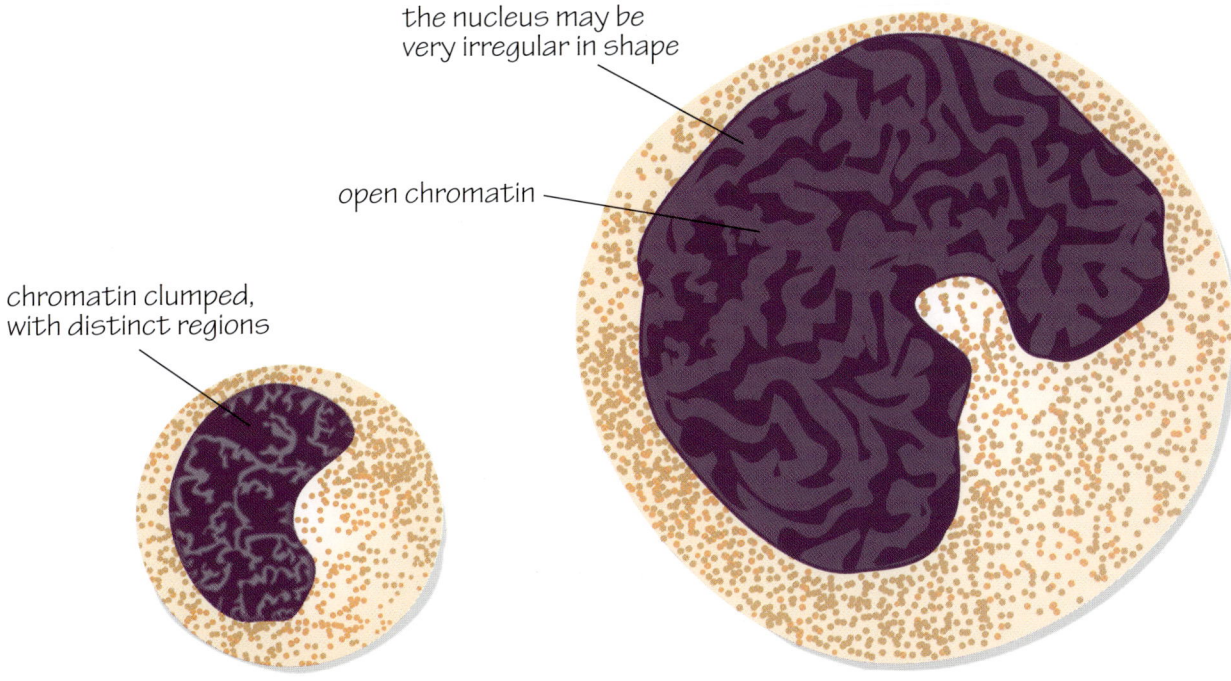

Normal Metamyelocyte

Giant Metamyelocyte

- chromatin clumped, with distinct regions
- the nucleus may be very irregular in shape
- open chromatin

Giant metamyelocytes may be 3 or more times normal size. They rarely circulate in the peripheral blood, presumably because they are too large to escape the bone marrow sinuses.

Granulocytic (Myeloid) Cells

Band Neutrophil, Giant (Bone Marrow)

SYNONYMS
giant stab

VITAL STATISTICS
- size .... 15 to 20 µm
- N:C ratio 1:3
- cell shape .... round to oval
- nuclear shape .... indented to more than half the nuclear width, C or S shaped
- chromatin .... loosely clumped, less condensed than normal band
- nucleoli .... none
- cytoplasm .... pale pink with many lilac granules

KEY DIFFERENTIATING FEATURES
increased size and decreased clumping of nuclear chromatin.

OTHER FEATURES
loss of nuclear-cytoplasmic synchrony
accompanying red blood cell changes (megaloblastic, oval macrocytes)

POTENTIAL LOOK-ALIKES
giant metamyelocyte
dysplastic myeloid precursors
normal band
normal metamyelocyte
monocyte
macrophage

ASSOCIATED DISEASE STATES AND CONDITIONS
vitamin B_{12} deficiency
folate deficiency
anti-metabolite therapy
alcoholism

Larger than normal (1.5 times the normal size or greater) bands with decreased chromatin clumping are seen in the marrow and the blood of patients where synthesis of DNA is compromised or abnormal. Such states include deficiency of cofactors for nucleotide synthesis such as vitamin B_{12} and folate deficiency and cases where the patient is receiving a nucleotide analog (such as 6-mercaptopurine) or a cofactor blocking agent (such as methotrexate). The recognition of giant band neutrophils and hypersegmented neutrophils strongly suggests that the marrow will demonstrate megaloblastic hematopoiesis.

Like giant metamyelocytes, giant bands may be 3 or more times normal size, as depicted in the illustration on the right. The nucleus seems to be too big for the cytoplasm; it is often irregular in contour, folded back on itself, and twisted into bizarre S and C shapes. The increased size reflects the over abundance of DNA material in a cell that has not divided in concert with cytoplasmic maturation. The nuclear chromatin is more open and resembles the almost "salami-like" changes seen in megaloblastic normoblasts.

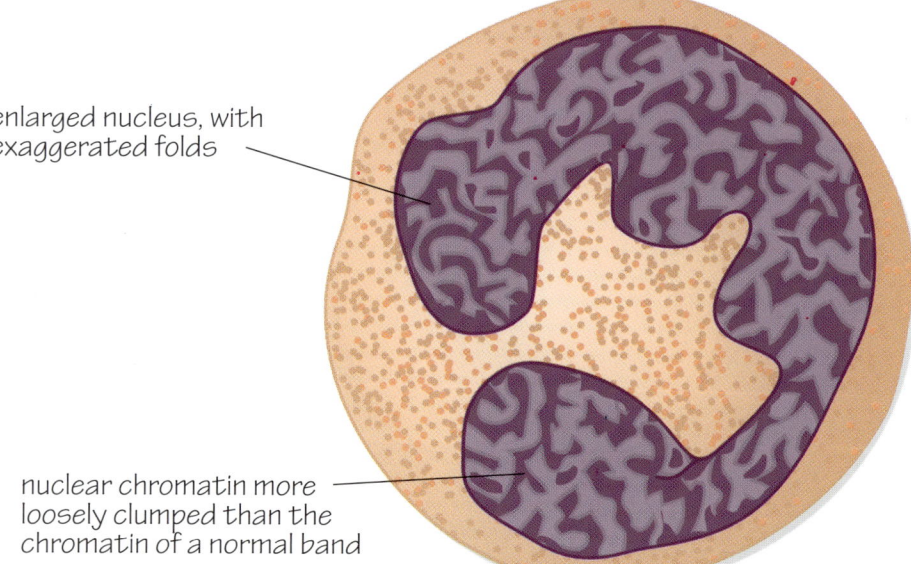

Giant Band

- enlarged nucleus, with exaggerated folds
- nuclear chromatin more loosely clumped than the chromatin of a normal band

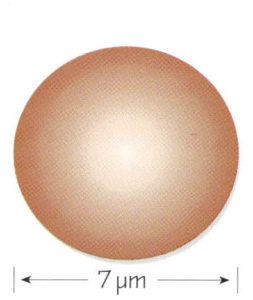

7 µm
size of normal red blood cell

HE-30, 1995 (Bone Marrow, Wright-Giemsa, X400)

Identification	Referee %	Participant %
Band, giant	89.2	61.5
Metamyelocyte, giant	7.1	9.8
Monocyte	-	14.6

The cell indicated by the arrow is a giant band. It is more than 1.5 times the size of normal myeloid elements. Compare it to the relatively normal metamyelocyte and band adjacent to the giant band on the side opposite the arrow. Giant metamyelocytes are also present. A good example is the largest cell next to the arrowed cell. Megaloblastic nucleated red cells are present at the 3 o'clock and 9 o'clock positions.

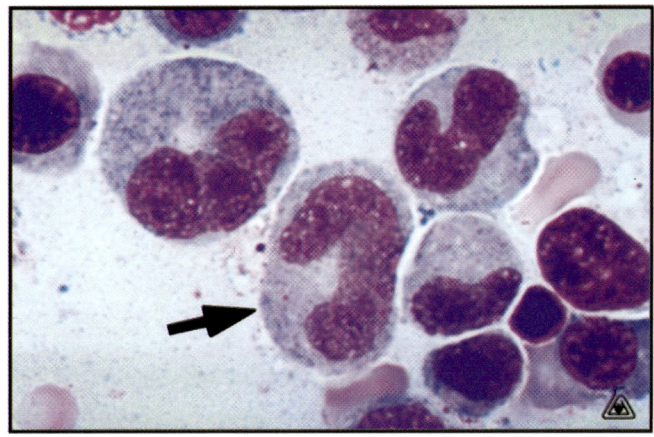

Comparison of Normal and Giant Neutrophilic Bands

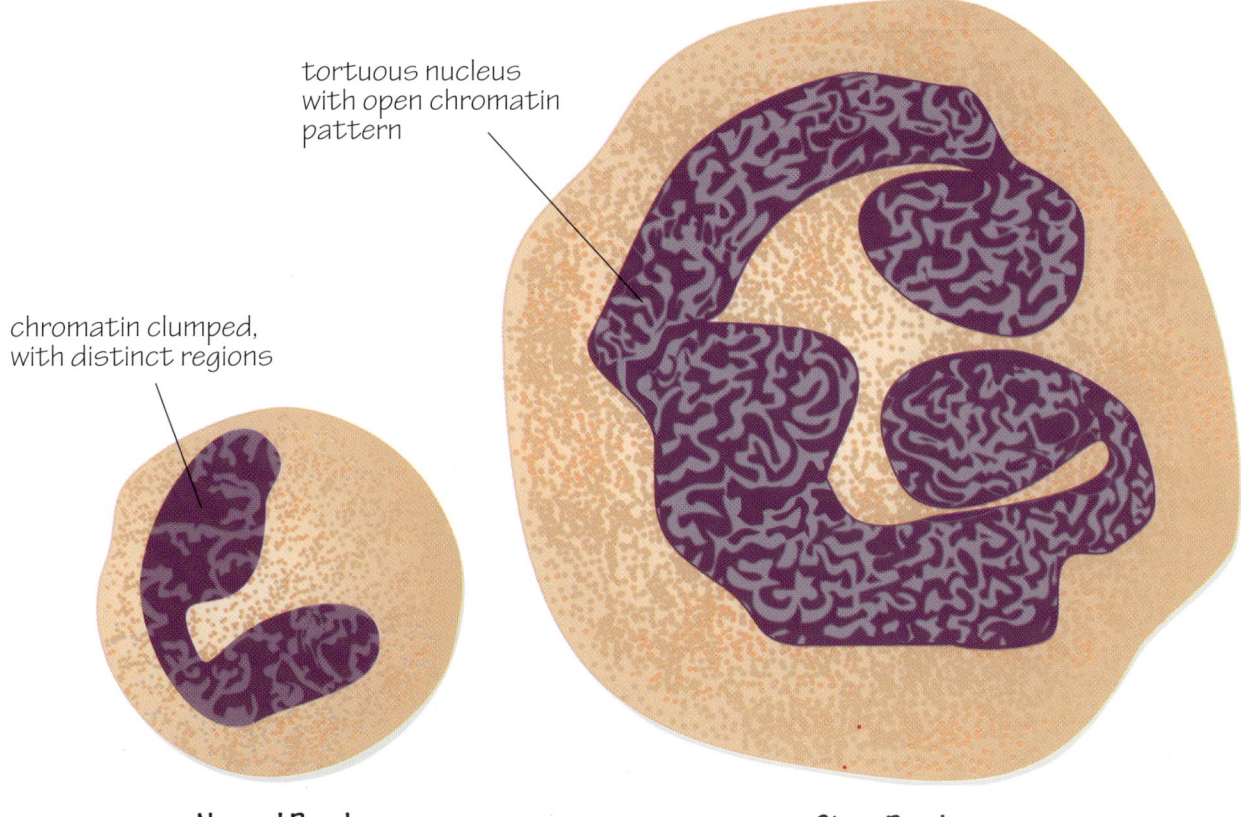

Normal Band — chromatin clumped, with distinct regions

Giant Band — tortuous nucleus with open chromatin pattern

Like giant metamyelocytes, giant bands may be 3 or more times normal size. They are too large to escape the bone marrow sinuses and therefore are only rarely found circulating in the blood.

Granulocytic (Myeloid) Cells

Hypersegmented Neutrophil

SYNONYMS
macropolycyte

VITAL STATISTICS
- size .... 1.5 to 2 µm
- N:C ratio 1:3
- cell shape .... round to oval
- nuclear shape .... segmented with six or more lobes
- chromatin .... clumped, less condensed than a normal neutrophil
- nucleoli .... none
- cytoplasm .... pale pink with many lilac granules

KEY DIFFERENTIATING FEATURES
increased size and increased lobulation

OTHER FEATURES
loss of nuclear-cytoplasmic synchrony
accompanying red blood cell changes (megaloblastic, oval macrocytes)

POTENTIAL LOOK-ALIKES
dysplastic neutrophils

ASSOCIATED DISEASE STATES AND CONDITIONS
vitamin B_{12} deficiency
folate deficiency
anti-metabolite therapy
alcoholism
rarely in sepsis, renal disease, myeloproliferative syndromes, and myeldysplastic disorders

Neutrophils that are a result of megaloblastic myelopoiesis are increased in size (because they have undergone fewer nuclear divisions during their development in the marrow) and have nuclei that demonstrate more than the normal number of lobes. To truly be defined as a hypersegmented neutrophil there should be at least six or more discrete lobes.

Hypersegmentation is the most unequivocal morphologic finding associated with megaloblastic hematopoiesis. It is indicative of impaired DNA synthesis. As noted previously, hypersegmentation means neutrophils with six or more nuclear segments (for proficiency testing purposes). In the bone marrow, this criteria can be relaxed when making a diagnosis of megaloblastosis. The majority of normal bone marrow segmented neutrophils have only two or three lobes. Therefore, a presumptive diagnosis of megaloblastosis can be made if >5% of the neutrophils have five or more nuclear segments or if the majority of neutrophils have 4 or more nuclear segments. Megaloblastic red cell morphology usually accompanies neutrophilic changes, but nuclear hypersegmentation may precede megaloblastic erythropoiesis.

Hypersegmented neutrophils are uncommon except in megaloblastic states, although they may rarely be seen as a congenital anomaly and in sepsis, renal disease, and myeloproliferative states.

Hypersegmented Neutrophil

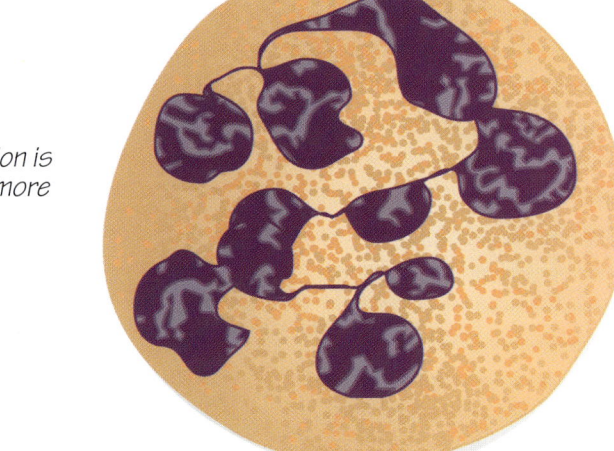

hypersegmentation is defined as six or more nuclear lobes

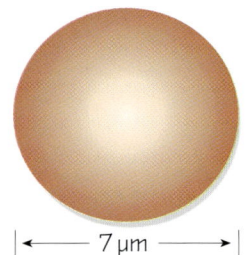

|← 7 µm →|
size of normal red blood cell

XH-32, 1994 (Blood, Wright-Giemsa, X400)

Identification	Referee %	Participant %
Hypersegmented neutrophil	100	92.9
Segmented neutrophil	-	5.2

The cell indicated by the arrow is clearly a segmented neutrophil; it has lilac granules in the cytoplasm and has a lobated nucleus. The lobes are connected by thin filaments. There are at least six lobes present; when a neutrophil has six or more lobes it is considered to be hypersegmented. Several oval macrocytic red cells are seen in the surrounding field.

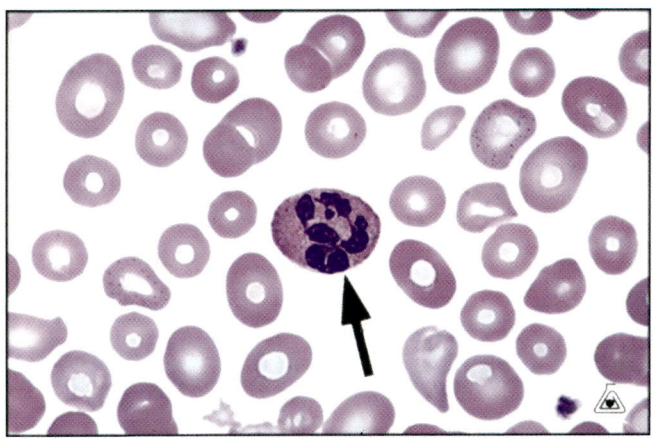

Hypersegmented Neutrophils

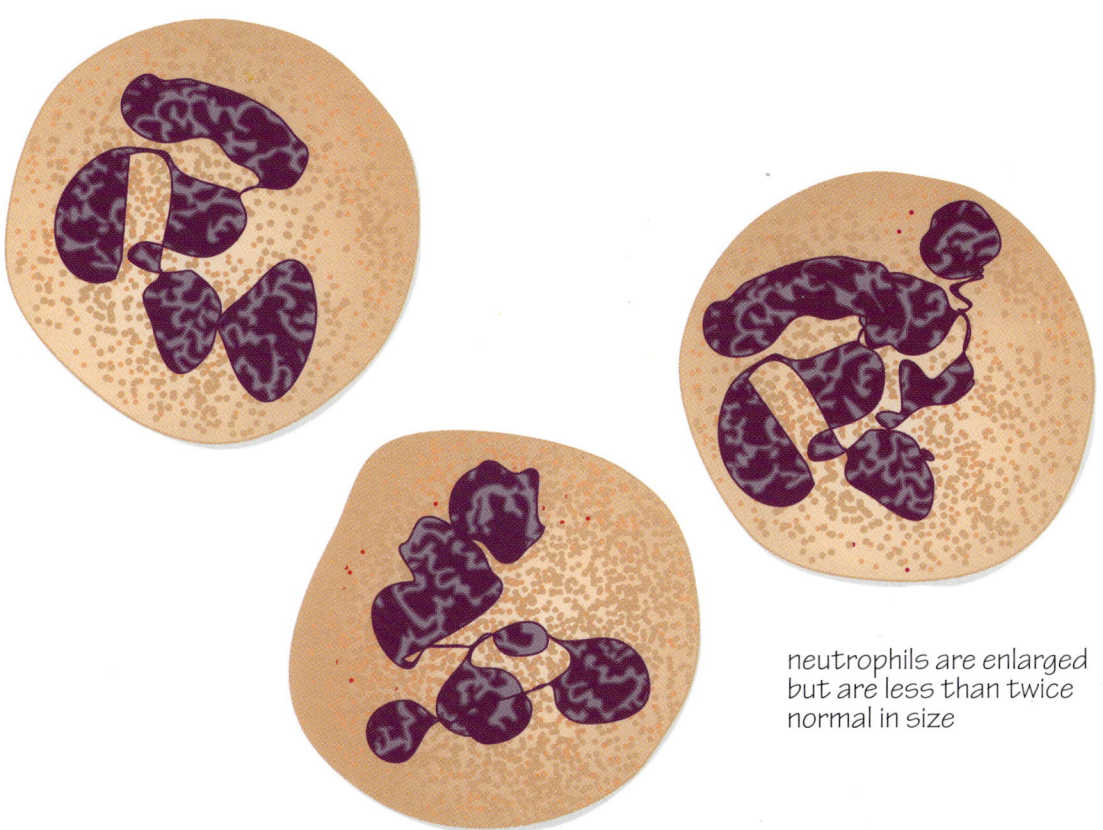

neutrophils are enlarged but are less than twice normal in size

Hypersegmentation is the most unequivocal morphologic finding associated with megaloblastic hematopoiesis. It is indicative of impaired DNA synthesis. In the bone marrow, hypersegmentation is suggested when one of the following is present: 1) neutrophils with six or more nuclear segments (this is the proficiency testing definition of hypersegmentation), 2) >5% of the neutrophils have five or more nuclear segments, or 3) most neutrophils have 4 or more lobes. (Since the majority of normal bone marrow segmented neutrophils have only two or three lobes, finding a predominance of cells with 4 or more is sufficient to warrant a presumptive diagnosis of megaloblastosis). Megaloblastic red cell changes usually accompany neutrophilic changes, but nuclear hypersegmentation generally precedes any megaloblastic erythropoiesis.

Granulocytic (Myeloid) Cells

Neutrophil with Dysplastic Nucleus/Agranular Cytoplasm

SYNONYMS
none

VITAL STATISTICS
- size .... 10 to 15 μm
- N:C ratio 1:3
- cell shape .... round to oval
- nuclear shape .... irregular segmentation
- chromatin .... clumped, similar to mature neutrophil; marked clumping in pseudo Pelger-Huët cell
- nucleoli .... none
- cytoplasm .... hypogranular form lacks neutrophil granules and has bluish color; pseudo Pelger-Huët form may have granules

KEY DIFFERENTIATING FEATURES
chromatin mature yet lobation irregular
lack of normal cytoplasmic granules

OTHER FEATURES
in some cases, hypergranulation or abnormal granules may be seen; pseudo Pelger-Huët forms are also a form of dysplasia

POTENTIAL LOOK-ALIKES
monocytes

ASSOCIATED DISEASE STATES AND CONDITIONS
myelodysplastic disorders
myeloproliferative syndromes

Dysplastic neutrophils are characteristic of myelodysplastic syndromes. Morphologically, the normal synchronous maturation of nucleus and cytoplasm is lost. In the cytoplasm, the primary and secondary granules are often decreased or absent, causing it to appear pale and bluish. The nucleus shows abnormal lobation with a mature chromatin pattern. Dysplastic neutrophils often manifest abnormal cytochemical reactivity; low to absent levels of myeloperoxidase or neutrophil alkaline phosphatase may be present. The dysplastic neutrophil may also exhibit functional deficits such as defective chemotaxis and bacterial killing.

For proficiency testing purposes, cells with Pelger-Huët nuclei are best defined as Pelger-Huët cells (discussed on page 58).

Various Dysplastic Neutrophils

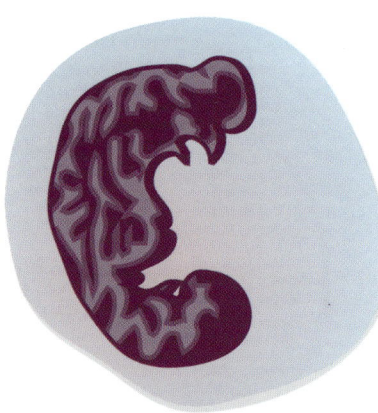
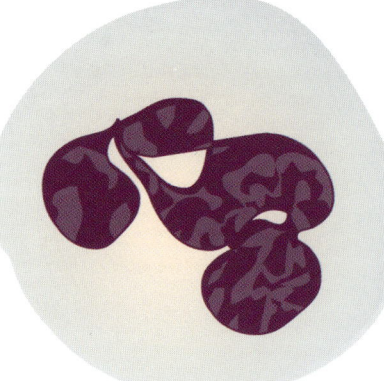

Hypogranular Neutrophils

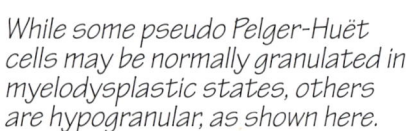

While some pseudo Pelger-Huët cells may be normally granulated in myelodysplastic states, others are hypogranular, as shown here.

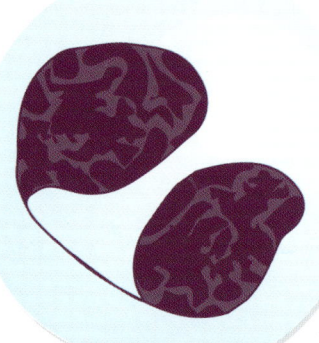
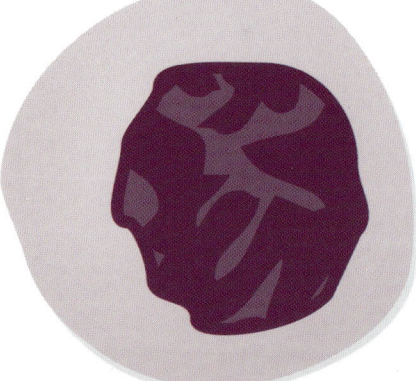

Pseudo Pelger-Huët Neutrophils

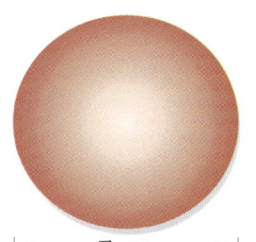

|← 7 μm →|
size of normal red blood cell

Granulocytic (Myeloid) Cells

H1-44, 1986 (Blood, Wright-Giemsa, X375)

Identification	Referee %	Participant %
Dysplastic neutrophil	88.2	42.1
Pelger-Huët neutrophil	-	2.8
Neutrophil necrobiosis	-	18

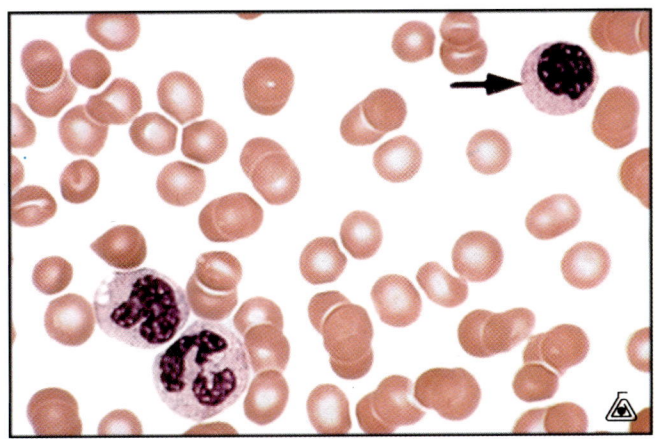

The cell indicated by the arrow has cytoplasm similar to the neutrophil in the lower left corner of the slide, but it has a rounded nucleus with clumped nuclear chromatin. The nucleus is not segmented, indicative of abnormal myelopoiesis, and is characteristic of dysplasia. The selection of Pelger-Huët neutrophil makes sense if one considers this cell an example of homozygous Pelger-Huët anomaly (cells with "pince-nez" nuclei are the result of heterozygous Pelger-Huët anomaly), but this idea cannot be supported in view of the fact that two normally segmented neutrophils are present in the same slide. (See Pelger-Huët discussion on page 58.)

H1-45, 1986 (Blood, Wright-Giemsa, X400)

Identification	Referee %	Participant %
Dysplastic neutrophil	70.6	43.5
Pelger-Huët neutrophil	-	2.6
Neutrophil necrobiosis	-	13.5

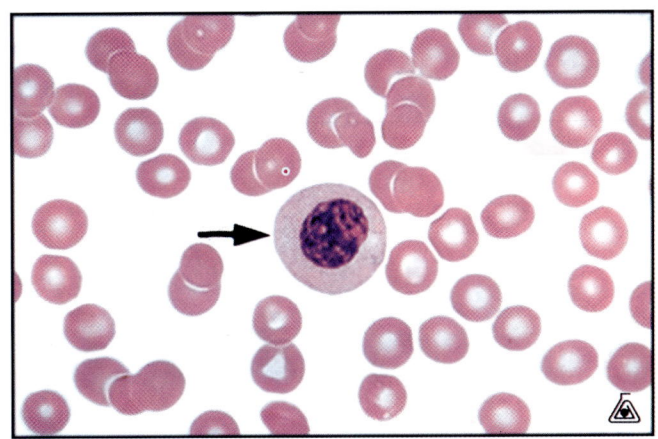

The cell indicated by the arrow is similar to one demonstrated above (HE-44, 1986). It has a granular cytoplasm characteristic of a neutrophil but an unsegmented nucleus. The red cells are not significantly abnormal.

HE-41, 1996 (Bone Marrow, Wright-Giemsa, X400)

Identification	Referee %	Participant %
Neutrophil with dysplastic nucleus/ hypogranular cytoplasm	65.4	50.3
Pelger-Huët neutrophil	23.1	22.6

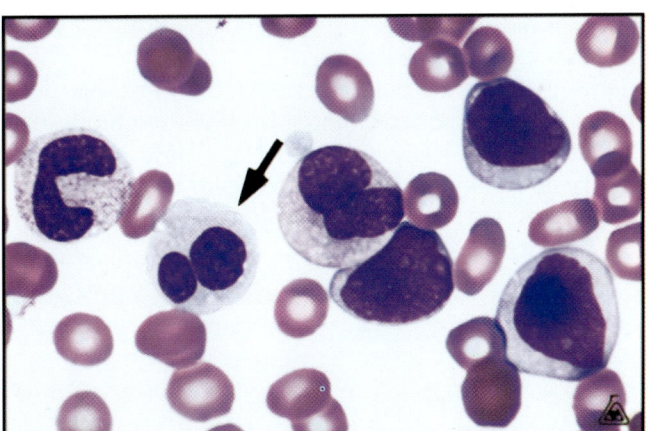

The cell indicated by the arrow is a dysplastic segmented neutrophil. The neutrophil has no apparent granules in the cytoplasm and a bilobed nucleus indicative of pseudo-Pelger-Huët change. Both identifications are acceptable. Note the presence of other neutrophil forms (band and cells with high N:C ratio and nuclei with open chromatin and nucleoli) which also are agranular. The patient had an evolving myelodysplasia.

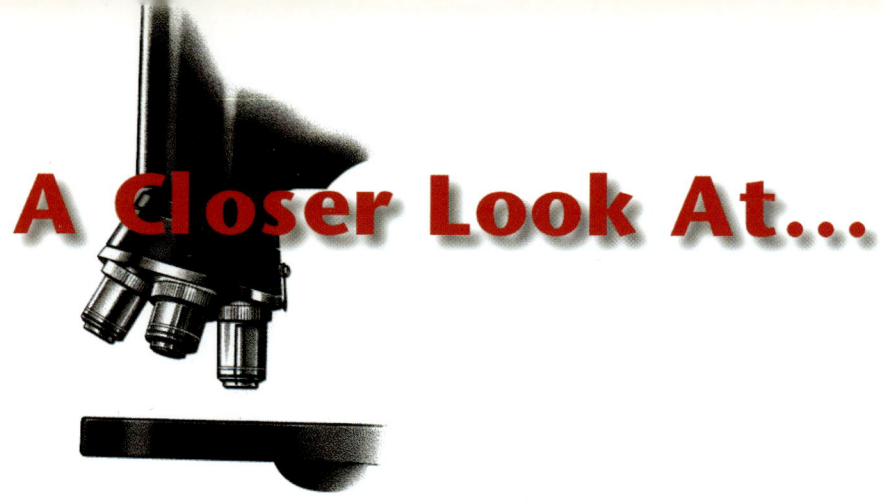

A Closer Look At...

Myelodysplastic Syndromes

The *myelodysplastic syndromes* are a heterogeneous and ill-defined group of hematologic disorders. They wax and wane over the course of years and roughly 25% of patients develop AML. For this reason, the myelodysplastic syndromes have been called "pre-leukemias." Hematology experts do not all agree on what constitutes pre-leukemia and what disorders should be given this moniker.

Part of the confusion centers on the difference between **dysplasia** and **neoplasia**. All the myeloproliferative disorders (like CML and AML) are neoplasias. The involved cells are malignant and derived from a single neoplastic stem cell.

Myelodysplastic syndromes, such as refractory anemia, are *pre-neoplastic.* Stem cells are abnormal but to a lesser degree. The end result is a mixture of normal and abnormal morphologies in the peripheral blood and bone marrow. Where dysplasia ends and neoplasia begins is difficult to determine. Qualitative and quantitative factors come into play.

Interestingly, the dysplasias often demonstrate more striking morphologic changes in the hematopoietic cells than is typically seen in AML. These qualitative dysplastic changes in the red cells, granulocytes, monocytes, and platelets are of primary importance in making a diagnosis of myelodysplasia. Table 1 on the next page lists some of the atypical or "dysplastic" features found in the different cells lines in myelodysplasias.

In an attempt to provide a framework for diagnostic uniformity, the French-American-British (FAB) cooperative group proposed a classification for hematopoietic disorders that precede the development of acute myelogenous leukemia. On the basis of morphology, the FAB group defined five different myelodysplastic syndromes:

Refractory anemia (RA)
Refractory anemia (RA) with ringed sideroblasts
Refractory anemia with excess blasts (RAEB)
Refractory anemia with excess blasts (RAEB) "in transformation"
Chronic myelomonocytic leukemia (CMML)

Each of these disorders may terminate in AML, but with varying propensity, as listed in Table 2.

The myelodysplastic disorders all show some of the morphologic abnormalities listed and specific criteria for each are well defined.

Table 1

Dysplastic Features of Hematopoietic Cells

Peripheral Blood
red cells: oval macrocytes, coarse basophilic stippling, polychromasia, dimorphic population, nucleated red cells (rosette nuclei)
granulocytes: degranulation, abnormally large granules, pseudo Pelger-Huët change, monocytoid change
monocytes: increase in number, granulocytic change, hyperlobulation of nucleus
platelets: giant forms, hypogranulation, bizarre shapes

Bone Marrow
red cells: megaloblastoid and megaloblastic erythropoiesis, nuclear budding, intranuclear bridges, nuclear budding, multinucleation, karyorrhexis, numerous Howell-Jolly bodies, intercellular contacts between cells, vacuolization of cytoplasm, irregular cytoplasmic contours, ring sideroblasts, excessive siderotic granules by Prussian blue staining
granulocytes: monocytoid change, degranulation, abnormally large granules, pseudo Pelger-Huët change, increased blast count
monocytes: increase in number, granulocytoid change
megakaryocytes: micromegakaryocytes, hyper- and hypolobation, abnormal clustering, paratrabecular location

Table 2

Frequency of Acute Leukemia Transformation in Myelodysplastic Syndromes

Refractory anemia (RA)	15%
(RA) with ringed sideroblasts	15%
Refractory anemia with excess blasts (RAEB)	30%
Chronic myelomonocytic leukemia (CMML)	40%
RAEB "in transformation"	100%

Pelger–Huët Anomaly

SYNONYMS
none

VITAL STATISTICS
- size .... 10 to 15 μm
- N:C ratio 1:3
- cell shape .... round to oval
- nuclear shape .... segmented with two equal lobes or round and not segmented
- chromatin .... clumped, denser than normal neutrophil
- nucleoli .... none
- cytoplasm .... pale pink with lilac granules

KEY DIFFERENTIATING FEATURES
"pince-nez" nuclei (two round lobes connected by a filament)

OTHER FEATURES
chromatin somewhat denser than normal neutrophil
granules in cytoplasm may be decreased

POTENTIAL LOOK–ALIKES
lymphoyctes
myelocytes
nucleated red blood cells (rarely)

ASSOCIATED DISEASE STATES AND CONDITIONS
true Pelger-Huët is a heritable condition
cells resembling Pelger-Huët (pseudo Pelger-Huët) may be seen in myelodysplastic states

The Pelger-Huët anomaly is an inheritable abnormality of nuclear segmentation. In heterozygotes, the nucleus has a characteristic bilobed appearance. Monolobated cells are also found. The homozogous state is extremely rare; most late phase neutrophils are monolobated. The various forms are illustrated below and on the next page.

The classic bilobed Pelger-Huët nucleus has a "pince-nez" conformation (two round or nearly round lobes connected by a single thin filament). The nuclear chromatin is generally denser than that of a normal segmented neutrophil.

In some cases of treated leukemia or myelodysplastic conditions the nucleus of neutrophils may have an appearance that resembles that seen in the heritable condition. They are called pseudo Pelger-Huët cells. Nuclear chromatin in these cells is very condensed, sometimes strikingly so. They are a form of neutrophil dysplastic maturation. The cells may also exhibit hypgranulation (see page 54 through 57).

Two other inherited neutrophil abnormalities are *Alder's anomaly*, discussed on page 302 and *May-Hegglin anomaly*, discussed on page 46.

Pelger-Huët PMN

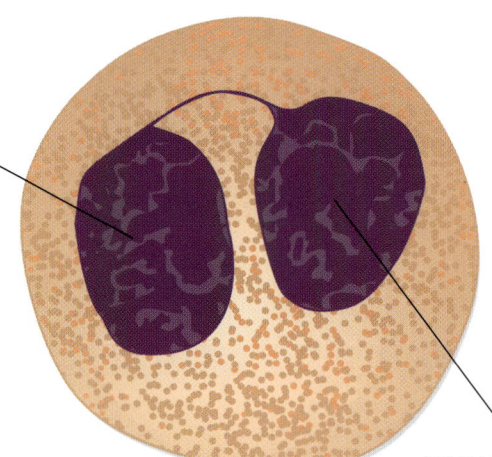

nucleus with closely approximated round nuclear lobes, resembling eye glasses (pince-nez)

pseudo Pelger-Huët neutrophils exhibit much more striking condensation of nuclear chromatin than normal segmented neutrophils

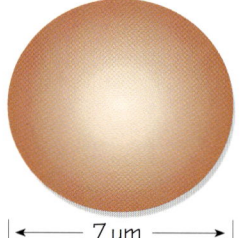

|← 7 μm →|

size of normal red blood cell

H1-06, 1984 (Blood, Wright-Giemsa, X400)

Identification	Referee %	Participant %
Pelger–Huët cell	81.3	71.6
Segmented neutrophil	12.5	25.2

The arrowed cell in the center of the field is a neutrophil with a Pelger–Huët nucleus. The cytoplasm contains lilac granules characteristic of a neutrophil. There are two nuclear lobes which are connected by a thin filament giving the nucleus a "pince-nez" appearance. By definition this is a segmented neutrophil, but when the majority of neutrophils have this characteristic appearance, a specific state is diagnosed (Pelger-Huët anomaly). The rest of the field demonstrates relatively normal red cells and platelets.

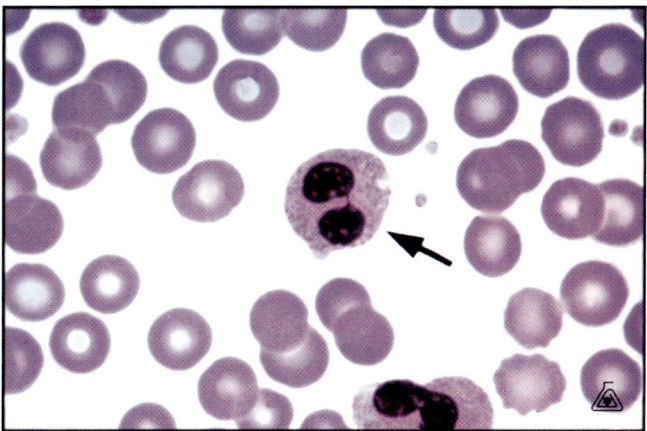

Pelger-Huët Anomaly Morphologic Variations

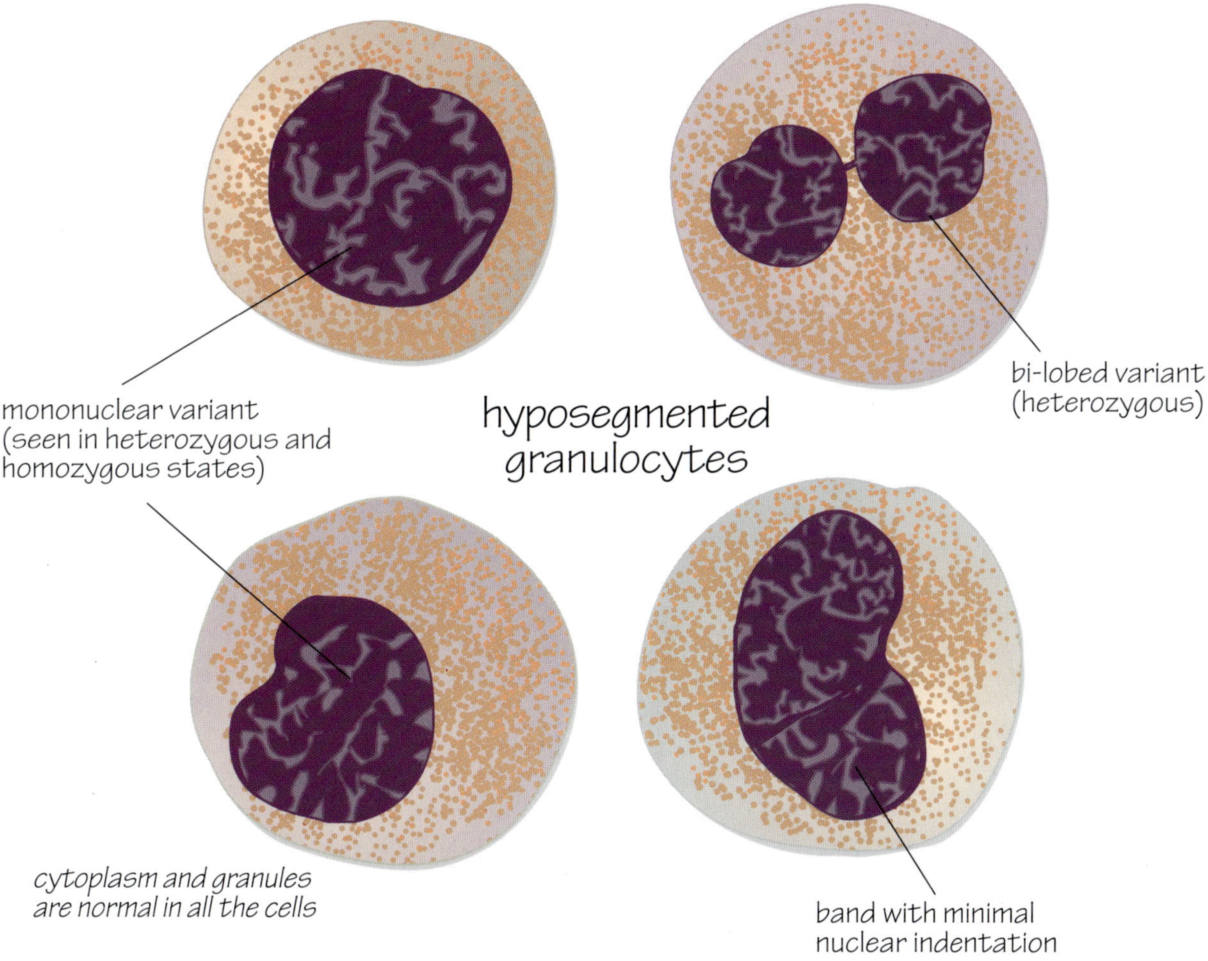

hyposegmented granulocytes

mononuclear variant (seen in heterozygous and homozygous states)

bi-lobed variant (heterozygous)

cytoplasm and granules are normal in all the cells

band with minimal nuclear indentation

Granulocytic (Myeloid) Cells

Erythrocytic Cells and Inclusions

Introduction	61
Erythrocyte (Normocytic, Normochromic)	62
Acanthocyte	64
A Closer Look At...How Acanthocytes Form	66
Bite Cell	68
A Closer Look At...Bite Cell Formation and Morphology	70
Blister Cell (Pre-Keratocyte)	72
A Closer Look At...Vacuolated Non-Nucleated Red Blood Cells	74
Echinocyte	76
A Closer Look At...Spiculated Red Cells	78
Fragmented Cell (Schistocyte, Helmet Cell, Keratocyte)	80
A Closer Look At...Microangiopathic Anemias	82
A Closer Look At...Diagnostic Morphology in MAHA and Heinz Body Anemia	84
Macrocyte (Oval or Round)	86
Microcyte (with Central Pallor)	88
Ovalocyte (Elliptocyte)	90
A Closer Look At...Hereditary Elliptocytosis	92
Polychromatophilic Red Cell (Non-Nucleated)	94
Sickle Cell	96
A Closer Look At...Sickle Cell Anemia	98
Spherocyte	100
A Closer Look At...Red Cell Membrane Loss and Spherocytosis	102
Stomatocyte	104
Target Cell	106
A Closer Look At...How Target Cells Form	108
Teardrop Cell	110
A Closer Look At...How Teardrop Cells Form	112
Reticulocyte (Supravital Stain)	114
Basophilic Stippling (Coarse)	116
A Closer Look At...How Basophilic Stippling Forms	118
A Closer Look At...Red Cell Inclusions	120
Heinz Body	124
A Closer Look At...How Heinz Bodies Form	126
Hemoglobin C Crystal	128
Hemoglobin H Inclusions (Supravital Stain)	130
A Closer Look At...Different Types of Precipitated Hemoglobin	132
Howell-Jolly Body (Wright-Giemsa Stain)	134
Howell-Jolly Body (Iron Stain)	136
A Closer Look At...How Howell-Jolly Bodies Form	138
Pappenheimer Bodies (Wright-Giemsa Stain)	140
Pappenheimer Bodies (Iron Stain)	142
A Closer Look At...How Pappenheimer Bodies Form	144
Red Cell Agglutinates	146
Rouleaux	148
A Closer Look At...Sticky Red Blood Cells	150

Introduction

Unlike white blood cells, normal circulating erythrocytes are not nucleated and are a relatively homogeneous population of cells dedicated to the same important task: delivering oxygen to tissues. Each enters the circulation slightly before it is fully mature, appearing as a larger, more basophilic non-nucleated cell without a mature erythrocyte's central pallor, when viewed with Wright-Giemsa stain. This is due to the small amount of RNA it still contains. Such a cell is called *polychromatophilic* because of its more heterogeneous staining when compared to a normal erythrocyte. It exists in this stage for 1 to 2 days before maturing to its adult form, and constitutes approximately 1% of the total number of circulating red cells, although this may vary somewhat: newborns and those who are recovering from a loss of blood have an increase in the number of these cells as an expected finding. To distinguish it from other large erythrocytes which have a pathologic cause, we take advantage of the polychromatophilic cell's retained RNA. This is done by staining the cell with a supravital stain such as New Methylene Blue which precipitates the RNA into a reticulum, or meshwork, pattern. Such cells are known as *reticulocytes*. Pathologic large erythrocytes do not demonstrate such a pattern when stained in this manner. Other types of non-nucleated erythrocytes found in the blood are almost always considered pathologic.

We have divided the non-nucleated red blood cells into three sections: *red cells defined by shape changes*, *red cell inclusions*, and finally, *a miscellaneous section* dealing with red cells that adhere to each other. This grouping allows the reader to compare and contrast similar morphologic abnormalities.

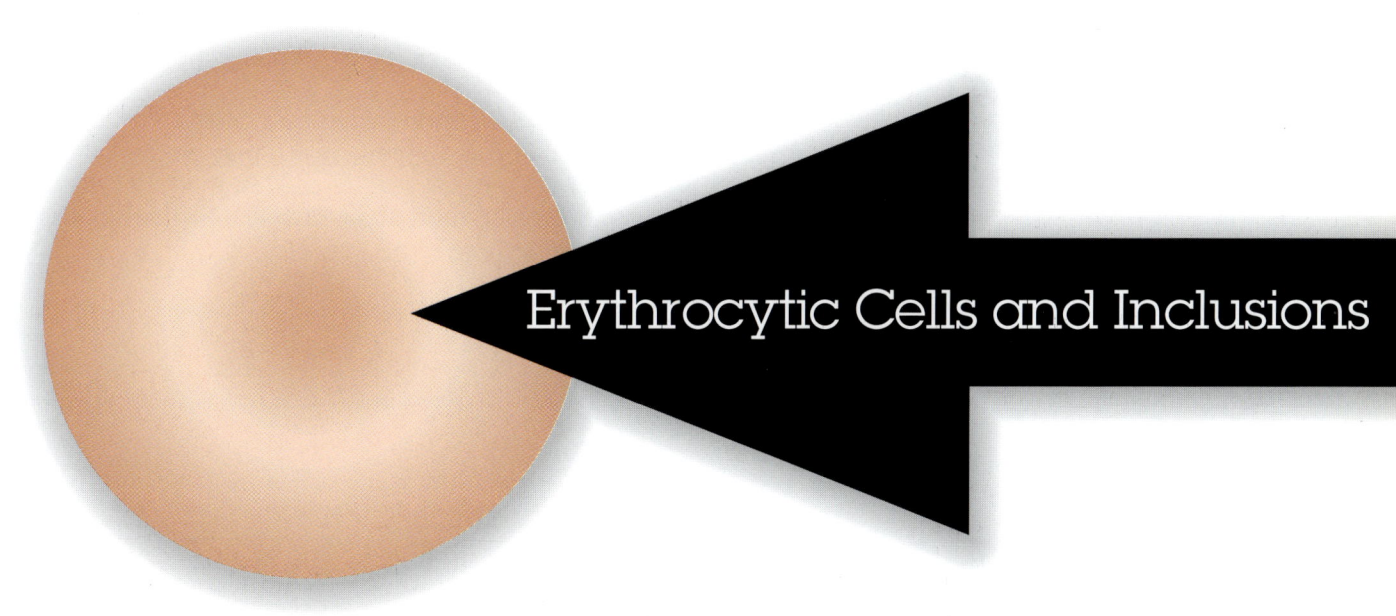

Erythrocytic Cells and Inclusions

Erythrocyte (Normocytic, Normochromic)

SYNONYMS
red cell, discocyte

VITAL STATISTICS
size .... 6.7 to 7.8 µm; MCV 80-100 fL
cell shape .... biconcave disc; round to slightly oval
cytoplasm .... eosinophilic, with central pallor, approximately one third of total diameter

KEY DIFFERENTIATING FEATURES
uniform round shape
central pallor occupying one third diameter of cell
no inclusions
lack of polychromasia

OTHER FINDINGS
normal red cells may or may not be found in association with other pathology; a mixture of normal and hypochromic red blood cells is called *dimorphism* or *partial hypochromia*; this picture is seen in iron deficiency partially treated with iron or transfused and in myelodysplasia, especially sideroblastic anemia

POTENTIAL LOOK-ALIKES
reticulocytes (polychromatophilic red cells)
red cells containing inclusions
macrocytes
other pathologic red cells

ASSOCIATED DISEASE STATES AND CONDITIONS
erythrocytes are the normal state
increased numbers of normal cells found in polycythemia

Erythrocytes are easily recognized by their round contour and bright red color with central pallor giving them a characteristic donut appearance in blood smears. They circulate in the blood as biconcave disks. Normal mature red blood cells measure 7.5 microns in diameter. The central pallor occupies about one third the diameter of the cell.

They are usually so numerous compared to white blood cells or platelets that they become background scenery. However, the normal circulating erythrocyte is the end product of a complex maturation process which occurs almost completely in the bone marrow and whose function is to deliver oxygen to cells. A red cell takes 7 days to develop in the marrow and then it circulates for 120 days before it is finally trapped in the spleen where it undergoes catabolism with eventual reutilization of its iron.

An erythrocyte contains hemoglobin which is composed of both heme and the protein globin. Heme carries the oxygen. It is composed of iron and protoporphyrin and is brightly colored (red). Globin is composed of 4 chains, 2 alpha and 2 beta. Normally, the alpha chain remains constant throughout life and the beta chain switches at various stages of development until the normal adult hemoglobin, hemoglobin A, is present as 97% of all hemoglobin by 1 year of age. If this hemoglobin production is abnormal (hereditary defect) severe pathology results. Decreased production of normal globin results in a thalassemia. Abnormal globin chain production (usually an amino acid substitution) results in hemoglobinopathy of which sickle cell anemia is probably the most famous example.

Most of the abnormal red cells described in this section are part of an anemia which may be due to any of several different causes (detailed in that cell's description); however, more than anemia may be responsible for some of these forms.

Normal Red Blood Cell

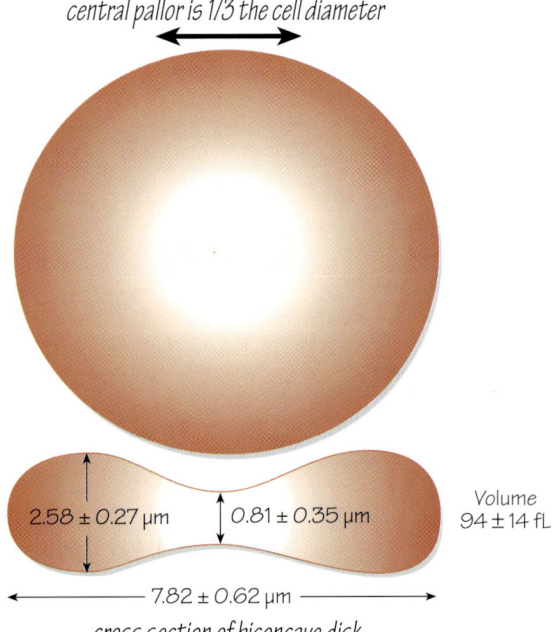

central pallor is 1/3 the cell diameter

2.58 ± 0.27 µm   0.81 ± 0.35 µm
Volume 94 ± 14 fL
7.82 ± 0.62 µm
cross section of biconcave disk

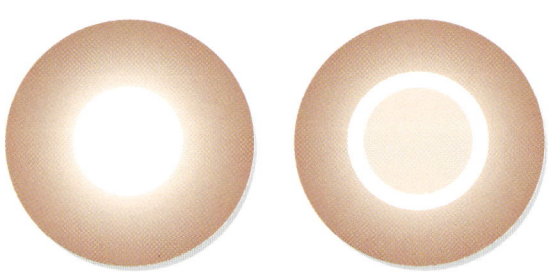

sharp cental pallor or rings of pallor are artifactual and reflect slow drying of smears

AH-04, 1990 (Blood, Wright-Giemsa, X400)

Identification	Referee %	Participant %
Erythrocyte, normal	85	72.5
Microcyte (with central pallor)	15	14.8

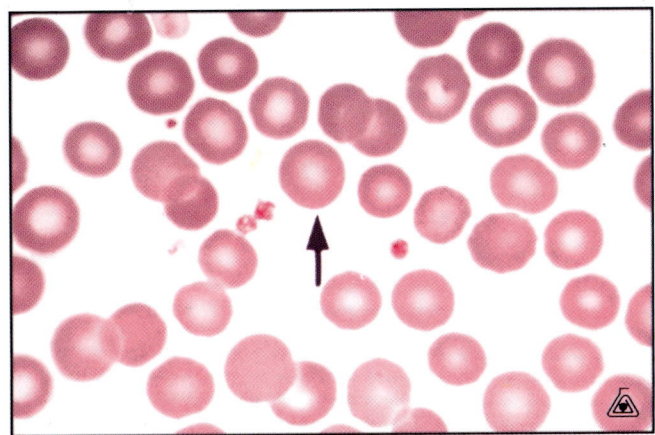

The round shape, central pallor approximately 1/3 of the cell's diameter, and the distinctive red color clearly identify this as an erythrocyte. The nearby platelets, with their central granule placement, are also normal. The identification of the arrowed cells as microcytic may have been inadvertent due to smaller erythrocytes present in this field. In fact, this sample was taken from a woman with hereditary sideroblastic anemia and demonstrates the dimorphic picture characteristic of that disorder.

H1-5, 1984 (Blood, Wright-Giemsa, X360)

Identification	Referee %	Participant %
Erythrocyte, normal	75	70.3
Macrocyte, oval or round	25	27.3

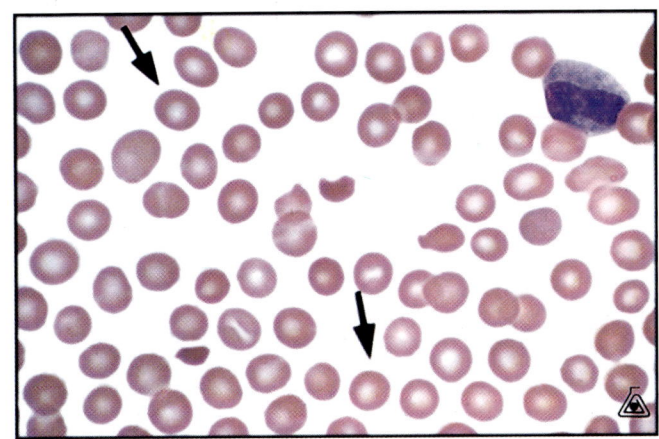

The two arrowed erythrocytes demonstrate central pallor and characteristic red color. Microcytes, for proficiency testing purposes, have increased central pallor, in contrast to microcytic spherocytes which lack central pallor. The arrowed cells have the normal amount of central clearing. Note, in contrast, the three fragmented cells (two in the central part of the field and one in the lower left) which do not have any characteristic size or shape and are also without central pallor. Platelets are decreased in this field. The sample was from an asymptomatic person with Pelger-Hüet anomaly.

HE-21, 1997 (Blood, Wright-Giemsa, X400)

Identification	Referee %	Participant %
Erythrocyte, normal	100	97.9

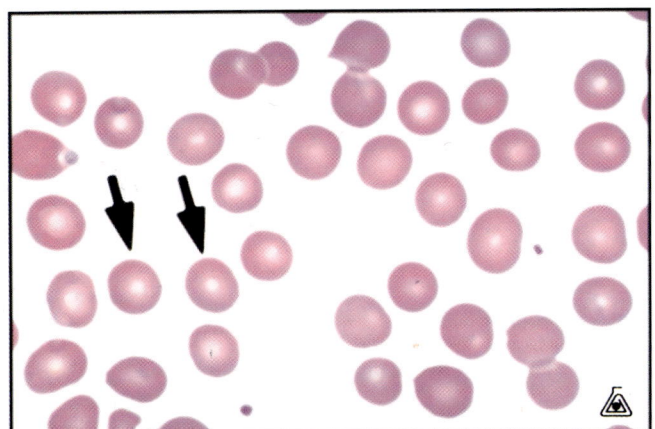

Each arrow points to a normal erythrocyte. The round shape and central pallor are distinctive; no inclusions are seen. This photomicrographic field is blood from a 28-year-old pregnant female with Hb AS (carrier state). A normal blood profile in Hb AS is the rule. She has an RBC = 4.21×10^{12}/L; Hgb = 12.6 g/dL; Hct = 37.9%; MCV = 90 fL; RDW = 14.0; WBC = 7.8×10^9/L; plt = 242×10^9/L.

Erythrocytic Cells and Inclusions

Acanthocyte

SYNONYMS
spur cell

VITAL STATISTICS
size .... smaller than normal RBC
appearance .... irregular projections of red cell membrane with a narrow base and sometimes knobby ends; the round center lacks central pallor

KEY DIFFERENTIATING FEATURES
3 to 20 irregular membrane spikes, unevenly distributed
no central pallor

POTENTIAL LOOK-ALIKES
echinocytes
schistocytes
microspherocytes

ASSOCIATED DISEASE STATES AND CONDITIONS
usually >10% acanthocytes
   abetalipoproteinemia (Bassen Kornzweig syndrome)
   homozygous hypobetalipoproteinemia
   advanced liver disease due to neonatal hepatitis, metastatic liver disease, Wilson's disease, cardiac cirrhosis, or alcoholism
   choreoacanthycytosis
   McLeod blood group phenotype
   In (Lu) blood group phenotype
usually <10% acanthocytes
   post splenectomy
   myeloproliferative disorders
   microangiopathic hemolytic anemia
   autoimmune hemolytic anemia
   sideroblastic anemia
   thalassemia major
   infantile pyknocytosis
   vitamin E deficiency
   neonatal period
   endocrine disorders (myxedema, panhypopituitarism)
   malnutrition (starvation, anorexia nervosa)
   large cell lymphoma
   psoriatic skin disorders

Acanthocyte comes from the Greek term for spike or horn. The shape results from poorly understood alterations in cell membrane lipid content and is irreversible. The most common cause is the post-splenectomy state.

The typical acanthocyte has 3 to 20 spikes with narrow bases and knobby ends. The projections are irregularly distributed over the surface. Acanthocytes have no central pallor and their spheroidal shape makes them smaller than normal red blood cells. They are usually easily distinguished from echinocytes (burr cells) which have central pallor and uniform smaller and blunter projections, evenly distributed over the surface. Transitional forms exist between acanthocytes and echinocytes which may blur these distinctions and make absolute diagnosis difficult. For CAP proficiency testing purposes, however, acanthocytes do not have central pallor.

A very rare acanthoycte may be encountered in otherwise normal blood films. They represent older, effete red blood cells approaching their extremes of life (120 days). Acanthocytes are readily found in post splenectomy states because of diminished removal of such poikilocytes. Large numbers are more characteristically seen in abetalipoproteinemia and advanced liver disease. Acanthocytes form due to derangement in the lipid content of the red cell membrane. In abetalipoproteinemia, the usual lecithin:sphingomyelin ratio is reversed. Sphingomyelin is more rigid than lecithin; it selectively expands the outer half of the lipid bilayer producing "wrinkles." In cirrhosis, the red cell membrane contains 40-70% excess cholesterol producing redundancy in the membrane. Bulges and excrescences develop. See *A Closer Look At...How Acanthocytes Form* on pages 66-67 for a more detailed discussion.

Acanthocytes

Spicules have a narrow base and are unevenly distributed. Most are sharp-tipped but some may be knobby.

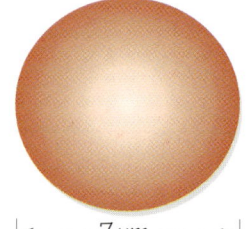

|← 7 µm →|
size of normal red blood cell

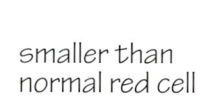
no central pallor

smaller than normal red cell

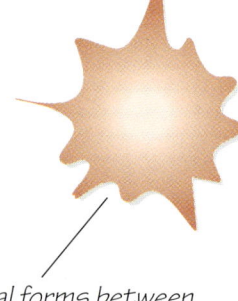

Transitional forms between acanthocytes and echinocytes may be seen. For CAP proficiency testing purposes, acanthocytes lack central pallor.

H1-31, 1983 (Blood, Wright-Giemsa, X360)

Identification	Referee %	Participant %
Acanthocyte	100	96.6

This is a case of abetalipoproteinemia. The patient presented with malabsorption, visual impairment, and ataxia. Hemoglobin was 12.5 gm/dL and cholesterol 48 mg/dL. The two arrowed cells are acanthocytes. The surface is distorted by small unevenly distributed spicules. Central pallor is lacking. The spicules are short, sharp, and have a narrow base. Other red cells in the field are acanthocytes, echinocytes and transitional forms between the two. Such diversity is often found in this disorder. For CAP proficiency testing purposes, acanthocytes lack central pallor while echinocytes have central pallor. The lone leukoycte in the field is a segmented neutrophil.

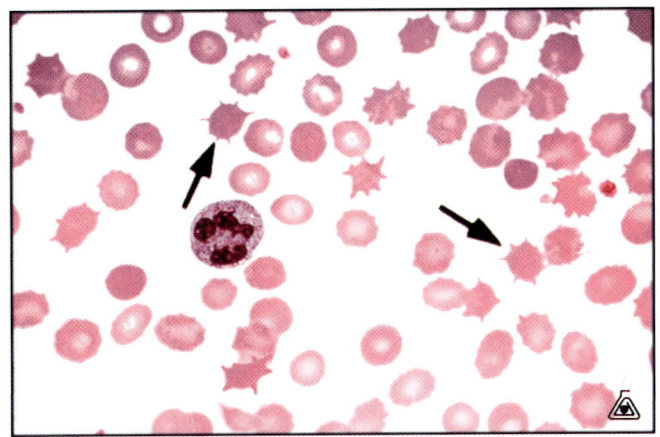

AH-28, 1990 (Blood, Wright-Giemsa, X400)

Identification	Referee %	Participant %
Acanthocyte	100	94.5

The patient has severe alcoholic liver disease. The arrowed cell is an acanthocyte. Notice the lack of central pallor and uneven surface projections. Echinocytes have central pallor and display more numerous, regular projections. Other spiculated cells in the field are echinocyte-acanthocyte hybrids; they have central pallor. The remaining red cells in the field are essentially normochromic-normocytic. Platelets are unremarkable.

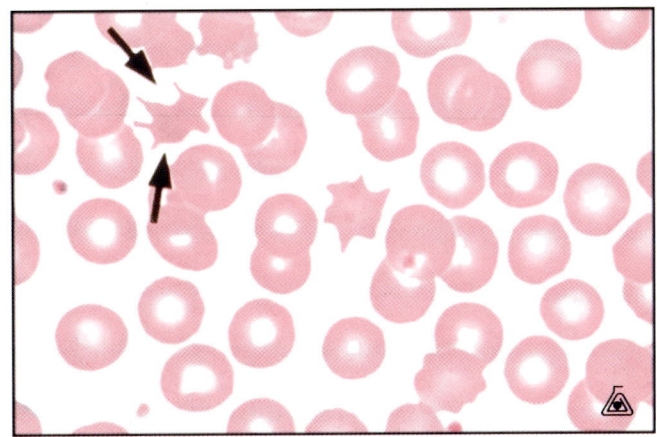

AH-26, 1990 (Blood, Wright-Giemsa, X400)

Identification	Referee %	Participant %
Acanthocyte	100	90

The patient is the same as that shown in AH-28, 1990, above. The arrowed spiculated cell is an acanthocyte. Once again, the cell lacks central pallor. The projections are irregular; they vary in length and are unevenly distributed. Some of the cytoplasmic spicules have knobby ends. The leukocyte in the right corner is a segmented neutrophil. Platelets are unremarkable.

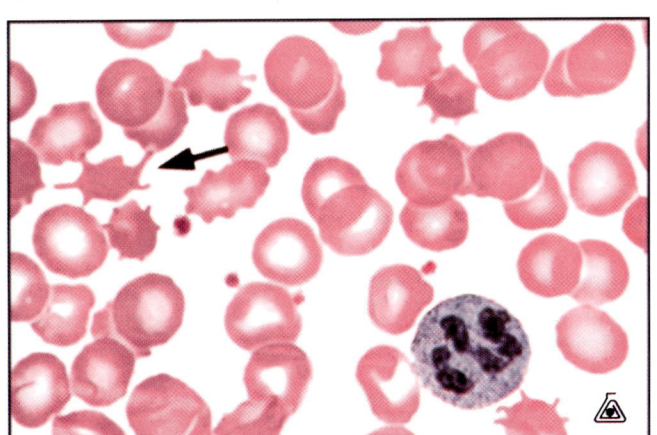

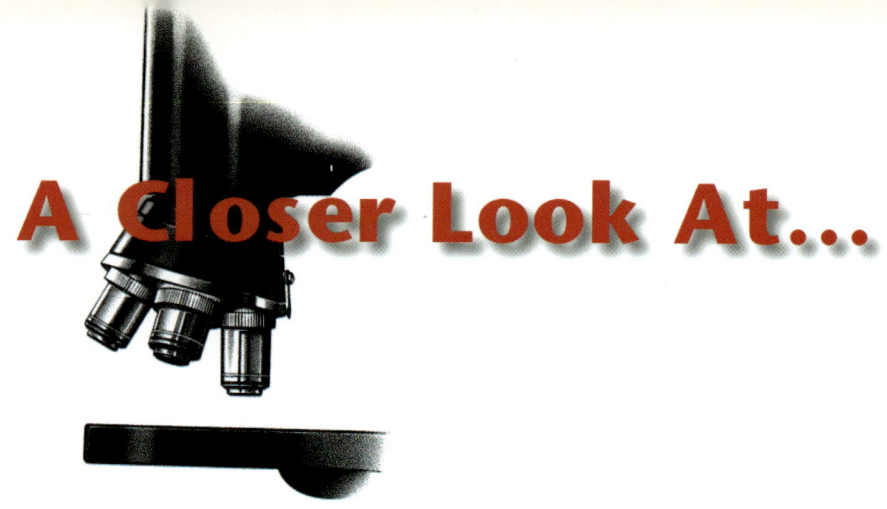

A Closer Look At...

How Acanthocytes Form

Acanthocytes are spheroidal dense red cells with multiple irregular thorny projections unevenly distributed over the surface. This change is irreversible and due to alteration of the lipid content of the red cell membrane. Small numbers of acanthocytes are most commonly seen post splenectomy. Large numbers are found in two types of disorders: abetalipoproteinemia and severe liver disease.

Abetalipoproteinemia is a very rare genetic disorder that results in defective hepatocyte secretion of apolipoprotein B (apo B). Without apo B, transport of triglycerides from the intestine to the liver is blocked. No VLDL, LDL, and chylomicrons enter the plasma. The small bowel fills with triglyceride droplets. Plasma cholesterol levels are less than 50 mg/dL.

Infants present in the first month of life with steatorrhea, diarrhea, and malabsorption of fat-soluble vitamins (D, A, K, and E). Progressive neurologic abnormalities develop along with blindness due to retinitis pigmentosa. Death usually occurs by age 30.

Anemia is mild and the life span of red cells is normal or slightly decreased. The blood contains 50% to 90% acanthocytes. Red cell precursors in the bone marrow are normal. The spiculated shape develops as the red cells age in the peripheral blood. Normal transfused cells also gradually transform into acanthocytes. The shape changes are irreversible.

Red cell membrane lipids are in equilibrium with plasma lipids. Sphingomyelin is a stable, immobile component of the red cell membrane. The lipid abnormalities in abetalipoproteinemia result in a marked increase in red cell membrane sphingomyelin and a decrease in lecithin. Sphingomyelin preferentially collects on the outer half of the lipid bilayer, selectively expanding it and resulting in irregular membrane projections. The underlying spectrin framework of the cells is not disturbed. The abnormal shape reduces the deformability of the red cell somewhat, but not to the degree seen in advanced liver disease. As a result, splenic sequestration and remodeling are minimal and hemolysis is mild.

Advanced liver disease, most commonly due to alcoholic cirrhosis, can lead to lipid abnormalities and the formation of acanthocytes. Unlike abetalipoproteinemia, the acanthocytes have a significantly shorter life span. They are much less deformable and are readily destroyed in the spleen. The resultant hemolytic anemia is progressive and severe. The term *spur cell anemia* is evoked for this condition.

The red cell membrane normally has a ratio of cholesterol to phospholipid of 1:1. As the amount of cholesterol increases, the surface area of the cell increases. The first step is the formation of broader and flatter cells which are seen as target cells in peripheral blood smears. In advanced cirrhosis, the damaged liver manufactures an abnormal high density lipoprotein (HDL) containing a large amount of free (unesterified) cholesterol. The abnormal HDL binds to the red cell membrane and functions as a lipid trap. Large amounts of free cholesterol accumulate in the outer half of the red cell membrane, disturbing the normal cholesterol:phospholipid balance. The excess cholesterol first forms target cells and then, as the amount of membrane increases even more, irregular projections and excrescences develop. In addition, the cholesterol damages the Na^+/K^+ pump and compromises cell deformity. The spleen continually remodels these cells, eventually producing a subpopulation of small spheroidal acanthocytes with short and sharp thorns. These cells are not deformable and eventually become trapped in the spleen and are destroyed.

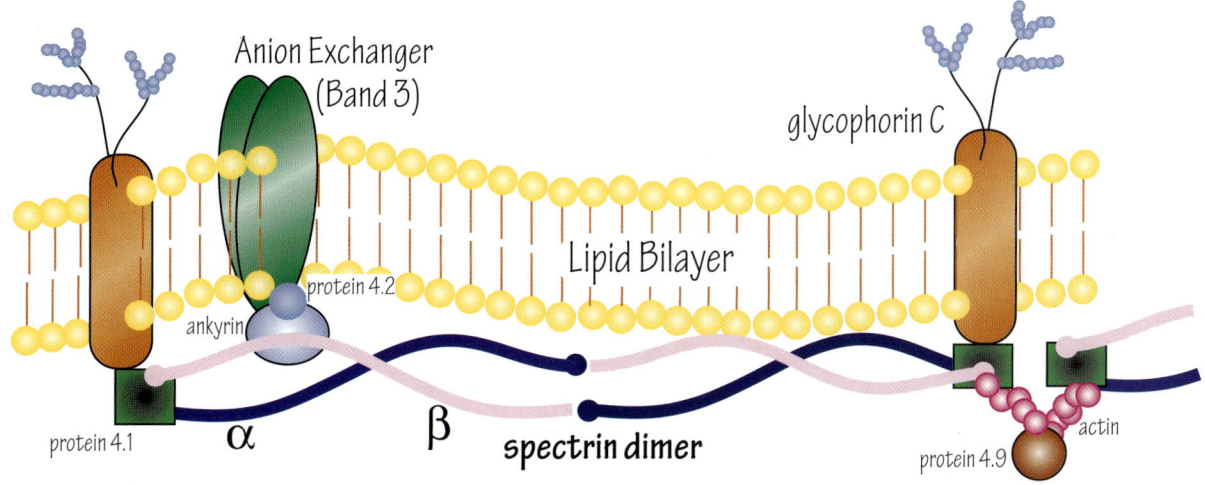

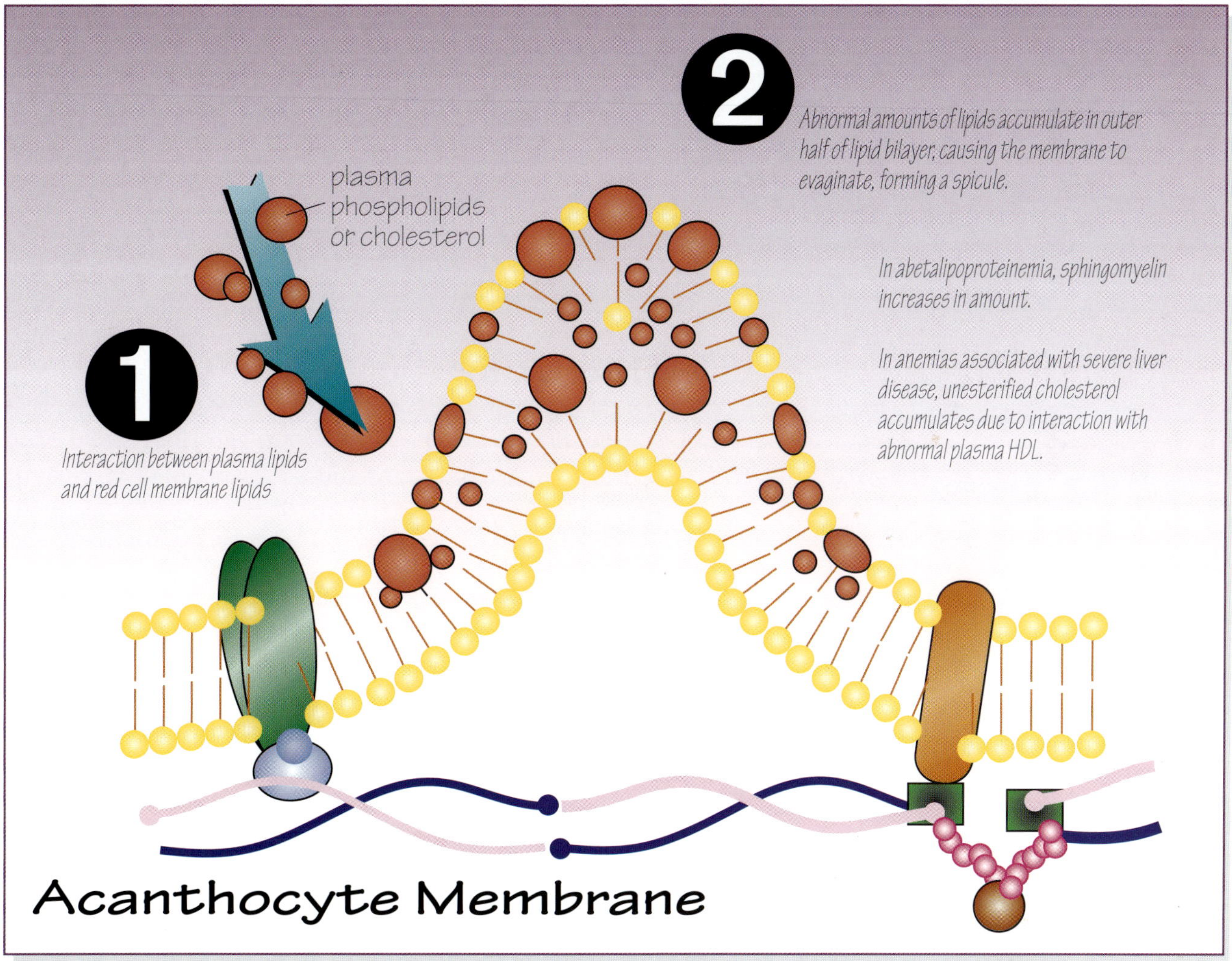

Bite Cell

SYNONYMS
cookie bite cell, degmacyte

VITAL STATISTICS
size .... normocytic to microcytic
cell shape .... varies, but characteristically shows peripheral "bites" taken out of the cytoplasm, with a somewhat scalloped membrane as the result
cytoplasm .... variably reduced, from small defects to an "apple core" poikilocyte

KEY DIFFERENTIATING FEATURES
peripheral defect of red cell membrane resulting in eythrocytes which look bitten

OTHER FINDINGS
spherocytes often also present, to variable degree

POTENTIAL LOOK-ALIKES
helmet type of fragmented cell

ASSOCIATED DISEASE STATES AND CONDITIONS
disorders associated with Heinz body formation:
   unstable hemoglobins
   chemical poisoning
   oxidant drugs
   G-6PD deficiency and other enzymopathies
   hemolytic anemia associated with severe alcoholic liver disease

The defect we term *bite cell* is seen in a subset of hemolytic anemias in which precipitated or denatured hemoglobin occurs. This is characteristically secondary to a defect in a red cell enzyme. When this abnormal erythrocyte traverses the spleen, the abnormally precipitated hemoglobin which is known as a Heinz body is removed. There is a residual deformity of the red cell which usually appears as though the cell has had a "bite" taken from it. How big a bite varies, being variously described as a *nibble*, *bite*, or even an *apple core* when large symmetrical defects occur in the midportion of the cell. More than one defective "bite" may be present in a cell. There are defects in this type of anemia which look just like the *helmet cell* poikilocyte of other anemias, so confusion may occur in some cases. These abnormal cells are eventually removed by the spleen.

The differences between the various types of bite cells are dicussed on page 70, *A Closer Look At…Bite Cell Formation and Morphology*. The underlying pathology leading to the bite morphology, namely the presence of Heinz bodies, are discussed on page 124.

Bite Cells

|← 7 µm →|
size of normal red blood cell

Erythrocytic Cells and Inclusions

H1-7, 1986 (Blood, Wright-Giemsa, X360)

Identification	Referee %	Participant %
Bite cell	87.5	81.8
Fragmented cell (helmet cell, schistocyte, keratocyte)	12.5	17.2

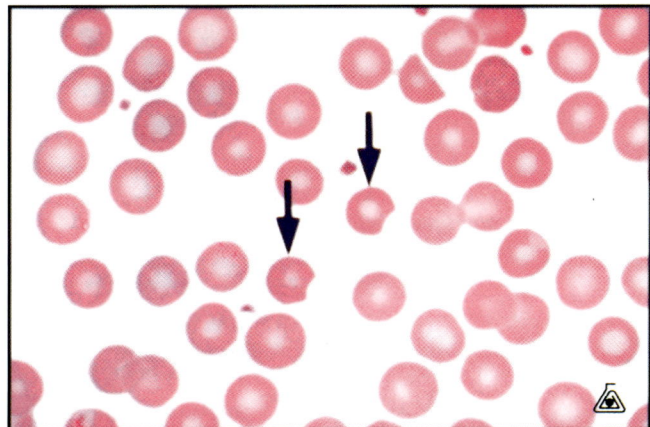

The photomicrograph is from the blood of a 17-year-old male who was treated for probable dermatitis herpetiformis (an itchy skin disease associated with sprue) with the drug 4,4' diaminodiphenylsufone (popularly known as Dapsone). Over the ensuing two months his hemoglobin dropped from 15.5 to 11.3 g/dL, then promptly normalized with discontinuance of the Dapsone. A diagnosis of drug-induced oxidant hemolysis was made. The two arrowed red cells are bite cells. The bites are small—too small to mimic a helmet cell (keratocyte). Such "nibble cells" as well as double bite cells and apple core cells are diagnostic of Heinz body anemia. The defect is the result of the spleen's function in removing abnormalities from red cells—in this case precipitated hemoglobin damage by excessive oxidation from Dapsone.

H1-8, 1986 (Blood, Wright-Giemsa, X360)

Identification	Referee %	Participant %
Bite cell	81.2	69.6
Fragmented cell (helmet cell, schistocyte, keratocyte)	18.8	28.2

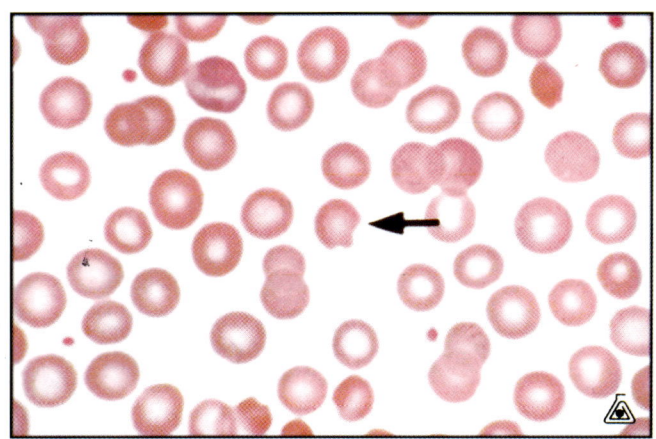

This case is from the same patient depicted above. The arrowed cell is a bite cell with two pieces missing from the cytoplasm. This is a so called "double-bite" cell. This type of morphologic change is diagnostic of Heinz body anemia. Small bites and apple-core forms are also diagnostic. Some bite cells may resemble helmet cells (below) and are not diagnostic of the presence of Heinz bodies. See *A Closer Look At…Bite Cell Formation and Morphology* on the next page and *A Closer Look At…Diagnostic Morphology in MAHA and Heinz Body Anemia* on page 84 for illustrations and a detailed discussion.

H1-4, 1986 (Blood, Wright-Giemsa, X360)

Identification	Referee %	Participant %
Bite cell	18.8	20.8
Fragmented cell (helmet cell, schistocyte, keratocyte)	81.2	78.6

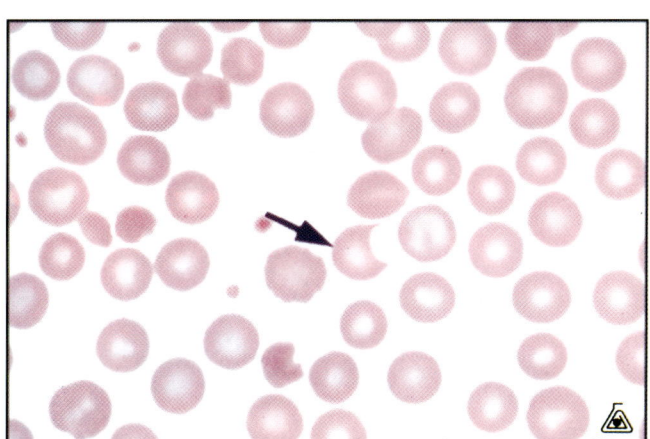

The case is from the same patient depicted in the above two photomicrographs. Morphologically, the cell is a *helmet cell* but it is really a *bite cell*. As depicted on the next page, cells with deep bites are indistinguishable from helmet cells. The decision as to when one designation ends and another begins is not completely defined and may be better seen in the context of surrounding cells. Given the drug history and the morphology of the cells seen in other fields, *bite cell* is a preferable designation. Without history or a supporting cast of classic bite cells, however, the arrowed cell could very well be called a *helmet cell*. The small, dense poikilocytes beneath and to the left of the arrow are compatible with hemolysis.

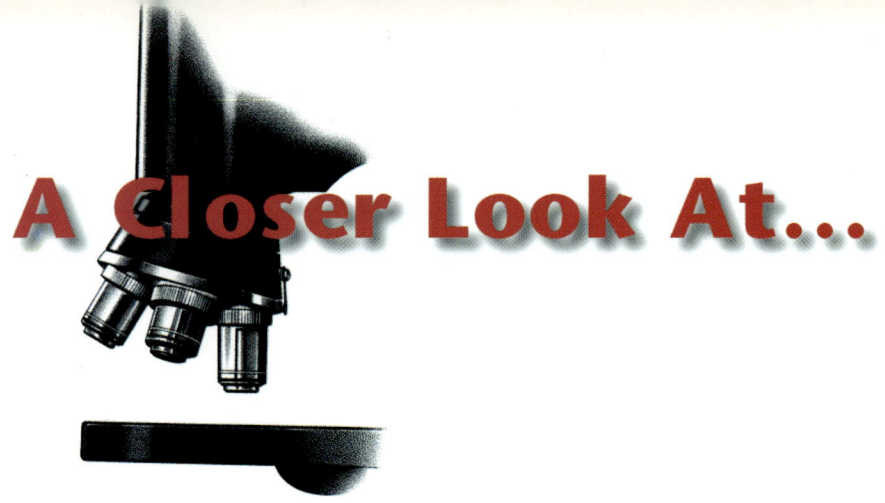

A Closer Look At...

Bite Cell Formation and Morphology

A bite cell is the term for a permanent change in an intrinsically abnormal erythrocyte. Its formation occurs as it circulates through the spleen's cords, as depicted in the upper illustration on the next page.

The erythrocytes are abnormal because they contain Heinz bodies, which are clumps of precipitated hemoglobin. (See *Heinz Body*, page 124 and *A Closer Look At...How Heinz Bodies Form*, page 126). The spleen's pitting function relieves the erythrocyte of its abnormal contents (Heinz bodies) but the erythrocyte may not completely mend the site; instead it retains the area of loss which is visible as a "bite." The cell's loss is variable, depending on the amount of precipitated hemoglobin which is removed, as well as the functional state of the spleen. These cells enjoy a range of descriptive terms, including *nibble*, *bite*, *helmet cell*, *double bite*, and *apple core* (see diagram, opposite). Such cells are quite valuable as morphologic clues in routine Wright-Giemsa blood film preparation in assessing the possibility of G6PD deficiency or an unstable hemoglobin. Spherocytes are very often found in association with bite cells, although somewhat surprisingly, in low numbers.

The various types of bite cells are illustrated in the lower drawing. Classic bite cells have small "nibbles" and are diagnostic of Heinz body anemia. Double bites may be either symmetrical ("apple core" forms) or asymmetrical. The morphology is also diagnostic of Heinz body anemia. The cells with one large "bite" cannot reliably be distinguished from helmet cells. This may create confusion because helmet cell-shaped poikilocytes (fragmented cells) are not unique to the spectrum of *bite cell anemia*. Helmet cells are often present in microangiopathic hemolytic anemias (MAHA) of various etiologies, such as severe burns, disseminated intravascular coagulation (DIC), and thrombotic thrombocytopenic purpura (TTP); other causes of helmet cell formation exist. In some instances it may be quite difficult to differentiate the cause based on laboratory findings alone and clinical correlation is required. The differences between MAHA and Heinz body anemia is further detailed in *A Closer Look At...Diagnostic Morphology in MAHA and Heinz Body Anemia* on page 84.

How Bite Cells Form

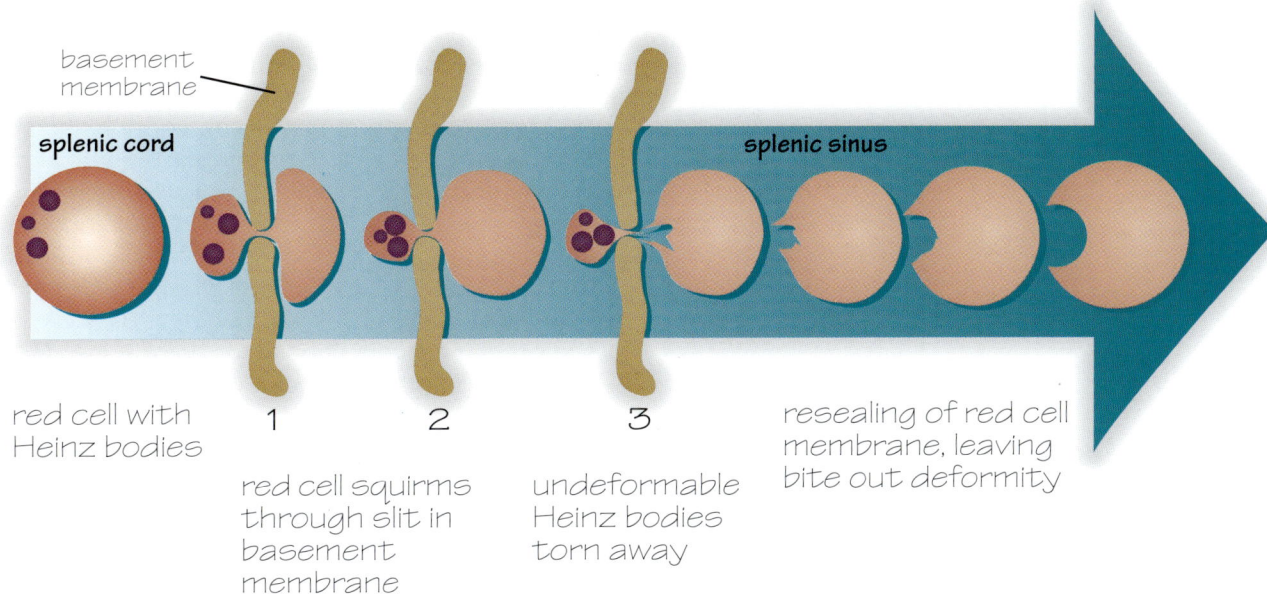

Types of Bite Cells

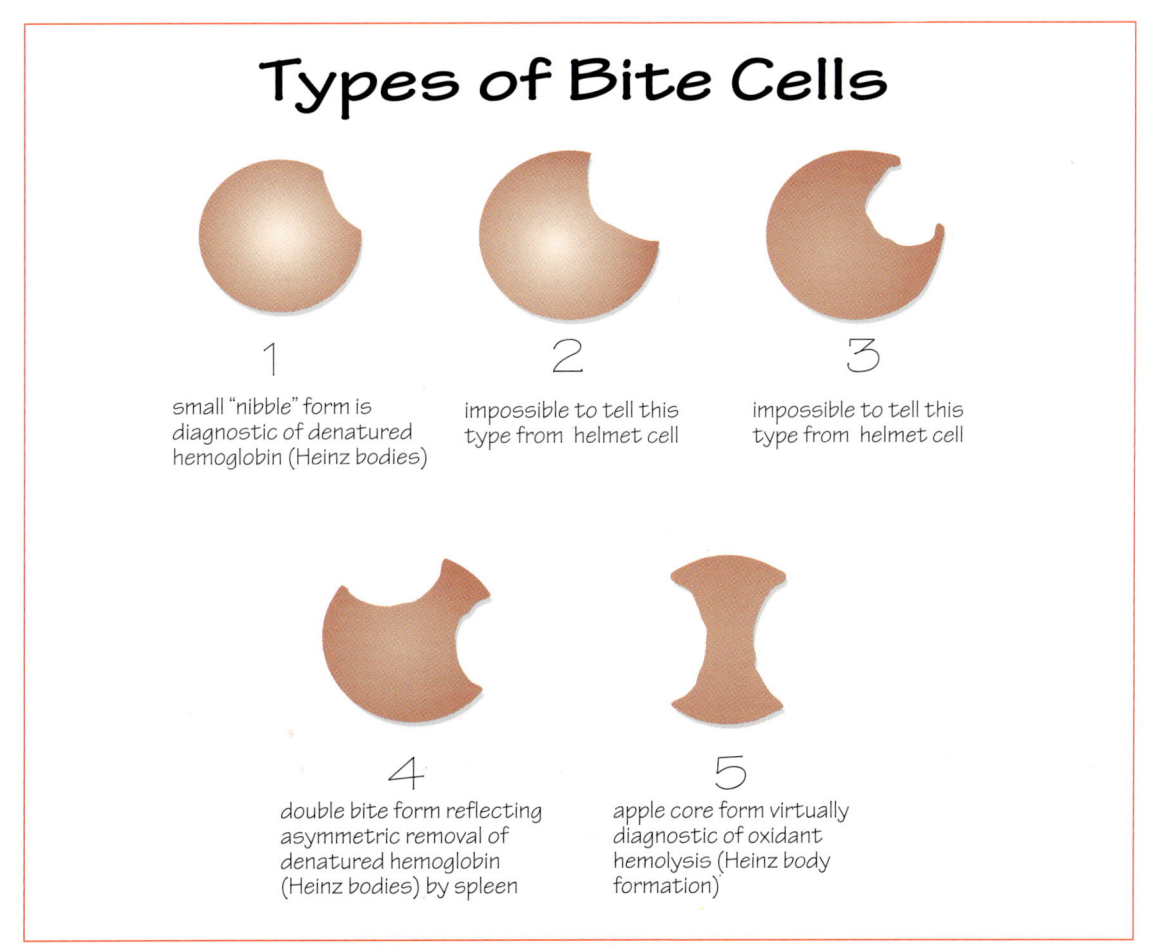

Blister Cell (Pre-Keratocyte)

SYNONYMS
pre-keratocyte, vacuolated non-nucleated red cell, hemi-ghost cell, eccentrocytes

VITAL STATISTICS
size .... 7.5-8 µm
cell shape .... round to more irregular
cytoplasm .... submembranous pseudo-vacuole(s), otherwise normochromic

KEY DIFFERENTIATING FEATURES
prominent eccentrically located "vacuole" in normochromic red blood cell (actually a pseudo-vacuole)
submembranous location
vacuole has a razor-sharp edge
single; rarely double

OTHER FINDINGS
peripheral smear may display evidence of red cell fragmentation, such as spherocytes and schistocytes, especially keratocytes
the pseudovacuole is sharply defined and appears to be a true vacuole by light microscopy, but electron microscopy demonstrates that opposing red cell membranes have actually fused after being disrupted; because all intervening hemoglobin is squeezed out, the fusion site does not stain and appears to be a hole in the red cell

POTENTIAL LOOK-ALIKES
bite cells
helmet (fragmented) cells
sickle cell (blister cell variant)
red cell containing hemoglobin C crystals
red cells in post-splenectomy state
artifacts

ASSOCIATED DISEASE STATES AND CONDITIONS
microangiopathic anemia

The abnormality present in an erythrocyte designated as a "blister" cell may be easy to overlook initially. Found in microangiopathic hemolytic anemia, where fragmented cells (poikilocytes) are present, they are part of that abnormal spectrum. The "blister" is, in fact, a pseudo-vacuole caused by the coming together again of membrane that was disrupted by a microcirculatory event such as a fibrin strand; there is no hemoglobin present between the resealed membranes and the remainder of the cell. These findings have been confirmed by electron microscopy. Sometimes the resealing of the membranes forms two smaller pseudo-vaculoes (see illustration on next page).

The pseudo-vacuole has a razor sharp edge. This is in contrast to another type of blister cell seen in sickle cell anemia. The margins of the latter have fuzzy edges that gradually blend the hemoglobinized and nonhemoglobinized portions of the red cell together. It is of interest that the term blister cell was first used to describe these sickle cell variants. Over time and with general usage, the term is now more commonly associated with the pseudo-vacuoles found in microangiopathic (MAHA) states. To help minimize confusion, *prekeratocyte* is a better term to use for the cells with pseudo-vacuoles caused by fibrin strand damage.

As the name implies, *prekeratocyte* is the forebearer of the *keratocyte*. A keratocyte occurs when the prekeratocyte's membrane bursts and thus it may resemble a helmet, bite, or horned cell. (see *A Closer Look At...Microangiopathic Anemias* on page 82). A careful search of the blood smear is important when a keratocyte is found, since blister cell connotes a microangiopathic process while bite/helmet cells without blister cells indicate an unstable hemoglobin or oxidant-induced hemolysis. Please refer to the *Bite Cell* entry on page 68 for discussion of the latter process.

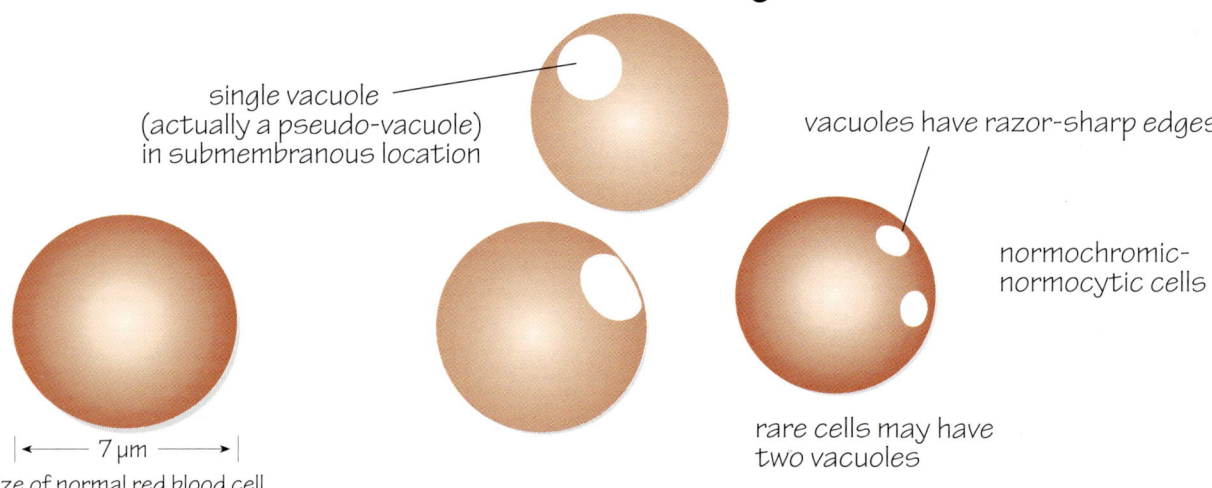

Pre-Keratocytes

single vacuole (actually a pseudo-vacuole) in submembranous location

vacuoles have razor-sharp edges

normochromic-normocytic cells

rare cells may have two vacuoles

7 µm — size of normal red blood cell

Erythrocytic Cells and Inclusions

HE-10, 1996 (Blood, Wright-Giemsa, X400)

Identification	Referee %	Participant %
Prekeratocyte (blister cell)	96.4	97.9
Echinocyte	3.6	0.1
Bite cell	-	0.7

This sample is from a 26-year-old male with severe abdominal pain. Hematologic values include a RBC of 6.89×10^{12}/L, Hgb of 13.1 g/dl; hematocrit of 42%; MCV of 61 fL, WBC of 7.9×10^9/L; and platelet count of 287×10^9/L. He has beta-thalassemia trait, which would explain the high red blood cell count with a very low MCV. The photomicrograph does not significantly demonstrate the target cells, ovalocytes, or basophilic stippling in beta-thalassemia trait. The arrowed cell is, however, a classic example of a blister cell. The membrane that was brought together to create the pseudovacuole below it is exquisitely fine; it is easy to see how this cell was named "blister." The cause of the blister cell was not stated but it is assumed to be related to the history of abdominal pain.

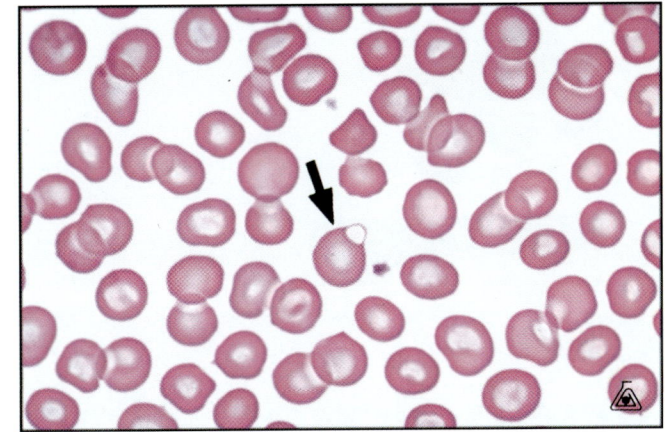

Pre-Keratocyte Formation

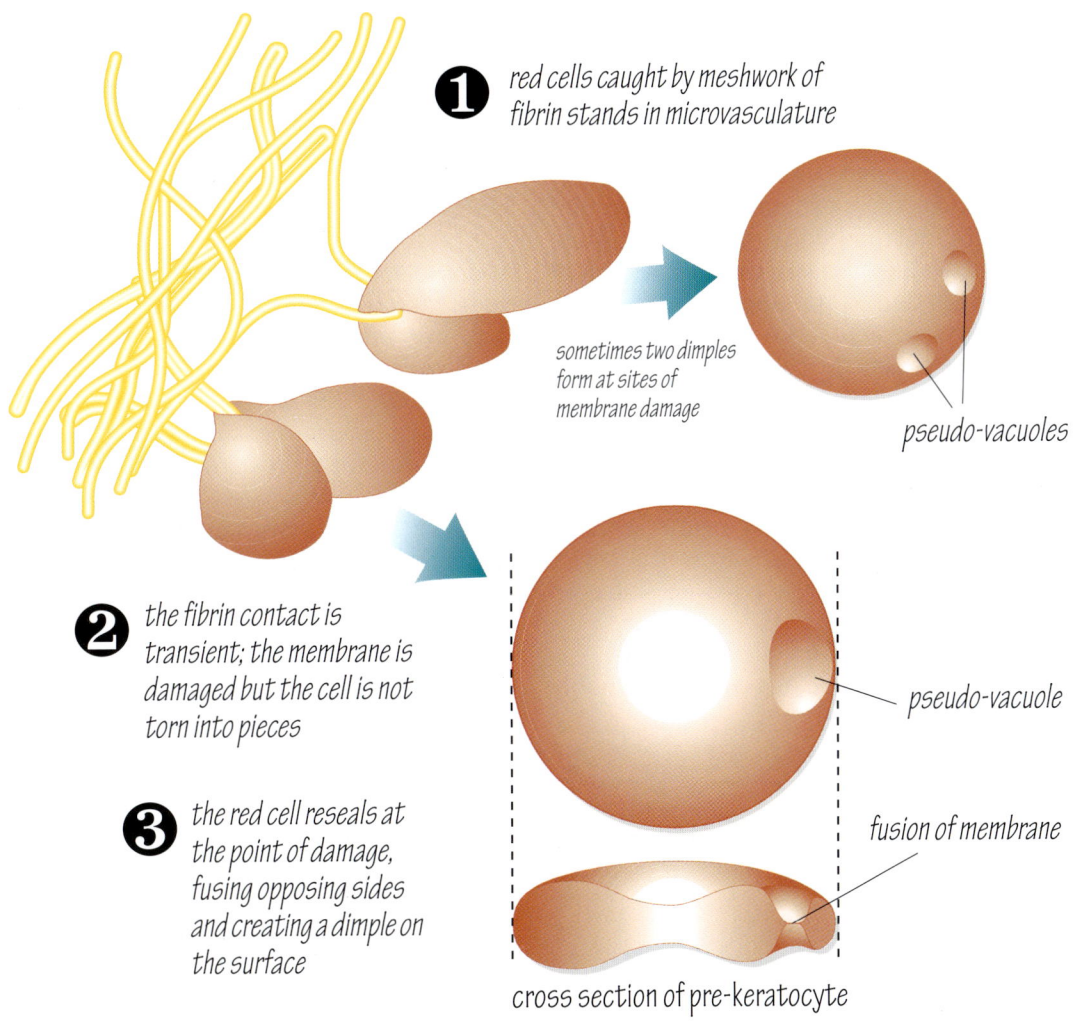

❶ red cells caught by meshwork of fibrin stands in microvasculature

sometimes two dimples form at sites of membrane damage

pseudo-vacuoles

❷ the fibrin contact is transient; the membrane is damaged but the cell is not torn into pieces

pseudo-vacuole

❸ the red cell reseals at the point of damage, fusing opposing sides and creating a dimple on the surface

fusion of membrane

cross section of pre-keratocyte

Erythrocytic Cells and Inclusions

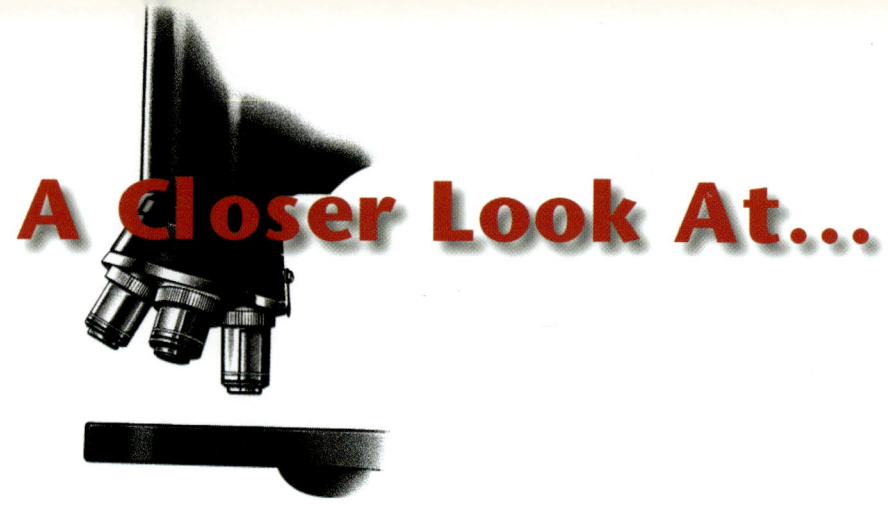

A Closer Look At...

Vacuolated Non-Nucleated Red Blood Cells

Vacuolated red blood cells may be caused by a variety of pathophysiologic events, the most common being the post-splenectomy state. Such vacuoles generally tend to be tiny and often multiple. Their margins are indistinct.

In a second variant of vacuolated cell, the vacuoles tend to be single (though occasionally double) and are crisply outlined. Such vacuoles are more apparent than real, since by electron microscopy they represent fusion of opposing membranes with exclusion of intervening hemoglobin. Red cells exhibiting such vacuoles are encountered in microangiopathic states, where they are believed to reflect juxtaposition and fusion of opposing membranes due to transient draping across fibrin stands in the microcirculation. (See *A Closer Look At...Microangiopathic Anemias*, page 82). Such cells have been referred to as *pre-keratocytes* since with continued circulation they tend to rupture, giving rise to two horns. The cell is then designated a *keratocyte*. It is of interest that keratocytes deriving from vacuole rupture are indistinguishable from other helmet cells in the microangiopathic state as well as from the larger nibbles associated with bite cell anemia exhibited in oxidant hemolysis.

A curious red cell encountered in sickle cell disease is associated with eccentrically located and presumably partially polymerized sickled hemoglobin. Such cells have been described as "blister cells." The margins of the resulting vacuole or blister are always fuzzy and indistinct, as opposed to the razor-sharp margins of the pseudo-vacuole in the pre-keratocyte.

Lastly, vacuoles in red cells may be artifactual, a product of high humidity and poor smearing. In this instance, the vacuoles are too crisply outlined. The margins are nearly refractile, indicative of trapped water droplets on top of the cell. Careful focusing can easily distinguish these imposters from the real thing.

A Footnote Regarding Terminology
Hematology monikers are sometimes not very precise. Historical precedent and common usage often overshadow accuracy. The terms associated with vacuolated non-nucleated red blood cells are a case in point. In the past, CAP proficiency challenges have used the term **blister cell** *to mean a* **pre-keratocyte.** *As discussed above, a blister cell should really refer to a specific type of sickle cell. Most textbooks, however, equate blister cell with pre-keratocyte. This atlas—acknowledging the force of general usage—follows suit but we would prefer participants keep the Greek term and avoid using blister cell altogether, at least when referring to changes associated with microangiopathic states.*

Vacuolated Non-Nucleated Red Blood Cells

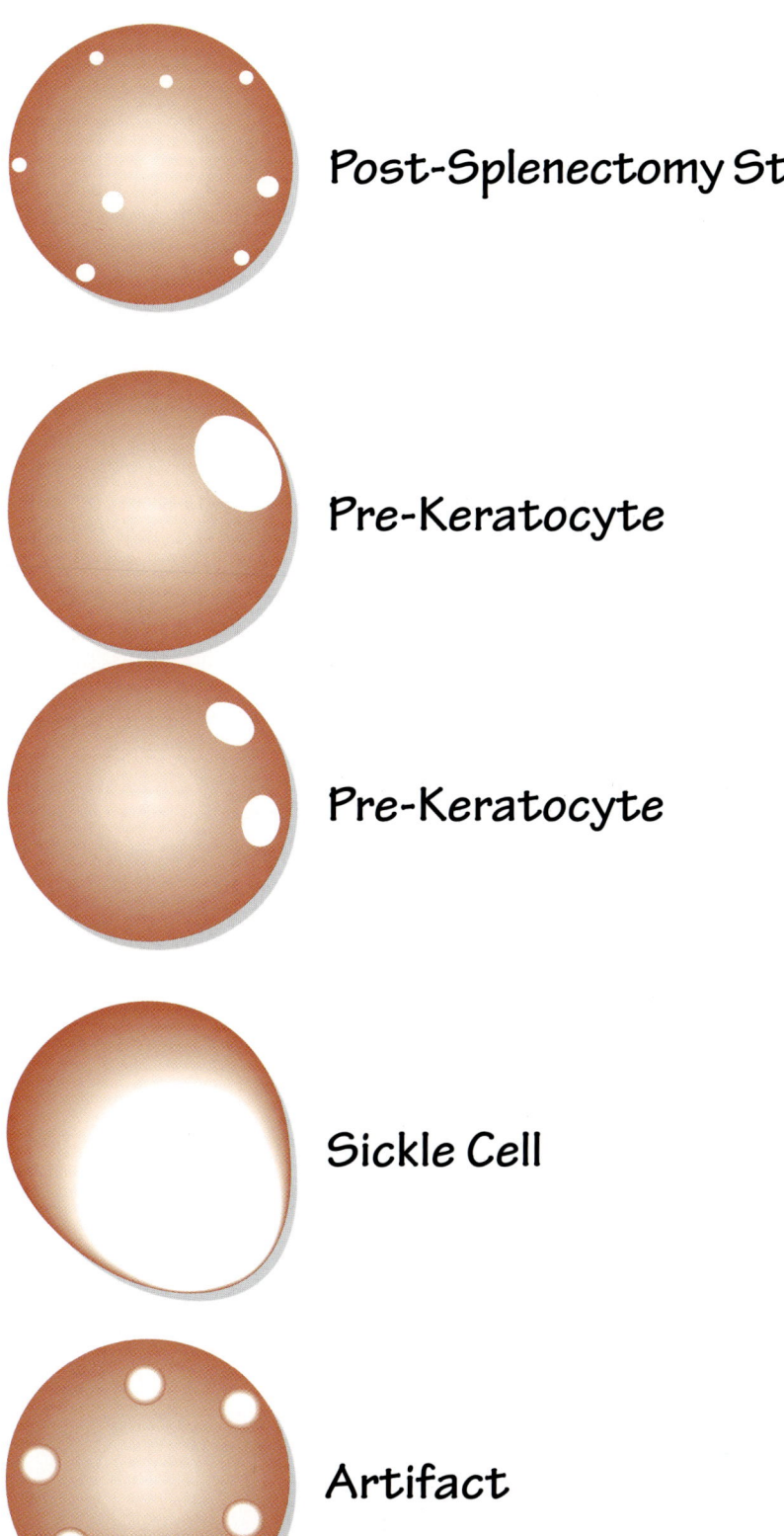

Post-Splenectomy State

Pre-Keratocyte

Pre-Keratocyte

Sickle Cell

Artifact

Echinocyte

SYNONYMS
burr cell, crenated cell

VITAL STATISTICS
size .... 6.7 to 7.8 μm diameter
cell shape .... even surface distribution of 10 to 30 short, blunt or pointed spicules
cytoplasm .... normochromic; retains central pallor

KEY DIFFERENTIATING FEATURES
evenly distributed, uniformly sized spicules
central pallor (unlike acanthocytes)

OTHER FINDINGS
Because echinocytes are most commonly an artifact due to pH changes in smear preparation, normal and abnormal red cells may undergo secondary transformation into their echinocytic counterparts; this produces hybrid cells such as echino-acanthocytes and sphero-echinocytes.

POTENTIAL LOOK-ALIKES
acanthocyte (spur cell)
non-specific poikilocytes found in iron deficiency

ASSOCIATED DISEASE STATES AND CONDITIONS
most common cause is an artifact of improperly prepared smears (slow drying, thick smears, aged blood) or "glass effect" (diffusion of basic substances from glass slide causing an elevated pH in the medium surrounding the cell)
rare causes include:
    uremia and chronic renal disease
    low potassium containing red blood cells
    bleeding peptic ulcer
    pyruvate kinase deficiency
    liver disease
    vitamin E deficiency
    hyperlipidemia
    myeloproliferative disorders
    heparin therapy
    immediately post-transfusion with aged or metabolically depleted blood

Echinocytes are spiculated red cells with 10 to 30 short, evenly spaced projections over the entire surface. They are usually the same size or slightly smaller than normal red cells. Unlike acanthocytes, the cells retain their central pallor. They are usually found in the center of a smear; increased surface tension at the extreme feather edge will flatten the cells and round off the projections.

The stages of echinocyte formation have been well documented, with the surface projections occurring first and the shape change next. Echinocytes are not the result of any inherited membrane abnormality. Several artifactual or physiologic environmental changes induce the transformation: increased pH, decreased albumin concentration, exposure to an anionic phenothiazine derivative, or the presence of lysolecithin. In each case, bumps form on the surface of the red cell. In some instances, the projections are due to preferential expansion of the outer leaflet of the plasma membrane lipid bilayer compared to the inner layer. The process is entirely reversible. If the environmental stresses become too severe or prolonged, the echinocyte irreversibly transforms into a sphero-echinocyte. Echinocytes may also become spherocytes as the spleen removes the projections.

Echinocytes are most commonly an artifact—the result of improperly prepared smears or the pH of the glass slide. In the occasional instance when the shape is not an artifact, echinoyctes are most commonly associated with severe renal disease (uremia). Burn patients may also on occasion show echinocytes. It is believed to relate to depletion of intracellular ATP or surface lipid accumulation.

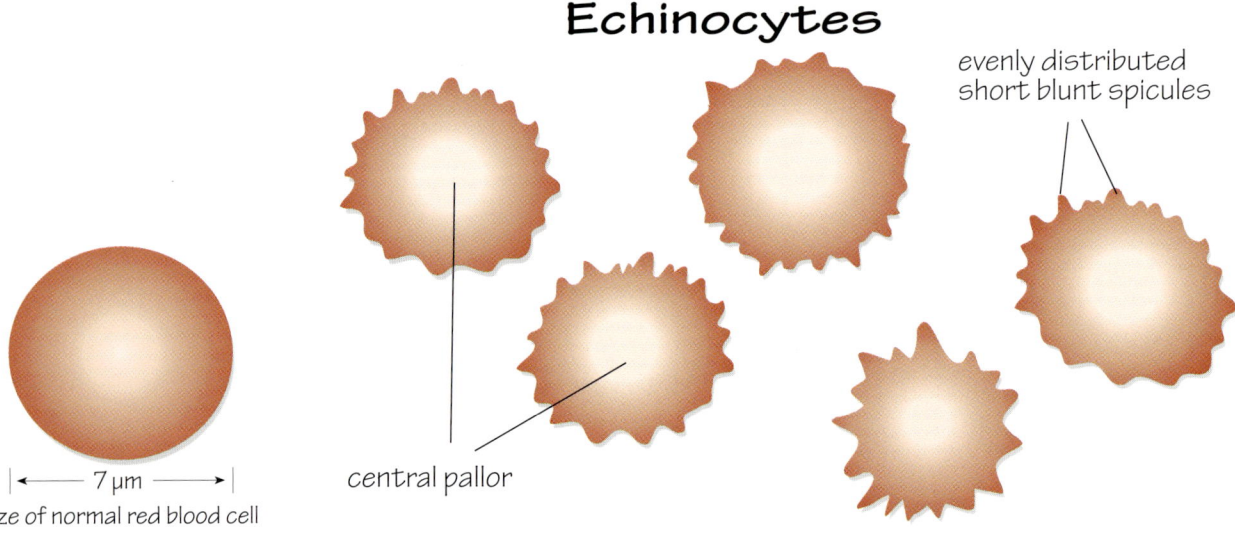

Echinocytes — evenly distributed short blunt spicules — central pallor — 7 μm size of normal red blood cell

H1-29, 1985 (Blood, Wright-Giemsa, X400)

Identification	Referee %	Participant %
Echinocyte	94.2	97.1
Spherocyte	5.9	-

The patient is a 66-year-old alcoholic with chronic pancreatitis, biliary tract obstruction and *E. coli* sepsis. WBC is 36.5 x 10^9/L; hemoglobin 14.7g/dL; hematocrit 41.8% and platelet count of 161,000 x 10^6/L. The red cell indices are normal. There are many echinocytes in this field. Note the uniformity of the short, blunt spicule projections. The cells all have central pallor, which helps to distinguish them from acanthocytes.

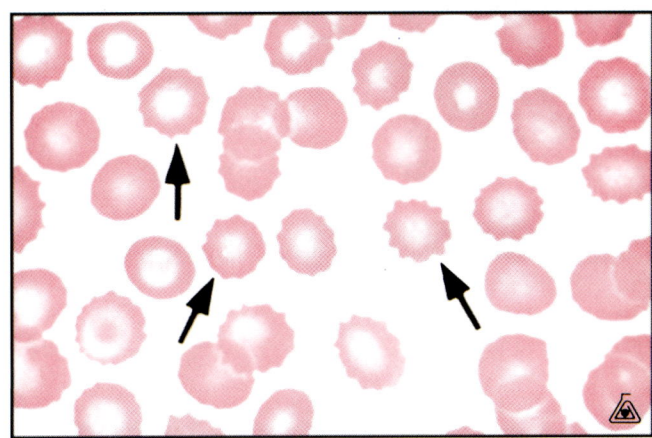

H1-34, 1985 (Blood, Wright-Giemsa, X400)

Identification	Referee %	Participant %
Echinocyte	94.1	96.5
Spherocyte	5.9	-

The patient is the same as the one above. Again, numerous echinocytes are depicted. The two arrowed cells have good central pallor. The numerous small surface membrane projections are very evenly distributed. Acanthocytes have fewer projections and lack central palor. The projections are usually much more irregular.

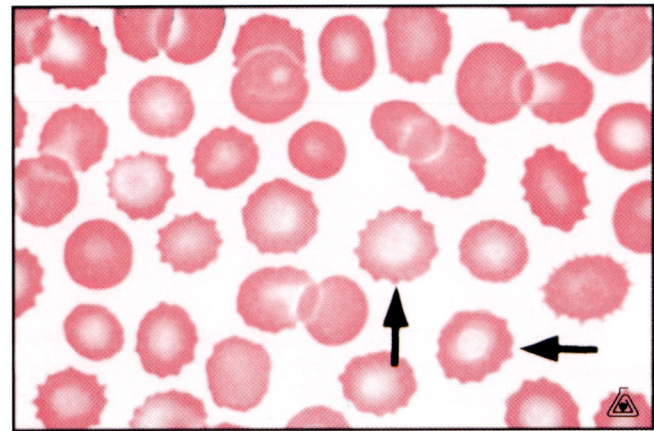

Erythrocytic Cells and Inclusions

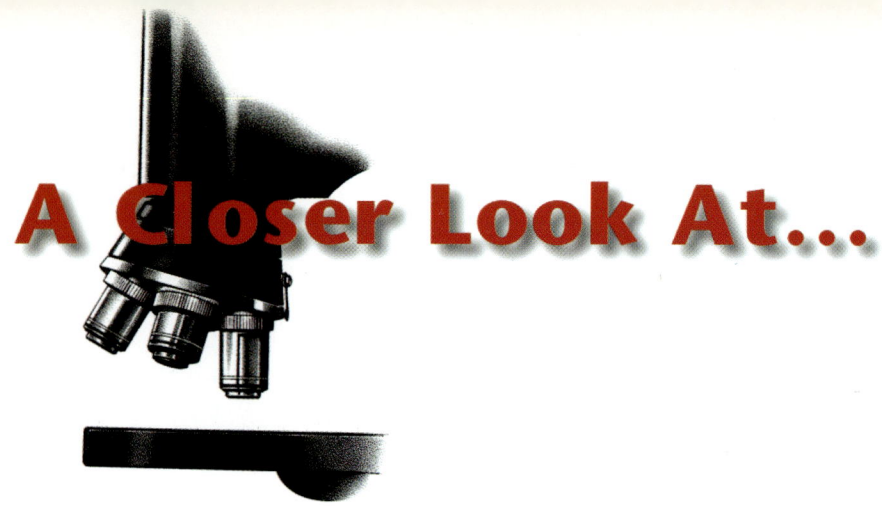

A Closer Look At...

Spiculated Red Cells

A spiculated red cell is a subset of the larger group of poikilocytes, or erythrocytes of abnormal shape. All of these forms have in common at least one pointed projection from the cell, and they all indicate a significant pathologic process (the only exception to the latter point is that echinocytes may be formed as an artifact of smear preparation). For a more detailed discussion of each abnormal form, please refer to the Table of Contents for their individual entries. It is important to also recognize that these pathologic processes are not confined to the hematopoietic system but are indications of disturbances in metabolism (abetalipoproteinemia, vitamin E deficiency, fat malabsorption) or function (myexedema, bleeding ulcer, burns), or may be associated with malignancy (gastric carcinoma, myeloproliferative disorders) or therapeutic interventions (heprin therapy, artificial heart valves).

As may be seen from the diagram on the opposite page, the formation of these abnormal erythrocytes is often related to a physical barrier which they must cross: the spleen, bone marrow, a partial (fibrin) barrier in a blood vessel, or an artificial heart valve. There are also intrinsic causes. When the red cell is inherently abnormal, as in sickle cell anemia (HbSS) for example, the sickled form of a red cell occurs under physiologic conditions which are not unduly stressful to normal erythrocytes. Thus spiculated red cells are an important finding when evaluating a blood smear.

Spiculated Red Cells

Cell Name (Synonyms)	Description	Associated Conditions
Acanthocyte Spur Cell	spheroidal cells with 2-20 spicules of varying length irregularly distributed over surface; no central pallor	abetalipoproteinemia parenchymal liver disease absent spleen starvation fat malabsorption myeloproliferative disorders myxedema panhypopituitarism retinitis pigmentosa rare neuromuscular disorders McLeod and In(Lu) phenotypes
Echinocyte Burr Cell	10-30 short, evenly spaced spicules; central pallor	artifact uremia gastric carcinoma bleeding ulcer liver disease pyruvate kinase deficiency vitamin E deficiency heparin therapy myeloproliferative disorders
Teardrop Cell Dacryocyte	single spicule forming a tear-drop shape	myelofibrosis myelophthisic anemia thalassemias
Sickle Cell Drepanocyte	sickle-shaped, pointed at both ends; dense cytoplasm	sickle cell disorders
Helmet Cell	large notch; may have projections at either end; if projections are long enough, the cell is designated a keratocyte (horn cell)	microangiopathic hemolytic anemia (DIC, TTP) heart-valve hemolysis severe burns Heinz body hemolytic anemia glomerulonephritis cavernous hemangiomas
Horn Cell Keratocyte	one or more notches with projections at either end	same as helmet cell
Schistocyte Fragmented Cell	fragmented cell with two or more points; no central pallor; helmet cell, horn cell and triangulocyte are specific examples	same as helmet cell

Erythrocytic Cells and Inclusions

Fragmented Cell (Schistocyte, Helmet Cell, Keratocyte)

SYNONYMS
schistocyte, helmet cell, triangulocyte, keratocyte, horn cell

VITAL STATISTICS
- size .... varies, usually microcytic
- cell shape .... varies from helmet to triangle to unclassifiable fragment
- cytoplasm .... smaller fragments lack central pallor; horn cells are normochromic

KEY DIFFERENTIATING FEATURES
irregularity of cell size and shape, with some shapes quite distinctive
small fragments lack any significant central pallor

POTENTIAL LOOK-ALIKES
bite cell
blister cell
sickle cells
non-specific poikilocytes associated with iron deficiency

ASSOCIATED DISEASE STATES AND CONDITIONS
microangiopathic anemia
severe burns
disseminated intravascular coagulation (DIC)
thrombotic thrombocytopenic purpura (TTP)
uremia
malignant hypertension
hemolytic uremic syndrome (HUS)

When an erythrocyte is distorted in shape, or partially disrupted, but not in a characteristically recognizable fashion, it is known by the general term *poikiloyte*. Poikilocytes may exhibit specific shape changes that are indicative of microangiopathic damage and in this case, the term *fragmented cell* can be used.

Fragmented red cells include *helmet cells*, *keratocytes* (horn cells), *trianglulocytes*, and a more all inclusive term, *schistocytes*. All these variants—except for keratocytes—share common features of irregular cell shape and lack of central pallor. Keratocytes have central pallor but helmet cells and the smaller red cell fragments typically do not. Small irregular cells with central pallor may well be due to microangiopathic hemolytic causes (when examined in context with other classic cell types), but they are not specific and can also be found in iron deficiency. They are best designated *non-specific poikilocytes*.

To conceptualize how fragmentation might occur, imagine a small blood vessel with interlacing fibrin strands across the lumen. As erythrocytes pass, they are randomly draped over/around such strands. The pressure of the flowing blood moves the cell forward, but it is haphazardly torn by the fibrin. The cells seal their torn edges and continue in the circulation. Eventually, of course, they are sequested in the spleen. Burn victims develop hemolytic anemia with fragmented cells; the latter are believed to occur as a result of spectrin denaturation by the heat. (See *A Closer Look At…Microangiopathic Anemias*, page 82).

Thus, the presence of fragmented cells indicates a significant pathologic process. They do not occur alone, but are a valuable adjunct in assessing the severity of the disease in which they occur.

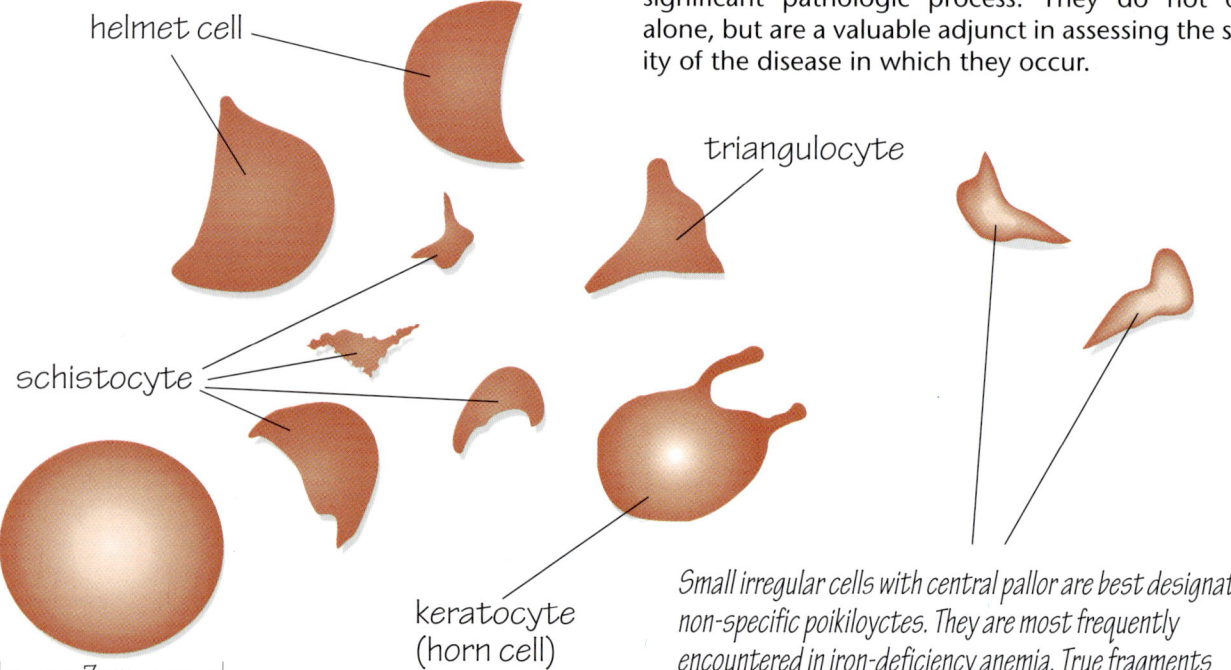

Fragmented Red Cells

Small irregular cells with central pallor are best designated non-specific poikiloyctes. They are most frequently encountered in iron-deficiency anemia. True fragments (schistocytes) lack any significant central pallor.

Erythrocytic Cells and Inclusions

HE-08, 1992 (Blood, Wright-Giemsa, X325)

Identification	Referee %	Participant %
Fragmented cell	100	97.7
Acanthocyte	-	1.1
Sickle cell	-	0.2

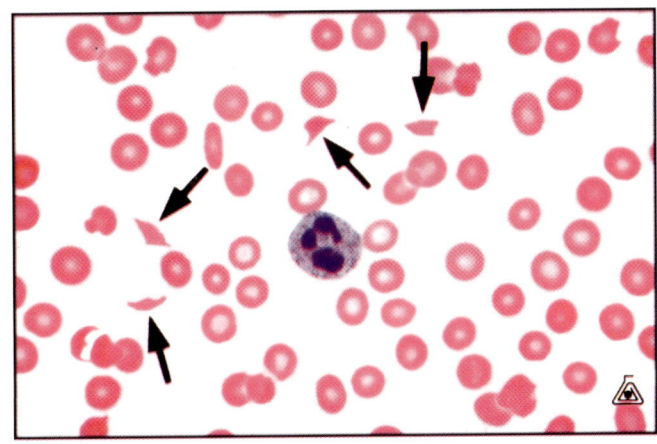

The arrowed cells demonstrate some of the shapes which schistocytes may take. Notice the lack of central pallor, which distinguishes these cells from the non-specific poikilocytes found in iron deficiency. The apparent decrease in erythrocytes is consistent with anemia and the lack of platelets with thrombocytopenia. This sample is from a child with hemolytic-uremic syndrome (HUS) in which a microangiopathic anemia is characteristic. Some speculate that HUS is the childhood counterpart of thrombotic thrombocytopenic purpura (TTP); however, TTP has neurologic manifestations and a more serious prognosis than HUS. The blood findings are similar in each disorder.

XL-25, 1986 (Blood, Wright-Giemsa, X375)

Identification	Referee %	Participant %
Fragmented cell	94.7	87.5
Acanthocyte	5.3	6

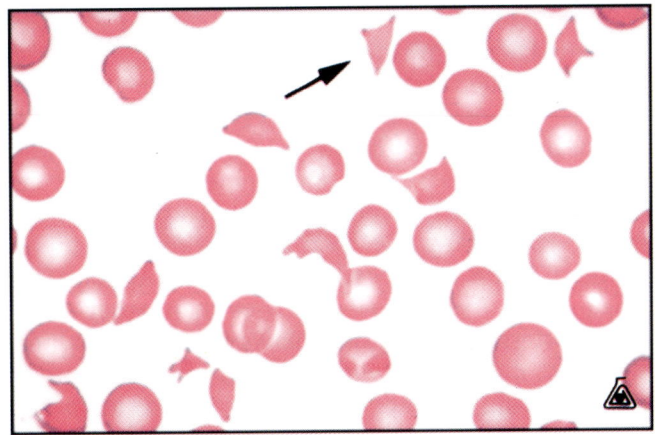

Although many fragmented cells are present they all vary in detail enough so that no specific name may be given to them. The arrowed cell most closely resembles a triangulocyte. An anemia is expected because of the decreased number of erythrocytes in this field. This is an example of microangiopathic hemolytic anemia. The non-fragmented erythrocytes are essentially normal.

HE-40, 1995 (Blood, Wright-Giemsa, X400)

Identification	Referee %	Participant %
Fragmented cell	100	98.3

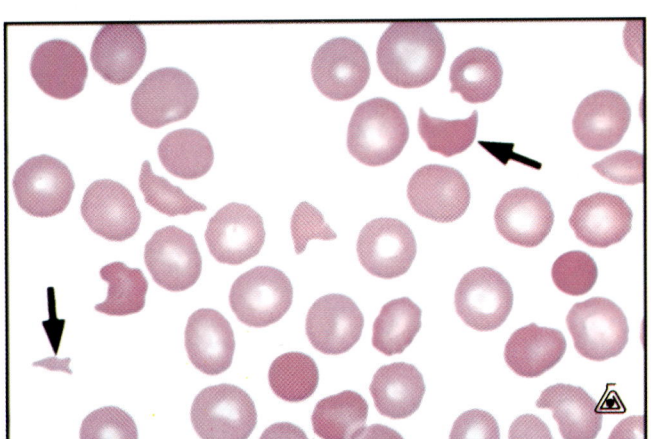

The two arrowed cells are fragmented cells. The presence of two spherocytes in the lower portion of the field and the apparent decrease in red cells lead one to suspect a microangiopathic anemia. This is a sample of blood from a 48-year-old female with anemia (Hgb 9.2 g/dL), thrombocytopenia (55 x 10^9/L) and leukocytosis (WBC 16.3 x 10^9/L). She complained of bloody diarrhea and abdominal pain; the ultimate diagnosis was thrombotic throbocytopenic purpura (TTP). Traditionally, a pentad of symptoms is present and makes the diagnosis of this syndrome: renal disease, fever, neurologic symptoms, thrombocytopenia, and microangiopathic hemolytic anemia. It is considered more a disorder of adults than children. Once associated with an 80% mortality rate, aggressive treatment with steriods and plasma exchange has greatly brightened the outlook for these patients. The etiology is believed to relate to endothelial cell damage from various causes and greatly increased platelet clumping.

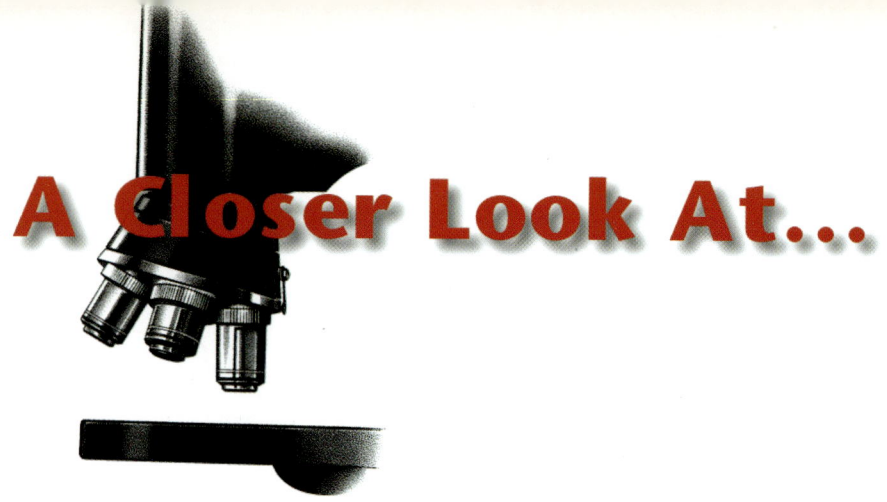

A Closer Look At...

Microangiopathic Anemias

As the name implies, the pathology causing this type of anemia occurs in blood vessels. The small vessels become the site of erythrocyte fragmentation when strands of fibrin begin to form a net, at least partially blocking the lumen. The fibrin originates from various pathologic states such as disseminated intravascular coagulation (DIC), severe burns, snake bites, septicemia, certain drugs, or thrombotic thrombocytpenic purpura (TTP); other causes exist. Even though the small vessels have a lower pressure than larger arterioles or arteries, the blood still flows with sufficient force such that the erythrocytes are damaged. They are (at least partially) caught on the fibrin strands in various ways and this results in different types of fragmented cells being formed (see diagram, opposite page). The fragmented cells include helmet cells, pre-karatocytes and keratocytes (horn cells) as well as irregular fragments without further definition (schistocytes). Spherocytes are also invariably formed. The spleen is instrumental in removing these fragmented cells.

However, some cells may lyse, releasing their hemoglobin within the vessel. If this occurs, then serum haptoglobin (a hemoglobin-binding protein) will decrease and eventually, when the haptoglobin is completely bound by the hemoglobin, free hemoglobin will be measurable in the plasma. Most patients will also demonstrate abnormalities in coagulation parameters, such as prolonged PT, PTT, and the presence of fibrin degradation products (FDP).

Similar morphologic variants are formed in large vessel diseases such as those of the heart and aorta. Though anemia resulting from lesions in these organs might more properly be termed *macro*angiopathic hemolytic anemia, the term microangiopathic anemia continues to be used in all settings, i.e., in both small and large vessel disease. A better, all inclusive designation would be *fragmentation anemias*. In an anemic patient, the morphologic hallmarks of a microangiopathic process are fragmented erythrocytes and spherocytes.

How Fragmented Cells Form

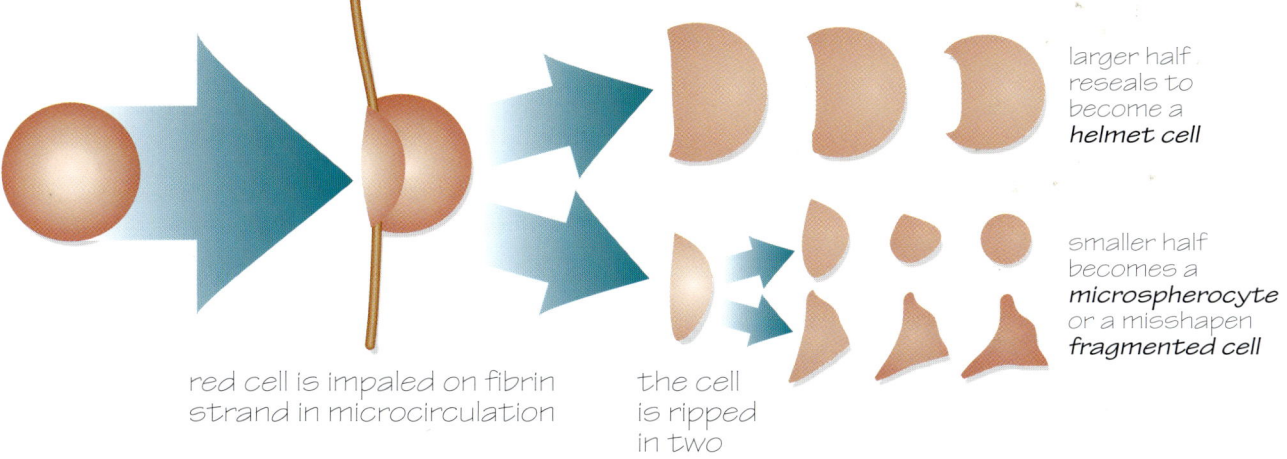

How Prekeratocytes Form

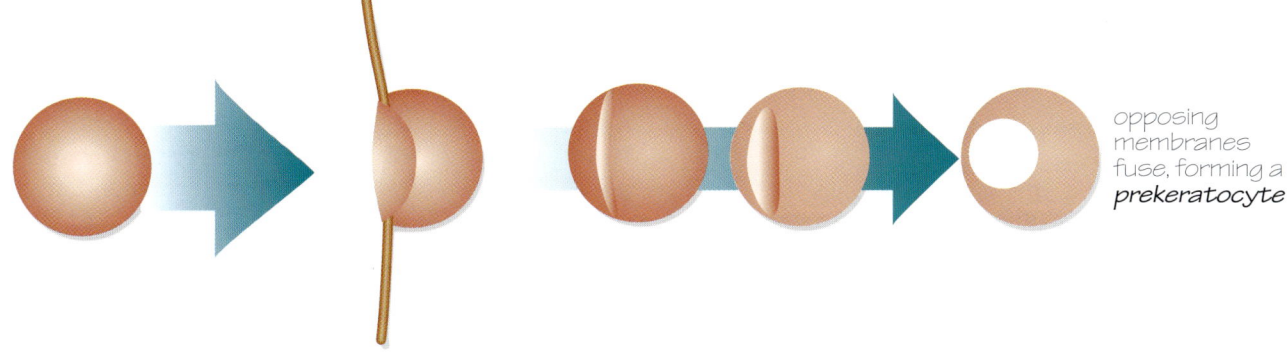

How Keratocytes Form

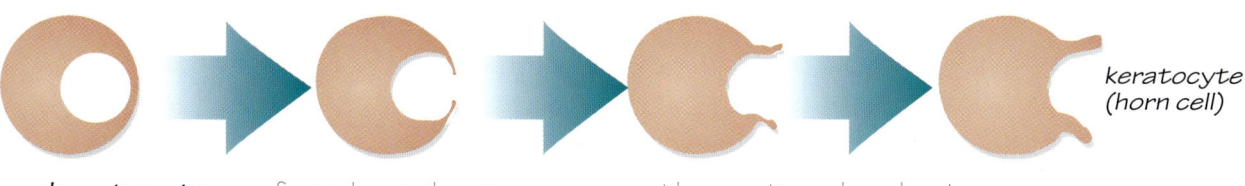

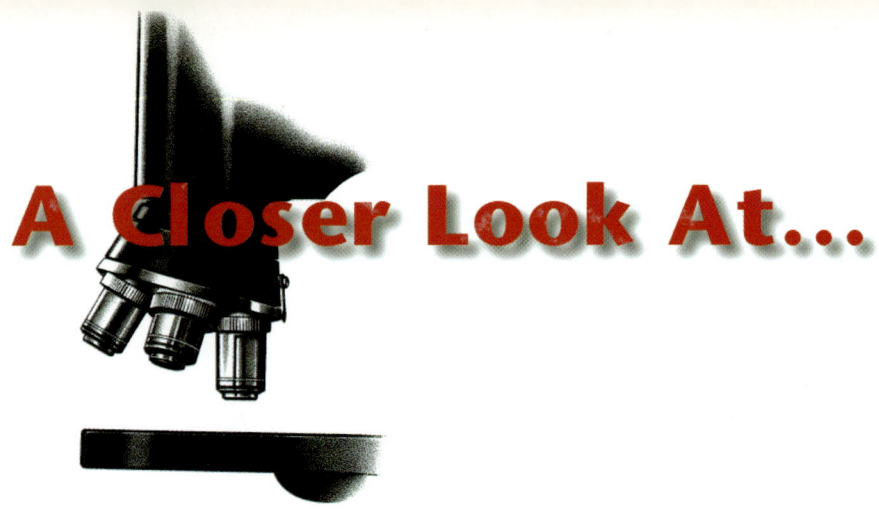

A Closer Look At...

Diagnostic Morphology in MAHA and Heinz Body Anemia

When considering the cause of a schistocyte in the blood, it is important to recall the pathophysiologic mechanism(s) behind its formation. The illustrations here (opposite page) divide schistocytes into three categories: microangiopathic hemolytic anemia (MAHA), Heinz body anemia, and a third category with cell shapes that could be present in either of the first two categories.

Microangiopathic hemolytic anemia has many causes (see entry for *Fragmented Cell*, page 80) but each cause has in common its effect on disrupted erythrocyte morphology because the small blood vessels are at least partially obscured by fibrin strands. Thus, there is an apparently haphazard "shearing" effect of the erythrocytes with the result being an unpredictable pattern of fragmentation. Spherocytes are usually found as well.

Heinz body anemia, in contrast, has a limited number of causes, and a narrower range of morphologic abnormalities (*Heinz Body*, page 124). The spleen removes the abnormality, precipitated hemoglobin, leaving a permanent defect in the cell (the "bite"). Depending on the number of Heinz bodies within the erythrocyte and on the functional state of the spleen, these bites leave a spectrum of misshapen red cells.

As the diagram on the right points out, certain morphologic changes are diagnostic of either MAHA or Heinz body anemia. Triangulocytes, small shistocytes lacking central pallor, pre-keratocytes, and keratocytes are all indicative of microangiopathic disease. Bite cells with small nibbles and slightly larger defects as well as double bite cells and apple core cells point conclusively to the presence of Heinz bodies. Ambiguous cells share morphology between these two distinctive groups. Helmet cells and keratocytes with short horns may resemble a bite cell with a very large defect.

Ambiguous cells need to be evaluated in the context of other cells. It is thus imperative to search the blood smear for as many morphologic findings as possible, so that the correct diagnosis may be made. Additional serum and blood tests may at times be required, however, before the diagnosis is made.

Comparison of Red Cell Morphology in Microangiopathic Hemolytic Anemia and Heinz Body Anemia

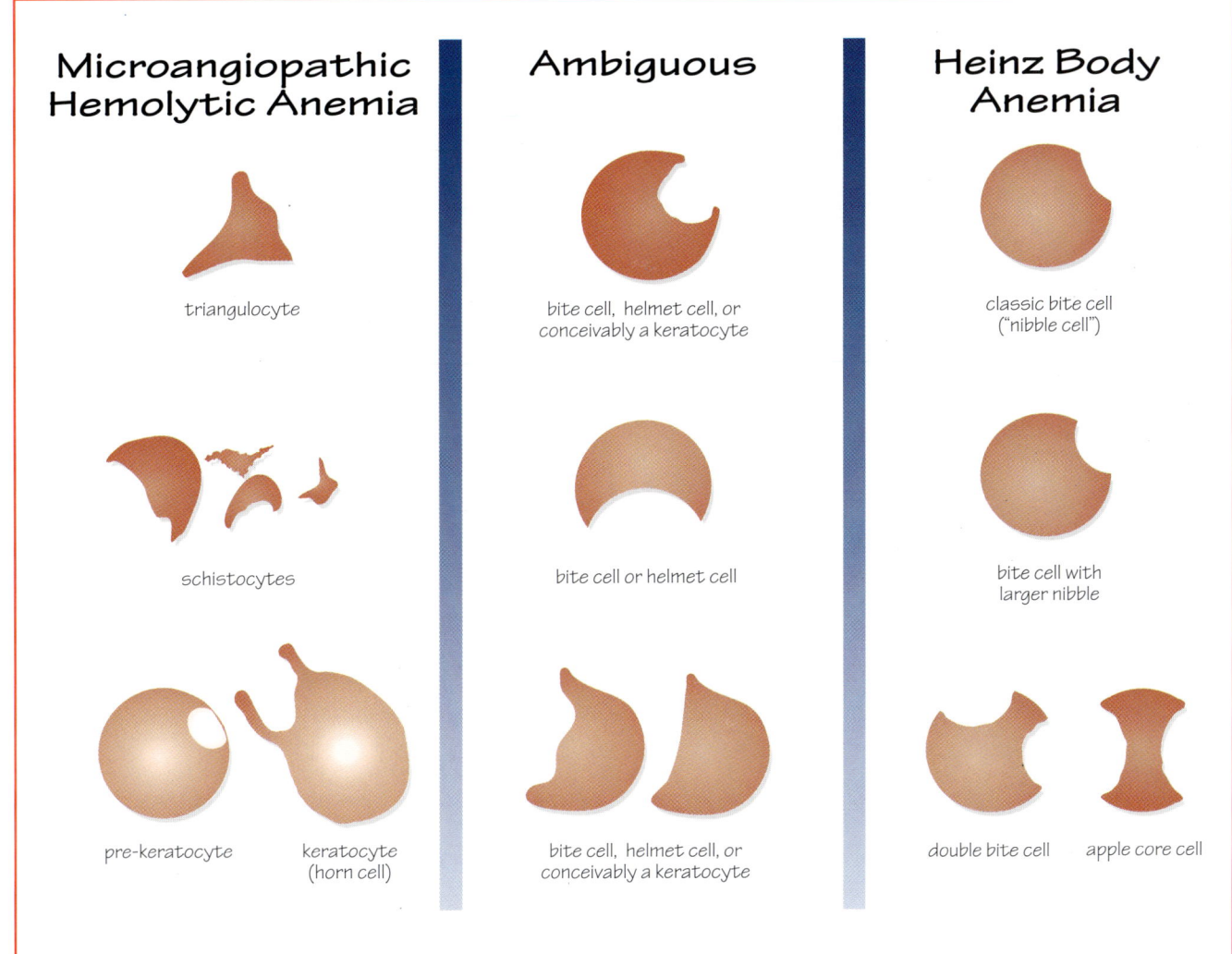

Macrocyte (Oval or Round)

SYNONYMS
macrocytic red cell; macro-ovalocyte (oval form)

VITAL STATISTICS
size .... greater than 8 μm diameter; MCV > 95-100 fL
cell shape .... oval or round
cytoplasm .... normochromic, but may sometimes be hypochromic; no polychromasia

KEY DIFFERENTIATING FEATURES
larger than normal red blood cell
round or oval shape; oval forms have sides that are not parallel to each other (unlike ovalocytes which are more rod-shaped and have hemoglobin concentrated at the ends of the cell)
normal hemoglobinization; no polychromasia

POTENTIAL LOOK-ALIKES
polychromatophilic red cells
giant hypogranular platelet
elliptocyte (ovalocyte)

ASSOCIATED DISEASE STATES AND CONDITIONS
oval macrocytes predominate in:
    vitamin B_{12} and folate deficiencies
    alcoholism
    aplastic anemia
    preleukemia and hematologic malignancies
    scurvy
    vitamin E deficiency
    chemotherapy
    chronic infection (TB, chronic pyelonephritis, etc.)
    Kwashiorkor
    inherited abnormalities of DNA synthesis
round macrocytes predominate in:
    post-splenectomy states
    liver disease
    conditions associated with reticulocytosis, such as response to hemorrhage, hemolytic anemias, and erythroblastosis fetalis (Rh incompatibility)
    hyperthyroidism and hypothyroidism (myxedema)
    hypopituitarism
    malaria
    neonatal macrocytosis

To earn the name of macrocyte, a red cell must be large—at least 8 μm in diameter on a blood smear or greater than 100 fL using an electronic counter. A macrocyte may be either oval or round, depending on why it has been produced. The hemoglobin concentration in macrocytes is normal but may be reduced if complications of the primary abnormality occur.

Round and oval macrocytes should be differentiated from polychromatophilic red cells (page 94). Polychromatophilic erythrocytes may be larger than normal red blood cells but they represent reticulocytes and not mature erythrocytes. As such, they have increased RNA giving the cytoplasm a gray-blue hue. Macrocytes lack significant amounts of polychromasia.

Ovalocytes (elliptocytes) may be mistaken for oval macrocytes. Elliptocytes are often longer than normal erythrocytes but they are significantly more narrow. The sides of the cells are nearly parallel, unlike the much more curved edges of oval macrocytes. Oval macrocytes are also much larger than ovalocytes.

The vital statistics listing to the left enumerates conditions in which either oval or round macrocytes predominate. Oval macrocytes are more clinically worrisome. They are most commonly associated with B_{12} or folic acid deficiency. Dietary deficiency, increased physiologic demand, or increased loss by malabsorption are the usual causes of deficits. Lack of either factor affects DNA synthesis in rapidly dividing cells with effects present in epithelia throughout the body as well as in blood cells. Megaloblastic anemia due to vitamin B_{12} lack or malabsorption may be more difficult to diagnose. When gastrointestinal abnormalities are present, the disease is called pernicious anemia. The cause is autoimmune in nature.

Abnormal red cell maturation (dyserythropoiesis) may also cause oval macrocytosis. Examples include chronic infection, hematologic malignancies, and aplastic anemia.

Round macrocytes are frequently associated with reticulocytosis, liver disease, hypothyroidism, and post-splenectomy states. Liver disease causes macrocytosis by addition of membrane lipids to the red cell.

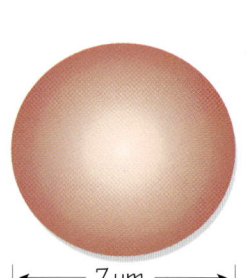

|← 7μm →|
size of normal red blood cell

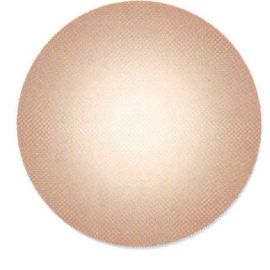

Round Macrocyte

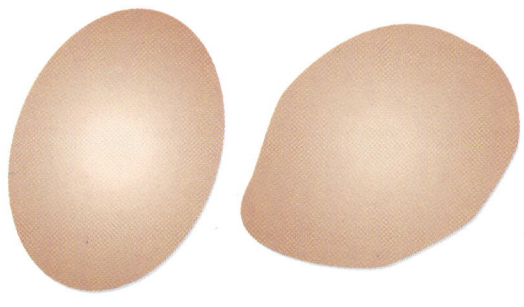

Oval Macrocytes

H1-43, 1989 (Blood, Wright-Giemsa, X400)

Identification	Referee %	Participant %
Macrocyte, round or oval	100	98.2

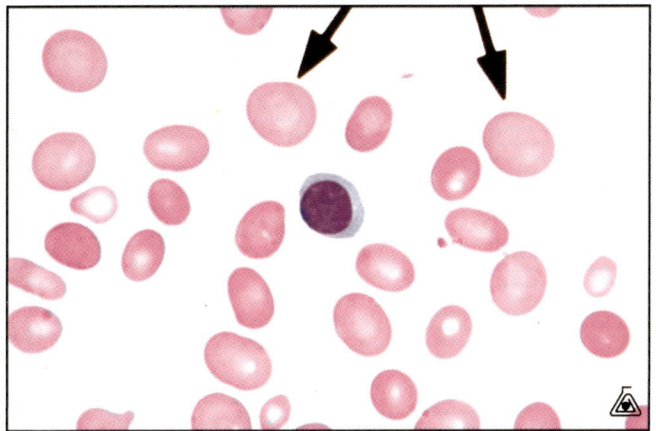

Each arrow points to a similar appearing erythrocyte, namely one that is large and oval. In this patient with full-blown pernicious anemia and a very low serum vitamin B_{12} level (<100 pg/mL) oval macrocytes would be expected. However, the difference between round and oval may be somewhat subjective. The small lymphocyte in the center of the field may be used to judge the size of the erythrocytes and indicates how very large some of these erythrocytes are. The presence of occasional small erythrocytes is also part of this disorder.

HE-09, 1995 (Blood, Wright-Giemsa, X400)

Identification	Referee %	Participant %
Macrocyte, round or oval	96.4	94
Ovalocyte	3.6	5

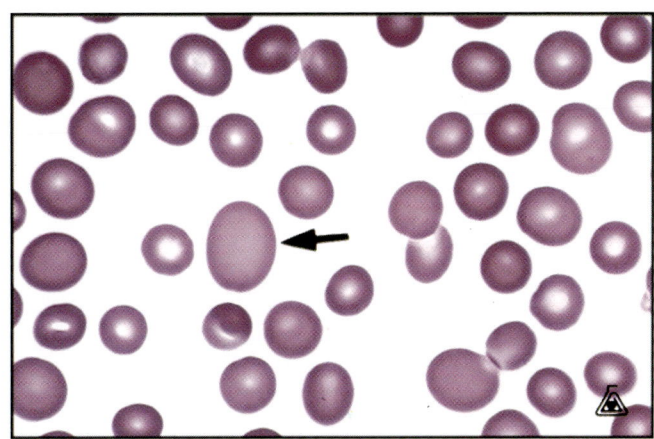

The very large erythrocyte indicated by the arrow is accurately termed a macrocyte. It is larger than the surrounding normal red cells and lacks polychromasia. The cell is not an ovalocyte (elliptocyte) which typically is more rod-shaped. The sides are nearly parallel and the cells have a much greater longitudinal axis length than transverse length. This photomicrograph reflects the reason why the MCV was 95 fL, since it is an average value for the anioscytosis shown here. This sample is from a 40-year-old female diagnosed with acute myeloblastic leukemia. Macrocytes in this condition may be considered stress erythrocytes.

HE-26, 1996 (Blood, Wright-Giemsa, X400)

Identification	Referee %	Participant %
Macrocyte, round or oval	100	99

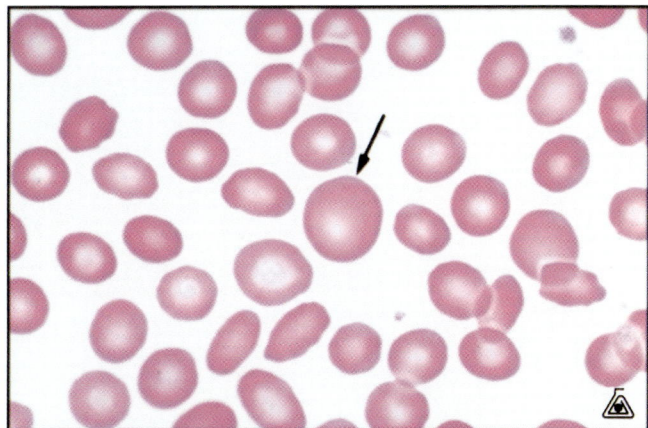

The arrowed cell is a macrocyte, even though there is no nucleated cell for comparison. However, the MCV is 101 fL, thus confirming the morphologic impression. The cell lacks any polychromasia; the hemoglobin staining is identical to the surrounding normal red blood cells. Since this sample is from a 47-year-old female scheduled for elective surgery, the significance of this isolated abnormality (other CBC parameters were described as normal) may have different causes, probably none of which is serious.

Microcyte (with Central Pallor)

SYNONYMS
microcytic red cell

VITAL STATISTICS
size .... < 6 µm; MCV < 80 fL
cytoplasm .... hypochromic, with central pallor greater than 1/3 of cell diameter

KEY DIFFERENTIATING FEATURES
small size
hypochromia (increased central pallor)
some cells contain so little hemoglobin that they are "ghost cells"

POTENTIAL LOOK-ALIKES
normal erythrocyte
echinocyte
micro-spherocyte

ASSOCIATED DISEASE STATES AND CONDITIONS
iron deficiency
thalassemia
lead poisoning

Microcytes are small erythrocytes measuring less than 6 µm in diameter or less than 80 fL when measured using electronic devices. For CAP proficiency testing purposes, the term "microcyte with central pallor" is used to designate cells that are hypochromic. They should be distinguished from micro-spherocytes, which have little or no central pallor (see page 100). Each is seen in very different clinical settings.

Usually, microcytes occur when there is a disturbance in the production of hemoglobin. Worldwide, iron deficiency is probably the most common cause. Thalassemias are also very common in certain parts of the world and are another common cause of microcytic anemia. By whatever mechanism, the production of a microcyte is the body's attempt to conserve oxygen-carrying capacity within the physical constraints of the circulatory system. It attempts to produce cells which can negotiate their way through the spleen and capillaries while still delivering as close to a normal amount of oxygen to tissues as possible.

Iron deficiency anemia is commonly caused by an inadequate dietary intake, remembering also that there is a fixed daily loss of iron normally; as well there are certain physiologic states (pregnancy, childhood growth) in which an increased demand for iron is normal. When blood is lost, either acutely or on a chronic basis, iron deficiency may result, unless replaced.

The inherited abnormality of hemoglobin synthesis which is generically termed thalassemia may not always produce a microcytic anemia. Usually alpha thalassemia minor and hemoglobin H disease are the major types associated with microcytic anemia or microcytosis, without other red cell changes.

Hypochromic Microcytes

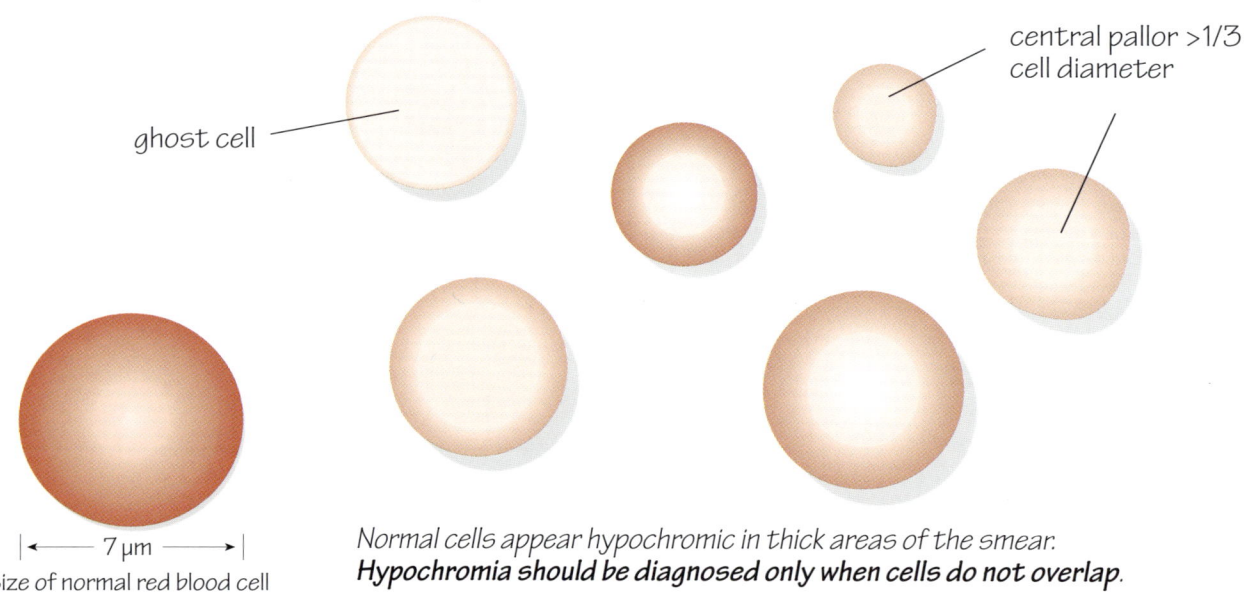

ghost cell

central pallor >1/3 cell diameter

|← 7µm →|
size of normal red blood cell

Normal cells appear hypochromic in thick areas of the smear.
Hypochromia should be diagnosed only when cells do not overlap.

Erythrocytic Cells and Inclusions

H1-46 1983 (Blood, Wright-Giemsa, X325)

Identification	Referee %	Participant %
Microcyte (with central pallor)	94.4	89.4
Erythrocyte, normal	5.6	2.2

Using the adjacent normal lymphocytes as a guide, the arrowed cell is clearly defined as a microcyte. The cell size is less than the diameter of the lymphocyte nucleus. The microcyte is hypochromic; central pallor is greater than 1/3 the diameter of the cell. The decreased number of red cells in this field indicates anemia, assuming that this is a representative field and not artifact. In this patient, who had been partially treated for malaria due to *Plasmodium vivax*, retreatment produced prompt hematologic normalization.

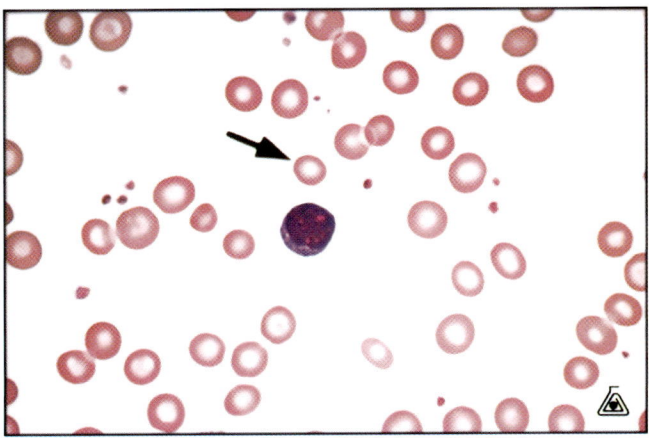

XL-63, 1986 (Blood, Wright-Giemsa, X400)

Identification	Referee %	Participant %
Microcyte (with central pallor)	100	69.9
Ovalocyte (elliptocyte)	-	24.9

The red cells in this field appear to be small. The arrowed cell is also obviously hypochromic. The presence of target cells, most notably in the upper right corner, raises the possibility of thalassemia. The Hgb was 11.9 g/dL, MCV 89 fL and MCH 30.5; no diagnosis for this patient was given, however. Although the arrowed cell is not perfectly round, the designation as elliptocyte by 24.9% of participants is disappointing because the more important finding of microcyte was missed.

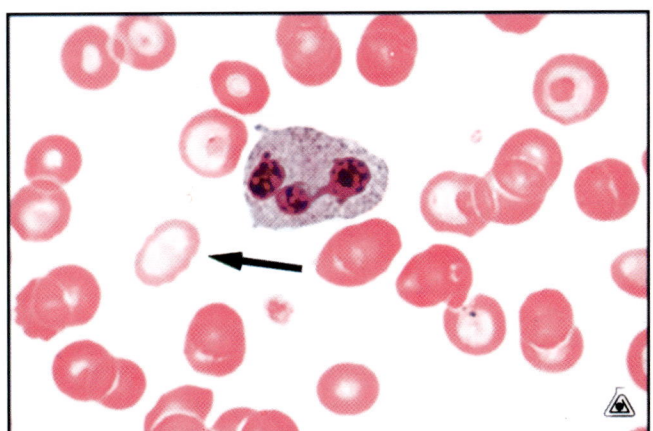

XL-44, 1985 (Blood, Wright-Giemsa, X400)

Identification	Referee %	Participant %
Microcyte (with central pallor)	100	94.6

The red cells in the field show a range of sizes. The arrowed red cell is definitely hypochromic and, like many other cells present, appears microcytic. This 75-year-old man was anemic (Hgb 10.5 g/dL) and had episodes of bronchopneumonia and urinary tract infection. It is easy to envision the development of an iron deficiency anemia in such a clinical setting: the small amounts of bleeding that may occur with lower urinary tract infection and bronchopneumonia coupled with poor diet when feeling ill add up to eventually produce anemia. The possibility of blood loss from other sources, especially an undetected malignancy, should also be kept in mind.

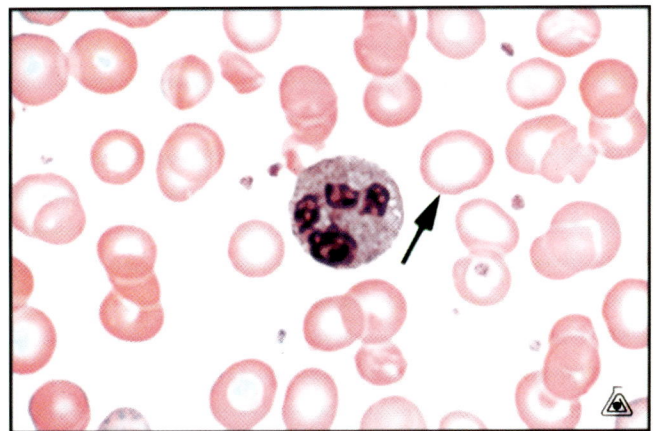

Ovalocyte (Elliptocyte)

SYNONYMS
elliptocyte, pencil form

VITAL STATISTICS
size .... variable; usually longer than normal red cell and much more narrow
cell shape .... elongate with round ends (pencil, cigar, egg shape)
cytoplasm .... normochromic; decreased to normal central pallor

KEY DIFFERENTIATING FEATURES
uniform, symmetrical rod shape; sides nearly parallel
polarization of hemoglobination, with preservation of central pallor

OTHER FINDINGS
some forms are more blunted and oval; there are stomatocytic and spherocytic variants of hereditary elliptocytosis (see A Closer Look At... page 92)
hemolytic/anemic subtypes have associated microelliptocytes, comma-shaped, and teardrop forms)
ovalocytes in excess of 10% suggest hereditary ovalocytosis (>25% is diagnostic)

POTENTIAL LOOK-ALIKES
teardrop cells
oval macrocyte

ASSOCIATED DISEASE STATES AND CONDITIONS
hereditary elliptocytosis (common, spherocytic, and stomatocytic subtypes)
megaloblastic anemia
myelophthisic anemia
thalassemia
congenital dyserythropoietic anemia
sideroblastic anemia
severe iron deficiency anemia
sickle cell anemia

Classic elliptocytes have a rod shape and nearly parallel sides. Hemoglobin is concentrated at the ends (so called "dumbbell distribution"). Other subtypes have more blunted ends or may be more oval. Some elliptocytes may superficially resemble oval macrocytes but they are never as large and they tend to be less oval.

Blood films from normal individuals may contain a rare ovalocyte (<1%). There are many diseases in which ovalocytes may be a component. Each disorder has its own characteristic set of findings, in addition to the presence of ovalocytes. Why or how ovalocytes occur is not precisely known in each instance, but may be theorized based on mechanism of disease, and its consequences.

The entity of *heredity ovalocytosis* (hereditary elliptocytosis) is well described and is due to an abnormality of erythrocyte skeletal membrane proteins. (See the following *A Closer Look At...* discussion on page 92). The disease may be broadly considered in the same category as hereditary spherocytosis. In constrast, however, poikilocytes are more often detected in hereditary ovalocytosis. It has been determined that more than 25% of red cells are ovalocytes in this disorder. There is speculation that hereditary ovalocytosis may be somewhat beneficial in that such cells are resistant to malarial infestation.

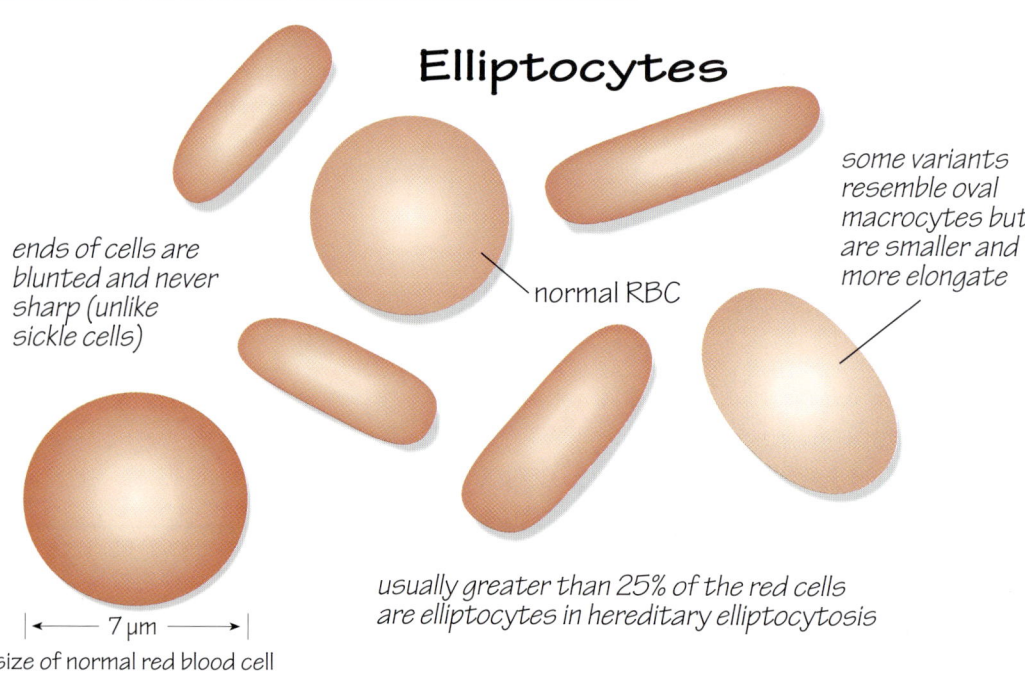

Elliptocytes

ends of cells are blunted and never sharp (unlike sickle cells)

normal RBC

some variants resemble oval macrocytes but are smaller and more elongate

|← 7 µm →|
size of normal red blood cell

usually greater than 25% of the red cells are elliptocytes in hereditary elliptocytosis

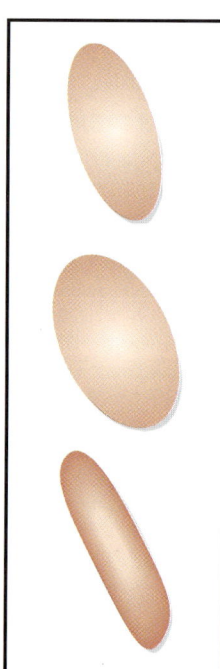

Elliptocyte Variants

XL-26, 1985 (Blood, Wright-Giemsa, X400)

Identification	Referee %	Participant %
Ovalocyte (elliptocyte)	100	97.9

The near unanimity reached by both referees and participants indicates the correct identification of ovalocyte. The sample is from a 24-year-old female with a hemoglobin of 14 g/dL and no known history of hereditary ovalocytosis. The arrowed cells well demonstrate the elongate, slim form of an ovalocyte with an area of central pallor also. Numerous other ovalocytes are present throughout the field.

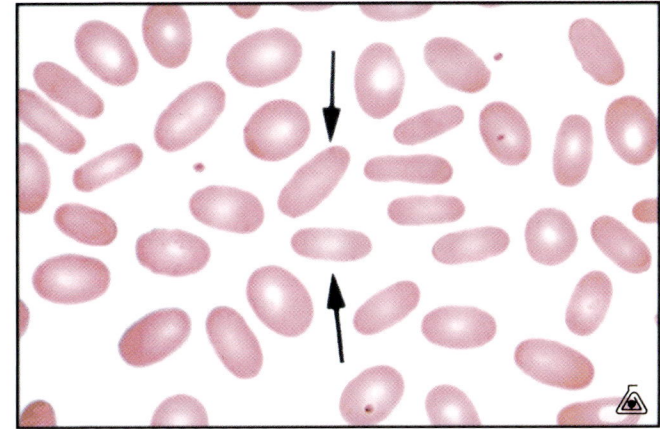

HE-9, 1996 (Blood, Wright-Giemsa, X400)

Identification	Referee %	Participant %
Ovalocyte (elliptocyte)	100	99.4

This blood film is from a patient with beta thalassemia trait. The arrowed red cell is an ovalocyte. In contrast to the other erythrocytes in this field, it is uniformly elongated with a smooth surface and small area of central pallor. The edges of the cell are nearly parallel and the ends are blunt. The occurrence of ovalocytes in thalassemia is well known.

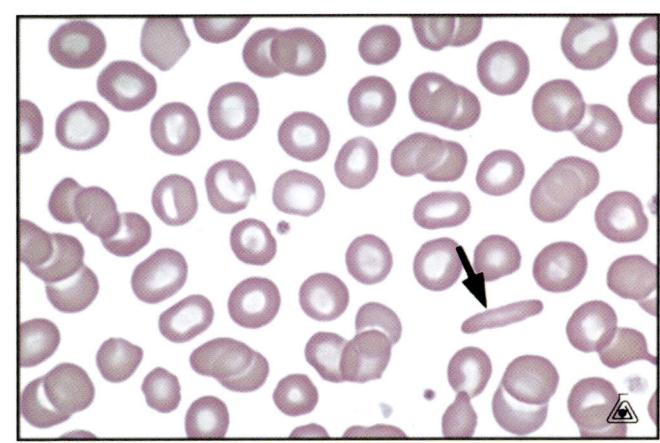

HE-22, 1993 (Blood, Wright-Giemsa, X320)

Identification	Referee %	Participant %
Ovalocyte (elliptocyte)	100	98.7

The ovalocytes from this 45-year-old female with a normal hemoglobin (14.0 g/dL) and MCV (87.5 fL) posed no problem in identification. The apparent variability in width may relate to technical factors, although their axial ratios (short/long axis) are each less than 0.75. It is assumed that their presence is a normal variation, since she had no family history of hereditary elliptocytosis and she was undergoing surgery for removal of a benign ovarian cyst. The neutrophil in the center of the field demonstrates *platelet satellitism*, discussed on page 206.

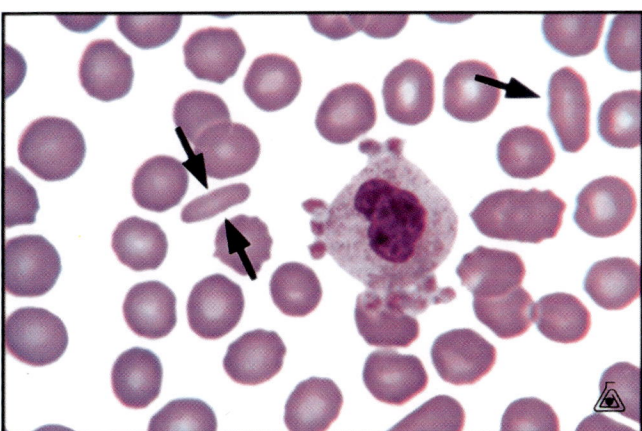

A Closer Look At...

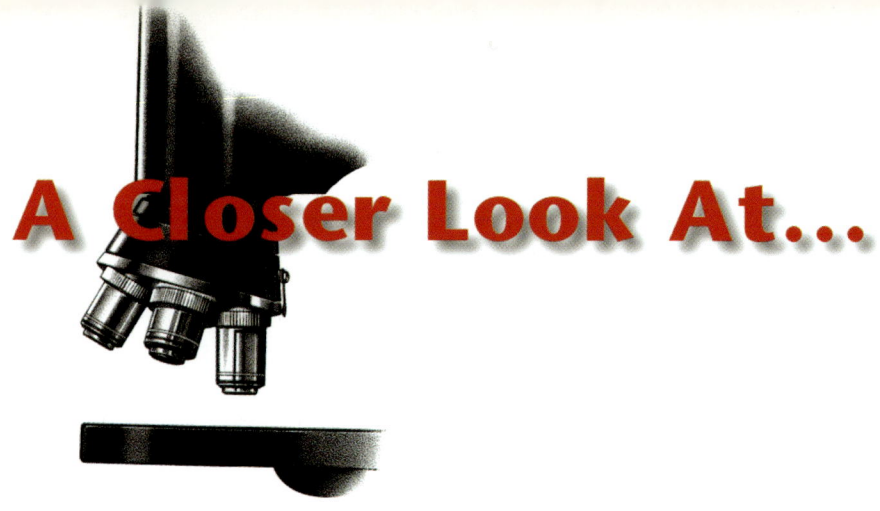

Hereditary Elliptocytosis

Hereditary elliptocytosis (HE) is one of a group of erythrocyte disorders which all have in common an intrinsic abnormality of the cell membrane and a variable degree of hemolytic anemia. Hereditary elliptocytosis is joined by hereditary spherocytosis (HS), hereditary pyropoikilocytosis (HPP, although clinically separate, it is really a subset of HE), hereditary stomatocytosis, hereditary xerocytosis, Rh-null disease, and paroxysmal nocturnal hemoglobinuria in this category. However, each also has its own unique set of findings and the interested reader is referred to any hematology textbook for further description.

The principal defect in HE involves horizontal membrane protein interactions. The different molecular abnormalities include a defect in the association of spectrin dimers, a deficiency of band 4.1 and dysfunction of ankyrin-3. Most have an autosomal dominant mode of inheritance.

Hereditary elliptocytosis is divided into three groups based on clinical severity and red cell morphology: *common HE*, *spherocytic HE*, and *stomatocytic HE*. The common HE occurs at highest frequency. The morphologic distinctions are illustrated below. Within this common HE group are six sub-types; mild HE is the most common subtype. It is characterized by a parent who also has mild HE, and mild to no hemolysis but the presence of at least 25% elliptocytic red cells; variations exist in certain families. Other important subtypes of common HE include hereditary pyropoikilocytosis and a form that in the first 2 years of life resembles HPP but then evolves as mild HE. Spherocytic HE, usually found in Northern Europeans or Japanese, is a hybrid of mild HE and HS. The balance of spherocytes and elliptocytes varies from patient to patient. Stomatocytic HE is restricted to Melanesians; the erythrocytes look like "shoe buckles" with two areas of central pallor bisected by a bridge of hemoglobin. Typical stomatocytes and blunt elliptocytes are admixed.

Because the inheritance of the membrane defect varies in the different groups of HE, so do their hematologic manifestations. The hemolysis and anemia may be minimal to obvious, as may the percentage of circulating elliptocytes (although they are usually plentiful). The spleen also plays a part in the manifestations of the disease; in some types of HE splenectomy ameliorates the hemolysis and thus the anemia. However, in mild HE and the infantile form, splenectomy has not proved to be beneficial.

Common HE	Spherocytic HE	Stomatocytic HE
oval and rod-shaped cells	fat ovalocytes and spherocytes	rounded ovalocytes; some are stomatocytic with longitudinal or transverse ridges
minimal to severe hemolysis	mild to moderate hemolysis	absent or mild hemolysis

Normal Red Cell Membrane

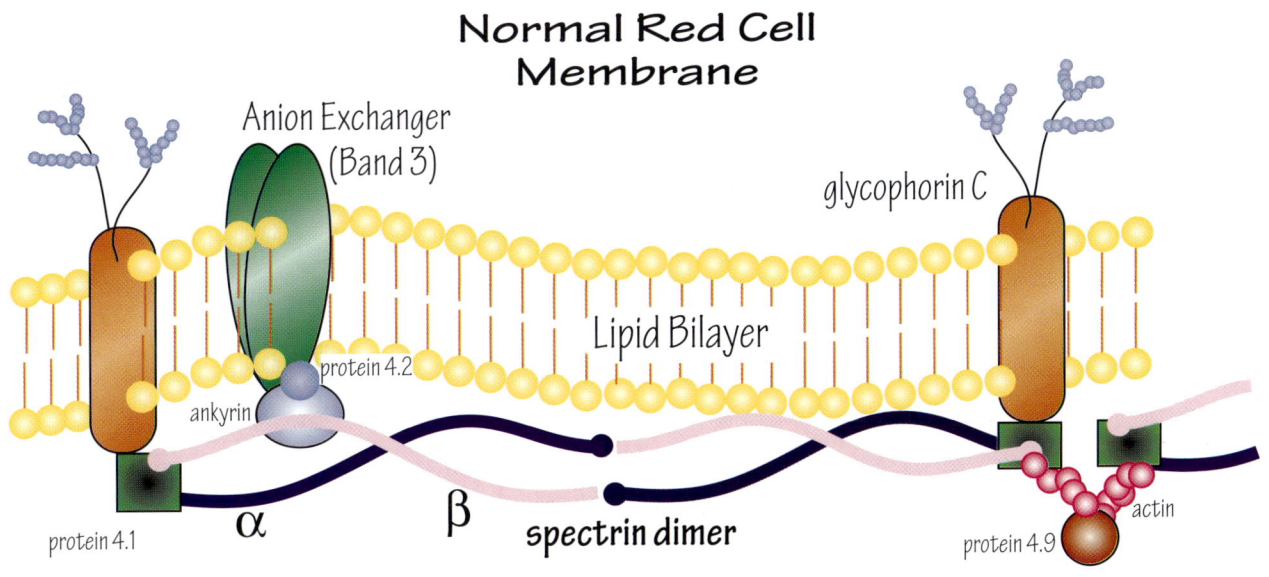

Hereditary Elliptocytosis

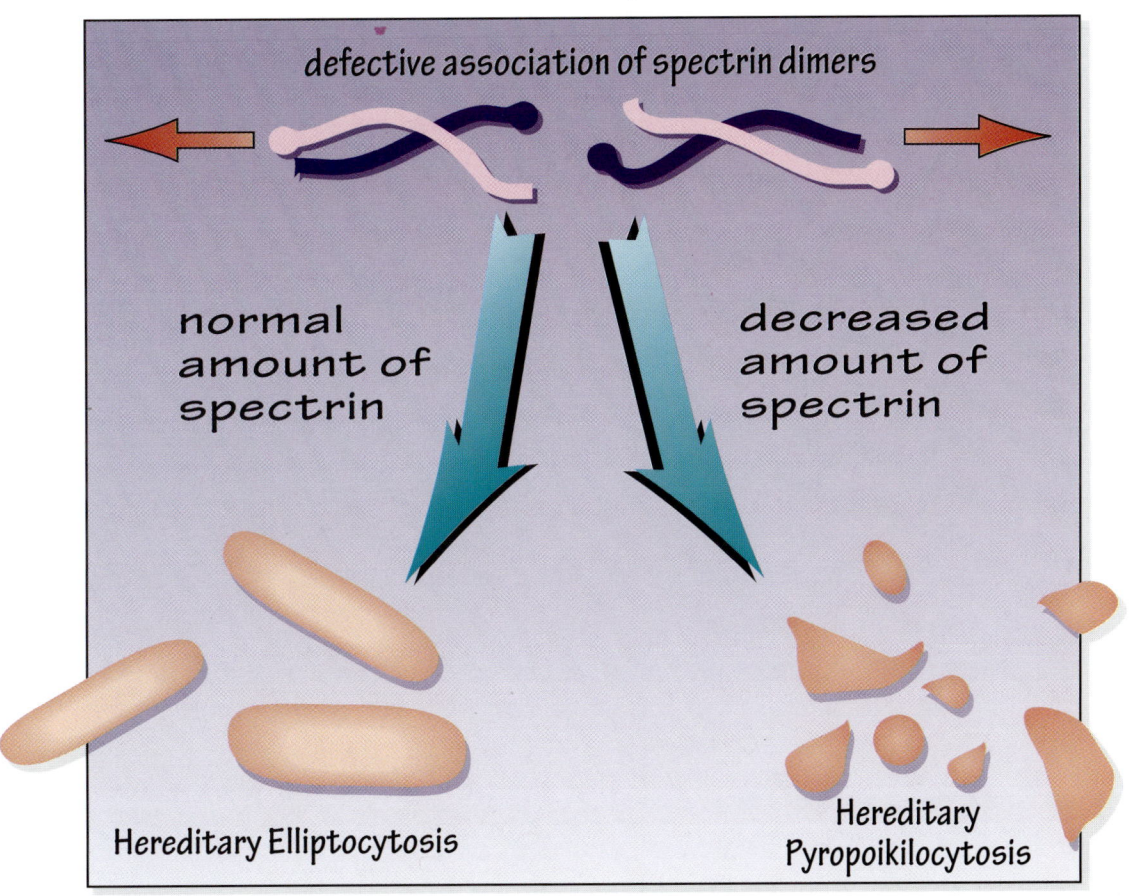

There are more than 80 different mutations in the red cell cytoskeleton. The most common molecular abnormality in hereditary elliptocytosis (HE) involves defects in spectrin-dimer self-association. Hereditary pyropoikilocytosis is a subtype of HE in which a spectrin defect is combined with a spectrin deficiency.

Polychromatophilic Red Cell (Non-Nucleated)

SYNONYMS
polychromatophils, reticulocyte (presumptive)

VITAL STATISTICS
- size .... slightly larger than erythrocyte
- cell shape .... round to slightly oval
- cytoplasm .... little or no central pallor; color is slightly more basophilic than that of an erythrocyte

KEY DIFFERENTIATING FEATURES
- size slightly larger than normal red blood cell
- slightly darker, gray-blue cytoplasmic coloration
- absent or significantly diminished central pallor

OTHER FINDINGS
- supravital staining reveals retained RNA (see *Reticulocyte*, page 114)

POTENTIAL LOOK-ALIKES
- round macrocytes

ASSOCIATED DISEASE STATES AND CONDITIONS
- newborns
- after acute blood loss
- recovery of marrow after cytoreduction (e.g., chemotherapy)

The very last portion of red cell maturation occurs in the circulation. This is where the polychromatophilic red cell matures from a reticulocyte into a normal red blood cell. A polychromatophilic red cell is an erythrocyte which still retains a small amount of RNA (ribonucleic acid). It is characteristically recognized in standard Wright-Giemsa stained blood smears as a cell without central pallor but which is somewhat larger and darker (basophilic) than an erythrocyte. These are the newest marrow contributions to the circulating population of erythrocytes. Approximately one percent of all circulating erythrocytes are replaced everyday, so a physiologic reticulocyte count is 1%. This hemostatic parameter is well controlled and therefore an increase in polychromatophilic cells (polychromasia is a shorthand word to describe this increase) is significant; it signals that the marrow is actively working at an increased rate to replace those erythrocytes which have been lost, most commonly by acute blood loss. However, an increase in polychromatophilic red cells may actually be normal at birth; it is not due to bleeding but rather is an indicator of the rate of hematopoiesis at this stage of life and normally decreases to adult levels within a week.

Since polychromasia may be more difficult to determine if a smear is poorly prepared or stained, a more definitive idea of erythrocyte homeostasis is given by the reticulocyte count (see *Reticulocyte*, page 114).

Normal and Polychromatophilic Red Cells

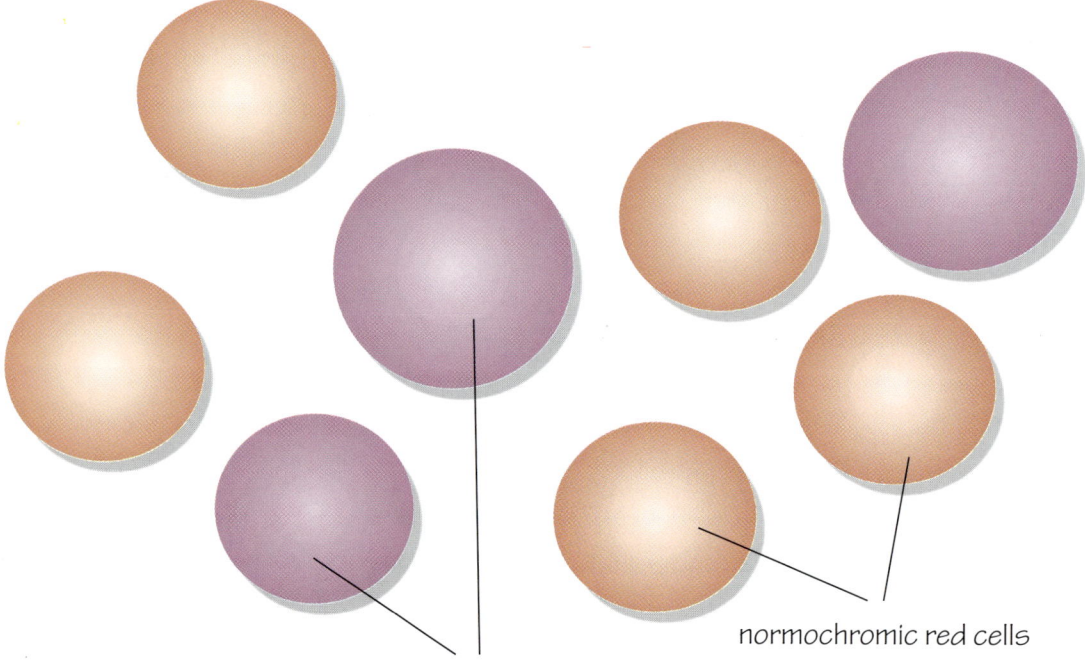

polychromatophilic red cells

normochromic red cells

Erythrocytic Cells and Inclusions

A-11, 1984 (Blood, Wright-Giemsa, X375)

Identification	Referee %	Participant %
Polychromatophilic red cell (non-nucleated)	100	89.8
Macrocyte, round or oval	-	3.6

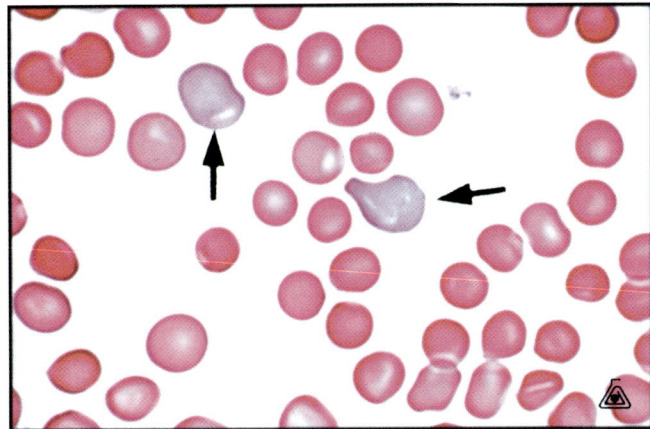

The two arrowed polychromatophilic red cells seen here are notable for their larger size and more basophilic color, when compared to the erythrocytes in the field. The cells are reticulocytes; the polychromasia is due to residual ribosomes within the cytoplasm. A reticulocyte is the stage of red cell maturation that begins just after extrusion of the nucleus. The cell matures for 48 hours in the marrow, then circulates in the blood. Hemoglobin production continues during this time. Once in the blood, the cell matures for another 24 hours, finally becoming a normal discoid erythrocyte after it has shed all of its ribosomes and cytoplasmic organelles. A reticulocyte stain would precipitate the ribosomes into a granular network (the "substantia filamentosa"). The cells are larger than normal but the term macrocyte is reserved for cells lacking significant polychromasia.

XL-24, 1986 (Blood, Wright-Giemsa, X400)

Identification	Referee %	Participant %
Polychromatophilic red cell (non-nucleated)	73.7	35.1
Macrocyte, round or oval	26.3	62.2

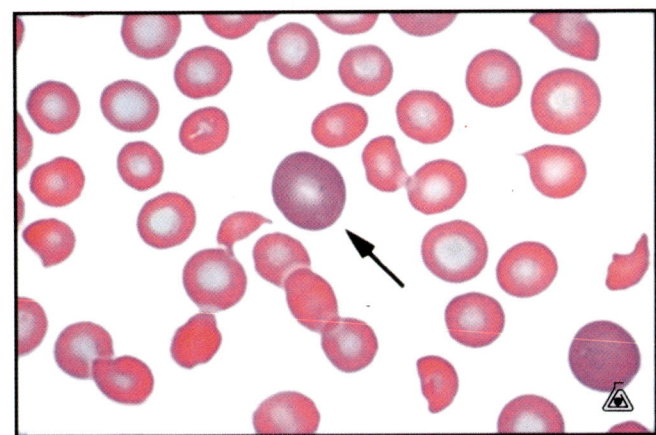

The polychromatophilic cell present in the middle of the field is certainly larger and more basophilic than the surrounding erythrocytes; another such cell is present in the lower right corner. The fragmented red cells scattered throughout the field coupled with these polychromatophilic cells, suggest that some type of hemolytic process is occurring. This patient was diagnosed with a microangiopathic hemolytic anemia. Polychromatophilic cells technically are macrocytic (i.e., large). For CAP proficiency testing purposes, however, the *macrocyte* ID should be used for cells without any polychromasia.

XL-74, 1987 (Blood, Wright-Giemsa, X400)

Identification	Referee %	Participant %
Polychromatophilic red cell (non-nucleated)	88.9	39.7
Macrocyte, round or oval	5.6	55.1

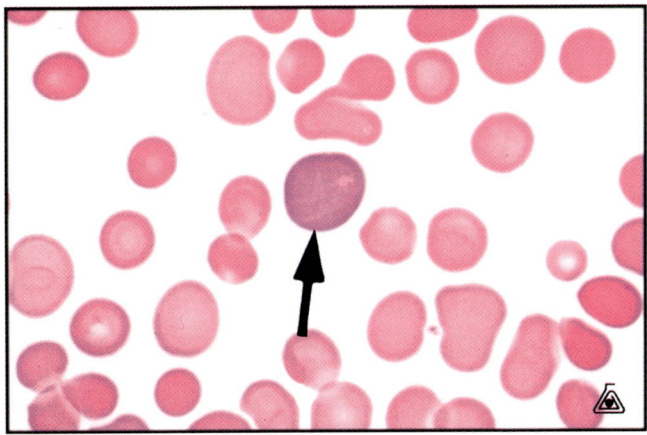

The diagnosis for this patient was a direct antiglobulin (Coomb's) positive anemia. The presence of polychromatophilic cells on Wright-Giemsa stain indicates an appropriate physiologic marrow response, since such cells are reticulocytes, the nearly mature erythrocyte. The arrowed cell is larger than normal red cells but they should not be designated *macrocytes*. Round or oval macrocytes are mature erythrocytes that display no significant polychromasia. The ability to distinguish a macrocyte and a polychromatophilic cell is important and at least partially dependent on the quality of the stain. The ability to tell a macrocyte from a polychromatophilic red cell may be the starting point for appropriate care in liver disease, bleeding, anemias, and vitamin deficiencies.

Sickle Cell

SYNONYMS
   drepanocyte

VITAL STATISTICS
   size .... variable; usually >10 μm
   cell shape .... sickle, with two pointed ends;
            may also be crescent-shaped,
            boat-shaped, filament-shaped,
            holly-leaf form, envelope cell
   cytoplasm .... normochromic to apparently
            hyperchromic; no central pallor

KEY DIFFERENTIATING FEATURES
   red cell having pointed ends, usually in crescent shape;
      rarely holly leaf or blister configuration
   very dense hemoglobin
   no central pallor

OTHER FINDINGS
   The blood in sickle cell anemia shows a normochromic, normocytic anemia as well as ovalocytes, target cells, polychromasia, basophilic stippling, nucleated red cells, and if autosplenectomy has occurred, Howell-Jolly bodies and Pappenheimer bodies; there is also a leukocytosis and thrombocytosis; modest eosinophilia is common; abnormal hemoglobin electrophoresis with an increase in Hb S and the presence of Hb F; Hb A_2 is normal but Hb A is absent

POTENTIAL LOOK-ALIKES
   fragmented red cells (schistocytes)
   ovalocyte (elliptocyte)
   hemoglobin C crystal
   malarial organisms (gametes)

ASSOCIATED DISEASE STATES AND CONDITIONS
   hemoglobin SS disease
   hemoglobin SC disease
   hemoglobin SD disease
   S-beta thalassemia

Sickle cells, also known as drepanocytes, are red blood cells deformed by rod-like structures of polymerized hemoglobin S. Sickle-shaped cells are found in the homozygous (SS) but not the heterozygous (SA) state.

Most of the deformed cells have a boat-shape or are thin crescents. They generally vary in length from 10 to 15 μm. Other deformities characteristic of sickle cell anemia include pointed ellipsoids, holly leafs, splinter shapes, envelope forms, and blisters. In the background are target cells, apparent hypochromic cells, Howell-Jolly bodies, and Pappenheimer bodies. The latter two inclusions are a consequence of auto-splenectomy. If the target cells are numerous, a diagnosis of S-C should be considered.

Blister cell variants have a dense crescent of hemoglobin within a ghost-like hypochromic membrane. This term is commonly used to refer to *pre-keratocytes* (see page 72) but in actuality it was first used to describe this type of sickle cell.

Sickle cell anemia is detailed in the following *A Closer Look At...* discussion on page 98. The mutant hemoglobin is the result of substitution of non-polar valine for polar glutamic acid at the sixth position of the A3 helix of the beta-globin chain. The shift in electrical charge markedly reduces the solubility of hemoglobin in the deoxygenated state. Deoxyhemoglobin S molecules tend to polymerize into rigid filaments. The cells then assume irregular crescentic shapes as the membrane is stretched by the polymers. The sickled cells may return to normal upon reoxygenization. Repeated sickling events lead to irreversibly sickled cells visible on air-dried smears. They are removed by the spleen, liver, and bone marrow. The number of these cells circulating is directly related to the severity of hemolysis.

Sickle Cells

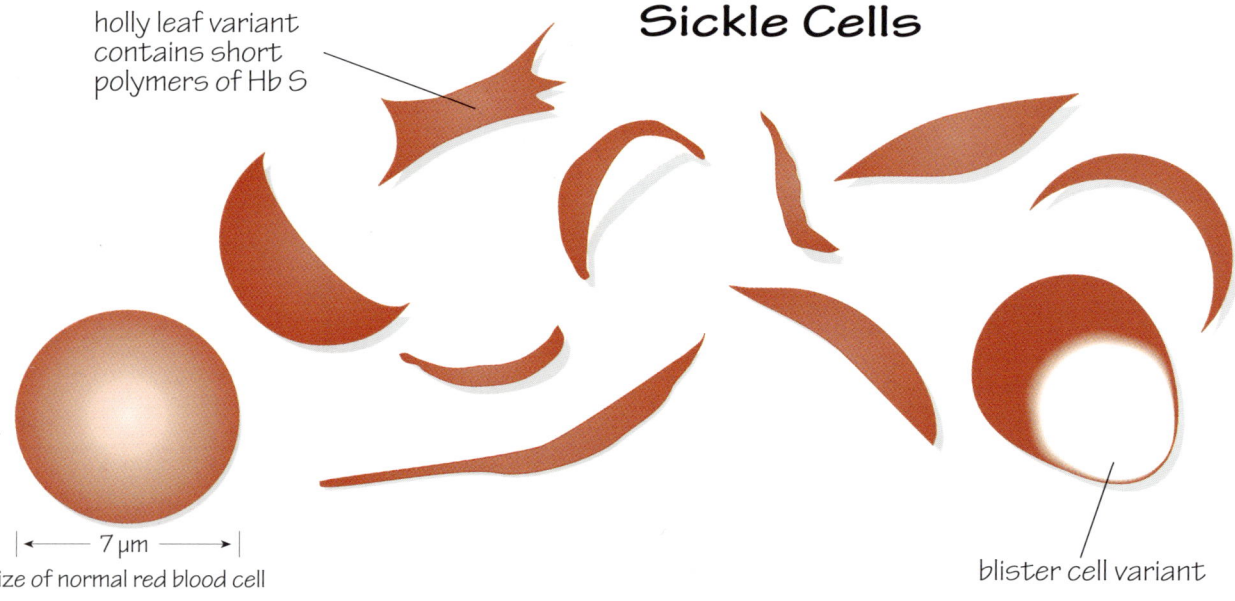

holly leaf variant contains short polymers of Hb S

|← 7 μm →|
size of normal red blood cell

blister cell variant

XL-62, 1985 (Blood, Wright-Giemsa, X340)

Identification	Referee %	Participant %
Sickle cell	100	99

The arrowed cell posed no identification problems. Indeed, with its thin elongate shape, pointed ends, and dense homogeneous appearance, the term sickle cell is readily invoked. Note also in this field the target cells, hypochromasia, and spherocyte. The patient was a 10-year-old black male with a leg ulcer.

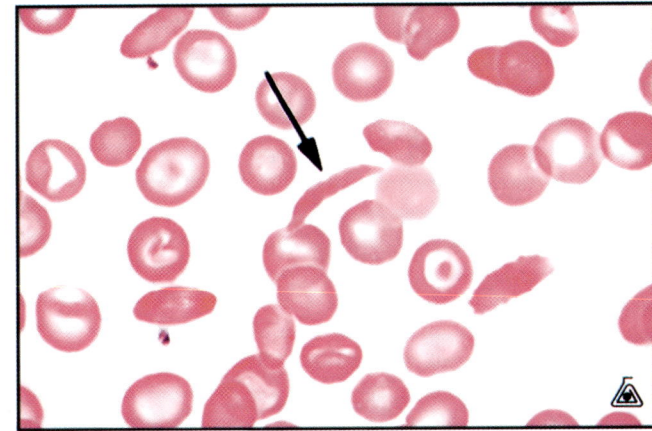

XL-26, 1987 (Blood, Wright-Giemsa, X360)

Identification	Referee %	Participant %
Sickle cell	100	99

Again, the arrowed cell was no identification problem. By the low number of red cells present, one may assume an anemia (Hgb = 6.5 mg/dL). Also of note are the classic findings of target cells, microcytes, spherocytes, and polychromatophilic cells (the latter indicating marrow response to the anemia; reticulocyte count = 7.5%). This 13-year-old black female with sickle cell anemia had chronic leg ulcers and cardiac murmurs as complications of her disease.

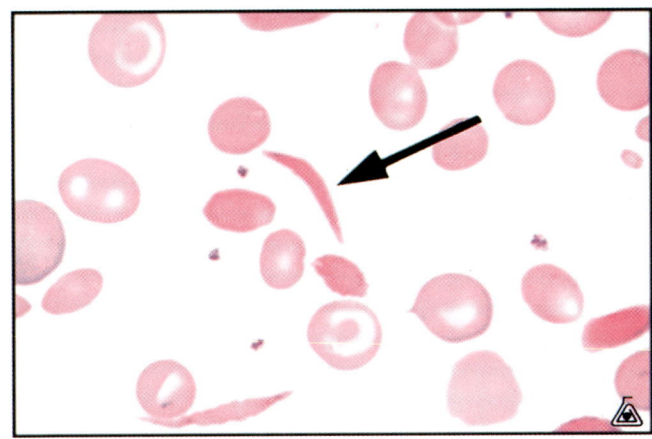

HE-42, 1993 (Blood, Wright-Giemsa, X500)

Identification	Referee %	Participant %
Sickle cell	100	99.5

The patient is a 25-year-old black, pregnant woman, with SC disease. The arrowed cell is markedly elongated with two pointed ends. It is a classic example of a sickle cell or drepanocyte. The cytoplasm contains dense hemoglobin and lacks central pallor. Another sickle cell is located in the upper left corner. Just beneath it is an envelope cell. There is a nucleated red blood cell in the lower right corner. From the number of erythrocytes present in the field, there is an assumed anemia. Sickle cells may be seen in sickle cell anemia, hemoglobin SC disease, SD disease, and S-beta-thalassemia, particularly when splenic function is compromised.

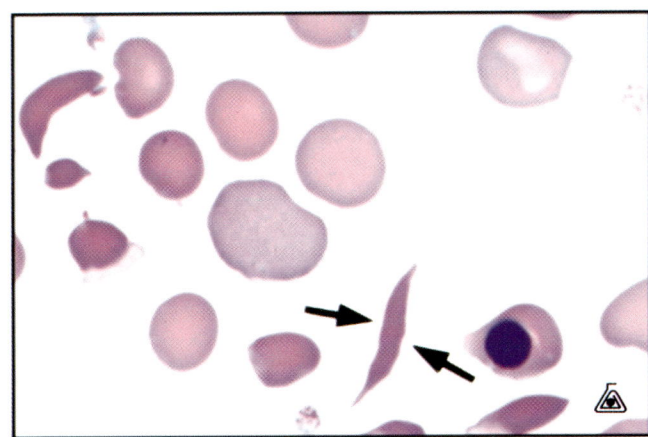

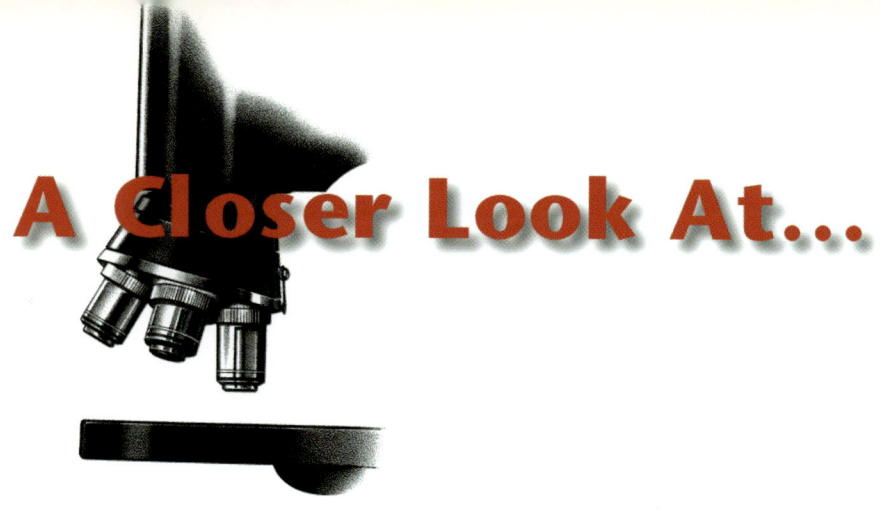

A Closer Look At...

Sickle Cell Anemia

Sickle cell disease is one of a group of inherited red cell defects collectively termed *hemoglobinopathy*. It is the most common inherited hematologic disease in the world today. The single substitution of one amino acid (valine instead of glutamine) at the sixth codon of the B-gene of hemoglobin results in the eventual polymerization of the hemoglobin which gives rise to the numerous complications characteristic of sickle cell disease. The facing page illustrates the process of hemoglobin polymerization and resultant disease.

The effects of sickle hemoglobin (HbS) occur under conditions of deoxygenation, when the HbS has less affinity for oxygen and polymerizes, or gels. Low pH (<7.2 may be sufficient), a high concentration of deoxy HbS (>20 g/dL), high temperature, and the presence of certain other abnormal hemoglobins (HbS, HbC, HbD, HbO Arab) also promote the formation of polymers, but deoxygenation is most important. As the polymerized hemoglobin increases in concentration, it gels; the gel will then contain tactoids which are crystals that polarize light and are described as boat-shaped, small and rigid. The polymers may dissolve with reversal of these factors (e.g., adequate oxygenation), but the body's physiology is such that polymerization will again invariably occur in the microcirculation. Eventually the red cell will become irreversibly sickled and then sequestered and destroyed. The number of such irreversibly sickled cells is fairly constant for an individual but does vary from patient to patient.

The hematologic findings are a direct reflection of this abnormal hemoglobin. There is an obvious hemolytic anemia with hemoglobin averaging 8 g/dL by 8 months of age. Hemolysis may be both intra- and extravascular, with a greatly increased rate of destruction. The morphologic abnormalities are many; most striking is the presence of the crescentic-shaped sickle cell as well as oval cells and cigar-shaped, boat-shaped, filament-shaped, holly-leaf shaped or envelope-shaped cells; numerous target cells are also present. The smear reflects the hemolysis in the form of polychromasia (reticulocytes average at least 10%), basophilic stippling and nucleated red blood cells. Once the spleen is no longer functional (autosplenectomy), Howell-Jolly bodies, Pappenheimer bodies and erythrocytes with pitted membranes appear; this usually occurs by age 5 or 6. Children with sickle cell anemia tend to retain their hemoglobin F longer than normal. Since hemoglobin F is protective against the effects of sickle cell anemia, with as little 4% moderating symptoms, the most severe manifestations of disease may not occur until after one year of age. The life-span of patients with sickle cell anemia, with aggressive supportive close care, is approaching normal.

Hemoglobin SS produces the full-blown disease. The carrier state, Hb AS, with a ratio of hemoglobin A:S of 60:40, has no symptoms normally; this is primarily due to the decreased polymerization effect of hemoglobin A. The blood is normal, or may show a few target cells. Diagnosis is made by hemoglobin electrophoresis. The erythrocytes may show sickling only with severe physiologic stress. Sickle cell trait individuals have a normal life span.

Hemoglobin S may also occur with other hemoglobinopathies, such as hemoglobin C (HbSC disease), HbD, HbO Arab, HbS-HPFH (hemoglobin S and hereditary persistence of fetal hemoglobin), HbS-Lepore, HbS-alpha thalassemia, and HbS-beta thalassemia. Each has somewhat unique manifestations, with less severe sickle cell manifestations in HbS-alpha thalassemia, HbSC disease, and HbS-beta thalassemia. However, others intensify the manifestations most notably HbS-D Los Angeles and HbS-O Arab disease.

Sickle Cell Formation

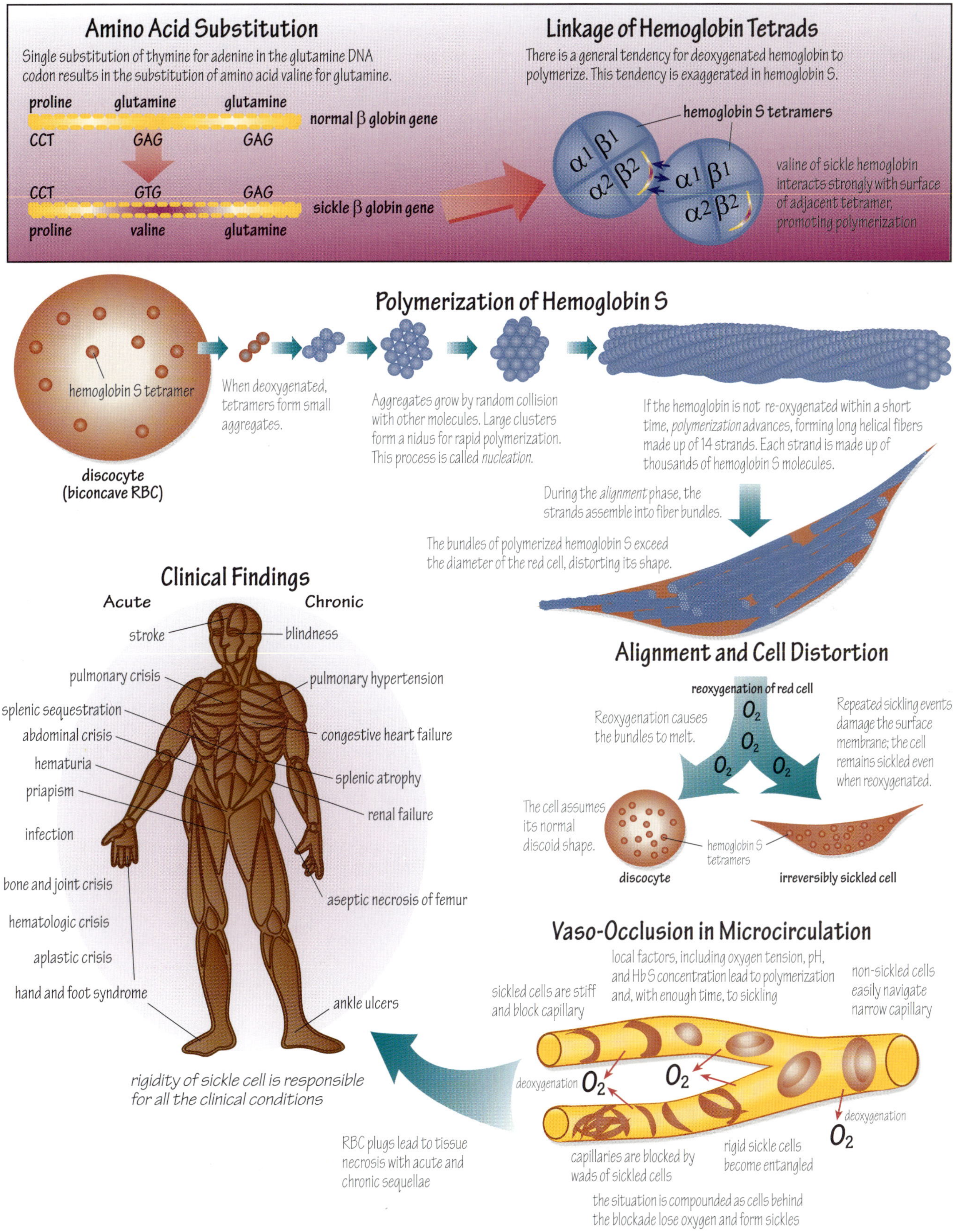

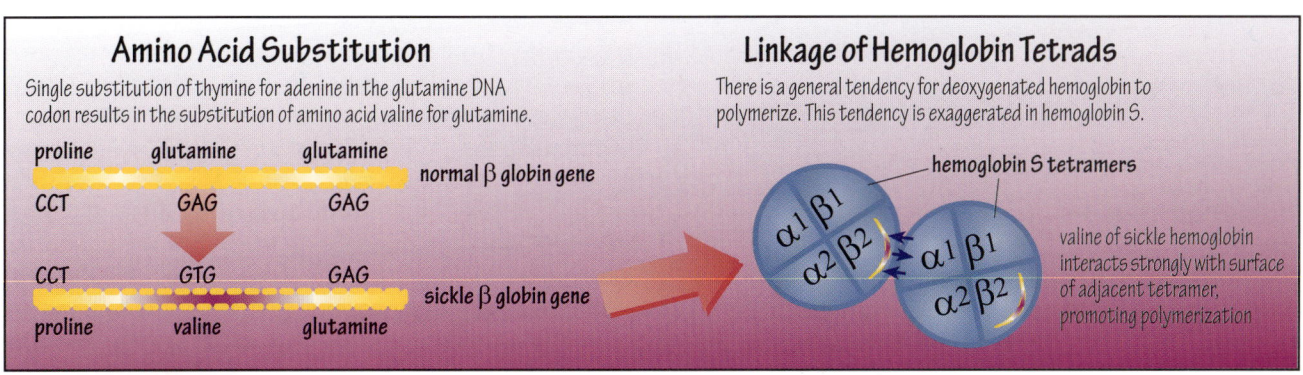

Spherocyte

SYNONYMS
none

VITAL STATISTICS
size .... slightly microcytic (< 6.5 μm diameter); MCV normal to slightly reduced
cell shape .... round, spherical
cytoplasm .... no central pallor; may appear hyperchromic

KEY DIFFERENTIATING FEATURES
lack of central pallor
smaller than normal erythrocyte

OTHER FINDINGS
artifactual spherocytes can be found at the extreme feather edge and outer margins of even the best prepared smears; they are more broad and pale than true spherocytes and often exhibit cornered margins

POTENTIAL LOOK-ALIKES
microcyte
polychromatophilic red cell
blister cells
various types of red cells containing polymerized or crystalized hemoglobin

ASSOCIATED DISEASE STATES AND CONDITIONS
hereditary spherocytosis
immune hemolytic anemias
thermal injury (e.g., burns)
microangiopathic hemolytic anemias

A spherocyte is an abnormal erythrocyte. It is round, thicker than normal, and without central pallor. It may be slightly smaller than normal, or sometimes much smaller (microspherocyte, defined as less than 4 μm in diameter). A spherocyte occurs as a consequence of membrane loss, thus resulting in a cell surface to cytoplasm ratio decrease. When the reduced surface membrane has been pulled taut over the constant volume of cytoplasm, the erythrocyte loses its biconcave shape and central pallor. This cell is rigid and cannot deform well enough to negotiate its way through small vessels or its most unforgiving inspector, the spleen. It is there removed from the circulation and catabolized, usually long before its normal 120 day life-span is over.

Spherocytes typically look undersized. MCV values vary widely, however, depending on the degree of reticulocytosis. If reticulocytes are few in relative number, the MCV is in the low-normal range. The question then arises if spherocytes are truly microcytic. Many authorities say no, although the appearance on blood films is one of microcytes.

Hereditary spherocytosis is an autosomal dominant disorder. It is the most prevalent hemolytic disease in persons of northern European ancestry. The cells have an intrinsic deficit of spectrin, the protein that forms the supporting scaffolding for the red cell membrane. Diagnosis depends on recognizing spherocytes that have little or no central pallor and that appear smaller than normal red cells. In 75-80% of cases they are quite numerous. The MCHC is higher than normal, usually between 36 and 40 g/dL. The high MCHC reflects mild cellular dehydration caused by a decreased K^+ and H_2O content.

The only other condition in which spherocytes are as numerous is in Coombs' positive hemolytic anemia. Causes of spherocytosis are discussed in the next *A Closer Look At...*section on page 102.

Artifactual spherocytes can be seen at the extreme feathered edge of all blood smears. The imposters are broad, pale, and often display cornered edges.

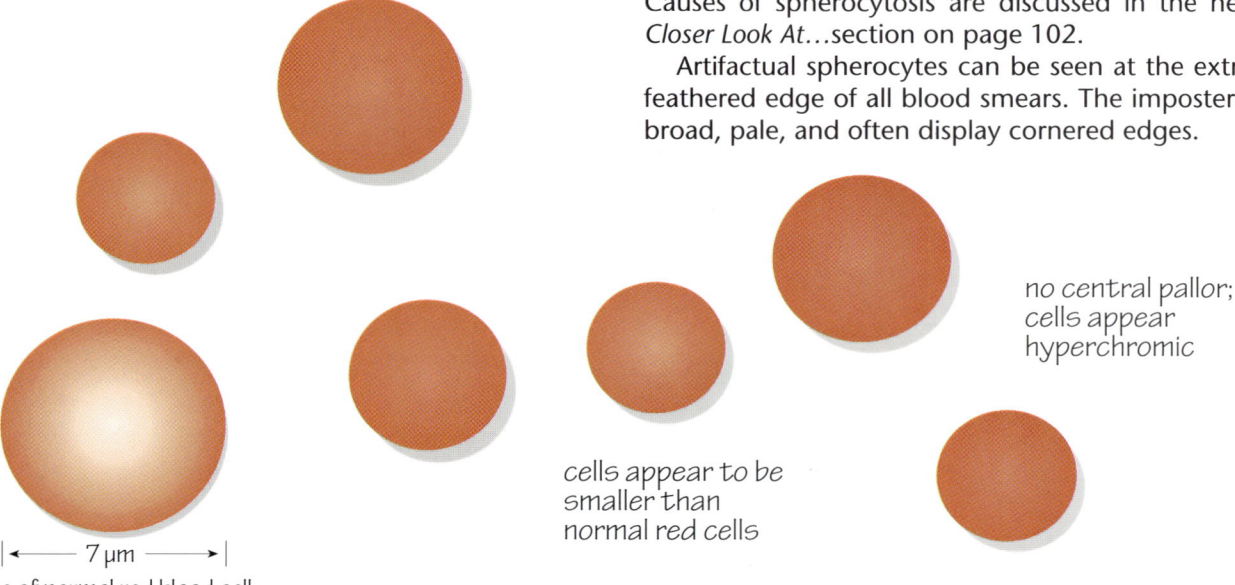

Spherocytes

no central pallor; cells appear hyperchromic

cells appear to be smaller than normal red cells

|← 7 μm →|
size of normal red blood cell

HE-45, 1993 (Blood, Wright-Giemsa, X400)

Identification	Referee %	Participant %
Spherocyte	40.7	57.1
Hemoglobin C crystal	37.0	28.6
Microcyte	14.8	10.6

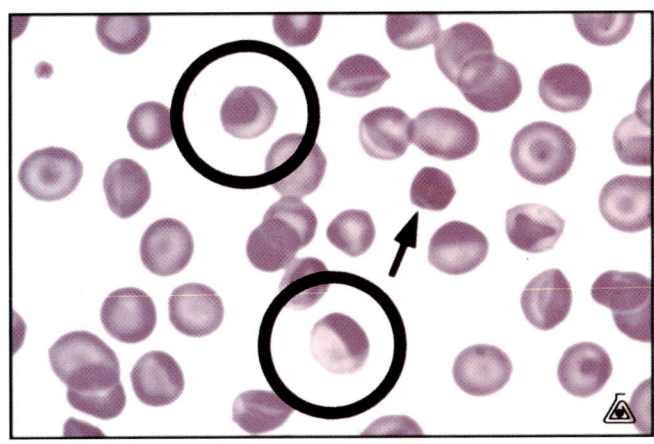

The arrowed cell is a spherocyte. It does appear smaller than many of the other erythrocytes in this field. Numerous target cells are also present. Please note the circled erythrocytes; they are erythrocytes with hemoglobin C crystals, a very important finding. They are examples of so-called *envelope forms*. Similar deformed red cells can also be seen in sickling disorders and thalassemia syndromes. The patient is a 25-year-old pregnant black female with a hemoglobin of 11.2 g/dL and an MCV of 74 fL. Hemoglobin electrophoresis confirmed hemoglobin SC disease.

XL-07, 1986 (Blood, Wright-Giemsa, X410)

Identification	Referee %	Participant %
Spherocyte	100	91.2
Erythrocyte, normal	-	5.8

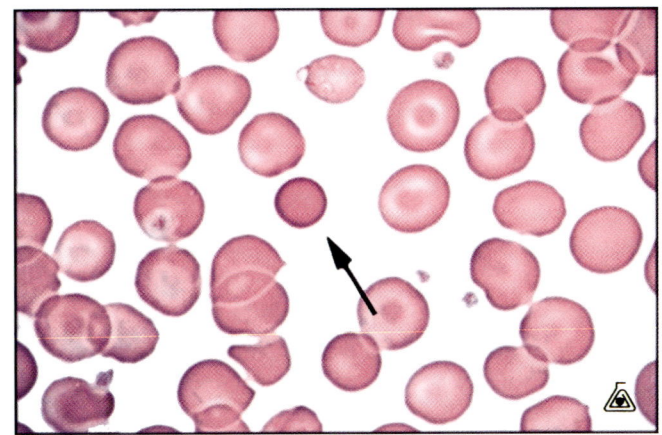

The arrowed spherocyte is not a problem in identification. Its dense, homogeneous, round red appearance makes it stand out in the field. The other finding of note is the many target cells. The spherocyte appears smaller than the surrounding red cells. Most students of hematology say that sperocytes are not microcytic; most examples have a normal MCV and are cup-shaped (not round) by scanning electron microscopy. However, when an erythrocyte is fragmented, and the small remnant "rounds up," it may appear small and round, without central pallor—a "micro" spherocyte. The discussion of spherocytes and micro-spherocytes will no doubt continue.

HE-09, 1994 (Blood, Wright-Giemsa, X400)

Identification	Referee %	Participant %
Spherocyte	100	96.5
Microcyte	3.4	2.9

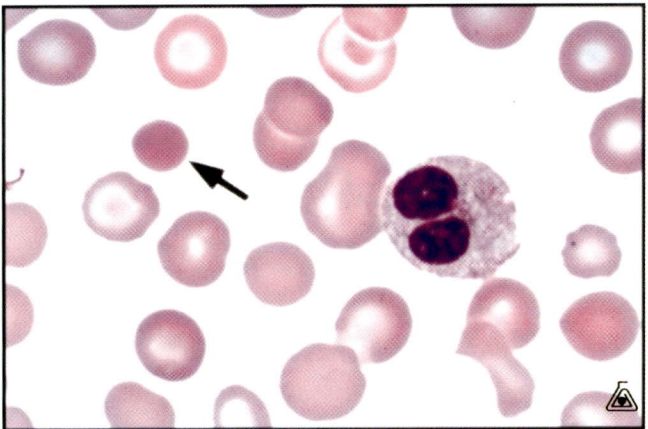

The arrowed cell is a spherocyte, with the typical appearance of such a cell. It is quite a bit smaller than the surrounding erythrocytes; the non-spherocytic erythrocyte to the right of the leukocyte is approximately the same size. Although both are small cells, the more important realization of spherocyte for the arrowed cell should take precedence. The small number of participants who identified the cell as a microcyte no doubt recognized the cell's abnormal size, but this is not a microcyte as normally defined since there is no central pallor. Likewise, since this erythrocyte is abnormal, the identification of erythrocyte does not apply. The sample is from a patient with the diagnosis of agnogenic myeloid metaplasia, a type of myeloproliferative disorder. The spherocyte most likely is the result of hemolysis, which may be seen in this disorder and is believed to be due to associated immune system abnormalities, including circulating immune complexes.

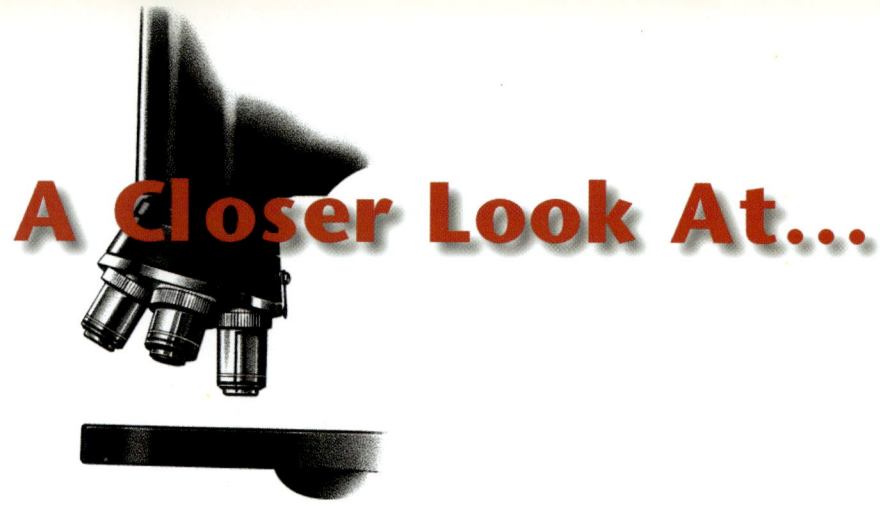

A Closer Look At...

Red Cell Membrane Loss and Spherocytosis

The mechanism of membrane loss may be either intrinsic to the cell, much as in *hereditary spherocytosis* (HS), or imposed from without, as in *immune hemolysis*. In hereditary spherocytosis, a lack of the membrane cytoskeletal component spectrin (and/or possibly, its abnormal function) results in a cell that is defective, leaks cations, and requires greater than normal amounts of energy for metabolism. This membrane defect is noted when the cell negotiates its way through the red pulp of the spleen, and the relatively acidic, hypoxic microenvironment exaggerates these cells' defect. Unable to deform adequately, they are eventually trapped in the splenic cords, where they are catabolized.

Hereditary spherocytosis, an autosomal dominant inherited disorder, is characterized by a mild, usually well compensated hemolytic anemia, eventual splenomegaly, mild jaundice, and pigmented gallstones secondary to the increased hemolysis. There may be familial clustering, but some cases appear to be sporadic. These patients are usually able to get along with minimal therapeutic intervention because their bone marrow can compensate for this increased hemolysis. A *crisis*, with marrow depletion, may occur with viral infection. Patients may eventually require splenectomy, which increases the red cell survival but does nothing to alter the inherent erythrocyte abnormality. Removal of the gallbladder due to an increase in pigment type of stones is frequently required, and may be needed at a young age. The osmotic fragility test is used to demonstrate the abnormal cells, with their reduced capacity to survive in hypotonic solutions.

Immune hemolysis, although quite different in etiology, treatment, and course, may share microscopic features with HS patients. Spherocytes are often quite numerous. Immune hemolysis may be due to a variety of causes, most commonly drugs. The classic offender is penicillin. Other types of antibody-induced hemolysis are red cell incompatibility as demonstrated by hemolytic disease of the newborn and hemolytic transfusion reaction. Lastly, immune hemolysis may be due to autoimmune hemolytic anemia. Although the etiology obviously varies for each, the final result is the production of antibody, either IgM or IgG isotype, which will cause complement-mediated intravascular red cell destruction in the former but extravascular erythrocyte removal with subsequent destruction in the latter. Immune hemolysis patients may clinically be very ill, with severe anemia, jaundice, and other diseases as well as the hemolysis. Thus, the presence of spherocytes in the blood indicates significant pathology.

Thermal injury and **microangiopathic hemolytic states** may also lead to spherocyte formation, as depicted on the facing page. Microspherocytes are commonly found in association with the fragmented cells typical of either disorder. They are never found as frequently as the spherocytes that typify hereditary spherocytosis, however.

Types of Membrane Loss Leading to Spherocyte Formation

Fibrin Strands

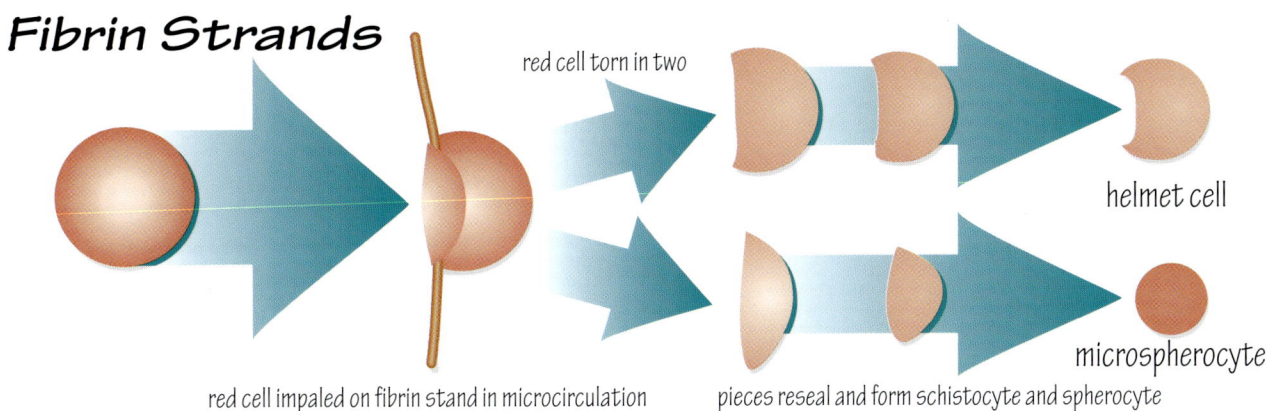

Thermal Injury

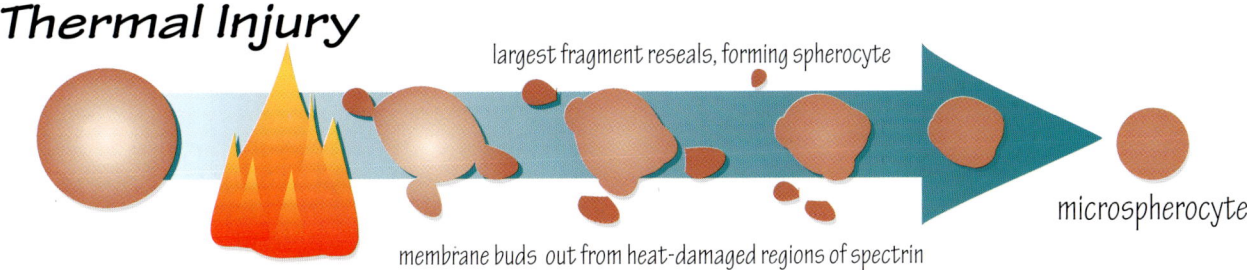

Intrinsic Abnormalities

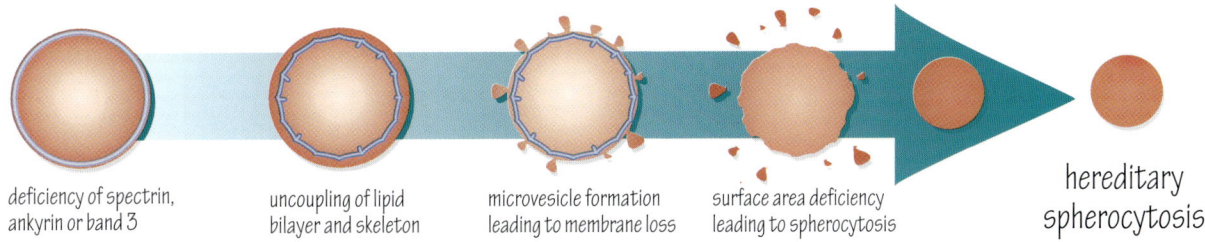

Immune Hemolysis

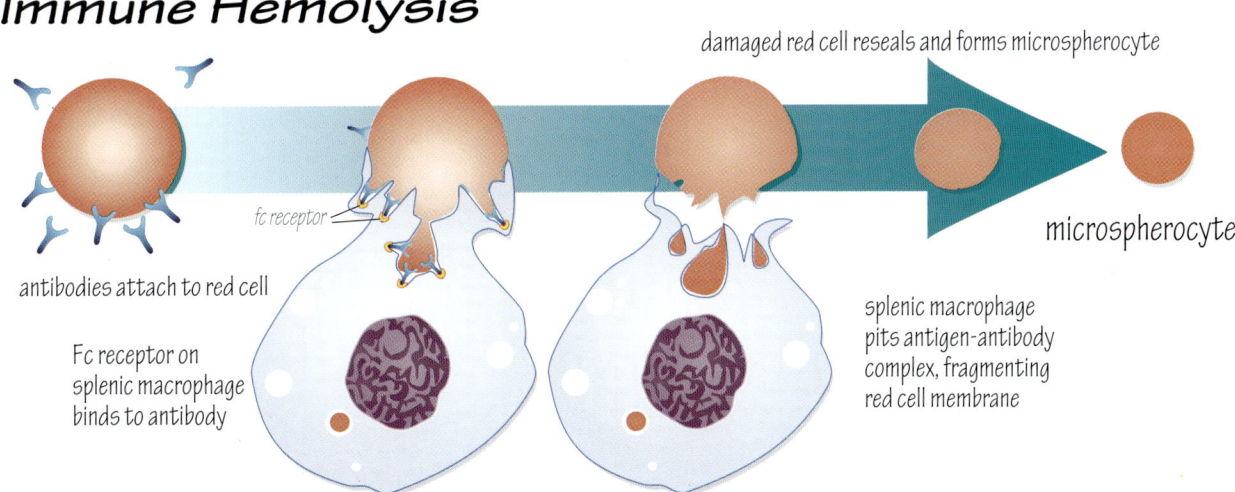

Stomatocyte

SYNONYMS
　hydrocyte

VITAL STATISTICS
　size .... normocytic
　cell shape .... round; uniconcave disc
　cytoplasm .... normochromic; central pallor appears slit-like, straight, fish-mouth, or curved rod-shaped; a few cells may have tripolar pallor creating cells that resemble sleigh bells

KEY DIFFERENTIATING FEATURES
　central pallor appears slit-like

POTENTIAL LOOK-ALIKES
　normal erythrocytes

ASSOCIATED DISEASE STATES AND CONDITIONS
　hereditary stomatocytosis
　Melanesian ovalocytosis
　hereditary hydrocytosis
　Rh null disease
　Tangier disease
　Stewart's syndrome
　cardiovascular disease
　carcinoma (some cases)
　alcoholic cirrhosis
　acute alcoholism
　obstructive liver disease
　phenothiazines
　artifact caused by slow-to-dry smears

In many respects, a stomatocyte is similar in appearance to a normal erythrocyte in its overall size, contour and staining characteristics. What sets it apart is its central area of pallor, which is slit-like instead of round. The formation of stomatocytes has been documented and found to occur at low (acidic) pH, when erythrocytes are exposed to agents such as cationic detergents, or with exposure to drugs such as phenothiazines. The erythrocyte first loses its central indentation on one side (which then becomes flat) but the depression on the other side increases, giving the appearance of a bow tie and then a cup. On smears the flattened cell shows its central area as more mouth-like. Such a cell will continue on to form a spherocyte.

Hereditary stomatocytosis is an autosomal dominant inherited hemolytic anemia with some resemblance to hereditary spherocytosis. There is an incompletely understood membrane defect which results in abnormal cation transport. The cells are not as sturdy as normal erythrocytes and show abnormality (increased) in the osmotic fragility test. Patients show a mild anemia with evidence of ongoing hemolysis. The stomatocytes may range from 10 to 50% of circulating erythrocytes. Splenectomy is reported to have variable results in controlling symptoms.

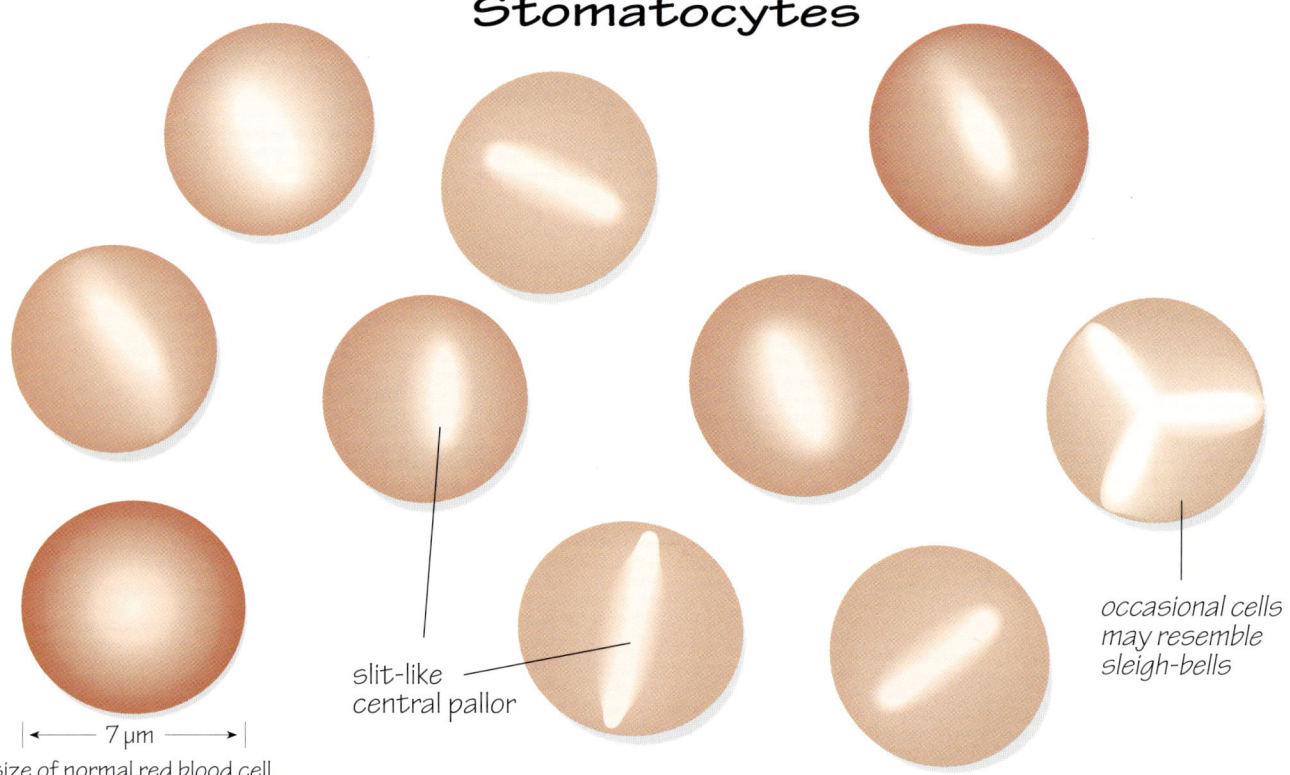

Stomatocytes

slit-like central pallor

occasional cells may resemble sleigh-bells

|← 7 μm →|
size of normal red blood cell

HE-23, 1995 (Blood, Wright-Giemsa, X400)

Identification	Referee %	Participant %
Stomatocyte	97.5	96.4
Erythrocyte, normal	2.5	1.6

The arrowed cell is a stomatocyte. In contrast to nearly all other erythrocytes in this field, the central pallor of the stomatocyte is elongate, giving the often-described "fish-mouth" appearance to this cell. It otherwise does not appear different from a normal erythrocyte in size, overall shape, or staining characteristics. The patient is a three-month-old boy with paroxysms of barking cough that suggests a diagnosis of either pertussis or whooping cough. The rare stomatocytes present on the smear should be considered artifactual in origin and not indicative of an inherited condition.

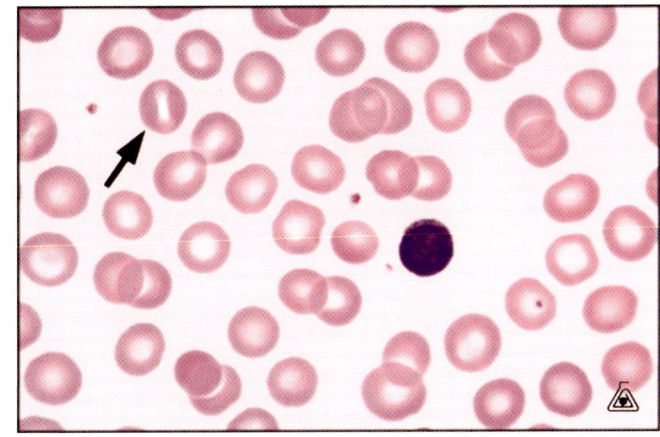

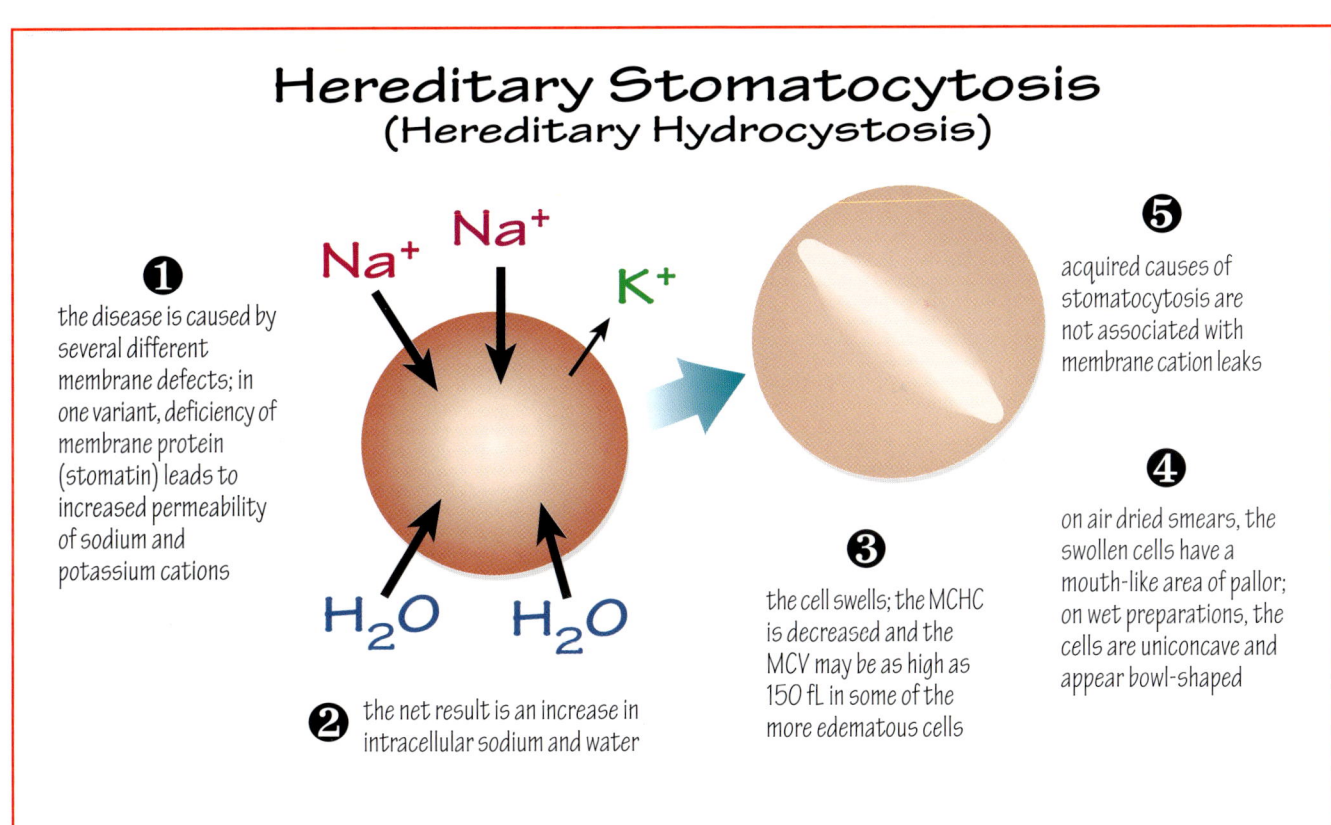

Erythrocytic Cells and Inclusions

Target Cell

SYNONYMS
  codocyte

VITAL STATISTICS
  size .... normocytic to slightly macrocytic
  cell shape .... round
  cytoplasm .... increased surface membrane to volume ratio results in a central darker hemoglobinized region within the area of central pallor; the result is the appearance of a target, bull's eye or "Mexican hat"

KEY DIFFERENTIATING FEATURES
  round cell with darker hemoglobinized region in middle of area of central pallor
  normocytic or slightly macrocytic

POTENTIAL LOOK-ALIKES
  normal erythrocyte
  microcyte
  various types of red cells containing polymerized or crystalized hemoglobin

ASSOCIATED DISEASE STATES AND CONDITIONS
  iron deficiency anemia
  thalassemia
  hemoglobinopathies (hemoglobin SS, C, SC, and E disease)
  post-splenectomy
  liver disease (especially obstructive jaundice)
  artifact of slow drying of blood smears or of samples with excessive EDTA anticoagulant (target cells appear numerous in some fields but rare in others)

The diversity of disease states in which target cells are found range from the serious inherited hemoglobinopathies to post-splenectomy; they may also be an artifact of smear preparation.

Target cells are quite distinctive in appearance, literally resembling their name, and in some respects may be considered the functional and morphologic opposite of spherocytes. Their formation results from an increased surface-to-volume ratio with the excess membrane "sinking" into the relatively less dense interior of the cell and then being pushed up at the cell's middle forming a bell-shape. This is the most efficient distribution of excess membrane. On a flat surface, the concavity becomes a central nipple of membrane into which hemoglobin redistributes. The denser center produces the targetoid appearance.

The cause of target cells may be broadly categorized as more membrane than normal (e.g., excessive membrane lipid deposition in liver disease) or less interior content than normal (e.g., thalassemia); in either case, the membrane:interior volume ratio of the erythrocyte is increased. Artifacts of air drying can also result in target cell formation. These various causes are discussed in the next section, *A Closer Look At…How Target Cells Form* on page 108.

Target cells demonstrate decreased lysis in the osmotic fragility test; their increased cell membrane allows greater intracellular fluid accumulation before lysis. Indeed, in some cases of B-thalassemia major, complete red cell lysis does not occur until they are incubated in distilled water (no saline).

Target Cells

|— 7 μm —|
size of normal red blood cell

increase in surface membrane relative to cell contents results in central condensation of hemoglobin

A-62 1986 (Blood, Wright-Giemsa, X400)

Identification	Referee %	Participant %
Target cell (codocyte)	100	99.4

This very striking example of a target cell is a straightforward identification. The central hemoglobinized area within the central pallor is unmistakable. This sample is from a 15-year-old black female who has no symptoms. Her hemoglobin shows the following: 11.9 g/dL, RBC 3.9 x 10^{12}/L, MCV 89 fL, MCH 30.5, WBC 6.5 x 10^9/L and platelets 220 x 10^9/L. The differential diagnosis would primarily include thalassemia and hemoglobinopathy. Hemoglobin electrophoresis is the confirmatory test.

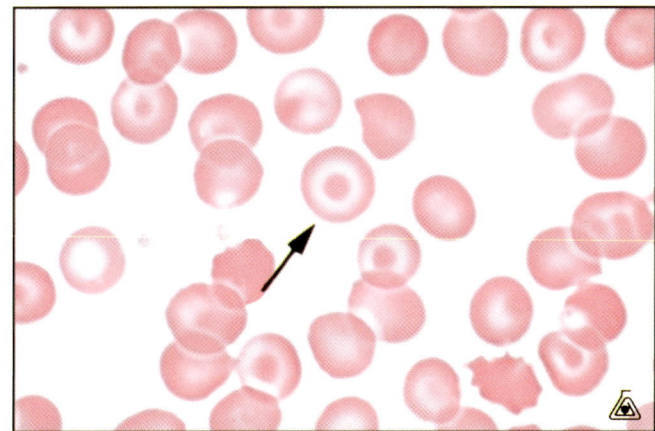

H-8 1979 (Blood, Wright-Giemsa, X360)

Identification	Referee %	Participant %
Target cell (codocyte)	99.5	100

The arrow points toward a small group of target cells. The central area of hemoglobinization is ringed by a clear area within the erythrocytes. Also in this photomicrograph are two nucleated red cells, a Howell-Jolly body (near the butt of the arrow), large erythrocytes with coloration suggesting polychromasia, and a possible spherocyte at the middle left edge. The central leukocyte is a segmented neutrophil.

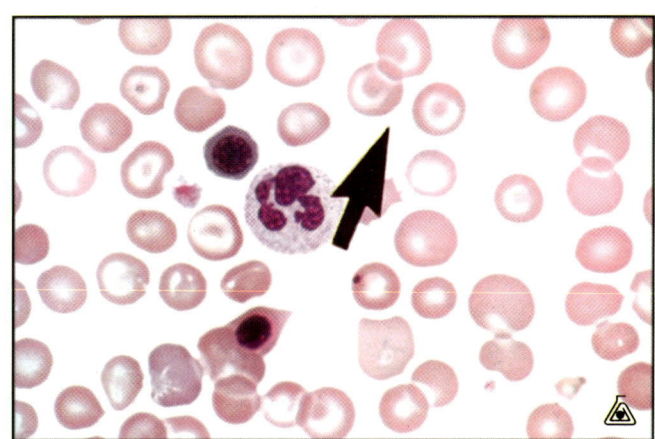

H-53 1980 (Blood, Wright-Giemsa, X400)

Identification	Referee %	Participant %
Target cell	100	99.5

The arrowed cell is a target cell. There are many such forms in this field. It appears, from the decreased number of erythrocytes present, that this person is anemic. The nucleated red blood cell present in the upper left corner of the field indicates there is a marrow response. Echinocytes are readily identified and there are hypochromic cells present as well.

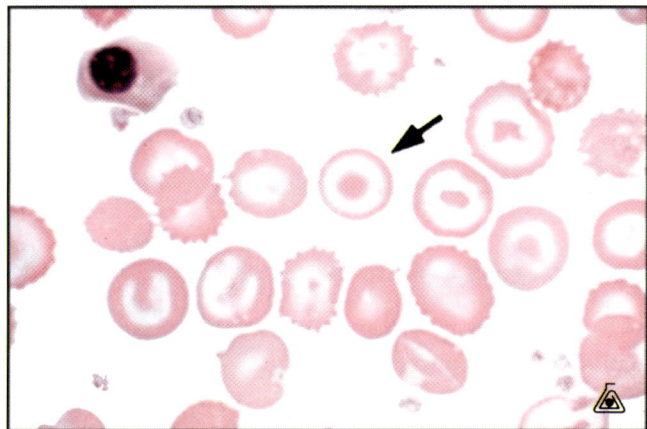

Erythrocytic Cells and Inclusions

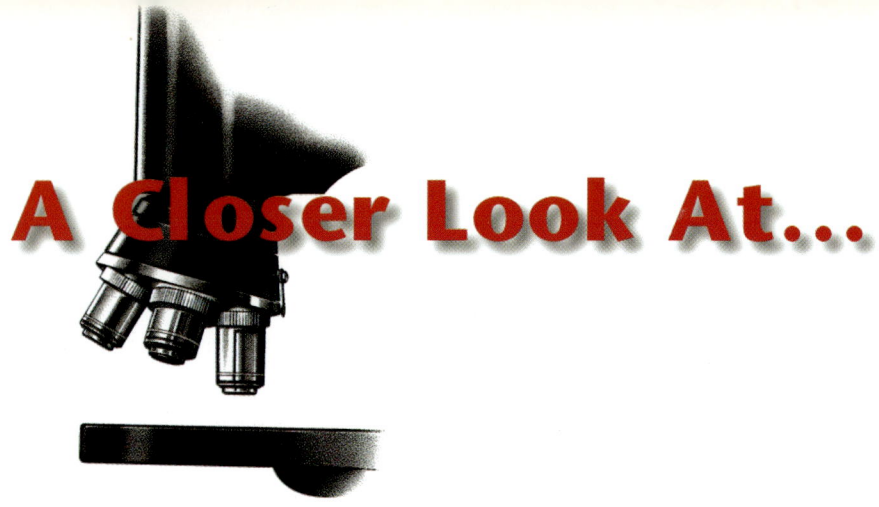

A Closer Look At...

How Target Cells Form

Target cells are also called codocytes, from the Greek term for "hat." In cell suspension, target cells have a morphology that has variously been referred to as a Greek helmet, Mexican hat, or bell-shaped.

The first illustration on the right shows normal and target cells as they appear fixed on a glass slide or circulating in the blood. They are divided into two types depending on the depth of their concavity. *Codocytes I* resemble soup plates; they have a shallow-concavity. *Codocytes II* have a deep concavity and resemble a hat. When they are spread out on a glass smear, the cells form a central "bump" of hemoglobin that gives them a target shape. This bump is due to that fact that the cells have more membrane than they should for the amount of hemoglobin inside.

Three groups of conditions are associated with target cell formation, illustrated in the second figure on the next page. It is important to remember that this grouping is a bit artifactual; target cell formation can be multifactorial.

In iron deficiency, thalassemia, and several hemoglobinopathies, the reduced hemoglobin content results in target cell formation. Depending on the disorder, other aberrant cells may be present. In sickle cell anemia, targets form due to a combination of asplenia and diminished solubility of hemoglobin S.

Abnormal plasma lipid composition can produce acquired membrane abnormalities. As discussed in the sections on acanthocytes (pages 64 and 66), the red cell membrane is a phospholipid-protein complex with about equal quantities of lipids and proteins. The lipids are in equilibrium with the surrounding plasma lipids. If the concentration of plasma lipids increases, the red cell membrane may acquire excess lipids. The result is an increase in the amount of membrane and therefore a relative decrease in hemoglobin content. Once again this results in an increase in the surface-to-volume ratio.

Liver disease can result in leptocyte, target cell, and acanthocyte formation. As plasma and therefore red cell membrane lipids increase, a leptocyte forms. Leptocytes are thin red blood cells with slightly more membrane than normal. They appear paler than normal red cells on blood smears and their center is colorless. As the membrane increases in amount, target cells form. In intrahepatic or extrahepatic *obstructive jaundice*, both cholesterol and phospholipids are increased in about the same proportion as that found in normal red cell membranes. The target cells are normocytic or macrocytic. In very severe liver disease—most commonly due to cirrhosis—large amounts of free cholesterol accumulate in the membrane, instead of both cholesterol and phospholipids. Projections and spikes form producing acanthocytes. The remodeling is helped along by the spleen. In *lecithin-cholesterol acyl transferase (LCAT) deficiency*—a rare autosomal recessive condition—cholesterol, phospholipids, and triglycerides accumulate in the blood. Large amounts of free (unesterified) cholesterol integrate into the red cell membrane producing target cells. After splenectomy, fragments of red cell membrane are no longer removed from reticulocytes. The excess membrane produces target cells.

Humidity and/or air drying of blood smears by waving them too slowly in the air (rather than using rapid arm movement or better yet, an electric fan) can produce artifactual target cells. Puddles of hemoglobin precipitate in the rim and center of the excessively broad and thin cells as water evaporates. Similarly, the very uniform targeting of hemoglobin C is due to central puddles of hemoglobin that form during drying because of decreased hemoglobin solubility.

Comparison of Target Cell Types

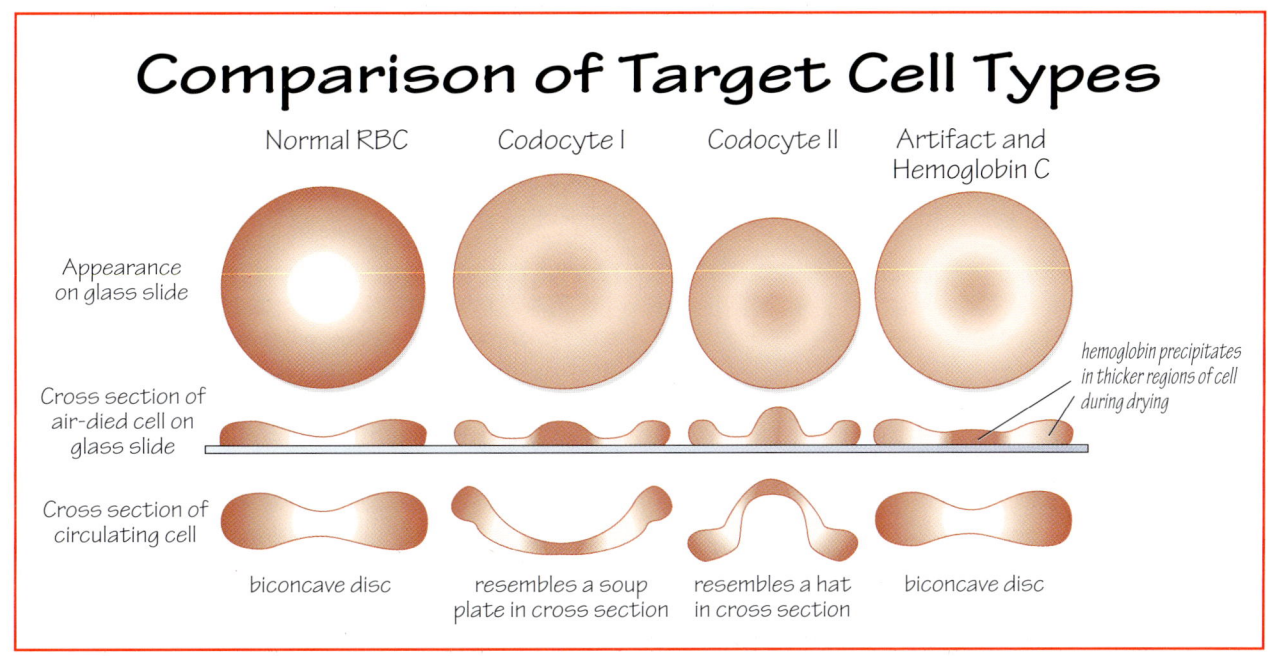

	Normal RBC	Codocyte I	Codocyte II	Artifact and Hemoglobin C
Appearance on glass slide				
Cross section of air-dried cell on glass slide				hemoglobin precipitates in thicker regions of cell during drying
Cross section of circulating cell	biconcave disc	resembles a soup plate in cross section	resembles a hat in cross section	biconcave disc

Three Causes of Target Cell Formation

Artifacts of Air-Drying and Hemoglobin Precipitation
Examples: high humidity, slow drying, and hemoglobin C

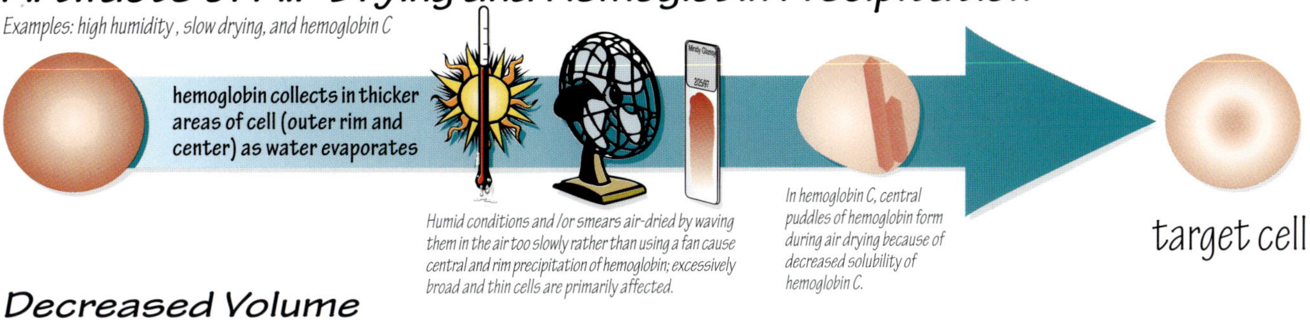

hemoglobin collects in thicker areas of cell (outer rim and center) as water evaporates

Humid conditions and/or smears air-dried by waving them in the air too slowly rather than using a fan cause central and rim precipitation of hemoglobin; excessively broad and thin cells are primarily affected.

In hemoglobin C, central puddles of hemoglobin form during air drying because of decreased solubility of hemoglobin C.

→ target cell

Decreased Volume
Examples: iron deficiency, thalassemia, and hemoglobinopathies (Hb S, E)

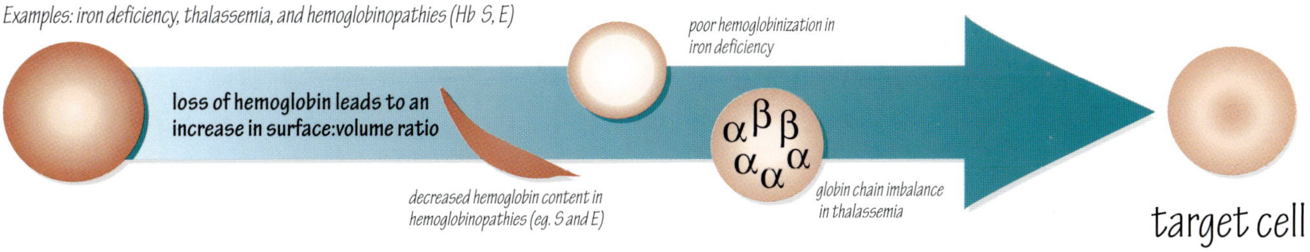

loss of hemoglobin leads to an increase in surface:volume ratio

decreased hemoglobin content in hemoglobinopathies (eg. S and E)

poor hemoglobinization in iron deficiency

globin chain imbalance in thalassemia

→ target cell

Increased Surface Membrane
Examples: liver disease (obstructive jaundice), LCAT deficiency, and asplenism

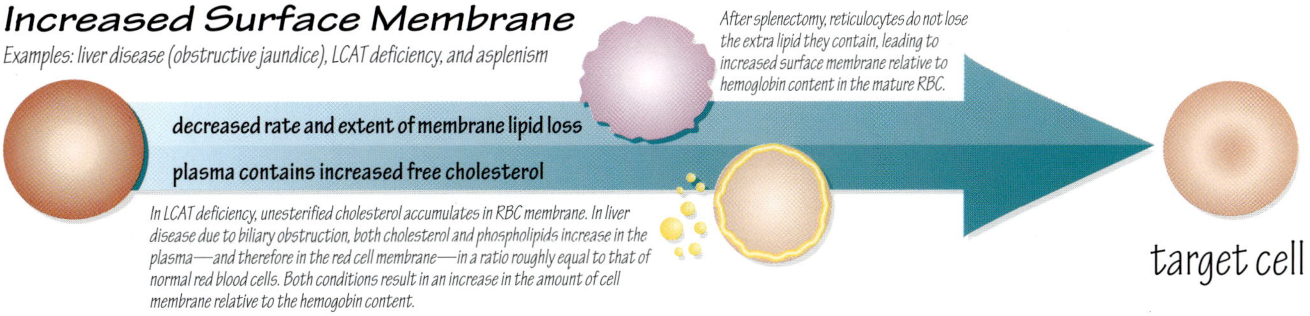

decreased rate and extent of membrane lipid loss

plasma contains increased free cholesterol

After splenectomy, reticulocytes do not lose the extra lipid they contain, leading to increased surface membrane relative to hemoglobin content in the mature RBC.

In LCAT deficiency, unesterified cholesterol accumulates in RBC membrane. In liver disease due to biliary obstruction, both cholesterol and phospholipids increase in the plasma—and therefore in the red cell membrane—in a ratio roughly equal to that of normal red blood cells. Both conditions result in an increase in the amount of cell membrane relative to the hemogobin content.

→ target cell

Erythrocytic Cells and Inclusions

Teardrop Cell

SYNONYMS
dacryocyte

VITAL STATISTICS
size .... microcytic to normocytic
cell shape .... teardrop or pear shape with a single, short or long, blunted or rounded end or tail
cytoplasm .... normochromic to hypochromic

KEY DIFFERENTIATING FEATURES
teardrop or pear-shaped red blood cell
unipolar tapered end with a blunt tip

POTENTIAL LOOK-ALIKES
oval macrocytes
ovalocytes
fragmented cells
sickle cells

ASSOCIATED DISEASE STATES AND CONDITIONS
myelofibrosis
myelofibrosis with myeloid metaplasia
pernicious anemia
anemia of renal disease
hemolytic anemia
thalassemia
bone marrow infiltration by hematologic or non-hematologic malignancy
artifact of slide preparation (usually all of the teardrop cells in an area are lined up, with tails pointing in the same direction)

Teardrop is the appropriate description for this abnormally shaped erythrocyte. One side of the cell is elongated with a blunt or round tip. The cell may also resemble a pear. The tip is never short and pointed, which is an artifactual change. Cell size is variable; most are normocytic but some are smaller than their normal counterparts. They may have increased or a normal complement of central pallor.

These cells are often associated with an abnormal spleen or bone marrow, where the erythrocytes must stretch to successfully negotiate their way out to the circulation. It may take minutes for the erythrocyte to move through abnormal splenic cords, and when this occurs over many circulations, the cell is permanently deformed. Likewise, an erythrocyte with an inclusion (such as may occur in thalassemia) may become teardrop-shaped when passing through splenic cords, since the abnormal hemoglobin will be pitted out when massed. In the bone marrow, a similar process for erythrocytes occurs as they travel through marrow sinuses. Thus, disease states with abnormal splenic (myelofibrosis with myeloid metaplasia, thalassemia, hemolytic anemia) or bone marrow function/structure (myelofibrosis, pernicious anemia, anemia of renal disease, infiltration of marrow by malignancy) demonstrate teardrop cells. Proof of the spleen's involvement in teardrop formation is their prompt disappearance after splenectomy.

An important caveat is that teardrop cells may also be artifactual due to an improperly made smear. It is usually obvious since there are many teardrops with their tails lined up, pointing in the same direction.

Teardrop Cells

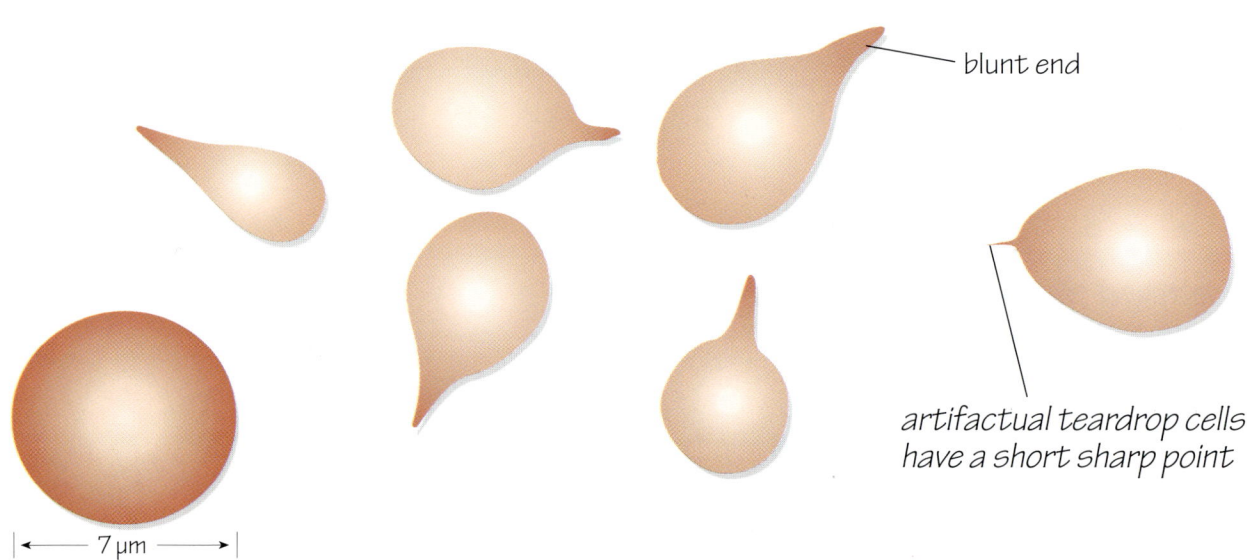

blunt end

artifactual teardrop cells have a short sharp point

7 μm — size of normal red blood cell

Erythrocytic Cells and Inclusions

XL-49, 1987 (Blood, Wright-Giemsa, X400)

Identification	Referee %	Participant %
Teardrop cell	100	99.1

The two arrowed teardrop cells are a straightforward identification. Notice the tapered end and the blunt tip. True teardrop cells never have short, pointed tails. This sample also indicates a decrease in erythrocytes (hemoglobin of 8.5 g/dL) and apparent microcytes. This 62-year-old man had a cough and difficulty breathing as well as a history of heavy smoking. This history raises the speculation of a primary lung malignancy with metastasis to the bone marrow as the cause of the circulating teardrop erythrocytes. The lone leukocyte in the upper right corner is a band neutrophil. Platelets are not remarkable.

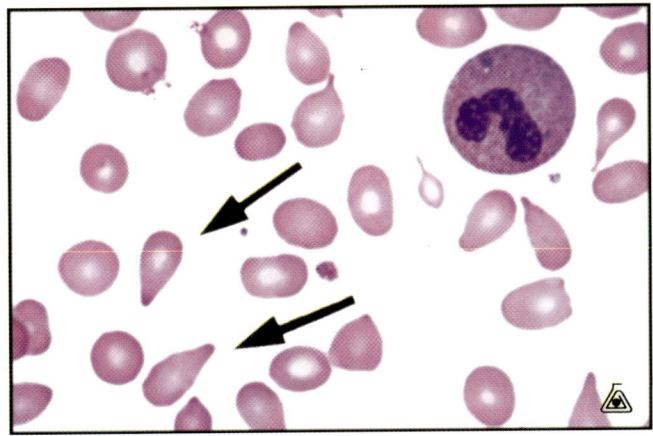

H-50, 1980 (Blood, Wright-Giemsa, X360)

Identification	Referee %	Participant %
Tear-drop cell	100	99.4

The arrowed teardrop cell poses no difficulty in identification. The cell has a long tail that is gradually tapered and ends in a blunt tip. In addition, the slide is also notable for a decrease in erythrocytes as well as the presence of microcytes and possibly stomatocytes; the latter may be artifactual in nature.

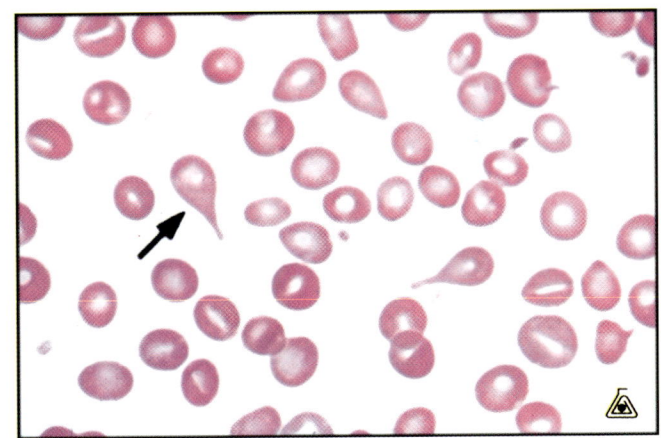

HE-39, 1994 (Blood, Wright-Giemsa, X400)

Cell	Referees %	Participants %
Teardrop cell (dacrocyte)	96.6	99.5

The teardrop cell is easily identified. Other abnormalities in this field include the following: microcytes, a fragmented cell, spherocytes, and macrocytes (erythrocytes at least as large as the normal lymphocyte at mid-field). All of these findings are compatible with the history of vitamin B_{12} deficiency in an 83-year-old female. Her initial hemoglobin was 5.0 g/dL, MCV was 132 fL, and she demonstrated increasing dementia and confusion. Of interest, she refused blood transfusion but allowed daily vitamin B_{12} injections; the smear was made on day 6 of treatment. Thus, the lack of polychromatophilic cells is somewhat surprising, although the hemoglobin had increased to 9.2 g/dL and the MCV fallen to 110 fL.

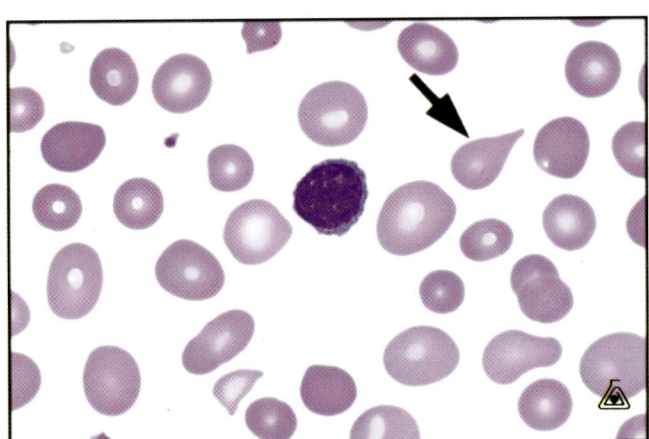

Erythrocytic Cells and Inclusions

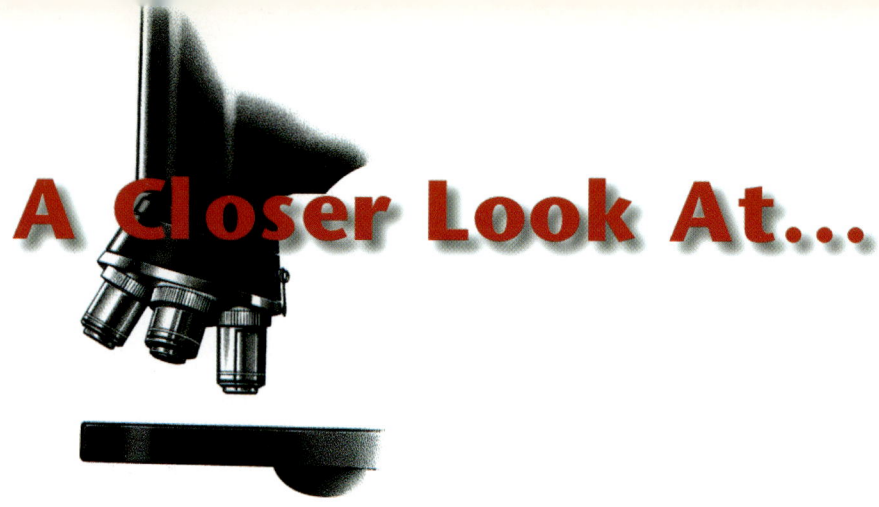

A Closer Look At...

How Teardrop Cells Form

In teardrop cell formation, as in the formation of many other poikilocytes, it is the erythrocyte's deformability that is severely challenged. In this case, it is not only the spleen, but also the bone marrow which must be successfully negotiated by a red cell which may or may not be normal. In addition, the spleen and/or bone marrow may itself be abnormal (e.g., idiopathic myelofibrosis), and cause such a prolonged transit time for the erythrocyte that its end result is a permanently deformed state. Thus, the distinctive teardrop-shaped erythrocyte is found in a wide spectrum of disorders, both primarily hematopoietic and those in which the bone marrow is secondarily involved.

It is a fairly straightforward concept to understand how teardrop cells are formed when they have an inclusion that is removed in the spleen or when an abnormality exists in splenic or marrow vasculature (see diagrams, opposite page). Non-deformable red cell inclusions, such as Heinz bodies or Howell-Jolly bodies, cannot pass through the narrow slits in the basement membrane separating the splenic cords and sinuses. The deformable red cell can squeeze through, and in the process of pulling and tugging several things can happen. First, the inclusion may be ripped from the cell, leaving a defect we recognize as a bite (see page 71). Second, the cell may reseal itself into a normal erythrocyte after the spleen pits out the inclusion. Third, the stretched red cell, working to free itself from the trapped inclusion, may become permanently deformed into a teardrop shape; this depends on the duration and degree of distortion the cell must endure. The latter process may create teardrop cells even when no inclusion bodies exist. This happens when the vasculature in the spleen and bone marrow is abnormal. Bone marrow fibrosis, for example, can distort the endothelial-lined sinuses to such a degree that normal red cells have a difficult time squeezing through. They may be stretched to an abnormal length for extended periods of time. It is inevitable that a small amount of red cell membrane is lost in the process. Repeated episodes lead to permanent tapering of the cell into a teardrop form.

Explaining the presence of teardrop cells in pernicious anemia may be a bit more complex. The macrocytes in this disorder have a large volume, much greater than normal erythrocytes. Thus, they are likely to intrinsically have a more difficult time in transit through both marrow and splenic sinuses, somewhat like an obese person putting on a pair of pants that are one size too small. By the time the macrocyte is finished traveling through the sinuses it has been permanently deformed, with a teardrop shape as the permanent signature of its difficult transit.

Two Causes of Teardrop Cell Formation

RBC Inclusion and Pitting Function of Spleen
Examples: Howell-Jolly bodies, Heinz-body anemias, and thalassemias (associated with alpha chain inclusion bodies and H bodies)

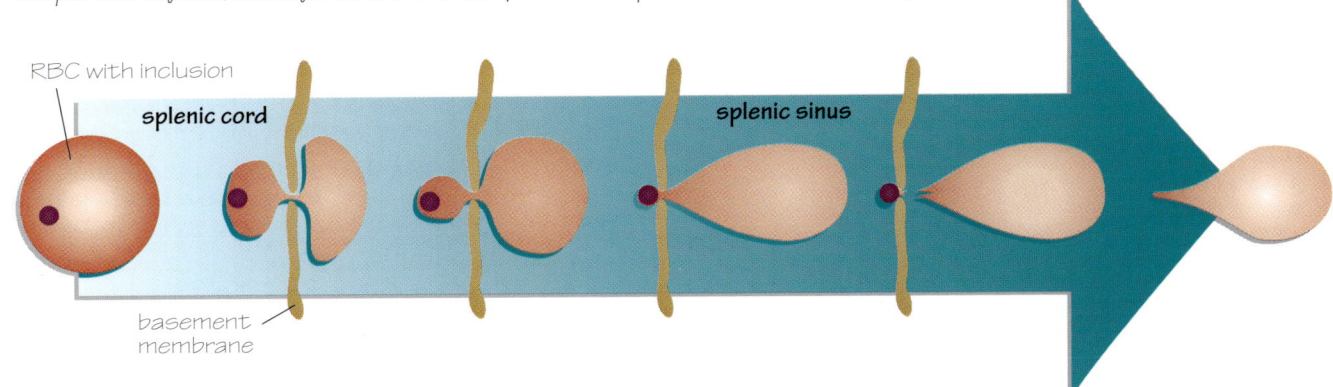

red cell containing inclusion squirms through slit in basement membrane that separates splenic cord and sinus

red cell stretched to abnormal length as end with inclusion is torn away; the degree and/or duration of distortion results in permanent damage to membrane

red cell loses its deformability at stretched end, forming teardrop shape

Normal RBC and Abnomal Vasculature in Spleen and Bone Marrow
Examples: idiopathic myelofibrosis (agnogenic myeloid metaplasia) and infiltrative myopathy (metastatic carcinoma to bone marrow)

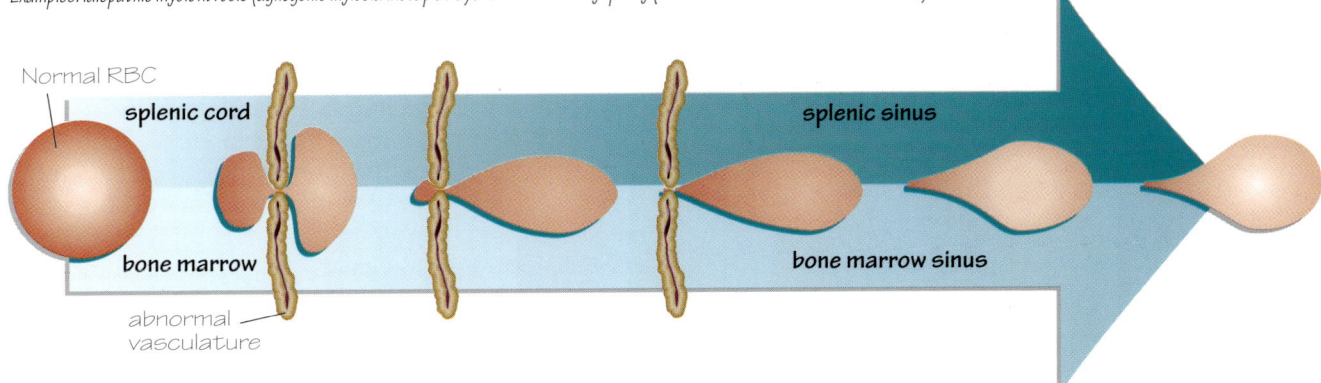

normal red cell attempts to squeeze through distored intermedullary vasculature of spleen and bone marrow

red cell stretched to abnormal length for long periods of time; a small amount of cell membrane is depleted as it finally squeezes through opening

repetition causes gradual loss of membrane leading to tapering and teardrop formation

Erythrocytic Cells and Inclusions

Reticulocyte (Supravital Stain)

SYNONYMS
none

VITAL STATISTICS
- size .... slightly larger than normal mature erythrocyte
- cell shape .... round
- cytoplasm .... blue to green, with precipitated RNA occurring as a dark network of varying amount

KEY DIFFERENTIATING FEATURES
- at least two dark purple granules visible after supravital staining (new methylene blue or brilliant cresyl blue)
- usually a network of dark fibrillar and granular material visible
- often larger than surrounding mature red cells

POTENTIAL LOOK-ALIKES
- Heinz bodies
- hemoglobin H crystals
- stain precipitate and dirt overlying red cell

ASSOCIATED DISEASE STATES AND CONDITIONS
- newborns
- after acute blood loss
- bone marrow stress conditions including various hemolytic anemias
- recovery of marrow after cytoreduction (e.g., chemotherapy)

The reticulocyte stage begins with the extrusion of the normblast nucleus and ends with the loss of cytoplasmic organelles. (See illustration page 165). As mitochrondria are dismantled and ribosomes degraded, the reticulocyte assumes a disk shape and circulates as a mature red cell.

Reticulocytes mature in the bone marrow for 48 hours and then in the blood for another day. On Wright-Giemsa stains, they have a bluish tinge (polychromasia). They are more accurately recognized using a supravital stain (for living, nonfixed cells), usually new methylene blue or brilliant cresyl blue, which stains the remaining RNA, golgi complex, and mitochondria in the cytoplasm. After staining, the ribosomes and organelles agglutinate into a network which varies with the age of reticulocyte; younger cells have a more pronounced "substantia reticulofilamentosa" which appears as granular deposits connected by a precipitated ribosomal meshwork of variable length. Reticulocytes normally represent about 1% of circulating erythrocytes.

Enumeration of such cells as a percentage of all red cells is the basis of the classical rectulocyte count, a valuable measure of red cell production in the bone marrow. Such testing may obviate the need for the more invasive bone marrow study and will indicate the appropriateness of the marrow's response to blood loss, response to chemotherapeutic agents, or other toxins.

Unfortunately, the accuracy of the reticulocyte count by manual methods is rather variable. This is due to many factors, from staining, to agreement on what actually constitutes a reticulocyte, to the method of counting. Additionally, the artifacts encountered in such testing may interfere. Automated methodologies do offer the prospect of not only increasing accuracy but also of determining the maturation of red cells (Maturation Index) and giving accurate absolute numbers of reticulocytes. In studies where such methodology was used, it was found predictive of marrow recovery after chemotherapy. The automation may involve use of a supravital dye or another, fluorescent dye, and enumeration by either electronic or laser light; the number of cells counted is much greater than a manual determination.

Reticulocytes (supravital stain)

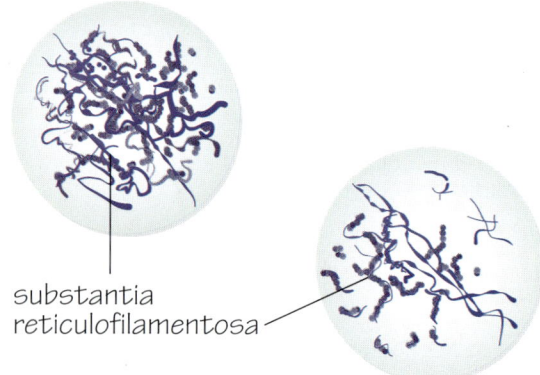

substantia reticulofilamentosa

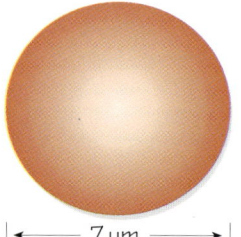

|← 7 μm →|

size of normal red blood cell

amount of precipitated RNA varies with the age of the reticulocyte

this is an older reticulocyte, with little RNA remaining

HE-42, 1995 (Blood, New Methylene Blue, X325)

Identification	Referee %	Participant %
Reticulocyte	100	98.7
Basophilic Stippling	-	0.5

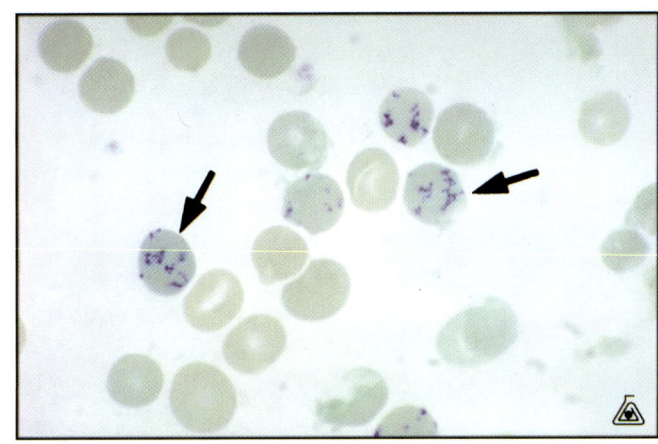

The patient history of chronic alcohol abuse and liver failure largely explains the given hemoglobin of 9.2 g/dL. The marrow was still able to respond to the anemia as evidenced by these reticulocytes. A supravital stain, to determine characteristics in living cells, must be used; new methylene blue was used here. Indicative of a late erythrocyte, this network is composed of a minimum of two of these purple-blue-black granules. Such granules are the remnants of the cell's hemoglobin production factory (mitochondria, Golgi complex, centriole, ribosomes). The arrowed cells do not represent basophilic stippling which is smaller (even smaller than hemoglobin H inclusions) and more punctate. Basophilic stippling is demonstrable with Wright-Giemsa stain as well as supravital stains.

H1-8, 1989 (Blood, Brilliant Cresyl Blue, X325)

Identification	Referee %	Participant %
Reticulocyte	77.8	68.4
Heinz body	16.7	18
Hemoglobin H inclusions	5.6	9.5

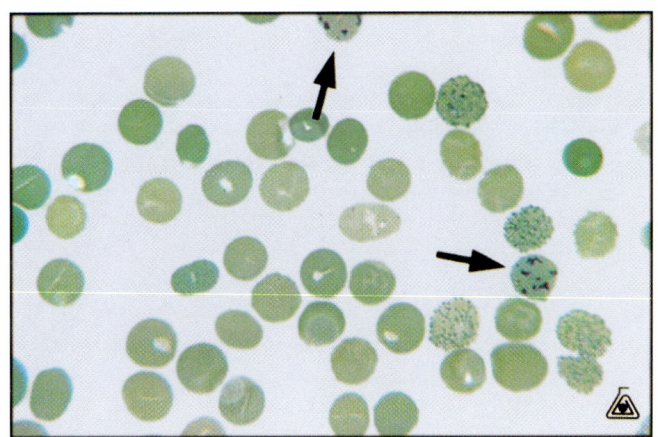

The patient is a Filipino male with hemoglobin H disease. This is a brilliant cresyl blue stain, a supravital stain that stains hemoglobin H inclusions, reticulocytes, and Heinz bodies. The two arrowed cells are reticulocytes. Compared to hemoglobin H inclusions, they are darker blue in color and appear as multiple medium-size granules in the interior of the cell, sometimes connected by a reticular network. Hemoglobin H inclusions are seen in other cells in the field; they are small, pale blue, and are evenly distributed, reminiscent of a "dimpled golf ball." Heinz bodies are much larger, darker blue, and are usually attached to the red cell membrane.

A-9, 1984 (Blood, New Methylene Blue, X325)

Identification	Referee %	Participant %
Reticulocyte	100	96.4

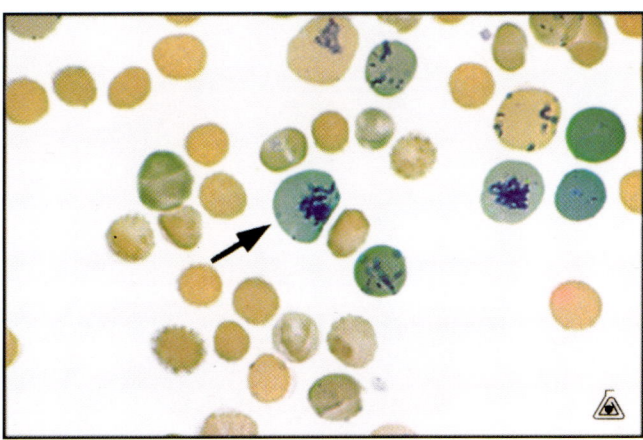

The large arrowed cell is a reticulocyte, stained with the supravital stain new methylene blue. Other similar cells are readily identified. They all contain a network of dark blue granular material representing precipitated RNA and other organelles. Young red cells, just after their nucleus is extruded, still contain the cytoplasmic machinery responsible for hemoglobin production. Reticulocytes mature in the bone marrow for approximately 48 hours before entering the blood stream. Maturation continues there for another 24 hours. Prior to removal by the spleen, these organelles are readily visible after supravital staining. The more "substantia reticulofilamentosa" that is present, the younger is the reticulocyte.

Basophilic Stippling (Coarse)

SYNONYMS
punctate basophilia

VITAL STATISTICS
size .... granulations of variable size, <0.5 µm in diameter
appearance .... deep blue or blue-gray; distributed throughout red cell cytoplasm
composition .... aggregated ribosomes and polyribosomes

KEY DIFFERENTIATING FEATURES
numerous small coarse granules
homogeneous distrubtion throughout red cell cytoplasm
deep blue or blue-gray color
easily seen after Wright-Giemsa staining (unlike fine stippling which is an artifact of drying and is more dust-like and almost imperceptible)

POTENTIAL LOOK-ALIKES
Pappenheimer bodies
stain precipitate and other artifacts
Howell-Jolly bodies
hemoglobin H inclusions
bacteria and fungi
karyorrhectic leukocytes

ASSOCIATED DISEASE STATES AND CONDITIONS
lead poisoning
thalassemia
refractory anemia
sideroblastic anemia
megaloblastic anemia (B_{12} or folate deficiency)
sickle cell anemia

Basophilic stippling consists of numerous, evenly distributed granules within the cytoplasm of red blood cells. The inclusions may be either fine or coarse.

Fine stippling is seen in reticulocytes and is an artifact of slow air drying. It is barely discernible in the red cell and is not of any clinical consequence. The red cell is usually larger and polychromatophilic compared to other normal cells in the field without stippling.

Course stippling, on the other hand, is clinically significant and suggests impaired hemoglobin synthesis. The punctation is readily visible and made up of relatively evenly distributed blue-gray granules. For CAP proficiency testing purposes, only coarse basophilic stippling should be identified.

Coarse stippling results from abnormal aggregates of ribosomes and polyribosomes in reticulocytes. In conditions such as lead intoxication and thalassemia, the altered reticulocyte ribosomes have a greater propensity to aggregate. Iron-containing mitochondria and siderosomes in the aggregates may further accentuate the stippling. The mechanics behind this process is detailed in the following *A Closer Look At...* section on page 118.

Coarse Basophilic Stippling

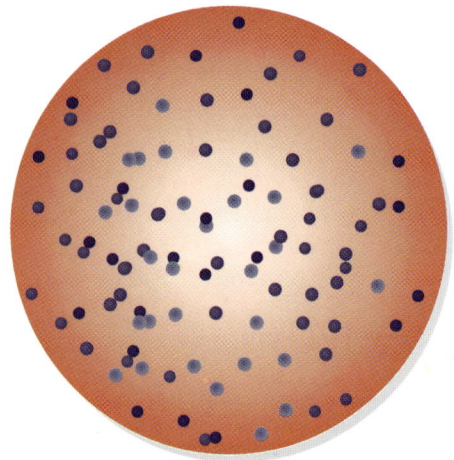

Fine Basophilic Stippling

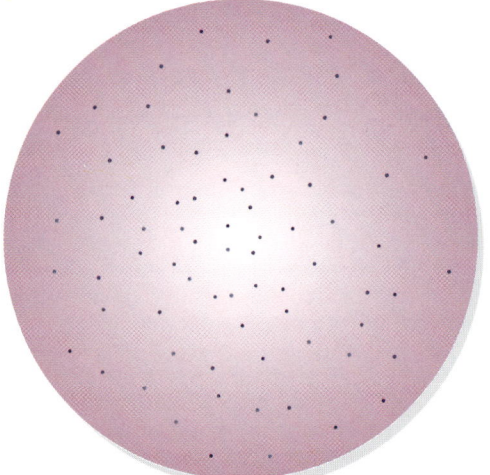

usually larger and polychromatophilic compared to normal red blood cell

HE-06 1996 (Blood, Wright-Giemsa, X400)

Identification	Referee %	Participant %
Basophilic stippling	100	98.5

The cell of interest is a red blood cell which demonstrates coarse basophilic stippling. The small red cell inclusions represents ribosomal RNA which is precipitated during staining. The coarse blue granules are distributed throughout the red cell cytoplasm in a random manner. Coarse stippling is associated with pathologic conditions such as thalassemia, hemoglobinopathies, heavy metal (lead) poisoning, and sideroblastic anemia.

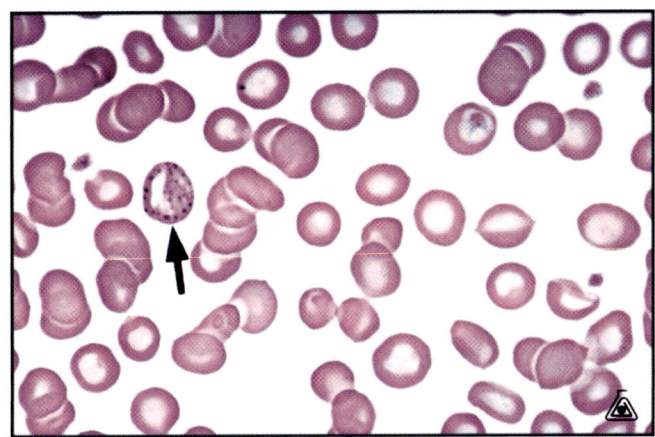

HE-37, 1996 (Blood, Wright-Giemsa, X400)

Identification	Referee %	Participant %
Basophilic stippling (coarse)	100	98.3
Pappenheimer body (Wright stain)	-	0.5

The case is from a 38-year-old female admitted to the hospital with abdominal pain, weakness, headache, and paresthesias. WBC = 6,800 x 10^6/L; Hgb = 7.8 g/dL; MCV 85 fL. A diagnosis of lead poisoning was made. The anemia of lead poisoning is usually normocytic but may be microcytic. Course basophilic stippling is readily identified. The arrowed cell contains numerous small, evenly distributed granular inclusions. A second stippled cell is located in the upper left corner. The inclusions are too numerous and evenly distributed to be Pappenheimer bodies.

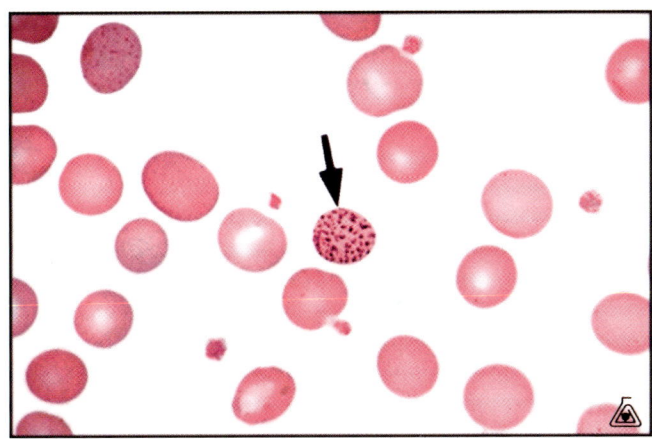

HE-08, 1994 (Blood, Wright-Giemsa, X400)

Identification	Referee %	Participant %
Basophilic stippling (coarse)	100	98.3
Reticulocyte	-	0.5
Pappenheimer body (Wright stain)	-	0.3

The case is from a 60-year-old female with agnogenic myeloid metaplasia (idiopathic myelofibrosis with myeloid metaplasia). The small arrowed red blood cell displays coarse basophilic stippling. The cytoplasm contains small, dark, blue-purple granules that are evenly dispersed. Pappenheimer bodies are small angular green-blue inclusions. They are single or form a small group. They are never as numerous or as evenly distributed as the granular inclusions of basophilic stippling. The leukocyte in the field is an abnormal megakaryocyte. The pink, granular cytoplasm forms small blunt projections. Nuclear chromatin is smudged and clumped. It is not a megakaryocyte nucleus because the cytoplasm is too abundant.

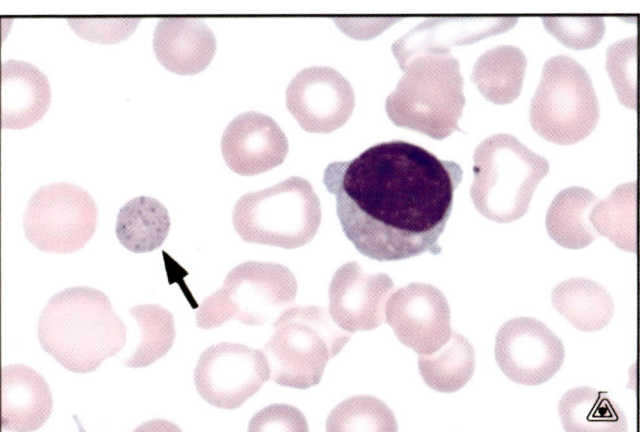

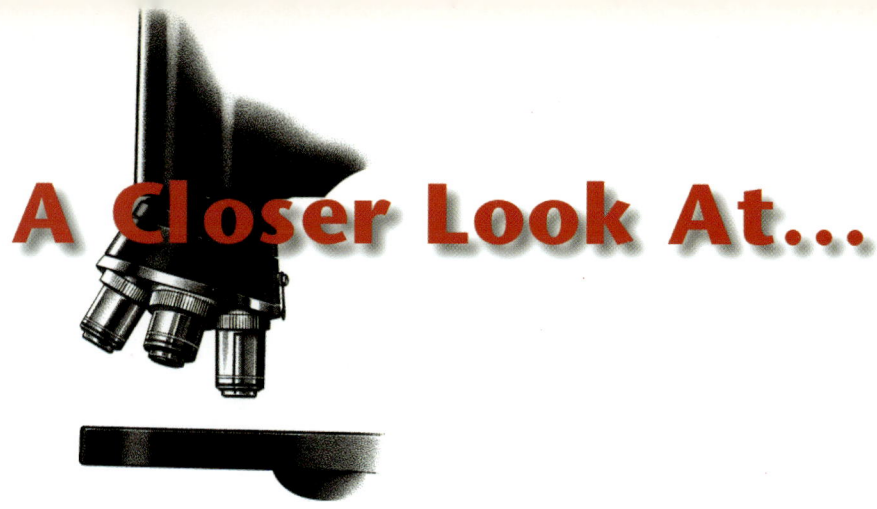

A Closer Look At...

How Basophilic Stippling Forms

Reticulocytes contain the machinery for hemoglobin production. With the nucleus gone, this machinery is no longer needed; it is gradually expelled over the next several days as the cell matures.

One component of the hemoglobin factory are RNA-containing ribosomes and polyribosomes. As the red cell matures, the RNA is broken down into nucleotides. Residual RNA is found only in the very youngest reticulocytes and then only in very small amounts.

In pathologic states, RNA degradation may be incomplete or the ribosomes themselves abnormal. If RNA degradation is impaired, red cells containing large amounts of RNA will be present in the circulation.

Wright-Giemsa stain is capable of precipitating RNA, but it is not very efficient at it and there is too little RNA in normal reticulocytes to produce any visible results. Supravital stains such as new methylene blue or brilliant cresyl violet can precipitate even very small amounts of RNA and thus are much better at staining and identifying reticulocytes.

In certain pathologic conditions, ribosomes are abnormal and the RNA degradation is imparied. If the amount of RNA is great enough, Wright-Giemsa staining can precipitate it and the result is coarse basophilic stippling.

Coarse basophilic stippling is never a normal finding and always indicates the presence of some form of abnormal hemoglobin production. Lead poisoning is the classic example.

Two Types of Basophilic Stippling

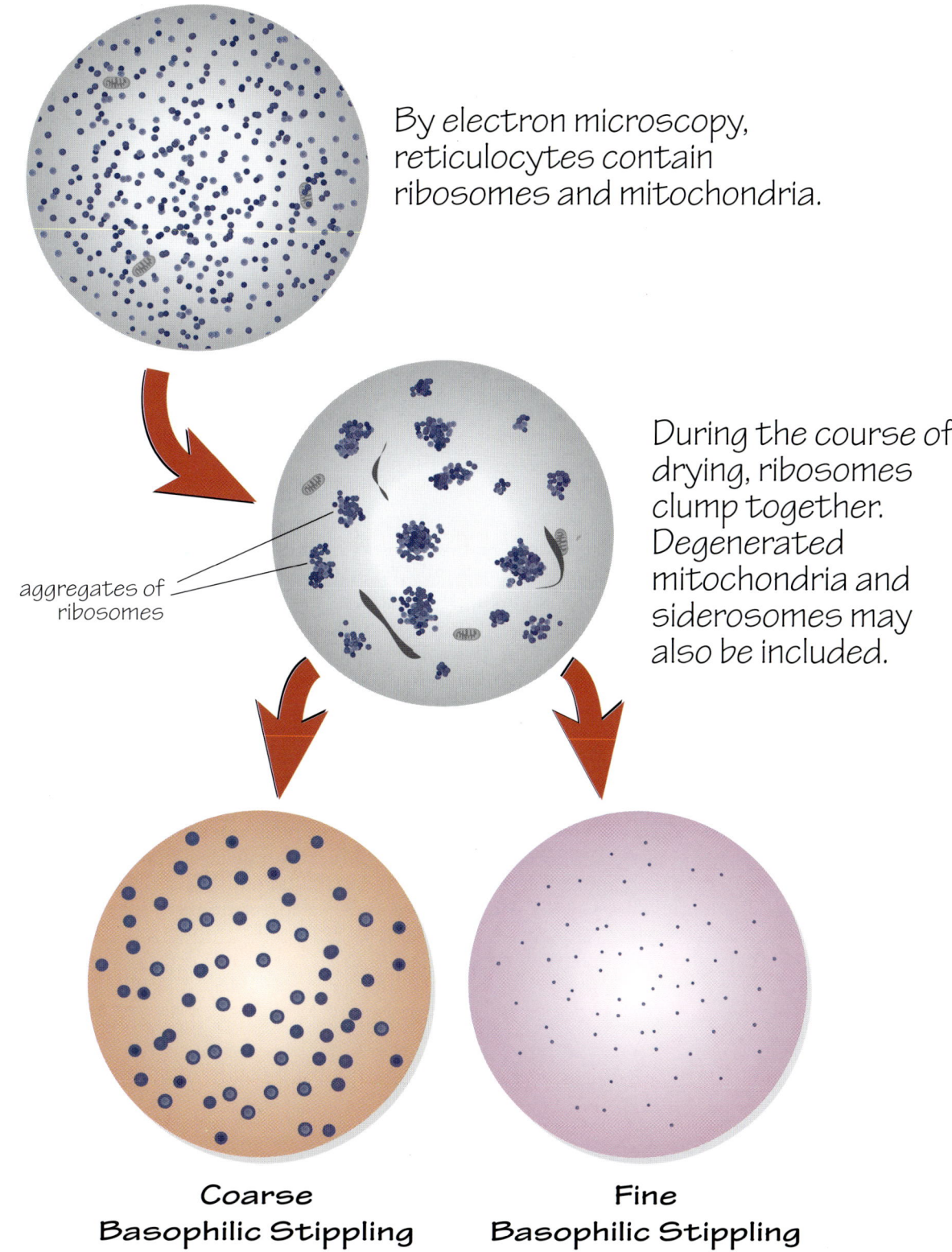

By electron microscopy, reticulocytes contain ribosomes and mitochondria.

During the course of drying, ribosomes clump together. Degenerated mitochondria and siderosomes may also be included.

aggregates of ribosomes

Coarse Basophilic Stippling

Fine Basophilic Stippling

In lead poisoning and thalassemia, the altered reticulocyte ribosomes have a greater propensity to aggregate, forming larger granules. This is referred to as *coarse basophilic stippling*. Iron-containing mitochondria in the aggregates may further accentuate the stippling.

Erythrocytic Cells and Inclusions

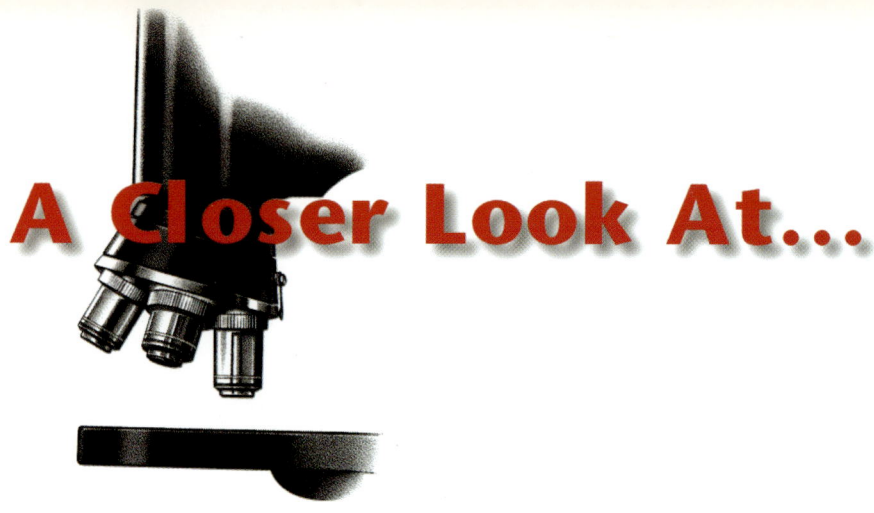

A Closer Look At...

Red Cell Inclusions

The various intraerythrocyte inclusions are compared and summarized in the table on the next page. Note that not all of the inclusions are visible by Wright-Giemsa staining; some require iron stain (siderocytes and sideroblasts) or supravital dyes (Heinz bodies, hemoglobin H, and reticulocytes) for visualization. The two pages following the table illustrate the differences between Wright-Giemsa and supravital staining. When identifying cells for CAP proficiency testing, note the stain used in the photomicrograph; that can be a helpful clue to diagnosis.

The majority of pathologic red cell inclusions are found primarily in young red blood cells (reticulocytes). The inclusions represent nuclear or cytoplasmic remnants derived from the latter stages of erythroid development in the bone marrow. Howell-Jolly bodies are nuclear fragments, Cabot rings are remnants of the mitotic spindle, basophilic stippling represents aggregates of ribosomes, and Pappenheimer bodies are iron-containing autophagosomes.

Prussian blue reaction is used to stain hemosiderin, ferritin, and iron-containing micelles blue. It identifies iron-containing inclusions called siderosomes in nucleated and non-nucleated red blood cells (called sideroblasts and siderocytes respectively). The stain also allows for the confirmation of Pappenheimer bodies and the identification of iron-containing micelles in mitochondria (the basis for ringed sideroblasts).

It is important to differentiate real intraerythrocyte inclusions from artifacts. Poorly made smears can result in stain precipitate, bubbles, and dirt on the slide that can mimic basophilic stippling, Howell-Jolly bodies, and Pappenheimer bodies. Platelets overlying red blood cells can be mistaken for malarial parasites (see page 292).

Comparison of Erythrocyte Inclusions

Inclusion	Constituent	Appearance Wright-Giemsa	Associated Clinical Conditions
Basophilic Stippling (coarse)	precipitate of ribosomes and polyribosomes	punctate blue granules	thalassemias, lead poisoning, myelodysplasias, sideroblastic anemias, congenital dyserythropoietic anemias
Howell-Jolly Body	nuclear fragment (DNA)	round blue granules, 1 μm in diameter, at periphery of cell; usually single but may be multiple (esp. in megaloblastic anemia)	hyposplenic conditions, absent spleen, severe hemolytic anemia, megaloblastic anemia
Pappenheimer Body	iron containing autophagosomes	blue-purple granules at periphery of cell, <1 μm in diameter, sometimes <0.5 μm; may form doublets; DNA stain (Feulgen) negative, iron stain positive	absent spleen, megaloblastic anemia, sideroblastic anemias, thalassemias, hemolytic anemias, congenital dyserythropoietic anemias
Siderosome	iron	usually invisible; designated Pappenheimer body if visible by Wright-Giemsa stain	normal finding in bone marrow; same conditions as Pappenheimer body
Heinz Body	denatured hemoglobin	invisible (visible with supravital stains only)	unstable hemoglobinopathies, oxidant drugs, severe alcoholic liver disease
H Bodies	denatured hemoglobin (excess β chains)	invisible (visible with supravital stains only)	alpha thalassemia (triple α gene deletion)
Alpha Chain Inclusion Bodies	denatured hemoglobin (excess α chains)	invisible (visible with supravital stains only)	beta thalassemia major
Cabot Rings	remnants of mitotic spindle	red-purple thread like rings	megaloblastic anemia, severe anemia, leukemia, lead poisoning, other causes of dyserythropoiesis
Crystals	hemoglobin C	dark pink to red rods; hexagagonal or pointed crystalloid structures	hemoglobin C, hemoglobin SC
Bacteria	bacteria	artifactual inclusion; bacteria adhere to surface of cell, but appear to be inside	sepsis; adherence to red cell membrane most pronounced in Bartonellosis
Parasites	variable	variable; see specific descriptions of malaria and babesia organisms	malaria, babesiosis
Mauer's Dots	malarial pigment	coarse violet granules that vary greatly in size	*Plasmodium falciparum* infection
Schüffner's Dots	malarial pigment	fine reddish granules	*Plasmodium vivax* infection
Nucleus	DNA	round or lobated, sometimes fragmented; rosette forms suggest dysplasia	stress erythrocytosis, myelodysplasias, myeloproliferative disorders, leukoerythroblastic conditions especially bone marrow fibrosis (myelophthisis)
Artifacts	variable (organisms, bubbles, dirt, stain, platelets, etc.)	variable; structures overlay red cells and mimic intracellular inclusions	no specific disease states; due to poorly made blood smears or improper air drying

Comparison of Wright-Giemsa and Supravital Staining of Selected Red Cell Inclusions

	Wright-Giemsa Stain	Supravital Stain
Reticulocyte		
Basophilic Stippling		
Pappenheimer Body		

Comparison of Wright-Giemsa and Supravital Staining of Selected Red Cell Inclusions

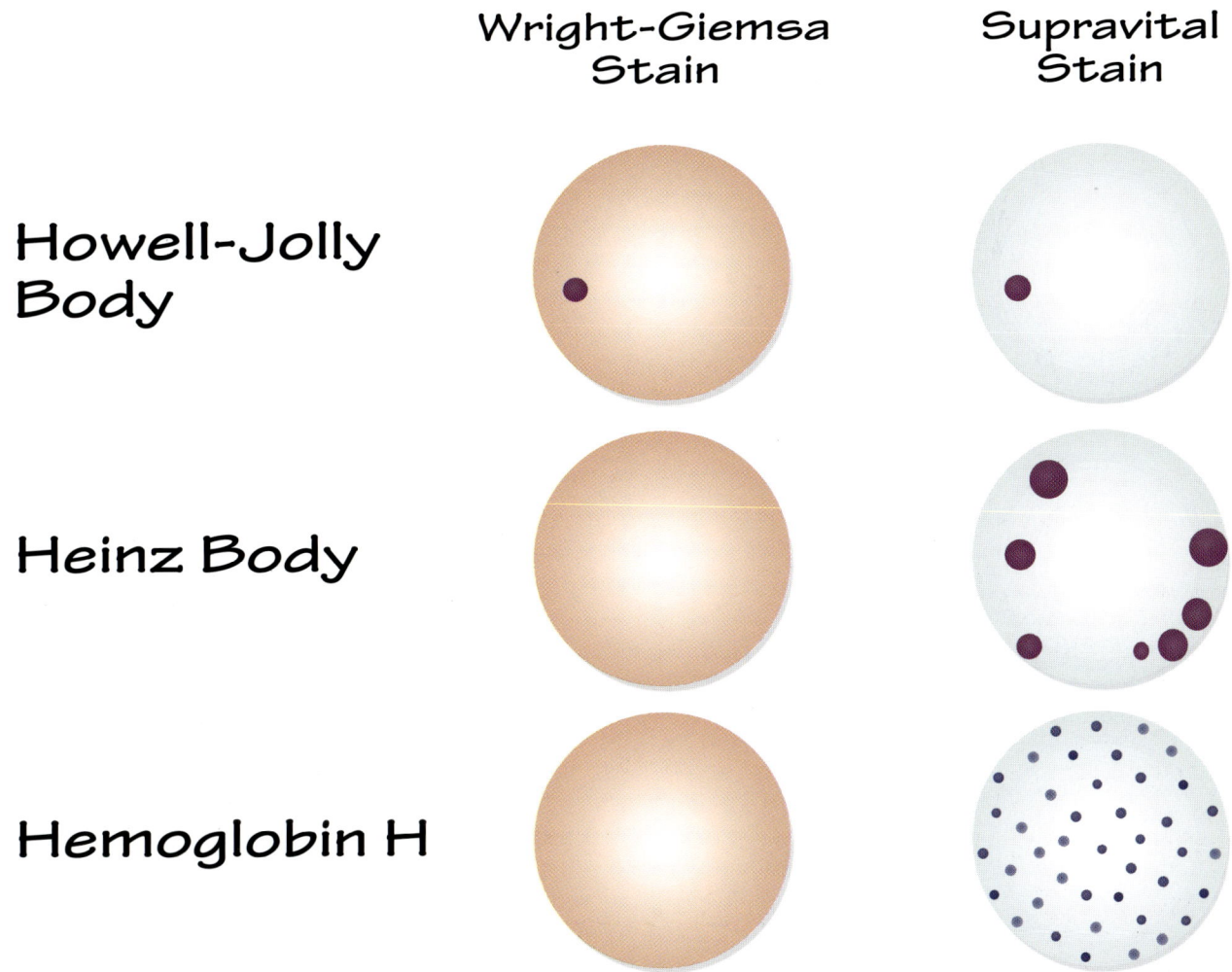

Erythrocytic Cells and Inclusions

Heinz Body

SYNONYMS
none

VITAL STATISTICS
size .... 1-3 μm or greater; size depends on rate of hemoglobin oxidation (if rapid as in G-6PD deficiency, bodies are small and numerous; if slow, as in oxidative drugs acting on normal RBCs, Heinz bodies form slowly and are larger and less numerous)
appearance .... spherical eccentrically located blue-purple RBC inclusion; visible only with supravital stains
composition .... denatured hemoglobin

KEY DIFFERENTIATING FEATURES
purple-blue round RBC inclusion not visible on Wright-Giemsa smears
visible only after supravital stains
bite cells suggest that Heinz bodies were present in those cells

POTENTIAL LOOK-ALIKES
Wright-Giemsa stained smears:
(Note: Heinz bodies are not visible with Wright-Giemsa but may be confused with these objects)
Pappenheimer bodies
basophilic stippling
Howell-Jolly body
nucleus of nucleated red blood cell
karyorrhectic leukocytes
parasites
bacteria and fungi
stain precipitate and other artifacts
Supravital stained smears:
H bodies
reticulocytes
alpha chain inclusion bodies

ASSOCIATED DISEASE STATES AND CONDITIONS
unstable hemoglobins
chemical poisoning
oxidant drugs
G-6PD deficiency and other enzymopathies (these disorders create a predilection for—but do not result in—Heinz body formation)
hemolytic anemia associated with severe alcoholic liver disease

Heinz bodies appear as large, single or multiple, blue-purple (depending on stain used) inclusions often attached to the inner surface of the red cell membrane. Depending on the disease, the Heinz body may consist of precipitated normal hemoglobin or structurally defective hemoglobin (unstable hemoglobin).

Heinz bodies are made visible by supravital stains such as crystal violet. (Note: crystal violet, gentian violet, and methyl violet are synonymous). Testing for pre-formed Heinz bodies with crystal violet must be done within one hour of venipuncture; after this time, Heinz bodies may form spontaneously in normal red blood cells. Classic Heinz bodies are not seen in Wright-Giemsa stained blood films. Bite cells are markers of their presence, however. (See page 68 and *A Closer Look At... Bite Cell Formation and Morphology* on page 70).

Heinz bodies are precipitates of denatured hemoglobin. They are primarily found in cases of hemolytic anemia due to "oxidant drug stress," such as following large doses of dapsone or phenazopyridine (e.g., Pyridium) or in the presence of unstable hemoglobins such as hemoglobin Zürich. On rare occasions, Heinz bodies may be found in the hemolytic anemia associated with severe liver disease. This is most likely due to abnormal enzyme activities involving the hexose monophosphate shunt and glutathione metabolism.

Supravital Stained RBC Containing Heinz Bodies

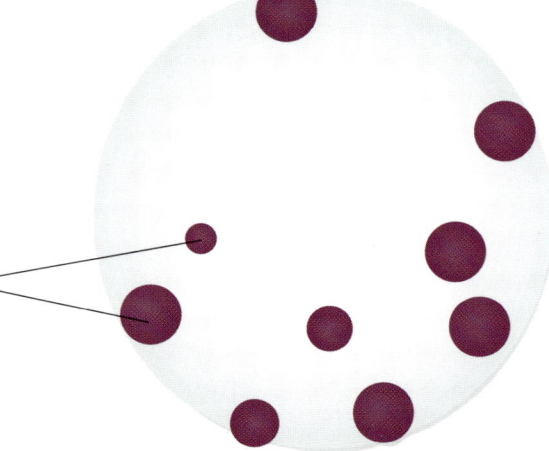

blue-purple inclusions visible only after supravital staining

inclusions are usually attached to plasma membrane and are most prevalent at the periphery of the cell

Heinz bodies should not be confused with hemoglobin H inclusions. These small round inclusions are morphologically much different from typical Heinz bodies. Excess β chains form tetrads, then precipitate when incubated with brilliant cresyl blue. The deposits are small and evenly distributed within the red cell, producing a "golf ball" appearance. Heinz bodies are larger, fewer in number, and localized.

The spleen is very efficient in removing Heinz bodies. The red cells are "pitted" rather than trapped or destroyed. In the process, bite cells or teardrop cells may be formed. After splenectomy Heinz bodies are more easily detected. This is especially true for unstable hemoglobin disorders. Heinz bodies are rarely seen prior to splenectomy.

The test for Heinz bodies is non-specific and has limited utility. Many clinicians think that it is less expensive or easiser to perform than a G-6PD assay or testing for unstable hemoglobin. This is not the case. Although it is important to be able to recognize Heinz bodies, the test itself should probably be retired from the laboratorian's armamentarium.

H-53, 1979 (Blood, Crystal Violet, X400)

Identification	Referee %	Participant %
Heinz body	85.7	71.4
Artifact	14.3	0.8
Siderocyte	-	5.2
Howell-Jolly body	-	1.4

All three cells in the field are red blood cells containing multiple Heinz bodies. These inclusions can vary in size from 1 to 3 μm. They are not visible by Wright-Giemsa staining alone and detection requires a supravital stain (crystal violet). Pappenheimer and Howell-Jolly bodies are both visible with Wright-Giemsa as well as crystal violet, but are morphologically distinct. Pappenheimer bodies would be much smaller (<1 μm). Howell-Jolly bodies are larger than Pappenheimer bodies but generally smaller than Heinz bodies. Circulating red blood cells containing this many Howell-Jolly bodies would be quite unusual.

HE-41, 1995 (Blood, Crystal Violet & Wright-Giemsa, X360)

Identification	Referee %	Participant %
Heinz body	91.7	92.2
Howell-Jolly body (iron stain)	4.2	0.6
Howell-Jolly body (Wright stain)	-	3.2
Reticulocyte	4.2	0.2
Pappenheimer bodies, presumptive (Wright stain)	-	1.3

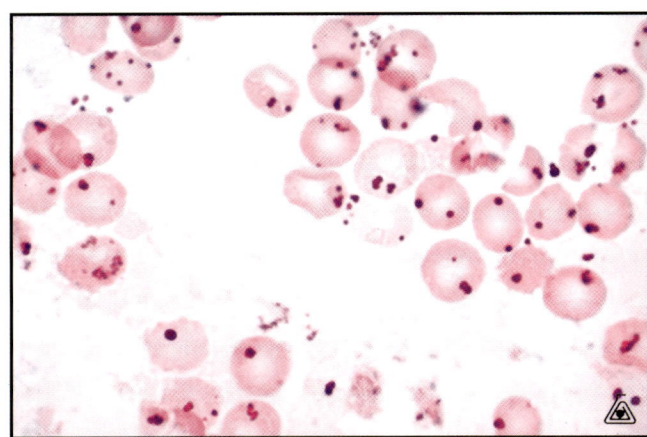

The blood smear has been stained first with crystal violet, then counter stained with Wright-Giemsa. The red cells demonstrate numerous Heinz bodies. They appear as large, single or multiple, blue-purple inclusions often attached to the inner surface of the red cell membrane. They characteristically are seen at the edge of the red cell, stuck to the interior of the membrane and protruding into the cytoplasm. Pappenheimer bodies, Howell-Jolly bodies, and stain precipitate all have different morphology or do not need supravital stains for visualization. Reticulocytes do not stain with crystal violet. (Both Heinz bodies and reticulocytes, however, are visible with brilliant cresyl blue, used to detect hemoglobin H).

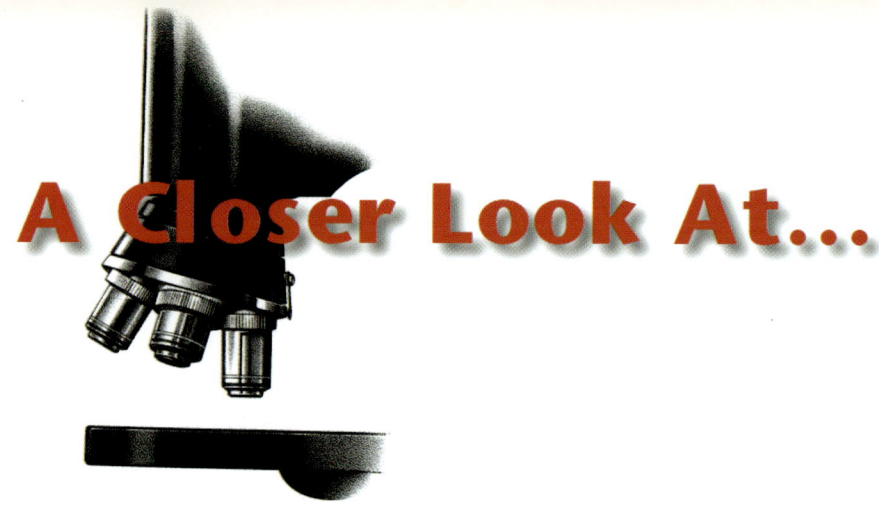

A Closer Look At...

How Heinz Bodies Form

Glucose within the red cell provides energy for all the various cell functions. A small amount is used in the oxidative hexose monophosphate (HMP) shunt to protect the cell from permanent oxidative injury. Certain metabolites within the red cell can oxidize sulfhydryl (-SH) groups on the hemoglobin molecule. Failure to reverse this process results in denaturation and precipitation of hemoglobin in the form of Heinz bodies. Severe oxidative stress can also damage the -SH groups in the red cell membrane leading to a leaky membrane.

During times of oxidative stress, the HMP shunt can normally accelerate 30-fold. Oxidant drugs such as phenylhydrazine produce enough free radicals and oxidative damage within the cell to overwhelm the HMP shunt. The formation, size, and number of Heinz bodies depend on the cell's capacity to safeguard hemoglobin. If the cell is completely overwhelmed, the Heinz bodies will be small and numerous. If the HMP shunt can keep up somewhat and oxidation is less severe, the Heinz bodies are larger and fewer in number.

G-6PD is an important enzyme in the HMP shunt. In G-6PD deficiency, the HMP shunt activity is curtailed and minor stresses can lead to Heinz body formation.

The *congenital Heinz body anemia*s are a group of disorders associated with altered stability of hemoglobin molecules. Amino acid substitutions in the hemoglobin molecule prevent it from maintaining a normal conformation. This leads to instability and denaturation. Disruption of the normal conformation may also affect the function of the hemoglobin molecule; unstable hemoglobins have a tendency to spontaneously oxidize to methemoglobin. Unlike the Heinz bodies characteristic of drug-induced hemolytic anemias, inclusions of unstable hemoglobins are unusually large and irregular. They are also more numerous in reticulocytes, unlike G-6PD deficiency in which reticulocytes are usually free of Heinz bodies.

The supravital stains used to identify Heinz bodies are of two types: one group induces precipitation of unstable hemoglobin while the other does not. Crystal violet stain indicates only the presence of Heinz bodies; it does not induce precipitation of unstable hemoglobin. Brilliant cresyl blue, on the other hand, causes the oxidative denaturation and precipitation of unstable hemoglobins. This stain is also used to detect hemoglobin H (β_4).

An oxidizing agent such as acetyl-phenylhydrazine may be used to stress the red cells to see how susceptible they are to Heinz body formation. Blood from a control and a patient are each mixed and incubated with the oxidizing agent at 37° C for 2 hours. Smears are then made and stained with crystal violet. Normal red cells contain fewer than five Heinz bodies each. In G-6PD deficiency, Heinz bodies are much more numerous. In evaluating the smears, cells with five or more Heinz bodies are considered positive. Normal controls have 0% to 30% positive cells whereas patients with G-6PD deficiency and unstable hemoglobinopathies have more than 45% positive red cells.

Heinz bodies attach to the red cell membrane and are removed along with a portion of the membrane as the cell traverses the spleen. The red cell is damaged in the process, producing *bite cells* and sometimes *teardrop cells* (see pages 70-71 and 112-113).

In general, looking for Heinz bodies is of limited value, especially in G-6PD deficiency. It is better practice to do specific tests for G-6PD deficiency or unstable hemoglobins. Such tests are widely available and less demanding of resources.

How Heinz Bodies Form

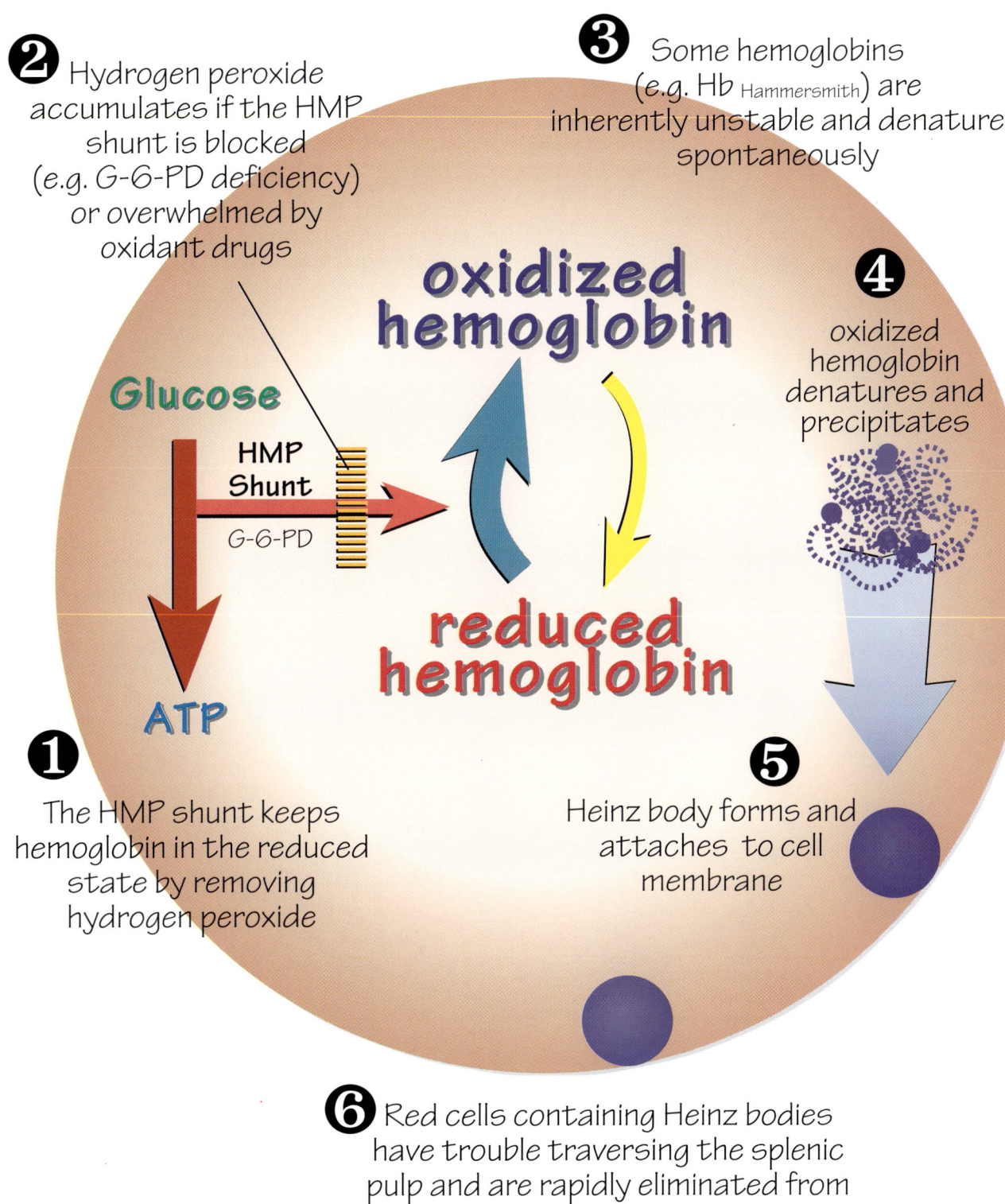

❷ Hydrogen peroxide accumulates if the HMP shunt is blocked (e.g. G-6-PD deficiency) or overwhelmed by oxidant drugs

❸ Some hemoglobins (e.g. Hb Hammersmith) are inherently unstable and denature spontaneously

❹ oxidized hemoglobin denatures and precipitates

❶ The HMP shunt keeps hemoglobin in the reduced state by removing hydrogen peroxide

❺ Heinz body forms and attaches to cell membrane

❻ Red cells containing Heinz bodies have trouble traversing the splenic pulp and are rapidly eliminated from the circulation

Hemoglobin C Crystal

SYNONYMS
none

VITAL STATISTICS
- size .... variable, since crystals may markedly distort the cell
- cell shape .... normal disc shape is distorted by the crystal; cytoplasm contains the crystal, which is a precipitate of hemoglobin C
- inclusion shape .... variable; classic example is an octahedral crystal reminiscent of the Washington monument; there is generally a clear area around the crystal

KEY DIFFERENTIATING FEATURES
- dense, angular crystalline forms of somewhat variable shape; may be rod-like, spherocytic, rhomboid, hexagon or rod resemble bird's wings
- red cell often pale or colorless

OTHER FINDINGS
- some of the red cells may be "envelope forms" which resemble a clam shell or clutch pocketbook; this type of crystal is also seen in thalassemias and sickling disorders

POTENTIAL LOOK-ALIKES
- sickle cell
- bite cell
- blister cell

ASSOCIATED DISEASE STATES AND CONDITIONS
- hemoglobin C disease (Hb CC)
- hemoglobin SC disease

The hemoglobin C crystals are distinctive but variable. The classic "Washington monument" appearance of a crystal distorts the cell shape and leaves most of the rest of the cell clear/colorless. This finding is virtually pathognomonic of hemoglobin C disease; it is only very rarely seen in C trait and SC disease. Dense spherocytic cells may also contain HbC. Other forms may resemble a bird's wings, rhomboid, hexagon, or rod. It is believed that these forms occur since the hemoglobin is abnormal and precipitates more readily, especially when exposed to the rigors of splenic circulation. Suspension of hemoglobin C-containing erythrocytes in a 3% sodium chloride solution overnight will precipitate crystal formation.

In splenectomized patients with homozygous C disease, up to 10% of the circulating cells will contain tetrahedral crystals. Crystals are rare or absent in non-splenectomized patients.

Hemoglobins may polyerize or crystalize. Crystals typically form discrete octahedral inclusions while polymers form long rigid strands. Unlike hemoglobin S polymers, hemoglobin C crystals are composed of oxyhemoglobin. The crystals "melt" when the cell is exposed to lower concentrations of oxygen. This explains why the cell can more readily navigate the narrow confines of the microvasculature and splenic cords compared to cells containing polymerized hemoglobin S. A mechanism distinct from crystal formation causes splenic destruction in hemoglobin C disease. Hemoglobin C is poorly soluble. An exuberant K+ pump dessicates the cell, bringing hemoglobin C close to precipitation. The cell stiffens, loses its deformability, and is entrapped by the spleen.

Hemoglobin C is one of the hemoglobinopathies, apparently originating in Africa, with a structural mutation at position 6 of the beta hemoglobin chain. Lysine

Hemoglobin C Crystals

octahedral crystals wrapped in a clear membrane are virtually pathognomonic of hemoglobin C disease (they are found rarely in C trait and SC disease)

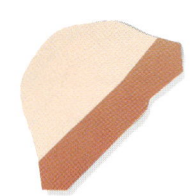
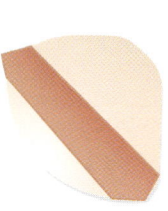
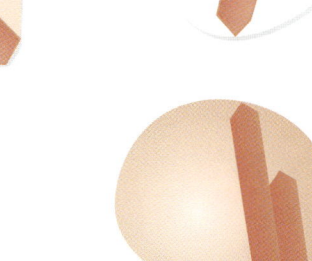

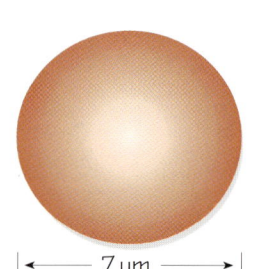

|←— 7 µm —→|
size of normal red blood cell

Erythrocytic Cells and Inclusions

replaces glutamic acid there and causes abnormal (lower) migration in routine hemoglobin electrophoresis. Worldwide, hemoglobin C is very common; it is estimated that in the United States, 2.4% of African Americans are Hb AC heterozygotes and 0.02% are Hb CC homozygotes.

Heterozygotes Hb AC is designated as hemoglobin C trait. Patients usually have no symptoms. The blood is remarkable for mild anemia and target cells. Studies indicate mildly shortened red cell survival but reticulocytes are not increased. Electrophoresis of erythrocytes shows 30-40% HbC, 50-60% Hb A, and a small increase in Hb A_2. If a patient has coexistent alpha thalassemia, the amount of Hb C is decreased in proportion to the number of defective alpha genes, since β^c globin chains have lower affinity for alpha globin.

Homozygous Hb CC is called hemoglobin C disease. This is manifested by mild to moderate hemolytic anemia, a marked increase in target cells, dense spherocytes, the presence of hemoglobin C crystals, and splenomegaly. These individuals have little in the way of symptoms with a normal lifespan and ability to handle infections the rule. Since they are affected by lifelong hemolysis, however, they have an increased incidence of pigment gallstones. Hemoglobin electrophoresis demonstrates almost all to be Hb C; there is no Hb A but there may be a small amount of Hb F. If a person has both alpha thalassemia and Hb CC, the Hb F may be increased.

Other combinations may occur with HbC. In addition to the above-mentioned alpha thalassemia, there may also be concomitant beta thalassemia or hemoglobin S. In SC disease, the individual has a course somewhat milder than in Hb SS disease.

H-38, 1979 (Blood, Wright-Giemsa, X400)

Identification	Referee %	Participant %
Hemoglobin C crystal	98.8	100

This is a beautiful example of a hemoglobin C crystal. The dense red color, rhomboid (Washington monument) shape, and the clear-appearing remainder of the cell are classic. Other findings of importance in this photomicrograph are the small, dense, round to rectangular shaped forms, assumedly Hb C crystals, and the many target cells present. Although this patient's history is not known, there is little other than a hemoglobinopathy containing Hb C that this could be.

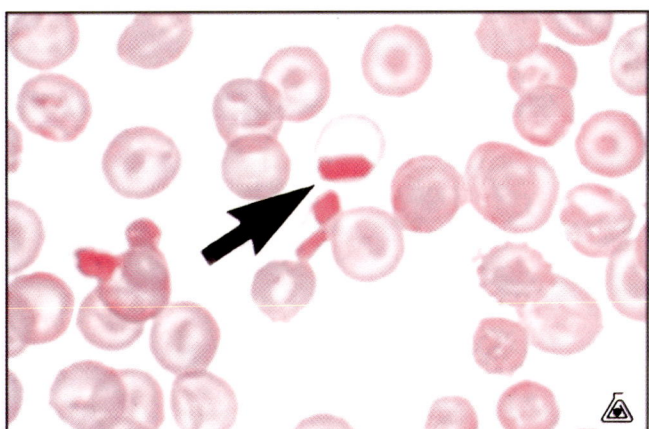

Hemoglobin H Inclusions (Supravital Stain)

SYNONYMS
H bodies

VITAL STATISTICS
- size .... <1 μm
- appearance .... small blue-purple granules, evenly distributed within RBC after supravital dye staining
- composition .... precipitated chains of beta hemoglobin (β_4 tetramers)

KEY DIFFERENTIATING FEATURES
small granular RBC inclusions numbering 20-50
even distribution
visible only with supravital stain (Brilliant Cresyl Blue)

OTHER FINDINGS
anemia, reticulocytosis, and target cells
abnormal hemoglobin electrophoresis with 5-30% Hb H and sometimes a trace of Hb Bart's

POTENTIAL LOOK-ALIKES
Wright-Giemsa stained smears:
(Note: H bodies are not visible with Wright-Giemsa but may be confused with these objects)
  Pappenheimer bodies
  basophilic stippling
  Howell-Jolly body
  nucleus of nucleated red blood cell
  karyorrhectic leukocytes
  parasites
  bacteria and fungi
  stain precipitate and other artifacts supravitally stained reticulocytes and Heinz bodies
supravital stained smears:
  Heinz bodies
  reticulocytes
  alpha chain inclusion bodies

ASSOCIATED DISEASE STATES AND CONDITIONS
hemoglobin H disease
myeloproliferative syndromes (acquired phenomenon)
erythroleukemia
refractory sideroblastic anemia

Hemoglobin H represents precipitated excess beta chains, seen only after supravital staining. The inclusions are small and have an even distribution that resembles the periodicity of dimples on a golf ball (hence the name "golf ball cells"). Hemoglobin H inclusions are related to Heinz bodies but they are not the same. The next section entitled *A Closer Look At...Different Types of Precipitated Hemoglobin* on page 132 details the differences.

The four types of alpha thalassemia correspond to deletions or mutations of one, two, three, or all four alpha globin genes. One gene deletion—so called *silent carrier state* or *α thalassemia minor, mild*—has little effect on hemoglobin levels. Red cell morphology is normal. The excess beta chains are not produced in sufficient quantity to damage the red cell.

Deletion of two genes—so called *α thalassemia minor, severe*—produces a spectrum of disease states that run the gamut from mild to marked anemia. The excess beta chains are more numerous and in some cases can precipitate within the developing red cell resulting in ineffective erythropoiesis.

Deletion of three genes produces hemoglobin H disease. The imbalance between alpha and beta genes is marked. The excess beta chains are not easily removed by normal proteolytic enzyme activity within the developing red cell. The chains arrange themselves into unstable tetramers (β_4), designated hemoglobin H. The tetramers are invisible by Wright-Giemsa staining.

Inclusions Seen After Brilliant Cresyl Blue Staining in Hemoglobin H Disease

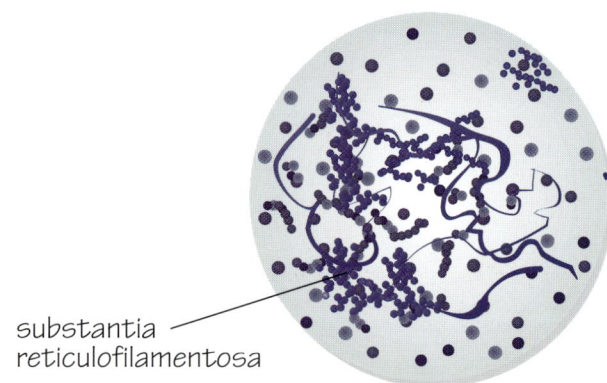

substantia reticulofilamentosa

H Bodies in Reticulocyte

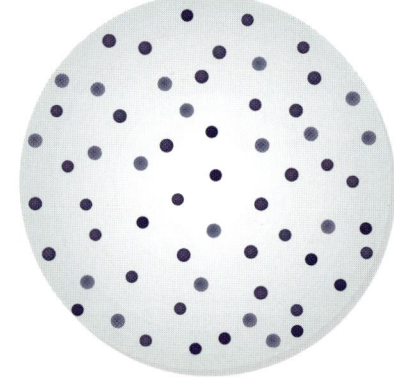

H Bodies in Mature Red Cell

Erythrocytic Cells and Inclusions

Hemoglobin H disease is most frequent in southeast Asia, the Mediterranean, and also the Middle East. Patients have mild to moderate anemia, marked microcytosis (e.g., MCV 55 fL), splenomegaly, and bone marrow erythroid hyperplasia. They are not overtly ill and usually have a normal life-span; they may come to medical attention only after severe infection, exposure to oxidant drugs, or during pregnancy. All show a fast migrating hemoglobin with electrophoresis. The circulating red cells are small and often misshapen or targeted. If the red cells are incubated with the supravital dye brilliant cresyl blue, the precipitated β_4 shows up as 20 to 50 evenly distributed small granules. The precipitated hemoglobin is bound to the red cell membrane. The hemoglobin H inclusions may be present in less than 50% of circulating erythrocytes. If splenectomy occurs, their percentage will markedly increase since the "pitting" function of the spleen is removed.

Deletion or mutation of all four alpha genes—*hemoglobin Bart's*—is not compatible with life. The fetus is either stillborn or dies within a few hours. The majority of the hemoglobin is composed of four gamma chain molecules (hemoglobin Bart's or γ_4). Bart's hemoglobin has a very high oxygen affinity. It is unsuitable as an oxygen transporter and the fetus dies of severe anemia and heart and respiratory failure. They have all the hematologic features of hemoglobin H disease (microcytic anemia, hemolysis, icterus, and splenomegaly) but they have 20-40% hemoglobin H. The rest is hemoglobin Bart's.

There is an acquired form of hemoglobin H associated with myelodysplastic syndromes and erythroleukemia. A neoplastic clone of red cells exhibits abnormal hemoglobin gene regulation. The vast majority (greater than 80%) of individuals are male and the finding may only be present in a subpopulation of the erythrocytes. The typical clinical and morphologic features of these acquired bone marrow disorders make them easy to distinguish from the congenital form of hemoglobin H.

Unfortunately, many lots of commercially available brilliant cresyl blue do not work effectively in the hemoglobin H test. When the test does work, it is important to remember that brilliant cresyl blue will stain any precipitable unstable hemoglobin, so care must be made to distinguish hemoglobin H inclusions form Heinz bodies. Heinz bodies are larger and less numerous, although also attached to the cell's surface. Hemoglobin H inclusions will also occur later (1 to 2 hours at 37° C incubation) than preformed Heinz bodies, which will appear as early as 10 minutes when incubated at room temperature. Hemoglobin H inclusions must also be distinguished from reticulocytes, which show larger precipitated masses with brilliant cresyl blue. In hemoglobin H disease, it would not be uncommon to find all three types of inclusions simultaneously. The different morphologies of these inclusions are illustrated in the drawing on the previous page.

H1-7, 1989 (Blood, Brilliant Cresyl Blue, X360)

Identification	Referee %	Participant %
Hemoglobin H inclusions	66.7	55.2
Reticulocyte	22.2	23.8
Heinz body	5.6	8.1

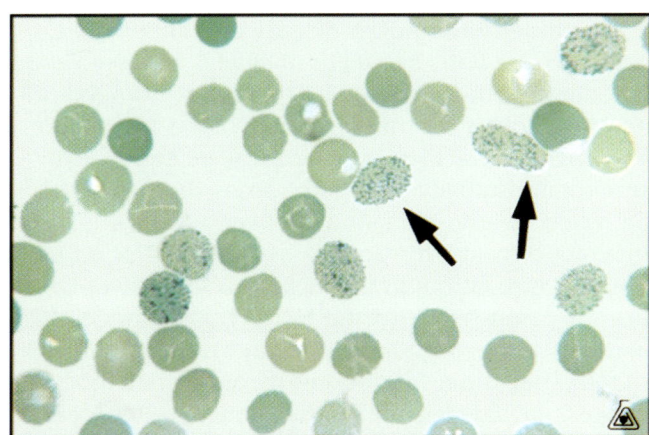

Supravital staining with brilliant cresyl blue (BCB) reveals numerous inclusions in the red blood cells. The two arrowed cells contain small, evenly distributed granular deposits. The inclusions are precipitates of excess beta hemoglobin chains, typically found in hemoglobin H disease. The small size and even distribution are reminiscent of the dimples on a golf ball. Compare the size and distribution to Heinz bodies, which are large, round, peripherally located dark blue inclusions (see pages 124-125). BCB stains reticulocytes and hemoglobin H inclusions. After 10 minutes of incubation at room temperature, only reticulocytes are visible. After 1-2 hours at 37°C, hemoglobin H inclusions become apparent. Reticulocytes are dark blue, uneven, clumped and medium-sized granules that are sometimes connected by a reticular network.

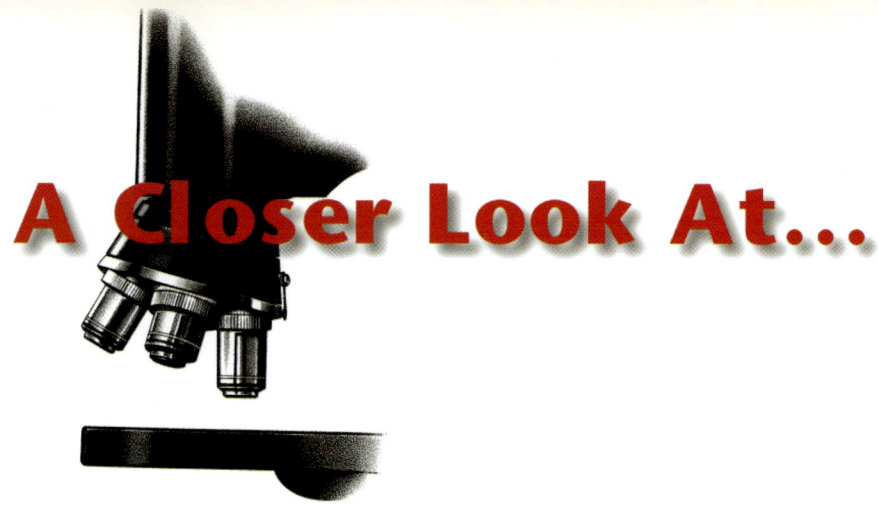

A Closer Look At...

Different Types of Precipitated Hemoglobin

Heinz bodies and H bodies, although both derived from hemoglobin, are distinctly different red cell inclusions. As discussed on page 124, Heinz bodies represent precipitated hemoglobin molecules due to either 1) severe oxidant drug reaction in normal individuals or in G-6PD deficiency or 2) unstable hemoglobins. The table below lists the more common drugs and chemicals associated with Heinz body formation.

The size and number of Heinz bodies varies with the ability of the body to handle the oxidative stress. If the red cell enzyme system can barely keep up, the Heinz bodies will be large and few in number. If the oxidative stress completely overwhelms an already weakened HMP shunt, as in G-6PD deficiency or in normal individuals if the amount of drug is excessive, the Heinz bodies will be small and numerous. Even the small variants of Heinz bodies are larger and lack the periodicity seen in hemoglobin H disease.

Unstable hemoglobin disease also known as *Congenital Heinz body hemolytic anemia* is an uncommon hereditary hemolytic disorder that is autosomal dominant. Hb Köln is the most common of the 130 variants. Various amino acid substitutions or deletions lead to structural instability that predisposes the hemoglobin molecule to auto-oxidation. Depending on the structural abnormality, the anemia may be mild or dangerously severe. Although the inclusions formed are identical in composition to the Heinz bodies induced by oxidant drugs, they are larger and more irregular in shape. They are also more numerous in reticulocytes, unlike G-6PD deficiency in which reticulocytes are usually free of Heinz bodies.

Heinz bodies attach to the inner surface of the red cell membrane, deforming the skeletal matrix. The rigid structures are excised as the cell navigates through the spleen producing bite deformities and teardrop cells (See *A Closer Look At...*sections on pages 70 and 112). Heinz bodies are most frequently observed in splenectomized individuals.

In the thalassemia majors the entire hemoglobin molecule does not precipitate. Instead, excess alpha or beta chains accumulate in the red cell cytoplasm. In hemoglobin H disease, a triple alpha gene deletion results in excess beta globin chains.

Beta thalassemia major, also known as homozygous β thalassemia or Cooley's anemia, is a rare congenital severe hemolytic anemia that can result in debilitation and premature death. Homozygous $β^+$-thal accounts for about 90% of cases while homozygous $β^0$-thal is responsible for most of the rest. The complete or near complete lack of beta chain production results in excess alpha hemoglobin chains. About 10% of the hemoglobin in marrow reticulocytes is made up of free α chains. The α hemoglobin chains lose the heme portion, undergo denaturation and oxidation, and precipitate. The number and distribution determine the severity of anemia. The aggregates of insoluble surplus

Representative Drugs and Chemicals Causing Heinz Body Hemolytic Anemia

Phenazopyridine
Flutamide
Dapsone
Acetanilid
Phenylhydrazine
Nitrofurantoin
Naphthalene

α chains deposit within the nucleus interfering with cell division and bind to the inner aspect of the red cell cytoskeleton. The inclusions damage the red cell membrane and limit egress from the marrow. The cells that do make it into the circulation are trapped by the spleen and further pitted and culled from the blood stream. Like Heinz bodies, the alpha chain inclusion bodies are visible by means of supravital stains but not Wright-Giemsa.

Alpha thalassemia associated with deletion of three of the four α globin genes results in hemoglobin H disease, discussed on the previous pages. These inclusions represent excess beta chains which arrange themselves into unstable tetramers ($β_4$), designated hemoglobin H. They are smaller than Heinz bodies and have an even distribution, likened to the dimples on a golf ball. Although similar in some respects, neither H bodies nor alpha chain inclusions are true Heinz bodies.

Disorders Associated with Precipitated Hemoglobin

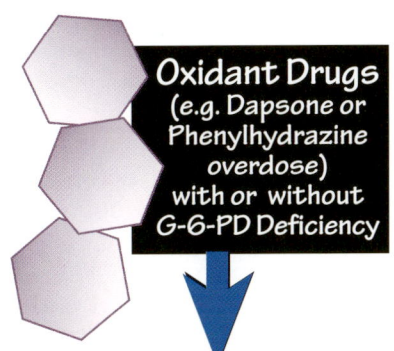

Normal Hemoglobin	Unstable Hemoglobin	Thalassemias	
denatured hemoglobin	spontaneous precipitation of unstable hemoglobin	β thal major — excess α chains	α thal (triple α gene deletion) — excess β chains
precipitation	precipitation	precipitation	precipitation

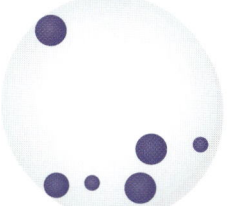 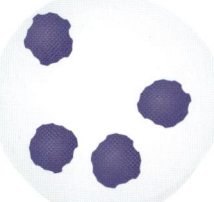 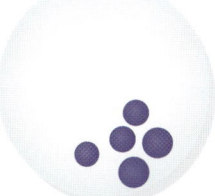 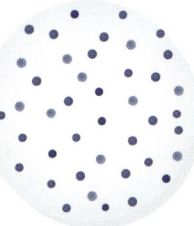

Heinz bodies   Heinz bodies   alpha chain inclusion bodies   H bodies

Howell-Jolly Body (Wright-Giemsa Stain)

SYNONYMS
nuclear fragment

VITAL STATISTICS
- size .... 1 µm; sometimes as small as 0.5 µm
- appearance .... round or oblong eccentrically placed purple-blue or blue-black red cell inclusion
- composition .... fragment of DNA

KEY DIFFERENTIATING FEATURES
- spherical blue-purple or blue-black intracytoplasmic red cell inclusion
- iron stain negative
- DNA stain positive (Feulgen stain)
- may be multiple, especially in myeloproliferative disorders and megaloblastic anemia

POTENTIAL LOOK-ALIKES
- Pappenheimer bodies
- basophilic stippling
- Heinz body (visible only after supravital dye staining)
- hemoglobin H inclusions (visible only after supravital dye staining)
- nucleus of nucleated red blood cell
- karyorrhectic leukocytes
- bacteria and fungi
- parasites
- stain precipitate and other artifacts

ASSOCIATED DISEASE STATES AND CONDITIONS
- very rarely seen in normal individuals
- hyposplenism
- asplenism
- severe hemolytic anemia
- megaloblastic anemia
- leukemia (some cases)
- congenital dyserythropoietic anemia

Howell-Jolly bodies are usually small round objects about 1 µm in diameter. They are larger than Pappenheimer bodies, are composed of DNA, and are formed in one of two ways, illustrated in the *A Closer Look At…Howell-Jolly Body Formation* section on page 138.

During the late phase of basophilic normoblast cell division, a chromosome may become separated from the mitotic spindle. When the nucleus is finally extruded, the chromosome may remain behind. The likelihood of this happening is increased if the nucleus contains more than the usual 4N number of chromosomes prior to cell division, such as in B_{12} or folate deficiency. Howell-Jolly bodies may also form in the process of karyorrhexis. A small nuclear fragment becomes separated from the main nuclear mass and is not expelled. Normally, the spleen removes any Howell-Jolly bodies but if the spleen is missing or hypofunctioning the erythrocyte inclusions may be readily found in the peripheral blood.

Small Howell-Jolley bodies may resemble Pappenheimer bodies. Howell-Jolly bodies are round and Pappenheimer bodies are angular. Both types of inclusions may be single or multiple. Pappenheimer bodies usually form tight clusters of inclusions in pairs or tetrads. Howell-Jolly bodies may be multiple as well. They may be grouped or dispersed and vary in size. An iron stain may be needed to confirm the morphologic impression. Howell-Jolly bodies are iron negative. See the next section, *Howell-Jolly Body (Iron Stain)*, on page 136.

Howell-Jolly Body Inclusions (Wright-Giemsa Stain)

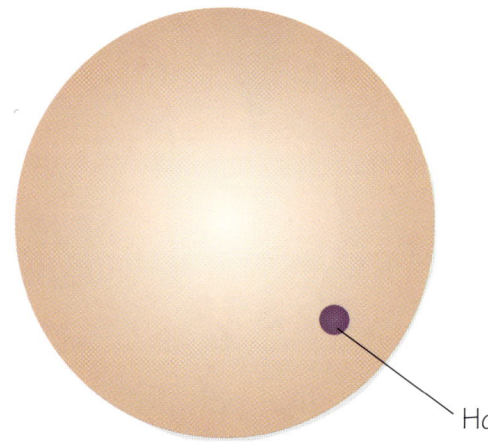

Howell-Jolly body

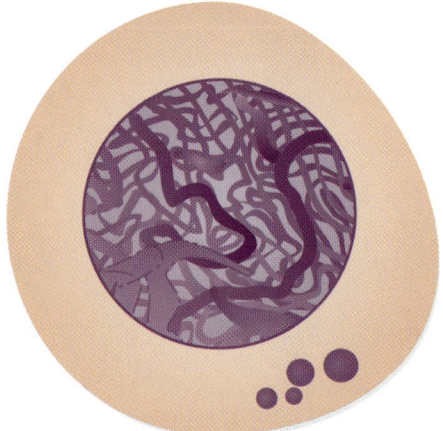

multiple Howell-Jolly bodies in nucleated red cell commonly seen in myeloproliferative syndromes and megaloblastic anemias

A-65, 1986 (Blood, Wright-Giemsa, X400)

Identification	Referee %	Participant %
Howell-Jolly body (Wright's stain)	87.5	88.5
Howell-Jolly body (iron stain)	12.5	8.2

The arrowed object is a Howell-Jolly body. This red cell inclusion is a nuclear fragment retained within the erythrocyte cytoplasm. It is usually manifested as a single, perfectly round, purple body 0.5 µm in diameter. Howell-Jolly bodies are most commonly seen in splenectomized patients, severe forms of megaloblastic and hemolytic anemias, and patients with hemoglobinopathies. The inclusions do not stain with iron.

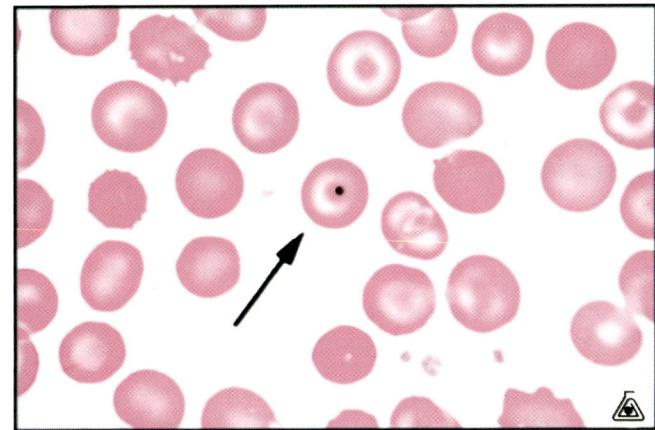

H-23, 1981 (Blood, Wright-Giemsa, X400)

Identification	Referee %	Participant %
Howell-Jolly body (Wright's stain)	100	98

The smear is from a patient with megaloblastic anemia. The arrowed red blood cell contains a single large round purple inclusion—a Howell Jolly body. The surrounding red cells contain smaller dark angular inclusions—Pappenheimer bodies. The size and shape differences between these two red cell inclusions are easily appreciated. Confirmatory iron stain would be positive in the Pappenheimer bodies but negative in the Howell-Jolly body. A DNA stain (Feulgen stain) would be positive in the Howell-Jolly body but not the Pappenheimer inclusions. Heinz bodies are round red cell inclusions composed of precipitated hemoglobin; they are invisible with Wright-Giemsa stain.

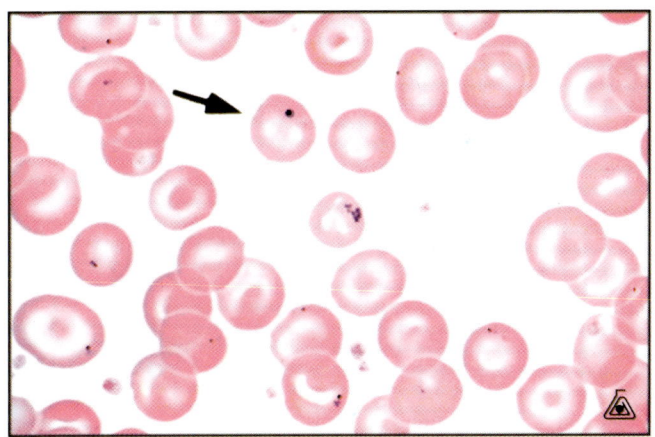

HE-22, 1987 (Bone Marrow, Wright-Giemsa, X360)

Identification	Referee %	Participant %
Howell-Jolly body (Wright's stain)	78.9	65.9
Howell-Jolly body (iron stain)	5.3	18.3
Siderocyte	15.8	18.3

This is a patient with partially treated megaloblastic anemia due to folate deficiency. The arrowed cell in the bone marrow is a non-nucleated red blood cell that contains multiple round fragments of DNA. These are Howell-Jolly bodies. They are too variable in size and shape as well as too large to be siderosomes (Pappenheimer bodies). Iron stain is negative but DNA stain is positive in Howell-Jolly bodies. Multiple Howell-Jolly bodies are typically seen in nucleated and non-nucleated maturing red blood cells in megaloblastic anemia and myelodysplastic conditions.

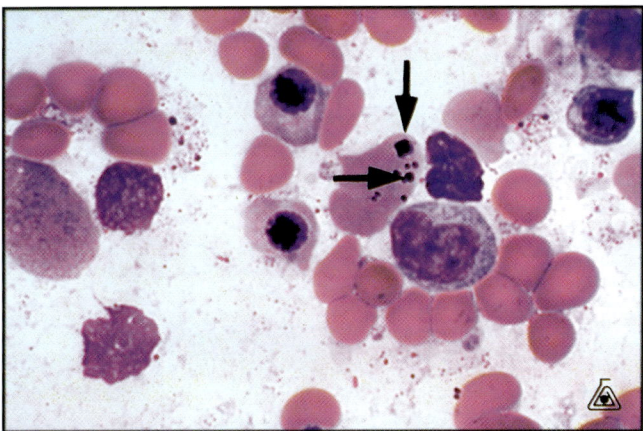

Howell-Jolly Body (Iron Stain)

SYNONYMS
nuclear fragment

VITAL STATISTICS
size .... 1 μm; sometimes as small as 0.5 μm
appearance .... round or oblong eccentrically placed pink red cell inclusion (color depends on counter stain)
composition .... fragment of DNA

KEY DIFFERENTIATING FEATURES
spherical intracytoplasmic red cell inclusion that is iron stain negative (does not stain blue)
may be multiple, especially in myeloproliferative disorders and megaloblastic anemia

OTHER FINDINGS
DNA stain positive (Feulgen stain)

POTENTIAL LOOK-ALIKES
Pappenheimer bodies (differentiate with iron stain)
nucleus of nucleated red blood cell
parasites
stain precipitate and other artifacts
karyorrhectic leukocytes
basophilic stippling (iron stain negative)
Heinz body (iron stain negative; visible only with supravital stain)
bacteria and fungi
hemoglobin H inclusions (iron stain negative; visible only with supravital stain)

ASSOCIATED DISEASE STATES AND CONDITIONS
hyposplenism
asplenism
severe hemolytic anemia
megaloblastic anemia
leukemia (some cases)
congenital dyserythropoietic anemia

As discussed in the section on *Howell-Jolly Body (Wright-Giemsa Stain)*, page 134, these red cell inclusions are composed of DNA. They represent either fragments of the nucleus that are retained within the red cell or aberrant chromosomes that have become separated from the mitotic spindle during cell division.

Howell-Jolly bodies do not contain iron and therefore do not stain blue with Perls' reaction (Prussian-blue iron stain). Typically, the counter stain used with the iron stain will stain DNA pink. In that case, Howell-Jolly bodies will stain the same pink color as the nuclei of leukocytes or nucleated red cells.

The chart on the next page shows various erythrocyte inclusions after iron staining. Only the inclusions in the middle row stain blue, indicative of the presence of iron. Depending on which counterstain is used, some of the inclusions are visible but they do not stain blue (such as basophilic stippling). Heinz bodies, hemoglobin H inclusions, and the substantia reticulofilamentosa of reticulocytes are invisible.

Howell-Jolly Body Inclusion (Iron Stain)

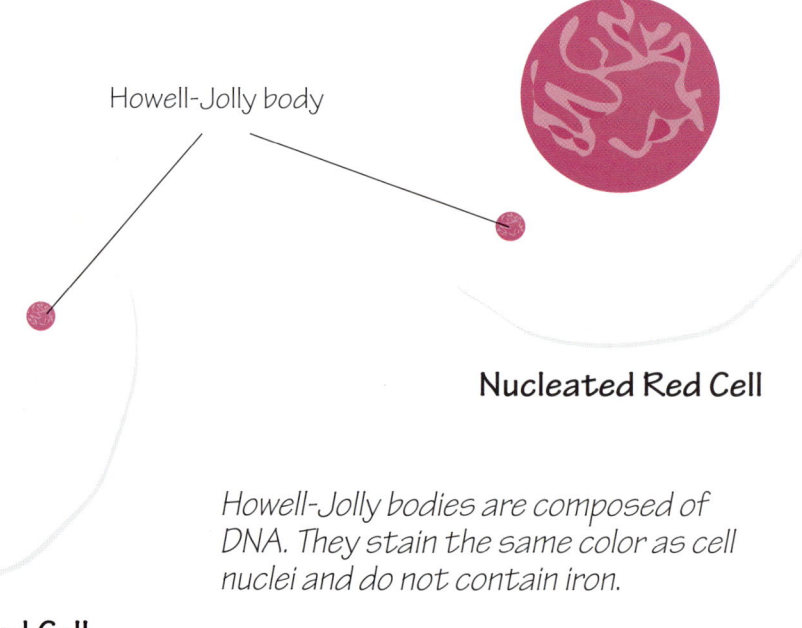

Howell-Jolly body

Nucleated Red Cell

Non-Nucleated Red Cell

Howell-Jolly bodies are composed of DNA. They stain the same color as cell nuclei and do not contain iron.

H-42, 1996 (Blood, Prussian Blue, X400)

Identification	Referee %	Participant %
Howell-Jolly body (iron stain)	84.6	80.3
Erythrocyte with overlapping platelet	7.7	3.2
Heinz body (supravital stain)	7.7	3.2
Pappenheimer bodies (iron stain)	-	4.9

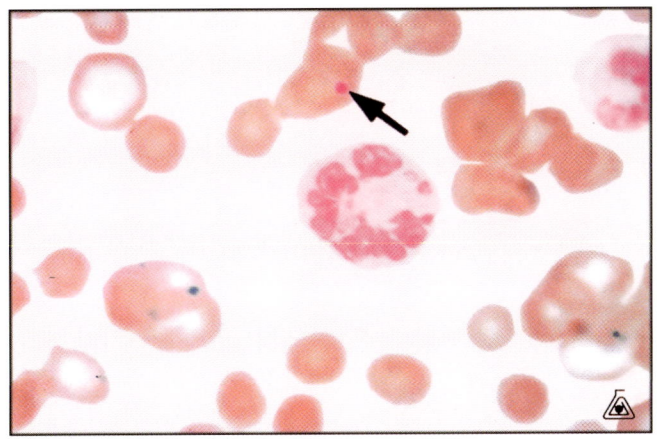

The patient has folate deficiency associated with chronic alcoholism. The photomicrograph is an iron stain (Prussian blue) of the peripheral blood. Keep in mind that after counterstaining, nuclear chromatin (DNA) stains pink and iron stains blue. The smear illustrated three morphologic features of megaloblastic anemia. In the center of the field is a hypersegmented neutrophil. The DNA of the nucleus stains pink; more than six lobes can be counted. The arrowed object is also pink and therefore is composed of DNA, not iron. This is a Howell-Jolly body. Lastly, siderocytes and Pappenheimer bodies are present. Pappenheimer bodies, like Howell-Jolly bodies are visible after Wright-Giemsa staining but they contain iron and not DNA; they therfore stain blue rather than pink. Pappenheimer bodies are smaller than Howell-Jolly bodies. Heinz bodies are usually larger than Howell-Jolly bodies and represent denatured hemoglobin. They are not visible with an iron stain but can only be seen with the help of supravital stains such as new methylene blue, Nile blue, crystal violet, or methyl violet.

Iron Staining of Various Red Cell Inclusions

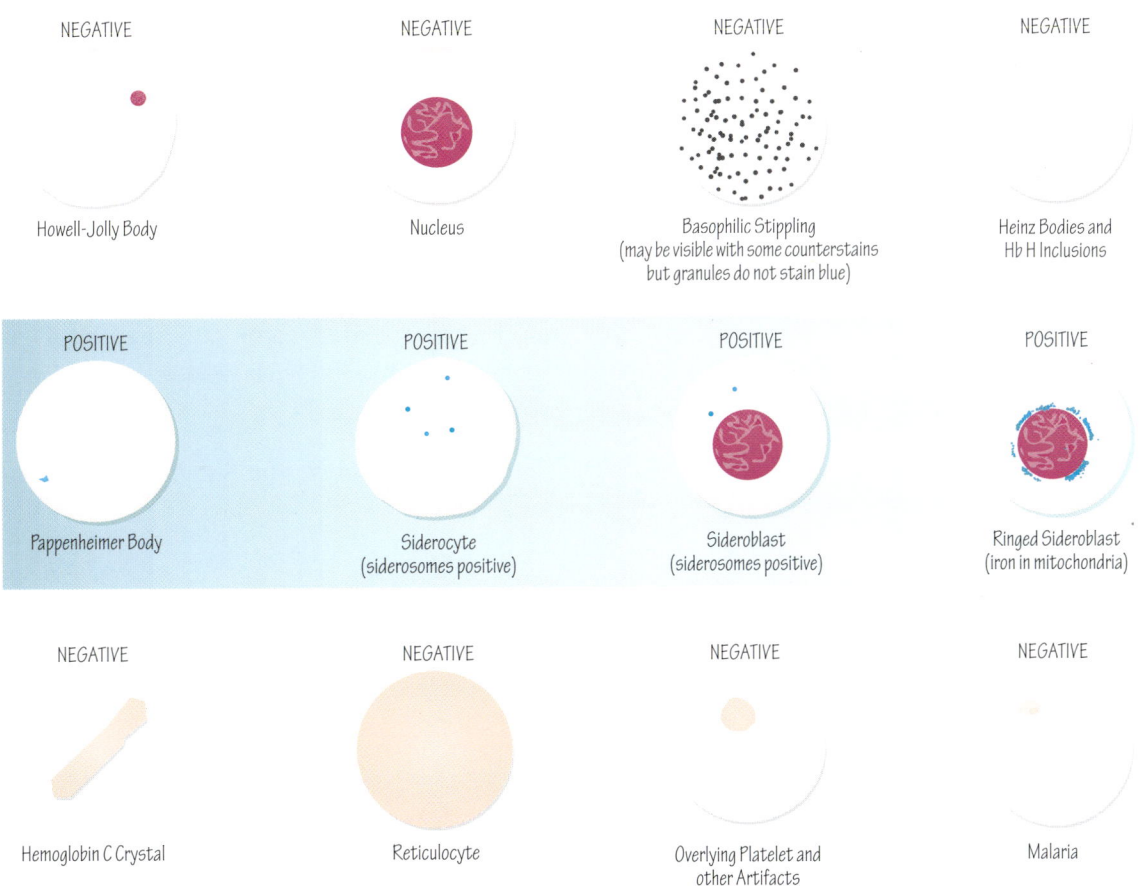

Erythrocytic Cells and Inclusions

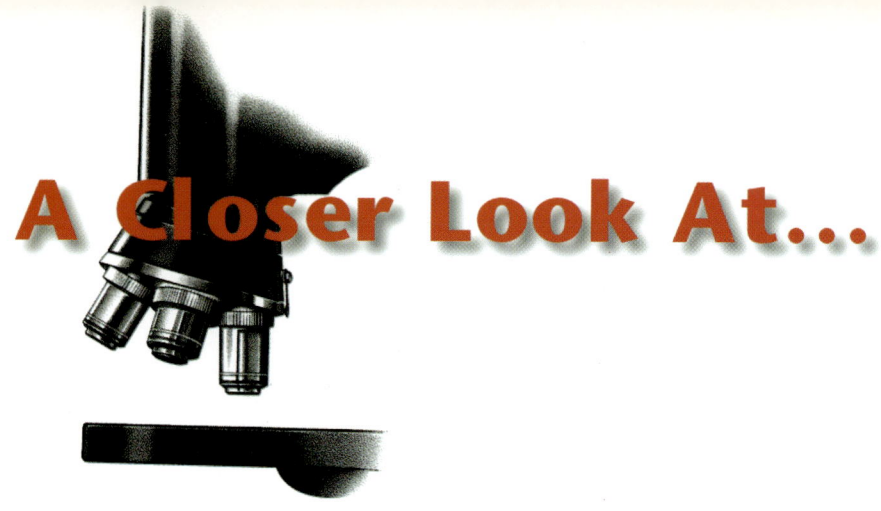

A Closer Look At...

How Howell-Jolly Bodies Form

The illustration on the right details the formation of Howell-Jolly bodies. They are derived either from chromosomes that have become separated from the mitotic spindle in the process of abnormal cell division or from small nuclear fragments produced by nuclear fragmentation (karyorrhexis).

During cell division, chromosomes are normally connected by threads of the mitotic spindle. In pathologic conditions, the chromosomes may become separated from the spindle and remain in the cytoplasm. This is most commonly seen in megaloblastic anemias. Here, there is maturation dyssynchrony between the nucleus and the cytoplasm. The cell undergoes fewer divisions and the number of chromosomes in the nucleus increases. The additional chromosomes are at greater risk of breaking loose from the spindle during mitosis. Several chromosomes may become separated; multiple Howell-Jolly bodies are often found in megaloblastic anemias.

In the second method, Howell-Jolly bodies form from DNA fragments. At the end of bone marrow erythropoiesis, the orthochromatic normoblast jettisons its nucleus to become a reticulocyte. The extrusion takes several minutes and occurs within the marrow. Sometimes the nucleus is ripped from the cell as it traverses the endothelial lining of the marrow sinuses. If this process is hurried, the nucleus may be irregularly shaped or fragmented as it squeezes into the blood stream. A few nuclear fragments may escape with the red cell. In hemolytic anemias, for example, circulating nucleated red blood cells may have irregularly lobated nuclei or fragments of nuclei. The smaller fragments are Howell-Jolly bodies.

Howell-Jolly bodies are very rare in normal individuals. Any small nuclear fragments in circulating red cells are quickly removed by the pitting action or enzymatic hydrolysis of the spleen. Some nuclear fragments may persist in the blood for hours or days, however. Howell-Jolly bodies are most commonly seen after removal of the spleen or in splenic atrophy or functional asplenia.

Howell-Jolly Body Formation

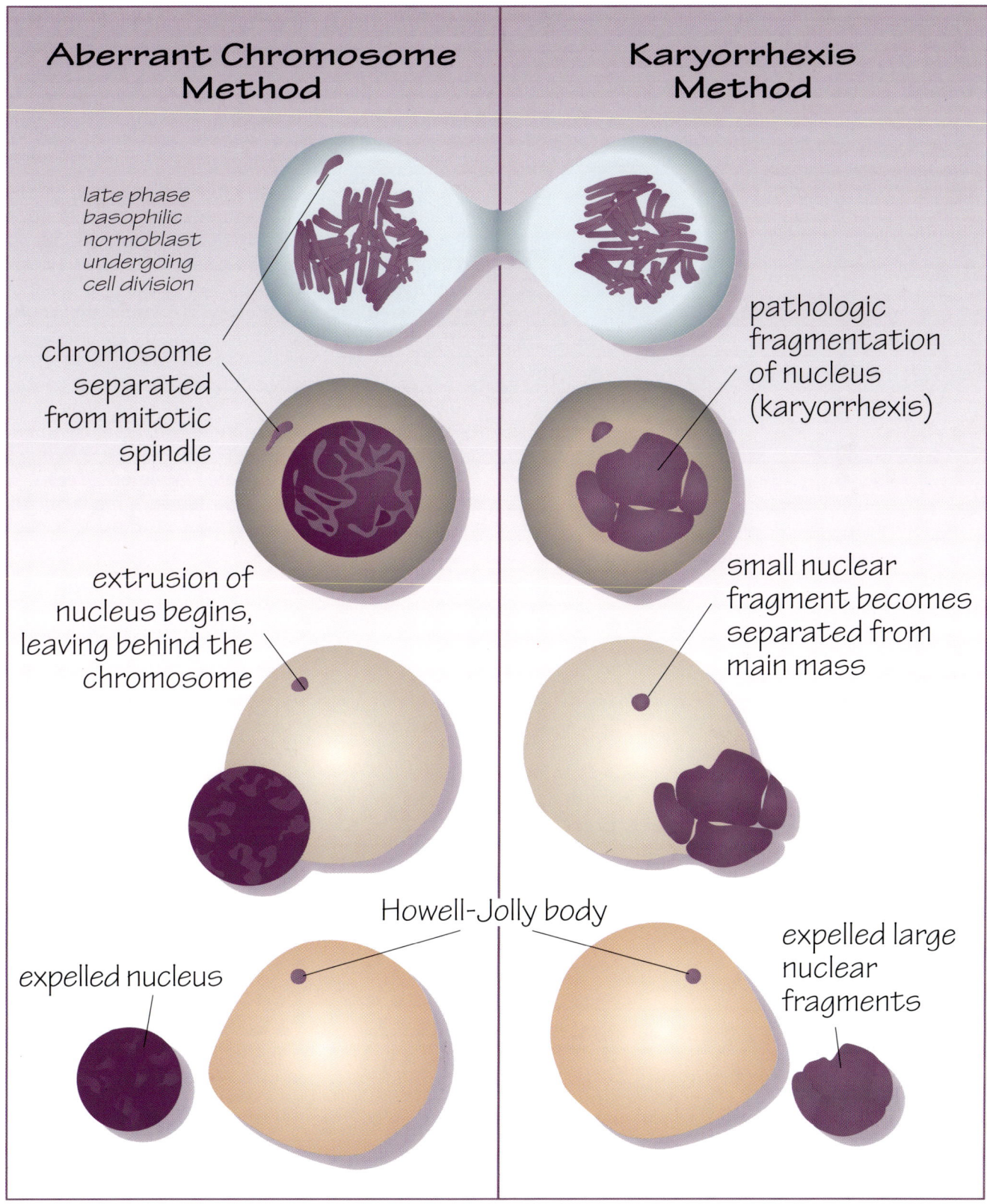

Pappenheimer Bodies (Wright-Giemsa Stain)

SYNONYMS
none

VITAL STATISTICS
- size .... usually less than 1 µm (sometimes <0.5 µm)
- appearance .... blue-purple granules with irregular, sharp edges
- composition .... secondary lysosomes composed of iron (non-heme) plus protein or iron-containing mitochondria

KEY DIFFERENTIATING FEATURES
- red cell inclusion visible on Wright-Giemsa stain
- usually found at periphery of cell
- one or two irregular small blue-purple-green granules; if multiple, they form irregular closely aggregated clusters
- iron stain is positive and confirmatory

POTENTIAL LOOK-ALIKES
- Howell-Jolly body (iron stain negative)
- Heinz body (iron stain negative; not visible by Wright-Giemsa stain; needs supravital stain)
- hemoglobin H inclusions (iron stain negative; not visible by Wright-Giemsa; needs supravital stain)
- basophilic stippling (iron stain negative)
- nucleus of nucleated red blood cell
- karyorrhectic leukocytes
- parasites
- bacteria and fungi
- stain precipitate and other artifacts

ASSOCIATED DISEASE STATES AND CONDITIONS
- sideroblastic anemias
- thalassemia
- megaloblastic anemias
- hemolytic anemias
- congenital dyserythropoietic anemias
- post-splenectomy states

Pappenheimer bodies are siderotic granules (iron-containing particles) that are visible on Wright-Giemsa stained smears. They are small, irregular basophilic deposits found in erythrocytes and nucleated red cells. The punctations are usually peripherally located and are either single or in doublets. They are less than 1 µm in size and thus are smaller than Howell-Jolly bodies. Wright-Giemsa stains the protein matrix of the granules. Prussian blue stain is also positive, indicative of the presence of iron.

Pappenheimer bodies are formed as the red cell discharges its abnormal iron-containing mitochondria. An autophagosome is created that digests the offending organelles. If the autophagosome is not discharged out of the cytoplasm or removed by the pitting action of the spleen, the inclusions will be visible on Wright-Giemsa stained blood films. Their true nature is confirmed with an iron stain. (Contrast this to Heinz bodies and Howell-Jolly bodies which do not contain iron.) See *A Closer Look At...How Pappenheimer Bodies Form* on page 144 for a more detailed discussion and illustration of the process.

Pappenheimer bodies are commonly seen in sideroblastic anemias, thalassemias, megaloblastic anemias, and in post-splenectomy states.

Pappenheimer Bodies

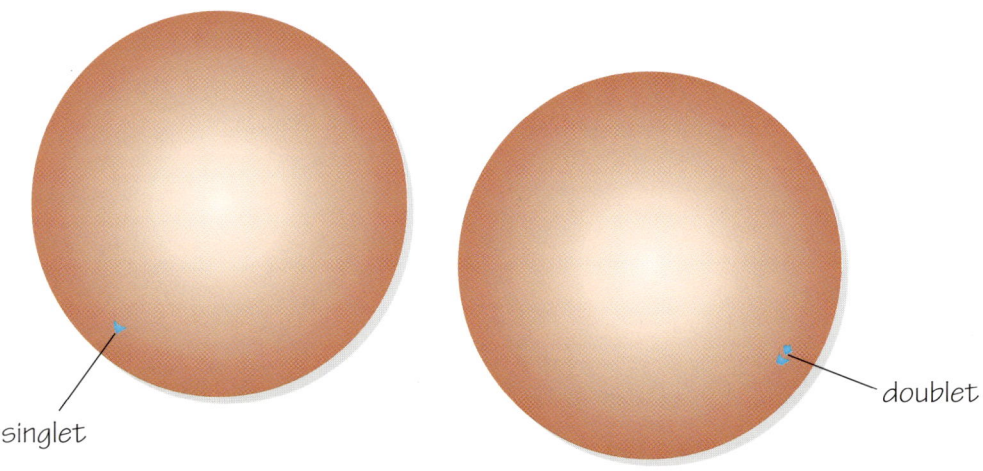

singlet

doublet

Erythrocytic Cells and Inclusions

H1-08, 1990 (Blood, Wright-Giemsa, X400)

Identification	Referee %	Participant %
Pappenheimer bodies	60	67.5
Howell-Jolly body	35	29

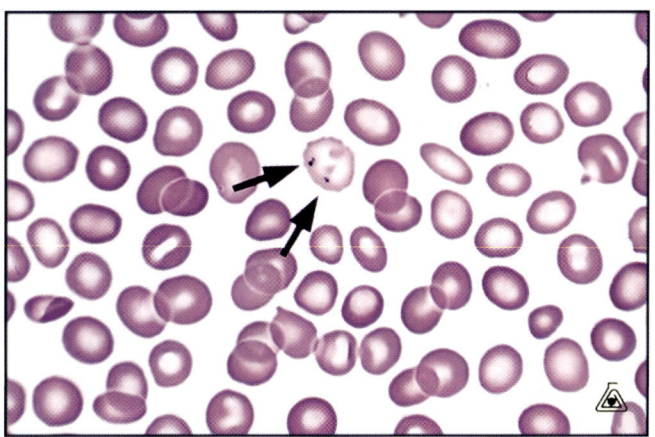

This is a case of hereditary sideroblastic anemia. The bone marrow showed erythroid hyperplasia and numerous ringed sideroblasts. The peripheral blood film depicted here demonstrates a dimorphic red cell population (a mixture of normal and hypochromic red cells). The two arrows point to small granular red blood cell inclusions. These are Pappenheimer bodies. The inclusions are not perfectly round; they have an angular outline. Iron stain is needed to confirm their true nature. The inclusions should not be confused with Howell-Jolly bodies, which are larger, round or oblong, and iron-stain negative. The Pappenheimer bodies in this field have a distinctly irregular morphology.

H-24, 1981 (Blood, Wright-Giemsa, X400)

Identification	Referee %	Participant %
Pappenheimer bodies	100	91
Heinz body	-	2.5
Howell-Jolly body	-	2.4
Basophilic stippling	-	1.4

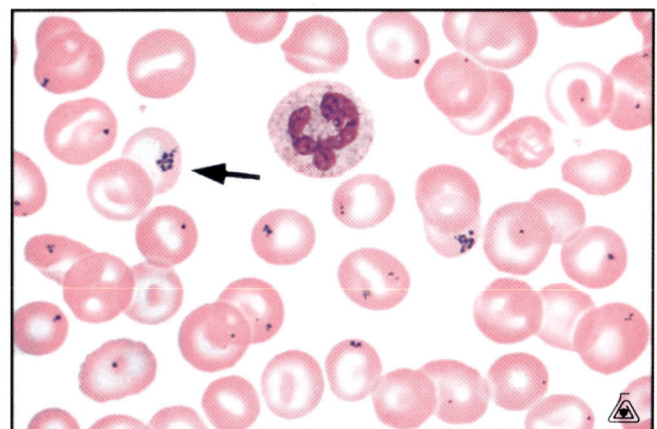

This is a case of megaloblastic anemia. Many of the red cells contain small, round or angular inclusions called Pappenheimer bodies. The arrowed cell contains multiple ones. These iron-containing red blood cell inclusions usually occur singly or in doublets. The arrowed cell contains three doublets. The corresponding iron stain of the smear is seen on page 143, case H-25, 1981. Other red cell inclusions can resemble Pappenheimer bodies. Howell-Jolly bodies are larger and not as angular. Coarse basophilic stippling is evenly distributed over the entire red cell. Heinz bodies are not visible with Wright-Giemsa; they require supravital staining.

Pappenheimer Bodies (Iron Stain)

SYNONYMS
none

VITAL STATISTICS
- size .... usually less than 1 μm (sometimes <0.5 μm)
- appearance .... blue granules with irregular, sharp edges
- composition .... secondary lysosomes composed of iron (non-heme) plus protein or iron-containing mitochondria

KEY DIFFERENTIATING FEATURES
usually found at periphery of cell
after iron staining, one or two irregular small blue inclusions; if multiple, they form closely aggregated clusters
iron stain is positive and confirmatory

OTHER FINDINGS
the inclusions are visible with Wright-Giemsa stain

POTENTIAL LOOK-ALIKES
normal iron inclusions in siderocytes and sideroblasts which are not visible on Wright-Giemsa stain (remember that Pappenheimer bodies are abnormal siderosomes that are visible on Wright-Giemsa stain)
Note: all of the following are iron-stain negative but may resemble Pappenheimer bodies on Wright-Giemsa smears
Howell-Jolly body
Heinz body (needs supravital stain)
hemoglobin H inclusions (needs supravital stain)
basophilic stippling
nucleus of nucleated red blood cell
karyorrhectic leukocytes
parasites
bacteria and fungi
stain precipitate and other artifacts

ASSOCIATED DISEASE STATES AND CONDITIONS
sideroblastic anemias
thalassemia
megaloblastic anemias
hemolytic anemias
congenital dyserythropoietic anemias
post-splenectomy states

Pappenheimer bodies are abnormal siderosomes. Unlike normal siderosomes found in siderocytes and sideroblasts which are composed only of iron, the pathologic iron-containing granules are composed of both a protein matrix as well as iron. The protein matrix is stainable by Wright-Giemsa and is thus visible on similarly-stained blood smears. The iron containing nature of the inclusions is confirmed with Prussian blue stain.

Pappenheimer bodies, as discussed on the previous page, are secondary lysomes (autophagosomes) made up of either iron-containing mitochondria or other organelles mixed with non-heme iron. The inclusion is irregular in shape and quite small, in contrast to the round and larger Howell-Jolly body. Pappenheimer bodies are either single or form a small cluster of two or four granules. These are peripherally located in contrast to the more diffuse nature of basophilic stippling.

Iron stain is needed to confirm the Wright-Giemsa stain appearance. The other types of abnormal red cell inclusions are all iron negative.

Pappenheimer Bodies (Iron Stain)

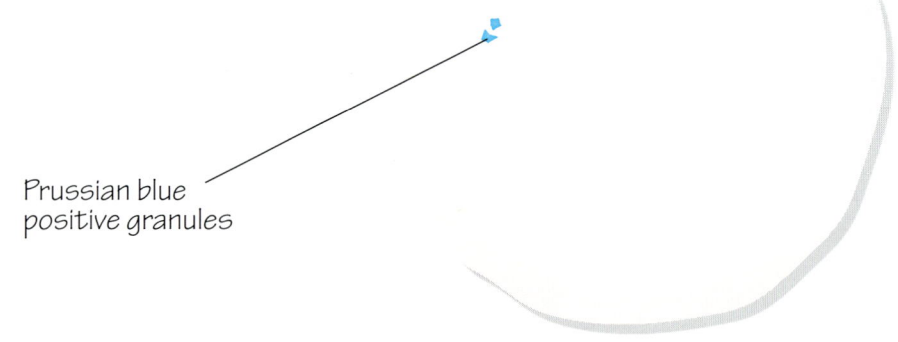

Prussian blue positive granules

H-25, 1981 (Blood, Prussian Blue, X400)

Cell Identification	Referee %	Participant %
Pappenheimer bodies (iron stain)	100	95.9
Sideroblast (iron stain)	-	2

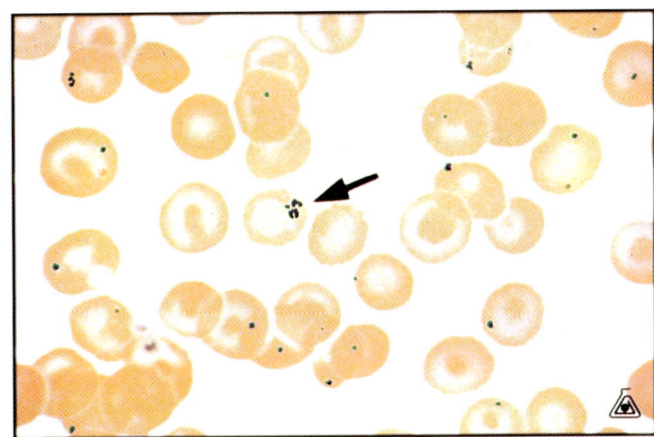

This is an iron stain. Many of the red blood cells contain small blue angular inclusions that are positive for iron. The arrowed cell contains multiple such inclusions, called Pappenheimer bodies. The corresponding Wright-Giemsa stain is seen in H-24, 1981 on page 141. Pappenheimer bodies are usually single but they may occasionally form small groups often arranged as doublets. Three doublets are found in the arrowed cell. Sideroblast is not a reasonable response, because sideroblasts must contain a nucleus as well as iron-positive inclusions.

HE-44, 1996 (Blood, split screen: Left, Wright-Giemsa, X400; Right, Prussian Blue, X400)

Cell Identification	Referee %	Participant %
Pappenheimer bodies (iron stain)	84.6	75.2
Howell-Jolly body	7.7	10
Sideroblast (iron stain)	3.8	1.5

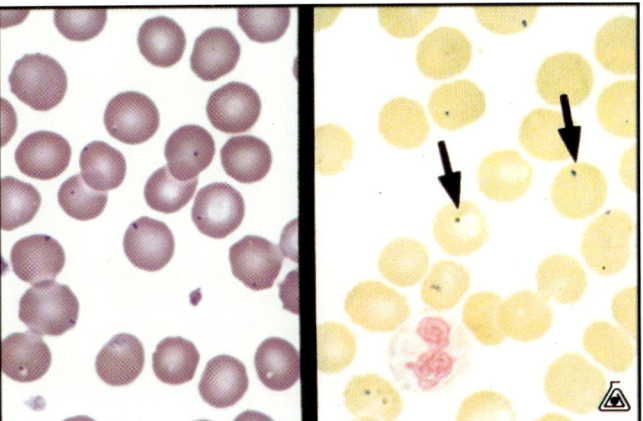

The split screen peripheral blood photomicrograph demonstrates a Wright-Giemsa stain on the left and an iron stain (Prussian blue) on the right. Numerous Pappenheimer bodies are seen on the Wright-Giemsa stain. The round dark punctations are single or in doublets. They are smaller than 1 µm, which is the size of most Howell-Jolly bodies. The small inclusions stain positively with Prussian blue, indicative of the presence of iron. Wright-Giemsa stain does not stain for iron, but rather the protein matrix which contains the iron. Therefore normal siderocytes (iron-containing non-nucleated red cells) are not visible with Wright-Giemsa. Iron-containing red cell inclusions are only seen after Wright-Giemsa staining when they are encased in a protein matrix. The inclusions are clearly not Heinz bodies because Heinz bodies are not visible by either Wright-Giemsa or iron stain. They are also not Howell-Jolly bodies which are composed of DNA and are iron negative.

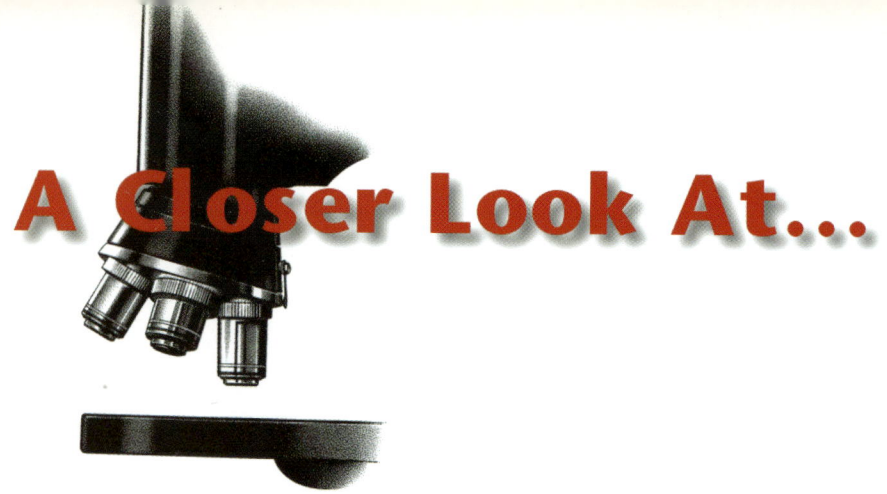

How Pappenheimer Bodies Form

The formation of Pappenheimer bodies is illustrated in the accompanying diagram. A reticulocyte is the last stage of red cell maturation in the bone marrow. The nucleus is gone and the cytoplasmic machinery used to manufacture hemoglobin is no longer needed. As a reticulocyte matures, the ribosomes and organelles progressively disappear. If the cell organelles are damaged or are pathologic in any way, they may elicit the formation of a digestive vacuole called an autophagosome. A delicate membrane surrounds the damaged organelles. Lysozymes join the vacuole and discharge their powerful enzymes inside, digesting the contents. The resulting protein aggregate may remain within the red cell or be discharged (a process called *exocytosis*). Once in the circulation, particles that remain in the red cell may be removed by the spleen. (This is called the "pitting function" of the spleen).

The process of autophagosome production occurs rarely in normal red cells, because the mitochondria, ribosomes, and other organelles are not pathologic. Consider the case of sideroblastic anemia, however. The mitochondria are damaged because they are full of iron. Autophagosomes form in an attempt to remove the offending organelles. The resultant red cell inclusions contain a mixture of protein and iron. The spleen attempts to remove them but if any remain, the small particles are clearly visible by Wright-Giemsa staining as Pappenheimer bodies. Because they also contain iron, Prussian blue stain (Pearls' reaction) is also positive.

How Pappenheimer Bodies Form

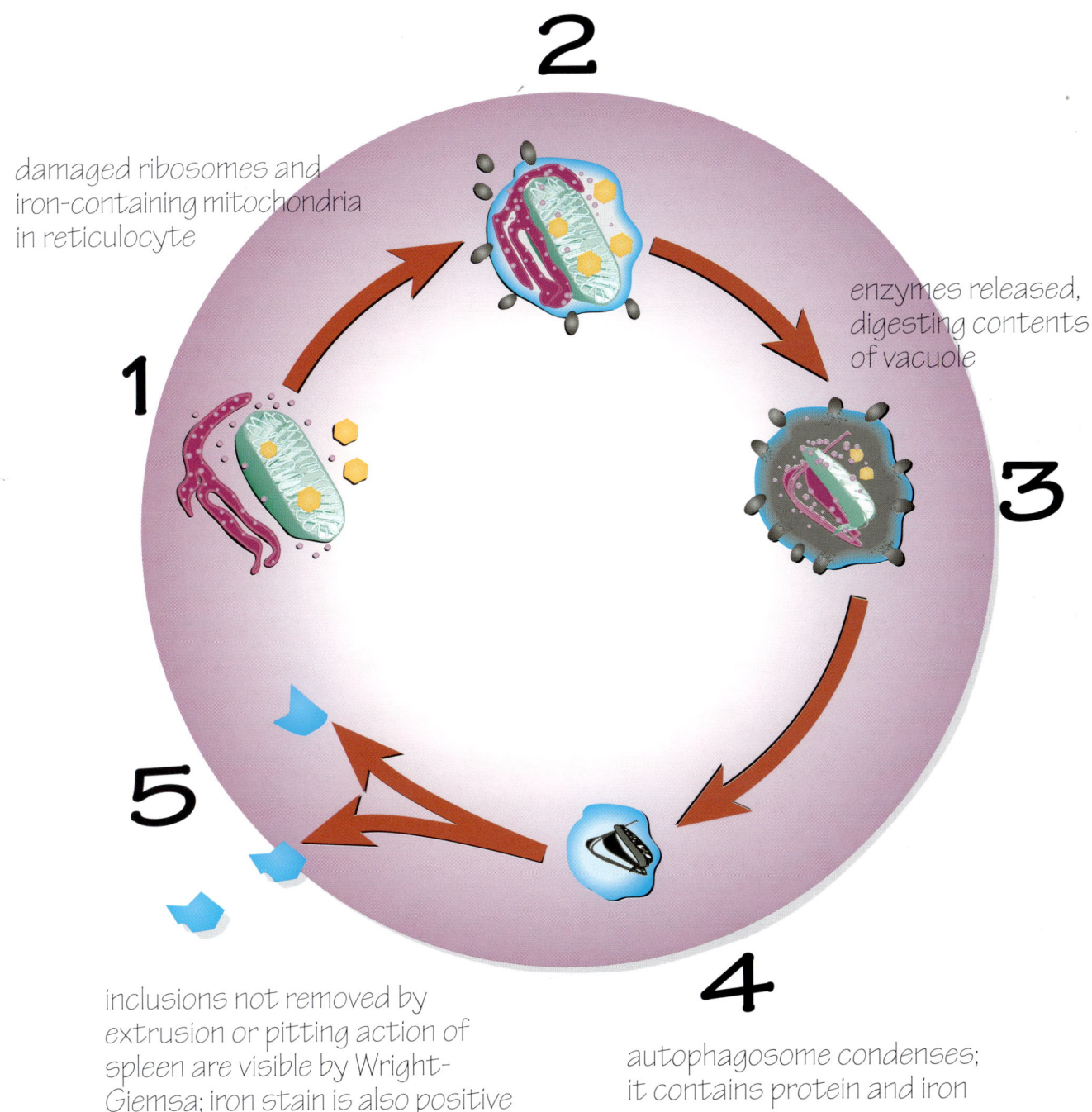

1. damaged ribosomes and iron-containing mitochondria in reticulocyte
2. vacuole surrounds organelles and lysozomes attach to its surface forming an autophagosome
3. enzymes released, digesting contents of vacuole
4. autophagosome condenses; it contains protein and iron
5. inclusions not removed by extrusion or pitting action of spleen are visible by Wright-Giemsa; iron stain is also positive

Red Cell Agglutinates

SYNONYMS
autoagglutination, red cell agglutination

VITAL STATISTICS
- size .... at least 14 by 14 µm, often greater
- shape .... irregular overlapping of red blood cells in a clump or cluster
- cytoplasm .... abundant, pink-red; central pallor may be present or can be obscured due to overlapping cells and look like spherocytes

KEY DIFFERENTIATING FEATURES
- clump or cluster of red blood cells overlapping in an irregular arrangement
- length and width of this arrangement is usually about the same

OTHER FINDINGS
- often associated with mild hemolytic anemia
- polychromasia and spherocytes can be seen
- may have artifactually decreased red blood cell count and/or increased MCV when sample is analyzed by automated instruments; this effect usually disappears with warming of the sample
- cases associated with malignant lymphomas or plasma cell dyscrasias may have blue proteinaceous background, anemia, thrombocytopenia and, rarely, circulating malignant cells

POTENTIAL LOOK-ALIKES
rouleaux

ASSOCIATED DISEASE STATES AND CONDITIONS
- cold autoimmune hemolytic anemia
- paroxysmal cold hemoglobinuria
- cold agglutinins without anemia
- malignant lymphomas associated with monoclonal IgM spikes (especially Waldenström's macroglobulinemia)
- plasma cell dyscrasias with monoclonal IgM paraprotein spikes

Red cell agglutinates are seen periodically in the hematology laboratory. This abnormality occurs when red blood cells cluster or clump together in an irregular mass in the thin area of the blood film. Usually, the length and width of these clumps are similar and one must distinguish this abnormality from rouleaux formation. True rouleaux also occurs in the thin area of the blood film. However, in contrast, rouleaux is a regular, linear arrangement of four or more red blood cells which resemble a "stack of coins," rather than an irregular clump of cells. Due to overlapping of cells in red cell agglutinates, individual red cells often appear to be spherocytes. This misperception is due to obscuring of the normal central pallor of the red cells in the clump.

Red cell agglutination is often associated with a factitously lowered red blood cell count when testing is performed on an automated hematology analyzer. This error results when red cells which are stuck together (i.e. doublets, triplets, etc.) are counted as a single cell and large clumps are ignored by the instrument. This same effect can increase the measured MCV. Since the hemoglobin is assayed after the red cells are lysed, it is not affected by agglutination. When the instrument calculates the MCHC, the falsely decreased red blood cell count and falsely elevated MCV can then lead to an erroneous MCHC which may be high or low, depending upon which measurement is affected to the greatest degree. An increased RDW (red cell distribution width) will also be seen in these cases.

Autoagglutination is due to cold agglutinins, most commonly an IgM antibody. Cold agglutinins can arise in a variety of diseases and are clinically divided into cases occurring after viral or *Mycoplasma* infections, cases associated with underlying lymphoproliferative disorders or plasma cell dyscrasias (cold agglutinin disease), and chronic idiopathic cases which are more frequently seen in elderly women. More detailed discussion of red cell aggregates comparing them to rouleaux is found in *A Closer Look At...Sticky Red Blood Cells* on page 150.

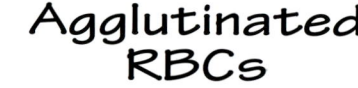

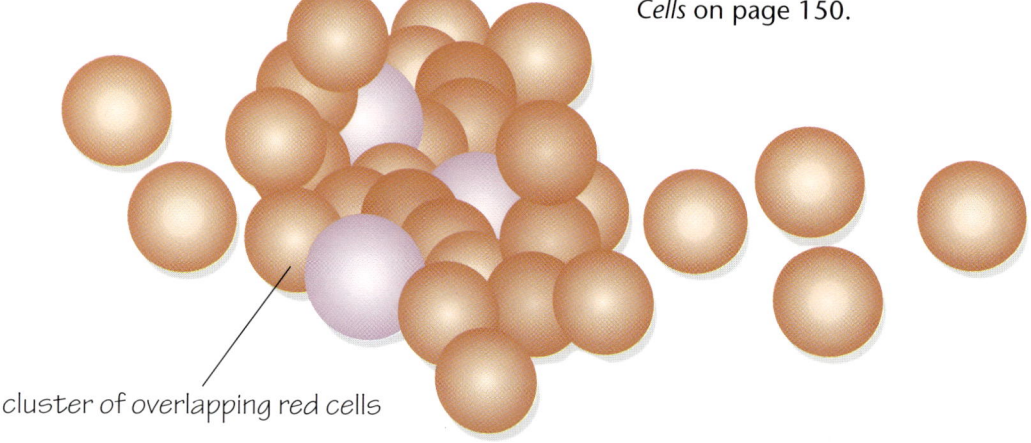

cluster of overlapping red cells

HE-26, 1997 (Blood, Wright-Giemsa, X160)

Identification	Referee %	Participant %
Red cell agglutination	100	97.8
Rouleaux	-	1.9

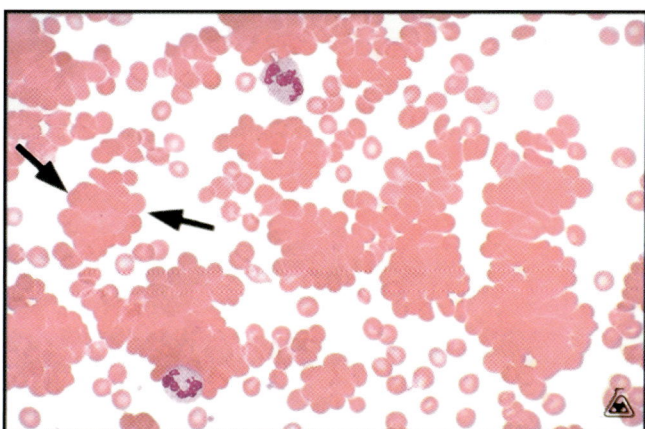

The arrowed object represents agglutinates of red blood cells. The width and length of the aggregate are about equal. This is in contrast to rouleaux in which the cells are linearly arranged in chains at least 4 cells long. Clumping or aggregation of red cells, often referred to as autoagglutination, usually indicates the presence of cold agglutinins. Cold agglutinins are anti-erythrocyte antibodies, usually IgM, that preferentially bind red cells at cold temperatures (4-18°C). Cold agglutinins are present in the sera of most healthy persons, but are usually in low titer. Elevated titers may arise as a complication of infectious diseases, most notably *Mycoplasma pneumoniae* infection. Monoclonal cold agglutinins are associated with B cell neoplasms. Cold agglutinins can activate the complement pathway on the cell membrane and induce hemolysis.

HE-26, 1995 (Blood, Wright-Giemsa, X400)

Identification	Referee %	Participant %
Red cell agglutination	100	98.8

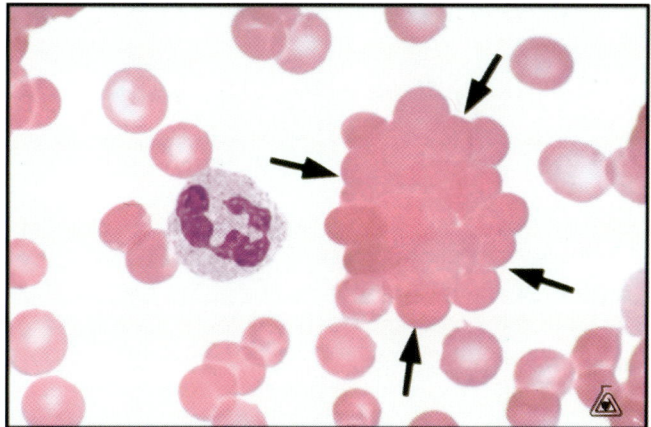

This blood film displays the typical appearance of red cell agglutination. The arrowed structure is an irregular clump of red blood cells which has an approximately equal length and width. The red blood cells in the clump appear to be spherocytes, but this misperception is secondary to overlapping of their cytoplasm. Scattered individual red blood cells are normochromic and normocytic with a few target cells. No platelets are visible. A single neutrophil is also seen.

Rouleaux

SYNONYMS
  none

VITAL STATISTICS
  size .... at least 7 by 18 µm, often greater
  shape .... linear arrangement of four or more red blood cells, simulating a "stack of coins"
  cytoplasm .... abundant, pink-red; central pallor may be present or can be obscured due to overlapping cells

KEY DIFFERENTIATING FEATURES
  linear arrangement of four or more red blood cells forming a "stack of coins" appearance
  length of arrangement is much greater than width and cells form a regular, uniform pattern

OTHER FINDINGS
  proteinaceous (blue staining) background
  artifactually decreased red blood cell count and increased MCV
  cases associated with liver disease may show anemia, target cells, acanthocytes, and thrombocytopenia
  cases associated with multiple myeloma or malignant lymphomas may have circulating malignant cells (plasma cells or lymphoma cells), anemia, and thrombocytopenia
  cases due to examination of thick area of blood film have no associated abnormal findings

POTENTIAL LOOK-ALIKES
  red blood cell agglutinates

ASSOCIATED DISEASE STATES AND CONDITIONS
  none, if noted only in the thick area of a blood film
  true rouleaux formation (in thin area of blood film):
    chronic liver disease with hypergammaglobulinemia
    malignant lymphoma
    multiple myeloma and monoclonal gammopathies
    chronic infections
    chronic inflammatory conditions

Rouleaux formation is a common artifact which can be observed in the thick area of virtually any blood film. This term describes the appearance of four or more red blood cells organized in a linear arrangement, which simulates a "stack of coins." The length of this arrangement (18 µm or more) will exceed its width (7-8 µm), which is the diameter of a single red blood cell. The central pallor of the red blood cells is generally apparent, but it may be obscured due to overlapping of the cell's cytoplasm. When noted in only the thick area of a blood film, rouleaux formation is a normal finding and not associated with any disease process.

True rouleaux formation is present when this artifact is seen in the thin area of a blood film. It is often associated with a proteinaceous, blue staining background. True rouleaux formation is due to increased amounts of plasma proteins, primarily fibrinogen or globulins. It is seen in a variety of infectious and inflammatory disorders associated with polyclonal increases in globulins and/or increased levels of fibrinogen. Rouleaux formation associated with monoclonal gammopathies can be seen in multiple myeloma and in malignant lymphomas such as Waldenström's macroglobulinemia.

Increased amounts of fibrinogen and globulins, which often have a net positive charge, attach to the negatively charged surface of the red cells. This protein binding results in neutralization of the red cell membrane's normal net negative charge that causes red cells to slightly repel each other and keep from sticking together. Thus, red cells coated with protein will tend to stick together and either rouleaux formation or red cell agglutination will result. The phenomenon is discussed in more detail in the following *A Closer Look At...* discussion on page 150.

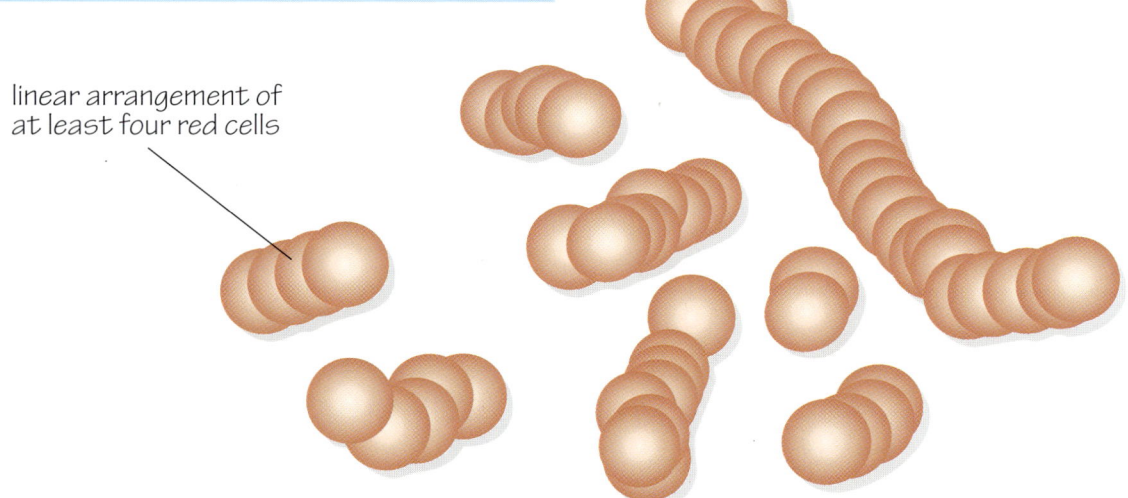

linear arrangement of at least four red cells

Rouleaux Formation

H1-30, 1986 (Blood, Wright-Giemsa, X375)

Identification	Referee %	Participant %
Rouleaux	88.9	96.5
Red cell agglutinates	11.1	3.2

This blood film illustrates the classic appearance of rouleaux formation. Scattered normal platelets are present. A single normal, mature lymphocyte is seen at the top of the field. The red cells are normochromic and normocytic. As shown in the arrowed structures, the red cells form a linear arrangement which resembles a "stack of coins." Depending on the degree of overlapping, central pallor can still be noted in some of the cells. This case is from a patient with multiple myeloma.

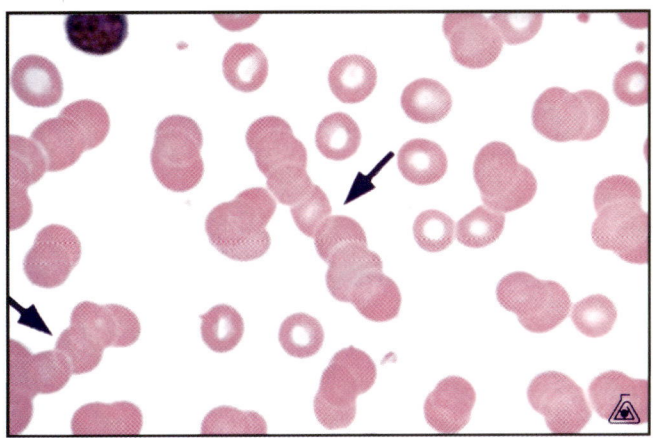

H1-29, 1986 (Blood, Wright-Giemsa, X375)

Identification	Referee %	Participant %
Rouleaux	72.2	72.3
Red cell agglutinates	27.8	27.5

This blood film again illustrates rouleaux formation. The red blood cells line up in groups of at least 4 cells. The linear pattern distinguishes the cells from the haphazard arrangement of agglutinated red cells. Red cell agglutinates have a width and length that are roughly equal; rouleaux formation is always considerably longer than it is wide. This case is from a patient with multiple myeloma. Elevated serum protein, primarily fibrinogen or globulins, decreases the electrical field around the cells, allowing them to loosely join together and form linear arrays. The lone leukocyte in the field is a segmented neutrophil.

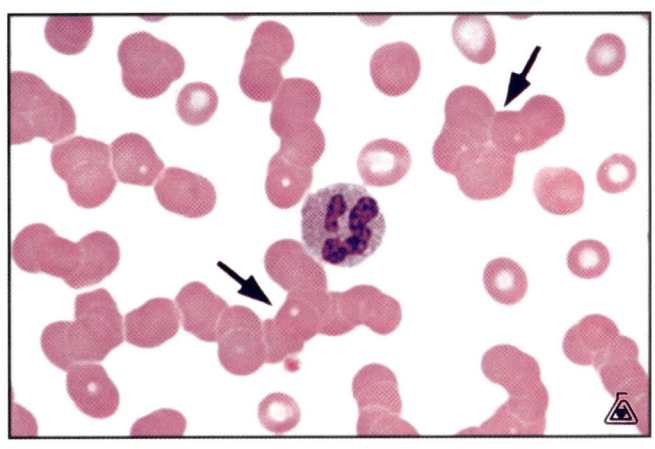

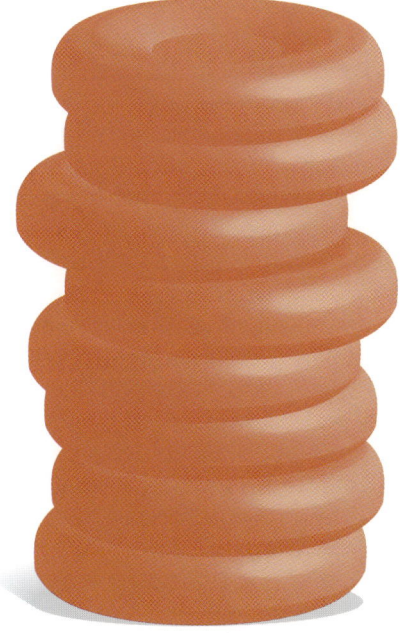

"stack of coins" configuration of red cells

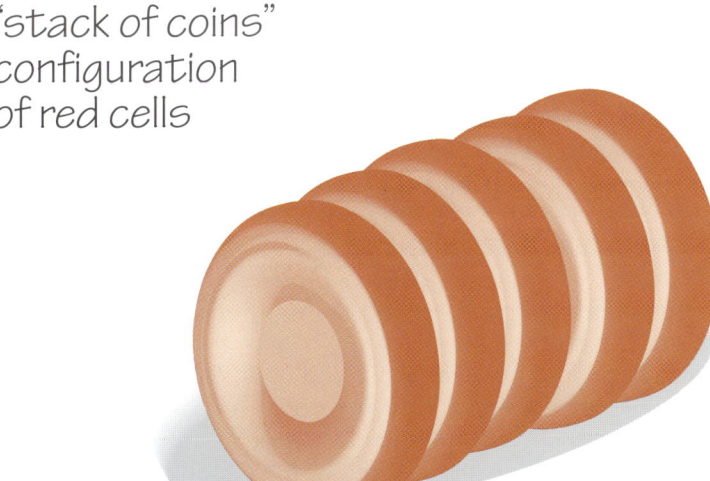

Erythrocytic Cells and Inclusions

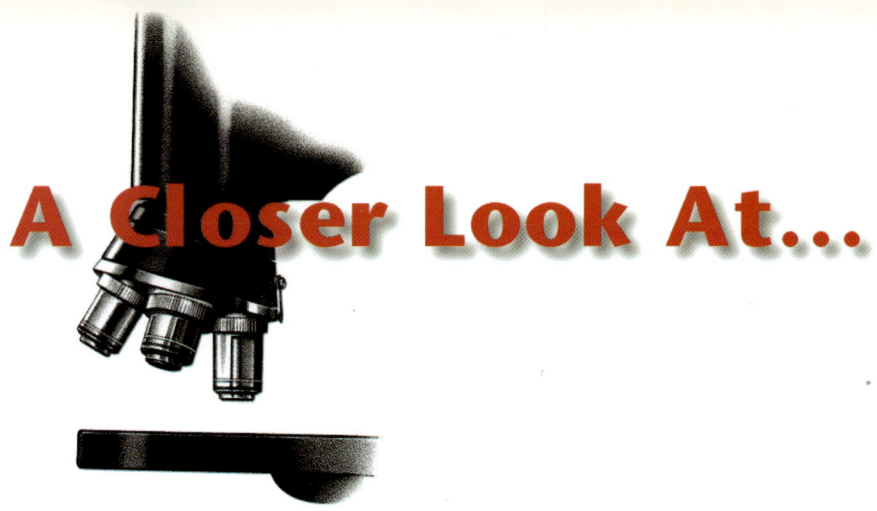

A Closer Look At...

Sticky Red Blood Cells

Normally, red blood cells will stick together in the thick area of the blood film, appearing as rouleaux formation or agglutination. A pathologic process is present only when these structures are found in the thin area of the blood film. Rouleaux formation and red blood cell agglutinates exhibit similarities, but differ in their morphologic appearance and causes. Rouleaux formation occurs when four or more red blood cells are organized in a linear arrangement with the length exceeding the width. Red blood cell agglutinates are clusters or clumps of red blood cells in an irregular mass. The length and width of these clumps are similar.

Both rouleaux formation and red cell agglutination can be associated with factitiously lowered red blood cell count and increased MCV when testing is done on an automated hematology analyzer. This error results when red cells that are stuck together (e.g. doublets or triplets) get counted as a single cell. Large clusters of red cells are often ignored by the instrument. This effect can also cause overestimation of the MCV. Since the hemoglobin is measured after the red cells are lysed, it is not affected by either disorder. When the instrument calculates the MCHC, the falsely decreased red blood cell count and falsely elevated MCV can frequently lead to an erroneously high or low MCHC, depending upon which measurement is affected to the greatest degree. An increased RDW (red cell distribution width) may also be seen.

Increased amounts of plasma proteins, mainly fibrinogen and globulins, are the cause of rouleaux formation. The proteins neutralize the negatively charged surface of the red blood cells. Instead of repelling each other, the red cells now bind together and form the linear arrangements of rouleaux formation.

Red blood cell agglutination is most commonly caused by IgM antibodies, called cold agglutinins. Clinically, they are classified as cases occurring after viral or Mycoplasma infections, cases associated with underlying lymphoproliferative disorders or plasma cell dyscrasias (cold agglutinin disease), and chronic idiopathic cases.

When cold agglutinins develop after infections caused by *Mycoplasma*, cytomegalovirus (CMV), Epstein-Barr virus (EBV), measles, or mumps, a mild hemolytic anemia is frequently observed. These cases of autoimmune hemolytic anemia demonstrate a positive direct antiglobulin test (DAT or direct Coombs' test) for anti-complement, but will be negative for anti-IgG. The IgM antibody is directed against the red blood cell I antigen in about 95% of cases. On occasion the antibody reacts with the fetal red blood cell i antigen. Anti-I activity is seen in cold agglutinins associated with *Mycoplasma* and most viral infections. Anti-i activity is associated with EBV infection.

Red cell agglutinates can also be found in cases of paroxysmal cold hemoglobinuria (PCH). This disease can exhibit a similar clinical pattern and may also occur after viral infections. In contrast, PCH is caused by an IgG antibody which binds to the red cells, paradoxically, at low temperature and then causes hemolysis when the blood is warmed to 37° C. Demonstration of this reaction in the laboratory is called the Donath-Landsteiner test. This antibody is usually directed against the red blood cell P antigen system.

Cold agglutinins associated with lymphoproliferative disorders and plasma cell dyscrasias are due to monoclonal production of an IgM paraprotein that also demonstrates anti-I activity. A small proportion of otherwise healthy individuals may have cold agglutinins. This chronic idiopathic form is more common in elderly women, and not associated with hemolysis.

Comparison of Red Blood Cell Agglutination and Rouleaux Formation

Zeta Potential

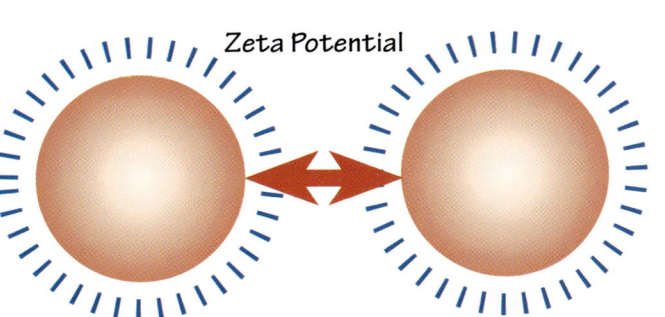

The negative charge of red cells is produced by the high sialic acid content of membrane.

Positive charges (cations) form an "ionic cloud" around the negatively charged red cells.

The difference in electrical potential between negative and positive charges is the **zeta potential**. This normally keeps red cells 25 nm apart.

Abnormal or Increased Plasma Proteins

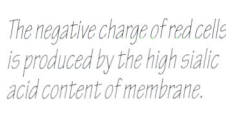

IgM Antibodies

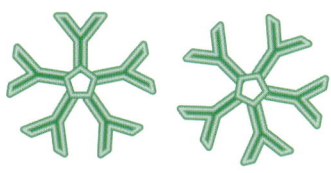

Non-Specific Aggregation

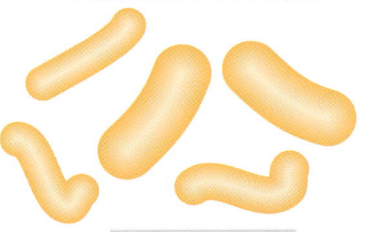

Proteins change surface charge of red cells, reducing zeta potential and allowing cells to loosely join together in rows.

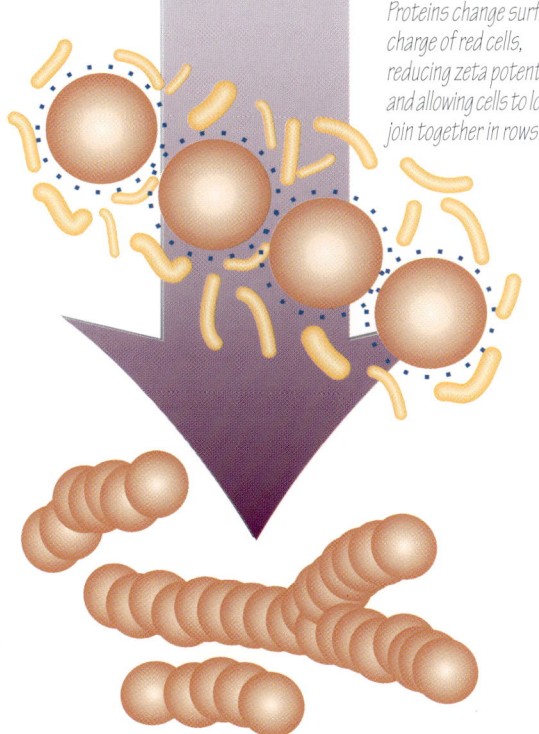

Specific Agglutination

IgM antibodies are large enough to span the zeta potential gap, forming a latticework that links the red blood cells.

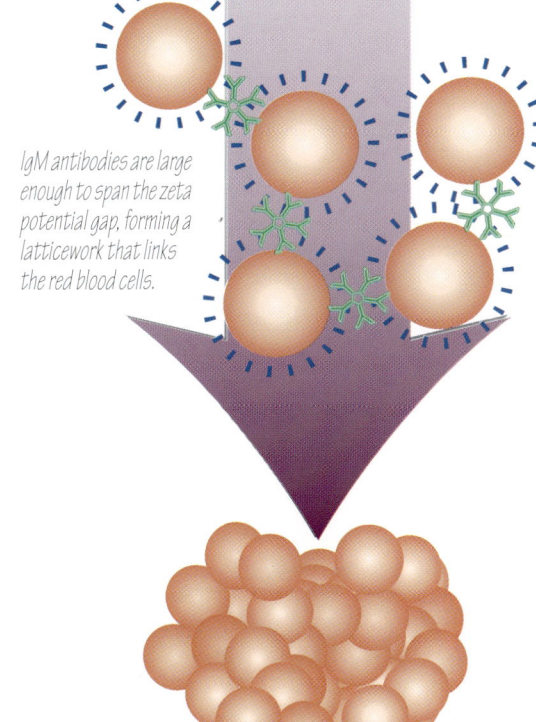

Erythrocytic Cells and Inclusions

Nucleated Red Cells

Introduction: Nucleated Red Cells 153
Pronormoblast (Bone Marrow) 154
   *A Closer Look At…*Red Cell Maturation and Cell Division 156
   *A Closer Look At…*Morphologic Keys to Identifying Early Normoblasts 158
Basophilic Normoblast (Bone Marrow) 160
Polychromatophilic Normoblast (Bone Marrow) 162
Orthochromic Normoblast (Bone Marrow) 164
Nucleated Red Cell, Megaloblastic (Bone Marrow) 166
   *A Closer Look At…*Megaloblastic Morphology 168
Nucleated Red Cell, Normal or Abnormal (Blood) 170
Nucleated Red Cell, Dysplastic (Bone Marrow) 172
   *A Closer Look At…*Megaloblastic vs. Megaloblastoid Erythroid Maturation 174
Sideroblast (Iron Stain) 176
   *A Closer Look At…*Sideroblasts and Siderocytes 178
Sideroblast, Ringed (Iron Stain) 180
   *A Closer Look At…*Hemoglobin Formation and Iron Utilization 182
   *A Closer Look At…*Formation of Ringed Sideroblasts 184

Introduction

The final product of red cell maturation, the anucleate biconcave disc is the result of a complicated maturation process that begins with a morphologically unrecognizable stem cell. The stem cell then becomes a lineage committed progenitor cell and enters the process of erythroid maturation. The first morphologically recognizable erythroid precursor is the proerythroblast. From there the maturation process continues through the basophilic, polychromatophilic, and orthochromatophilic normoblast stages until an anucleate cell leaves the bone marrow and is present in the circulation for approximately 120 days.

There are many factors that can impact this process resulting in both quantitative and qualitative abnormalities of the maturing erythroid cell. Some of these, such as megaloblastic, megaloblastoid, and dysplastic changes, are morphologically recognizable. The pages that follow will outline the morphologic appearance of normal erythroid precursors as well as several examples of what can occur when the normal maturation process is interrupted. In reviewing the College of American Pathologists proficiency testing data, it is clear that the interobserver reproducibility of red cell categorization has been a problem over the years. This portion of the atlas is an attempt to provide classic examples and discuss some of the criteria that can be used to increase the consensus of erythroid cells at various stages of maturation.

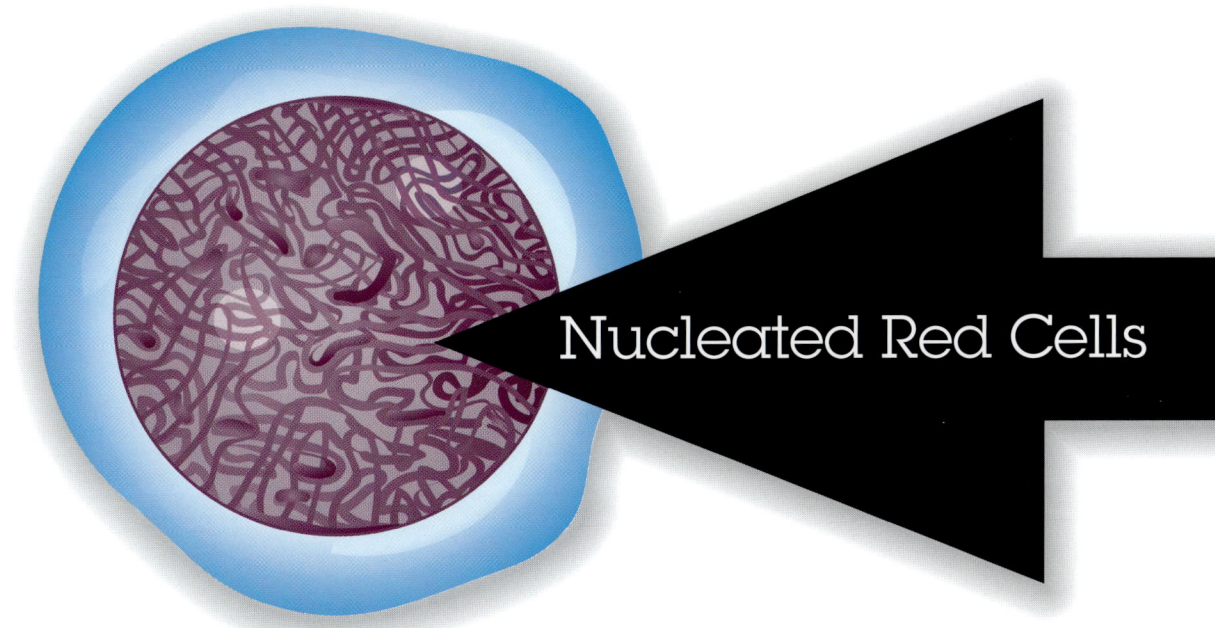

Pronormoblast (Bone Marrow)

SYNONYMS
rubriblast, erythroblast, proerythroblast

VITAL STATISTICS
size .... 17–24 μm
N:C ratio 8:1
cell shape .... round or oval
nuclear shape .... round or oval
chromatin .... finely reticulated (granular)
nucleoli .... prominent; one or more
cytoplasm .... scanty, pale blue, agranular

KEY DIFFERENTIATING FEATURES
large size
immature chromatin pattern with prominent nucleoli
pale blue cytoplasm with perinuclear halo

OTHER FINDINGS
cytoplasmic vacuoles may be seen in cases of ethanol abuse, chloramphenicol therapy, riboflavin deficiency, hyperosmolar coma, phenylalanine deficiency and copper deficiency

POTENTIAL LOOK-ALIKES
other blasts (myeloblasts, lymphoblasts, plasmablasts)

ASSOCIATED DISEASE STATES AND CONDITIONS
normal bone marrow cell
increased numbers may be found in:
  erythroid hyperplasia
  AML (erythroleukemia, FAB M6)
  parvovirus infection (usually with intranuclear inclusions)

Pronormoblasts are the most immature cells in the erythroid series. They are normally confined to the bone marrow where they comprise <3% of the nucleated erythroid cells. In cases of acute erythroid leukemia they may rarely be found in the peripheral blood. The normal proerythroblast is a large cell, 17 to 24 μm in diameter. The nucleus occupies 80% of the cell and is round to slightly ovoid and contains one or more prominent nucleoli. The chromatin is finely reticulated and parachromatin is sparse and indistinct. As the cell matures, the chromatin becomes thicker and more "beady." This gradually obscures the nucleoli. The cytoplasm stains light blue and does not contain granules. It usually appears as a thick band around the nucleus. A perinuclear halo corresponding to the Golgi apparatus is usually evident.

In pathologic states the pronormoblast can have dysplastic, megaloblastic and lobulated nuclear forms. The most extreme examples occur in acute erythroleukemia (FAB M6/DiGuglielmo's syndrome). In this condition erythroid "gigantoblasts" with hyperlobated nuclear features may be seen. The abnormal proerythroblasts found in acute erythroid leukemia will have a "block" pattern of PAS reactivity. Normal erythroid cells are PAS negative. (See page 173).

Pronormoblast

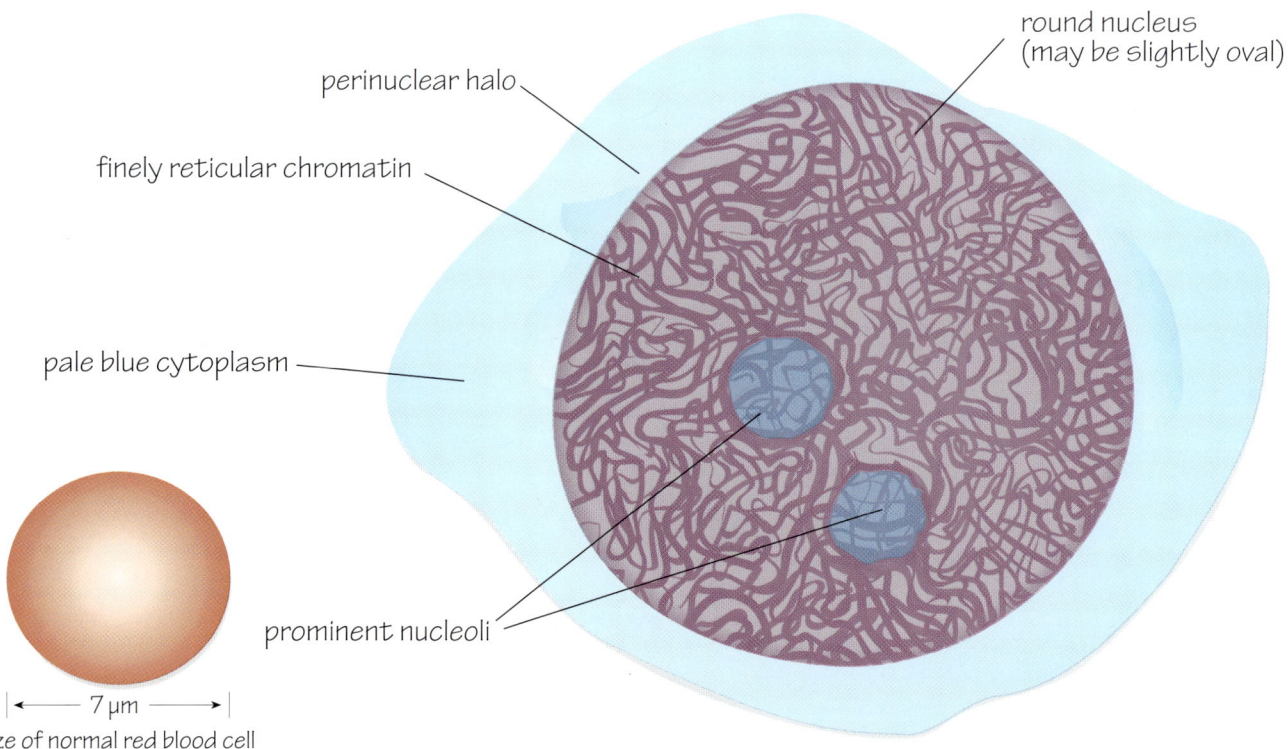

round nucleus (may be slightly oval)
perinuclear halo
finely reticular chromatin
pale blue cytoplasm
prominent nucleoli

7 μm
size of normal red blood cell

H1-46, 1989 (Bone Marrow, Wright-Giemsa, X350)

Identification	Referee %	Participant %
Pronormoblast	100	96.7

The arrowed cell is a pronormoblast. The cytoplasm is more deeply basophilic than usual. The N:C ratio is high. The chromatin pattern is immature. In this field there are increased numbers of erythroid precursors as one would see in a case of erythroid hyperplasia.

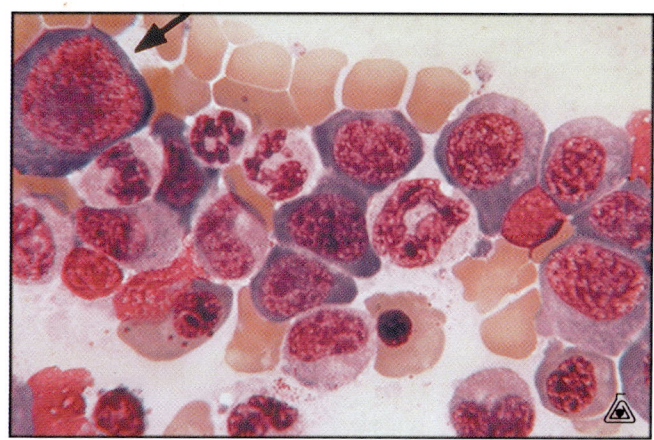

HE-45A, 1996 (Bone Marrow, Wright-Giemsa, X210)

Identification	Referee %	Participant %
Pronormoblast	56	61
Basophilic normoblast	16	31

The low power view of this bone marrow demonstrates erythroid hyperplasia with all stages of erythroid maturation present. The two large arrows are pointing to the largest cells in the field, which are pronormoblasts. These youngest of developing nucleated red blood cells are slightly late in their stage of maturation, evidenced by the cytoplasm which is somewhat darker than that of prototypic pronormoblasts. The nuclear:cytoplasmic ratio is high and the chromatin immature. Several pale nucleoli are visible. The presence of nucleoli and absence of thick, rope-like areas of chromatin condensation characterize this cell as a pronormoblast rather than a basophilic normoblast.

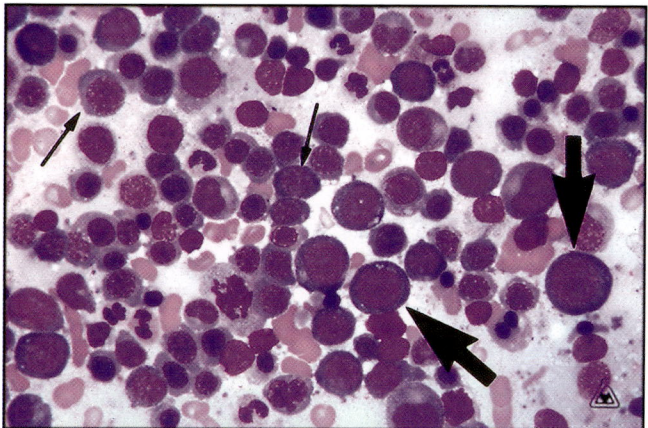

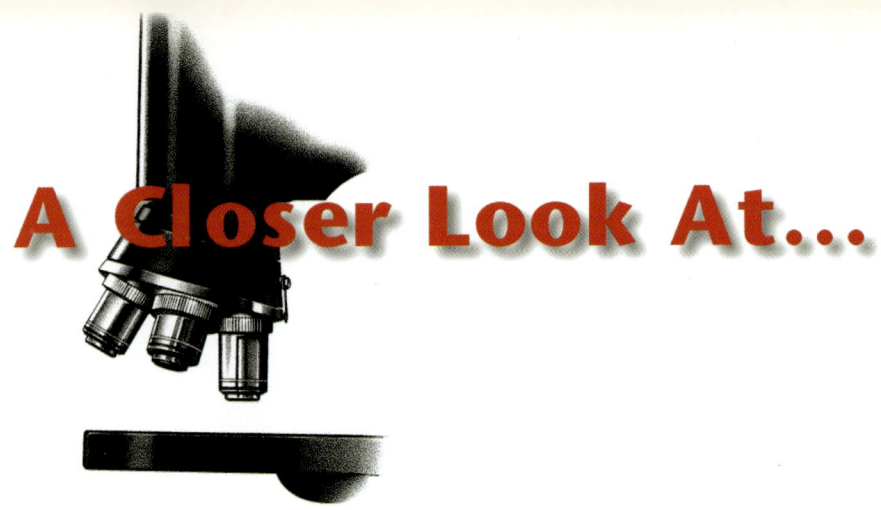

A Closer Look At...

Red Cell Maturation and Cell Division

Hematopoiesis begins from the pluripotential stem cell which gives rise to a progenitor cell which is lineage committed. The initial proliferation and maturation of the early stem cells and erythroid progenitor cells is stimulated by general cytokines such as GM-CSF, IL-3, IL-1. The later divisions of the committed erythroid stem cell are driven primarily by erythropoietin. The first morphologically recognizable erythroid cell derived from the erythroid progenitor cell is the *pronormoblast*. In normal hematopoiesis, the pronormoblast undergoes nuclear and cytoplasmic maturation resulting in nuclear condensation, cytoplasmic hemoglobinization, reduction in cell size, and eventual nuclear extrusion. The result is an anucleate red blood cell (reticulocyte) that undergoes further maturation in the bone marrow and peripheral blood to finally tranform into a mature erythrocyte.

Nuclear and cytoplasmic changes are appreciated during the various stages of erythropoiesis. In the early stages, the pronormoblast nucleus is large and consists of immature delicate chromatin with one or two nucleoli. In this immature stage, the nucleoli contain large amounts of RNA. As the cell matures, the nucleoli become less distinct, with the chromatin condensing to form coarse strands and clumps with open parachromatin spaces and DNA nucleolus-associated heterochromatin is present.

The cytoplasm of basophilic normoblasts is rich in organelles and stains deeply basophilic owing to the large amounts of cytoplasmic RNA. Over time the level of cytoplasmic RNA decreases and the degree of cytoplasmic hemoglobinization increases. The cytoplasm gradually shifts to orange or pink.

The pronormoblast, basophilic normoblast, and polychromatophilic normoblast are capable of cell division. Seven days are required for maturation of erythroid cells to the late polychromatophilic stage. Over a three-day period, the late polychromatophilic normoblast matures through the orthochromatophilic stage, extrudes its nucleus, and becomes a reticulocyte which is then released into the peripheral blood. The small amount of residual cytoplasmic RNA present in a reticulocyte is visible with vital stains such as new methylene blue. Once released into the circulation, the mature red cell has an average life span of 120 days.

Red Blood Cell Maturation & Cell Division

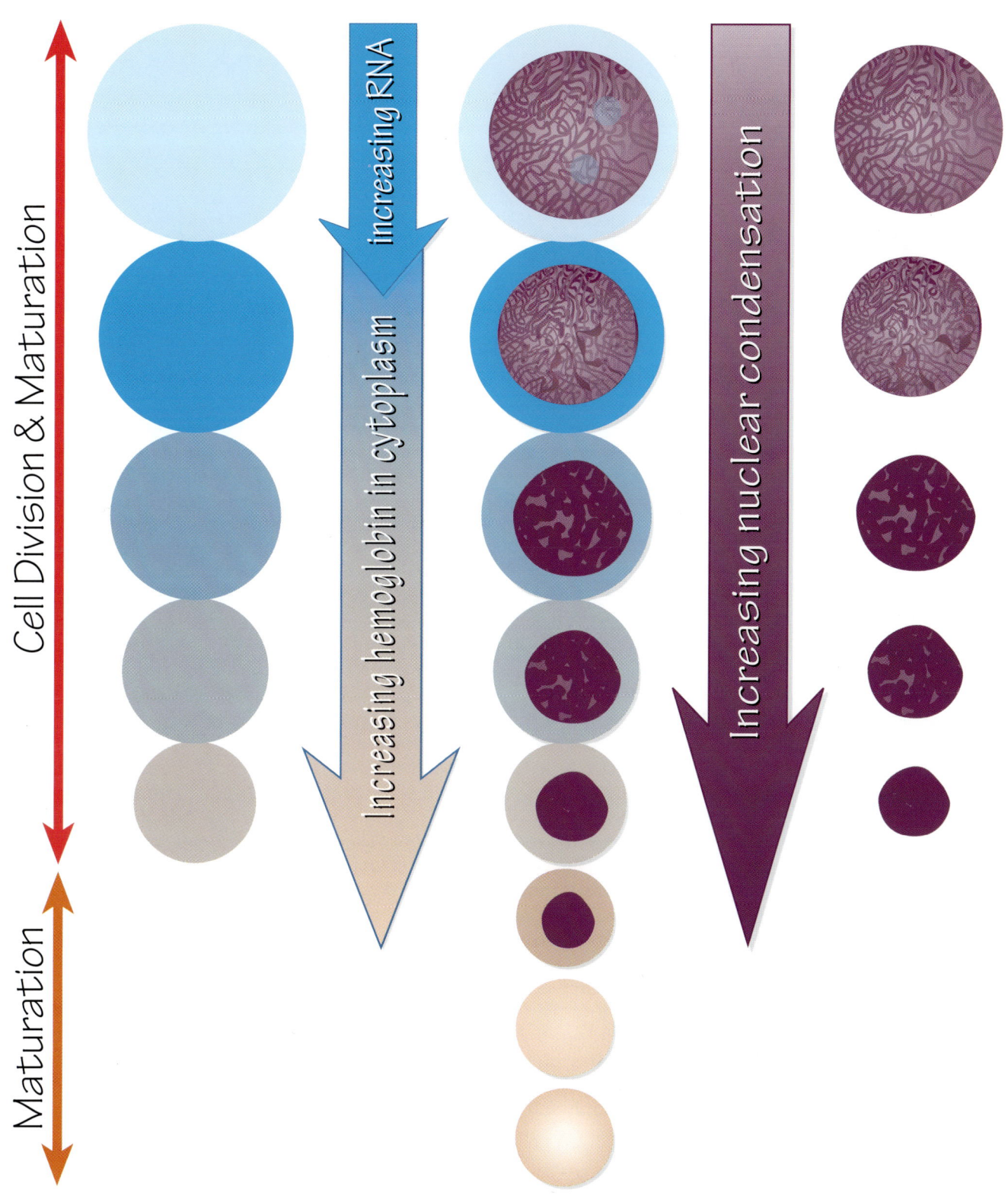

Nucleated Red Cells

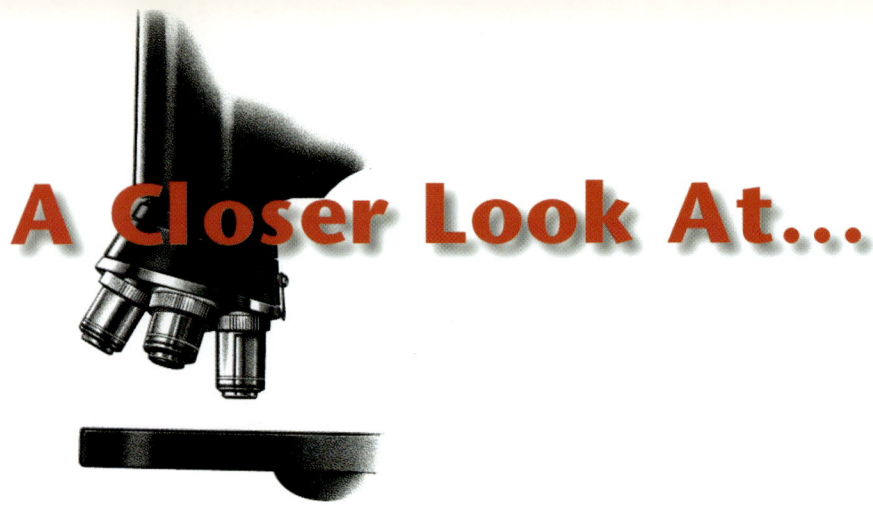

A Closer Look At...

Morphologic Keys to Identifying Early Normoblasts

Identification of the various normal stages of red cell maturation has proven to be particularly problematic in hematology proficiency tests. After reviewing referee and participant responses over the years and the photomicrograph discussions, it is clear that we have not been morphologically consistent. Part of the problem is a lack of clear criteria. Textbooks—not just CAP authors—do not agree on what are the crucial points of differentiation. Some emphasize cytoplasmic staining while others nuclear chromatin pattern. There is disagreement as to whether nucleoli are found in basophilic normoblasts. This exercise is an attempt to more precisely articulate our current views and define the critical morphologic requirements for each stage in red cell development.

The illustration on the next page stresses the three most important differential criteria needed to correctly identify developing erythrons: **cell size**, **cytoplasmic staining**, and **nuclear chromatin clumping**. It is divided into three columns. To the left are highly stylized drawings of prototypic early normoblasts. They are meant only to provide key points to help the morphologist develop an identification algorithm. The center column lists morphologic criteria for the cells. The last column is composed of photomicroscopic examples which have not been used in proficiency testing challenges. Some of colors in the photomicrographs are not correct due to limitations in the printing process. The royal blue cytoplasm of the basophilic normoblasts is a case in point.

It is important to emphasize that any morphologic description is only a snapshot of reality. Some cells are difficult to classify because they exhibit features that meld two maturation stages. In those cases, we tend to shade our identification to the more mature form.

Pronormoblasts have pale blue cytoplasm and are large cells (17-24 µm in diameter). As in all maturation stages, the nucleus is nearly perfectly round; it is never folded or anglular. The chromatin is lacy and blast-like; there should be no clumping. Nucleoli are prominent and have a punched out appearance.

Early basophilic normoblasts show a hint of chromatin clumping as chromocenters begin to form. The strands are thicker and begin to obscure the nucleus. The cytoplasm takes on more RNA and is intensely basophilic producing a royal-blue color. This is darker than the cytoplasm of pronormoblasts.

Late basophilic normoblasts have thick chromatin strands with more prominent chromocenters giving a beaded appearance. Prominent chromatin clumping is never a feature, however. The cytoplasm takes on a hint of gray as hemoglobin begins to accumulate and alter the coloration.

Polychromatophilic normoblasts display distinct chromatin clumping as well-defined chromocenters appear. The cytoplasm is now well hemoglobinized giving it a gray-blue (early) or pink-gray (late) variegated appearance.

Orthochromic normoblasts have pink orange cytoplasm and dramatic chromatin clumping. The cytoplasm should closely resemble that of the adjacent non-nucleated red cells and the nucleus is often eccentric or in the process of being extruded.

Identification of Early Normoblasts

Key Morphologic Features

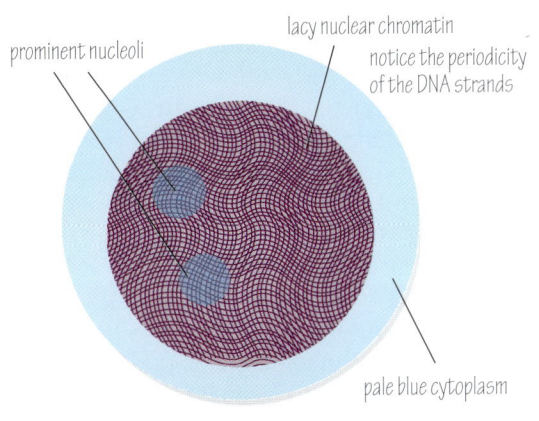

Pronormoblast
- prominent nucleoli
- lacy nuclear chromatin / notice the periodicity of the DNA strands
- pale blue cytoplasm

Pronormoblast
- large size (17-24 μm)
- round or oval nucleus
- lacy, evenly distributed chromatin
- prominent nucleoli
- pale blue cytoplasm

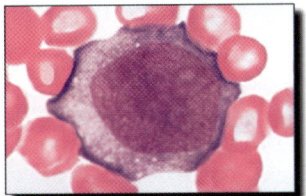
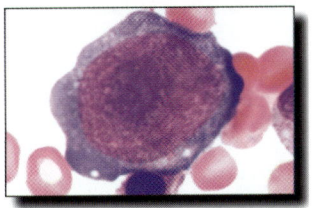

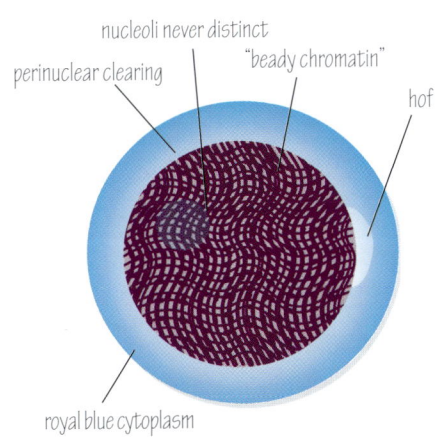

Basophilic Normoblast
- nucleoli never distinct
- perinuclear clearing
- "beady chromatin"
- hof
- royal blue cytoplasm

Basophilic Normoblast
- intermediate size (10-17 μm)
- round nucleus
- open, "beady" chromatin without significant clumping
- nucleoli visible in early forms, less conspicuous in later forms as chromatin strands thicken
- cytoplasm intensely basophilic giving a royal blue color; later cells may have a slight gray tint due to early hemoglobin production
- slight clearing around nucleus
- paranuclear clear area (hof)

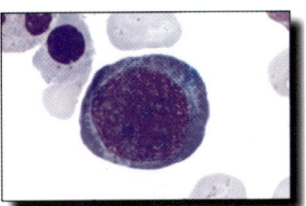
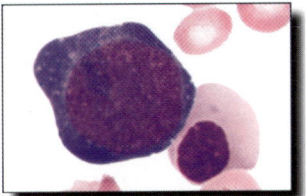
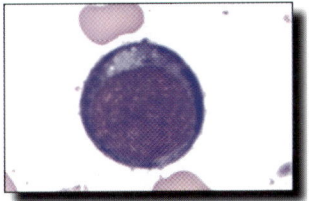

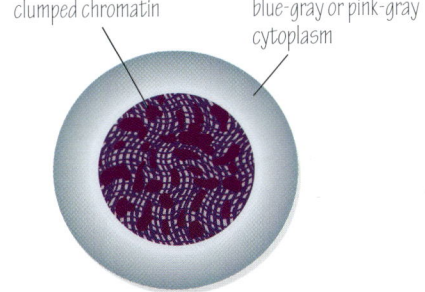

Polychromatophilic Normoblast
- clumped chromatin
- blue-gray or pink-gray cytoplasm

Polychromatophilic Normoblast
- smaller size (10-15 μm)
- round nucleus
- clumped chromatin; prominent chromocenters
- nucleoli not visible
- blue-gray ("dishwater blue") to pink-gray cytoplasm

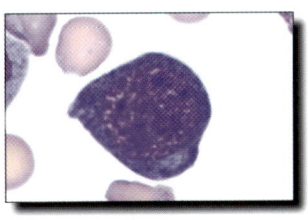
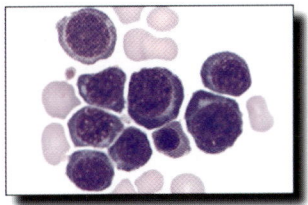

early and late polychromatophilic normoblasts

Basophilic Normoblast (Bone Marrow)

SYNONYMS
prorubricyte

VITAL STATISTICS
- size .... 10 to 17 μm
- N:C ratio 6:1
- cell shape .... round to oval
- nuclear shape .... round to oval
- chromatin .... open chromatin with thickened strands ("beading"); no significant clumping
- nucleoli .... barely visible in early forms; absent in later forms as chromatin strands thicken
- cytoplasm .... deeply basophilic (royal blue color); slight gray appearance in later cells

KEY DIFFERENTIATING FEATURES
- "beady" chromatin pattern
- deeply basophilic cytoplasm (royal blue)
- faint or absent nucleoli

POTENTIAL LOOK-ALIKES
- immature plasma cells
- lymphocytes

ASSOCIATED DISEASE STATES AND CONDITIONS
- normal bone marrow cell
- increased in various causes of erythroid hyperplasia

Basophilic normoblasts are smaller (10 to 17 μm in diameter) than pronormoblasts, but similar in cellular and nuclear shape. Normally they comprise 6-8% of the nucleated erythroid cells in the marrow. The chromatin of the basophilic normoblast is open but the strands are thickened or "beady." Pronormoblast nuclei display open chromatin without any condensation or thickening of the strands. The nuclei of large or early basophilic normoblasts may reveal single nucleoli. As the cell matures, the chromatin thickens and nucleoli are no longer visible. Basophilic normoblasts have more cytoplasm than pronormoblasts. It is typically intensely basophilic, producing a royal blue appearance. As the amount of hemoglobin increases, late cells may have a very slight gray color. If too gray, the cell is best classified as a polychromatophilic normoblast.

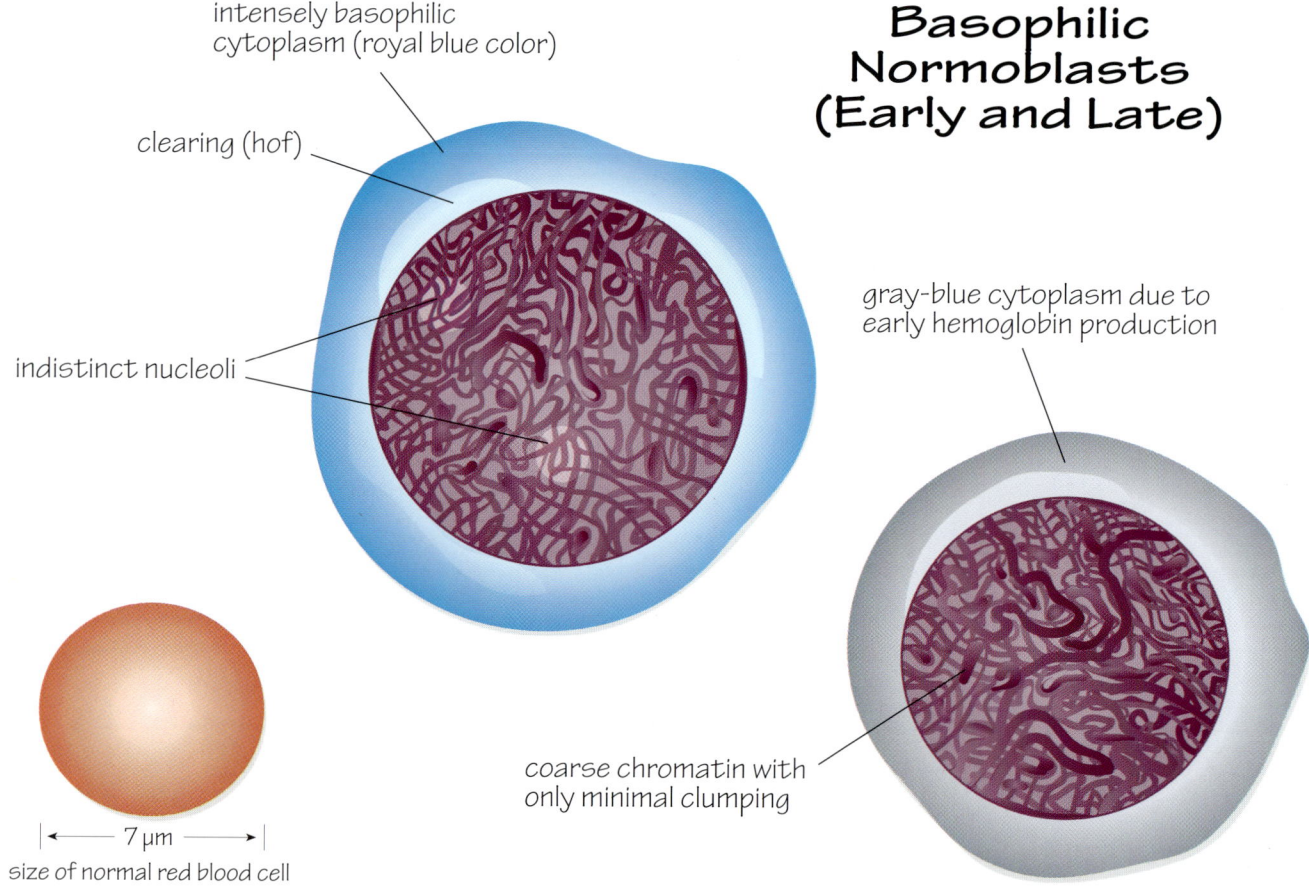

Basophilic Normoblasts (Early and Late)

- intensely basophilic cytoplasm (royal blue color)
- clearing (hof)
- indistinct nucleoli
- gray-blue cytoplasm due to early hemoglobin production
- coarse chromatin with only minimal clumping
- 7 μm — size of normal red blood cell

HE-46, 1996 (Bone Marrow, Wright-Giemsa, X400)

Identification	Referee %	Participant %
Basophilic normoblast	40	36.8
Nucleated red cell, megalobastic	60	32

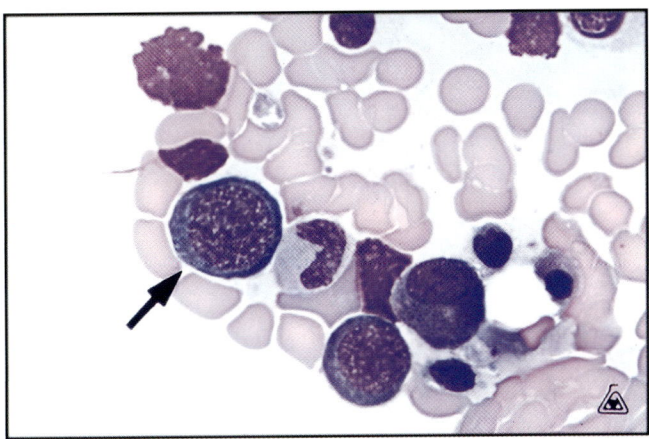

The arrowed cell is a basophilic normoblast. The nuclei of basophilic normoblasts have thick strands of chromatin, obscuring nucleoli. As these cell mature, the chromatin strands become thicker and chromocenters more pronounced. When the clumping is prominent, the term polychromatophilic normoblast is appropriate. The clumping in the arrowed cell is significant enough that polychromatophilic stage should also be considered. Megaloblastic change is difficult to recognize in early maturing erythroid cells. When it is present there should be nuclear to cytoplasmic dyssynchrony. At the basophilic normoblast stage of maturation this would be depicted by very immature, blast-like chromatin. The cell depicted here clearly exhibits nuclear chromatin clumping.

HE-50, 1996 (Bone Marrow, Wright-Giemsa, X400)

Identification	Referee %	Participant %
Basophilic normoblast	36	26.1
Pronormoblast	24	48.1
Megaloblastic nucleated red cell	40	15.5

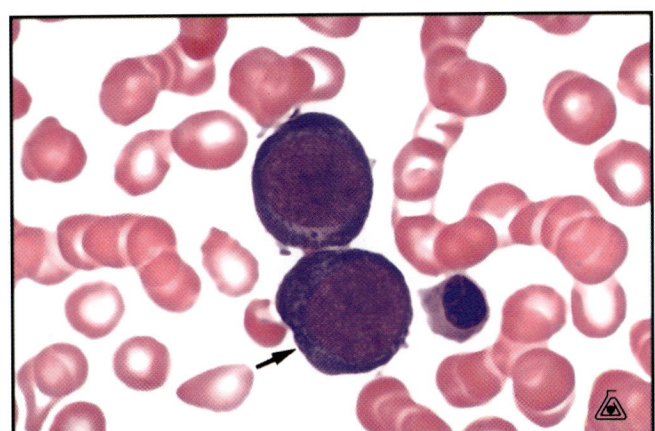

The two dominant cells are basophilic normoblasts. Each nucleus has open chromatin with slight thickening that obscures nucleoli; only faint outlines or lighter zones of chromatin suggest their presence. The cytoplasm of classic basophilic normoblasts should be intensely basophilic. These two cells have slightly gray cytoplasm, indicating a little more hemoglobin content than is usual. Pronormoblasts are larger with pale blue cytoplasm and very prominent nucleoli. Megaloblastic pronormoblasts and basophilic normoblasts are difficult to distinguish from their normal counterparts. Unless additional history is available or surrounding cells support the diagnosis, megaloblastosis should not be used as a defining term for any nucleated red cell earlier than a polychromatophilic normoblast.

Polychromatophilic Normoblast (Bone Marrow)

SYNONYMS
rubricyte

VITAL STATISTICS
size .... 10 to 15 μm
N:C ratio 4:1
cell shape .... round or oval
nuclear shape .... round or oval, may be centrally or eccentrically placed
chromatin .... clumped
nucleoli .... absent
cytoplasm .... ranges from blue-gray to pink-gray

KEY DIFFERENTIATING FEATURES
clumped chromatin with absent nucleoli
variation in color of cytoplasm from blue-gray to pink-gray

POTENTIAL LOOK-ALIKES
plasma cell
lymphocyte
orthochromic and basophilic normoblasts

ASSOCIATED DISEASE STATES AND CONDITIONS
normal finding in bone marrow
increased in various causes of erythroid hyperplasia

Polychromatophilic normoblasts are round or ovoid cells like their precursors, but are slightly smaller (10 to 15 μm in diameter). The nucleus is round and centrally or eccentrically located. The chromatin is clumped and parachromatin is distinct, sometimes giving a cartwheel appearance. Nucleoli are absent. A perinuclear halo is visible. The cytoplasm is abundant and stains as admixtures of blue-gray to pink-gray, depending upon the relative proportions of RNA and hemoglobin present. The N:C ratio is approximately 4:1. This is the last red cell progenitor that is capable of dividing.

Polychromatophilic normoblasts present the most varied morphology of any of the nucleated red cell stages in the bone marrow. At one end of the spectrum are cells that display mild nuclear chromatin clumping and basophilic cytoplasm; these cells resemble basophilic normoblasts. Rather than royal blue, the cytoplasm has more gray in it due to the early accumulation of hemoglobin. This gives the cell a "dishwater-blue" appearance. The subtle differences between basophilic normoblasts and early polychromatophilic normoblasts are illustrated on page 159.

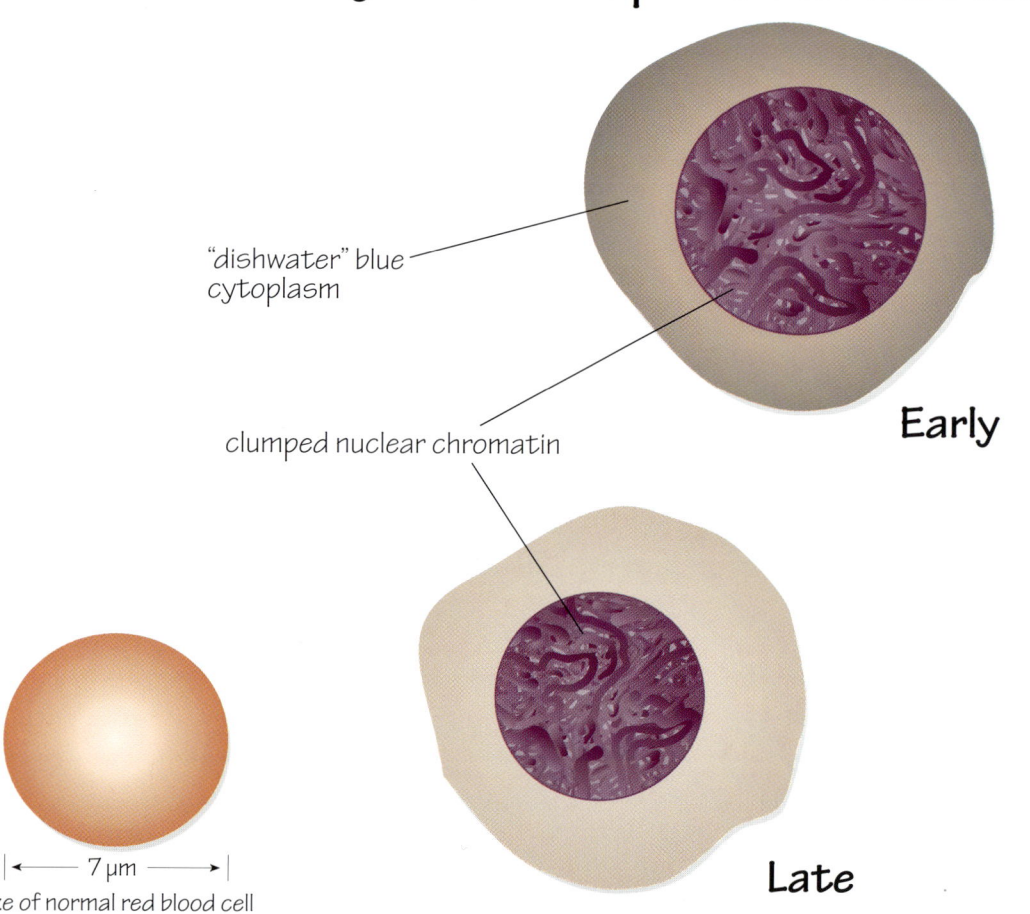

Polychromatophilic Normoblasts

"dishwater" blue cytoplasm

clumped nuclear chromatin

Early

Late

|←— 7 μm —→|
size of normal red blood cell

At the other end of spectrum are the late-phase, more mature cells that resemble orthochromatophilic normoblasts. These erythroblasts have more abundant hemoglobin in their cytoplasm and display a pink-gray color. The nucleus at this stage is much more condensed and exhibits clumps of chromatin; lighter areas of parachromatin are still visible. It is not a dark, homogeneous, and pyknotic mass. The nucleus should not be extruding from the cytoplasm, a feature normally reserved for orthochromatophilic erythroblasts.

The "cart-wheel" appearance of chromatin and blue-gray cytoplasm in early cells may be confused with plasma cells. In comparison to plasma cells, the polychromatophilic normoblasts tend to have greater numbers of "clumped areas" that reflect the more numerous chromocenters that are present. In addition, plasma cell nuclei tend to be smaller and eccentrically located. In comparison, the plasma cell cytoplasm is copious, opaque blue-gray, and may contain vacuoles of immunoglobulin.

H1-32, 1989 (Bone Marrow, Wright-Giemsa, X400)

Identification	Referee %	Participant %
Polychromatophilic normoblast	67	61
Orthochromatophilic normoblast	28	26

The arrowed cells are polychromatophilic normoblasts. The cytoplasm is pink grey with an N:C ratio of approximately 4:1. The nuclear chromatin is clumped and nucleoli are not evident. Areas of parachromatin are still present and stain pink. Precise identification of where a specific cell is in the process of erythroid maturation is somewhat artificial. The orangeophilic cytoplasm of the arrowed cells suggest late polychromatophilic or orthochromatophilic stages of differentiation. However, the prominent parachromatin and nonpyknotic nucleus causes the appropriate identification to be that of a polychromatophilic normoblast.

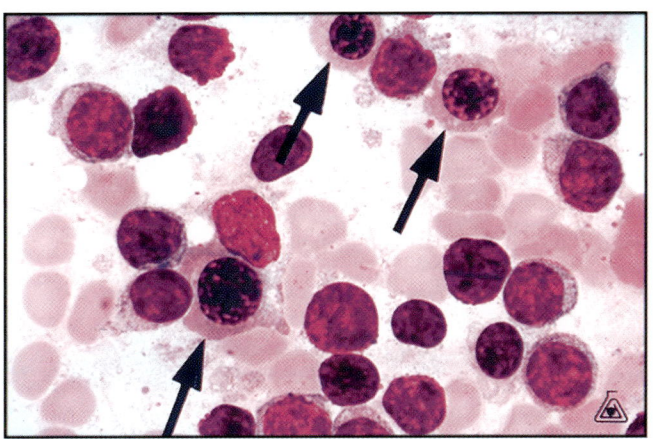

HE-45B, 1996 (Bone Marrow, Wright-Giemsa, X210)

Identification	Referee %	Participant %
Polychromatophilic normoblast	20	14.7
Basophilic normoblast	48.8	56.1
Pronormoblast	16	9.9

The two small arrows point to early polychromatophilic normoblasts. Neither cell exhibits any megaloblastic or dysplastic morphology. Most of the participants and referees favored an identification of basophilic normoblast. Basophilic normoblasts have royal blue cytoplasm. Sometimes the cytoplasm has a darker more basophilic rim at the periphery. A lighter perinuclear halo may be present. The nucleus is round and contains dark purple coarse strands with minimal clumping. Polychromatophilic normoblasts have coarse nuclear chromatin with distinct clumping. The cytoplasm is less intensely blue, reflecting increased hemoglobin content. The two arrowed cells display distinct chromatin clumping, more than the typical basophilic normoblast. The cytoplasm is not as basophilic as a typical basophilic normoblast; it has a sort of "dishwater-blue" appearance.

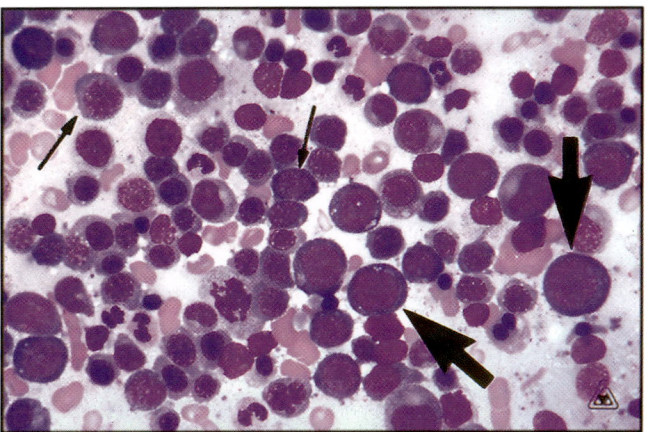

Orthochromic Normoblast (Bone Marrow)

SYNONYMS
  metarubricyte

VITAL STATISTICS
  size .... 8 to 12 µm
  N:C ratio 1:2
  cell shape .... round to oval
  nuclear shape .... round to oval
  chromatin .... pyknotic, dense; may be eccentrically placed, extruding or fragmented
  nucleoli .... absent
  cytoplasm .... pink-orange; very little basophilia; may be nearly the same color as surrounding non-nucleated red blood cells

KEY DIFFERENTIATING FEATURES
  dense, pyknotic nucleus
  uniform pink orange cytoplasm with minimal or absent basophilia
  the uniform staining and lack of significant basophilia distinguish the cell from polychromatophilic normoblasts which have variegated coloration and more significant basophilia

OTHER FINDINGS
  the nucleus can be partially extruded or fragmented

POTENTIAL LOOK-ALIKES
  necrobiotic polymorphonuclear granulocytes
  late phase polychromatophilic normoblasts

ASSOCIATED DISEASE STATES AND CONDITIONS
  normal bone marrow cell
  increased in various causes of erythroid hyperplasia

Orthochromic normoblasts are round to ovoid cells and smaller (8 to 12 µm in diameter) than polychromatophilic normoblasts. The nucleus is also very small, often pyknotic and sometimes appears as a homogeneous mass of dense chromatin. It is often eccentrically placed and at times may be extruding or fragmented. The cytoplasm is greater in relative amount than in the polychromatophilic normoblast and usually stains pinkish-orange with little basophilia. The cytoplasmic color is uniform, unlike the variegated coloration of the polychromatophilic normoblast. The N:C ratio is approximately 1:2. Together with polychromatophilic normoblasts, they normally represent 90% of the nucleated erythroid cells found in the bone marrow.

Orthochromic normoblasts are the last maturation stage of the nucleated red blood cell series. The nucleus undergoes pyknotic degeneration as the chromatin condenses into an almost homogeneous mass. At this stage, the cell can no longer divide. The cytoplasm contains nearly its full complement of hemoglobin, but it is rarely exactly the same color as mature erythrocytes. It is, however, distinctly more acidophilic than the polychromatophilic normoblast stage.

After the nucleus is extruded, the cell becomes a reticulocyte. The two methods of nuclear shedding are illustrated on the next page. Both occur with roughly the same frequency. Some orthochromic normoblasts lose their polyribosomes and other organelles at the same time the nucleus is shed. Supravital stains cannot distinguish these newly formed red cells from mature red cells, since they lack any substantia reticulofilamentosa (see page 114).

Orthochromic Normoblast

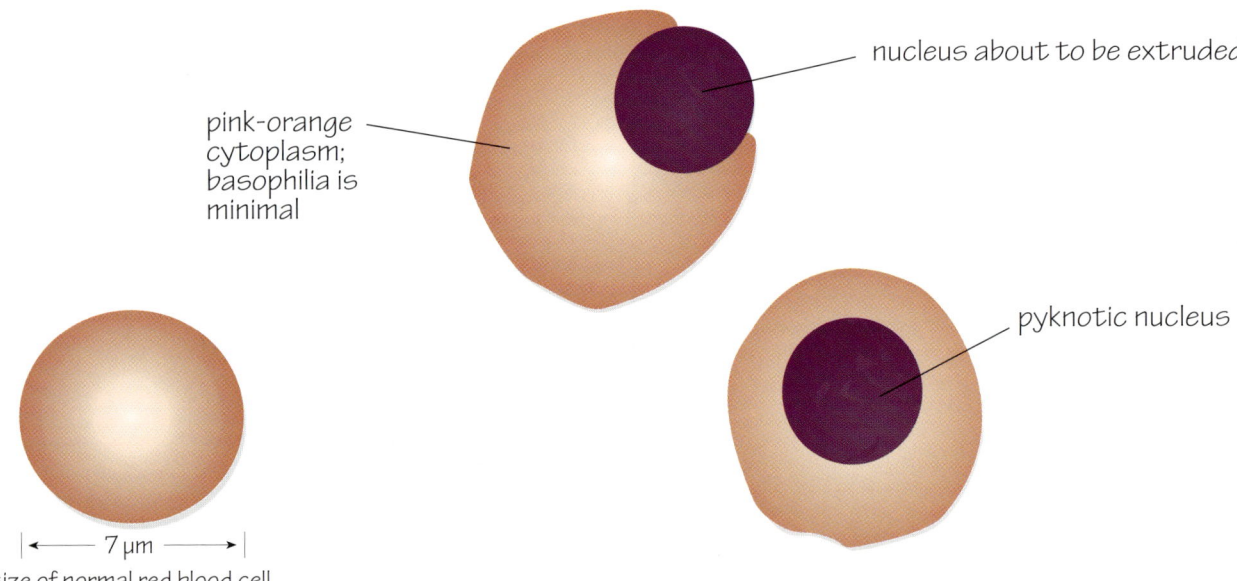

nucleus about to be extruded

pink-orange cytoplasm; basophilia is minimal

pyknotic nucleus

|← 7 µm →|
size of normal red blood cell

Nucleated Red Cells

H-52, 1981 (Bone Marrow, Wright-Giemsa, X400)

Identification	Referee %	Participant %
Orthochromic normoblast	86	94

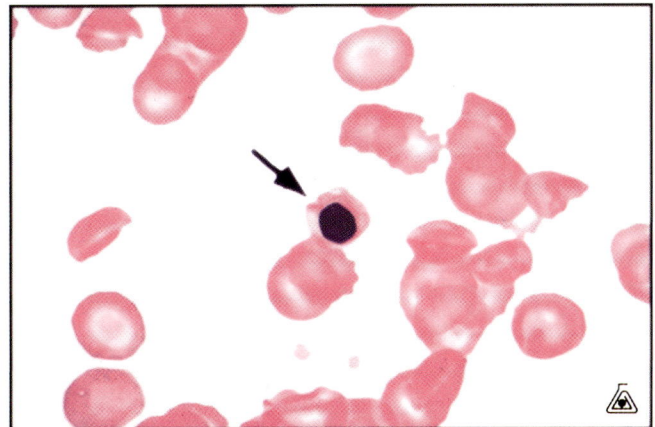

The arrowed cell is an orthochromic normoblast. The nucleus is eccentrically located, very dense and nearly pyknotic; it is about to be extruded. Once the orthochromic normoblast loses its nucleus, it becomes a reticulocyte. The cytoplasm is pink to slightly polychromatophilic, similar in staining to the neighboring non-nucleated red cells. The color is uniform and lacks the variegated appearance of polychromatophilic normoblasts. In order to distinguish these two cell types, compare the cytoplasm to the surrounding non-nucleated red blood cells. If the cell cytoplasm is nearly identical or slightly more basophilic and the nucleus is pyknotic or almost so, the nucleated erythrocyte is an orthochromic normoblast. If the cytoplasm is more blue-gray to pink-purple and the chromatin clumped, it is best designated a late-phase polychromatophilic normoblast.

Transformation of Orthochromic Normoblasts into Reticulocytes

The orthochromic normoblast is the last maturation stage of the nucleated red cell series. The cell sheds its nucleus to become a reticulocyte in one of two ways. Both methods occur with approximately the same frequency.

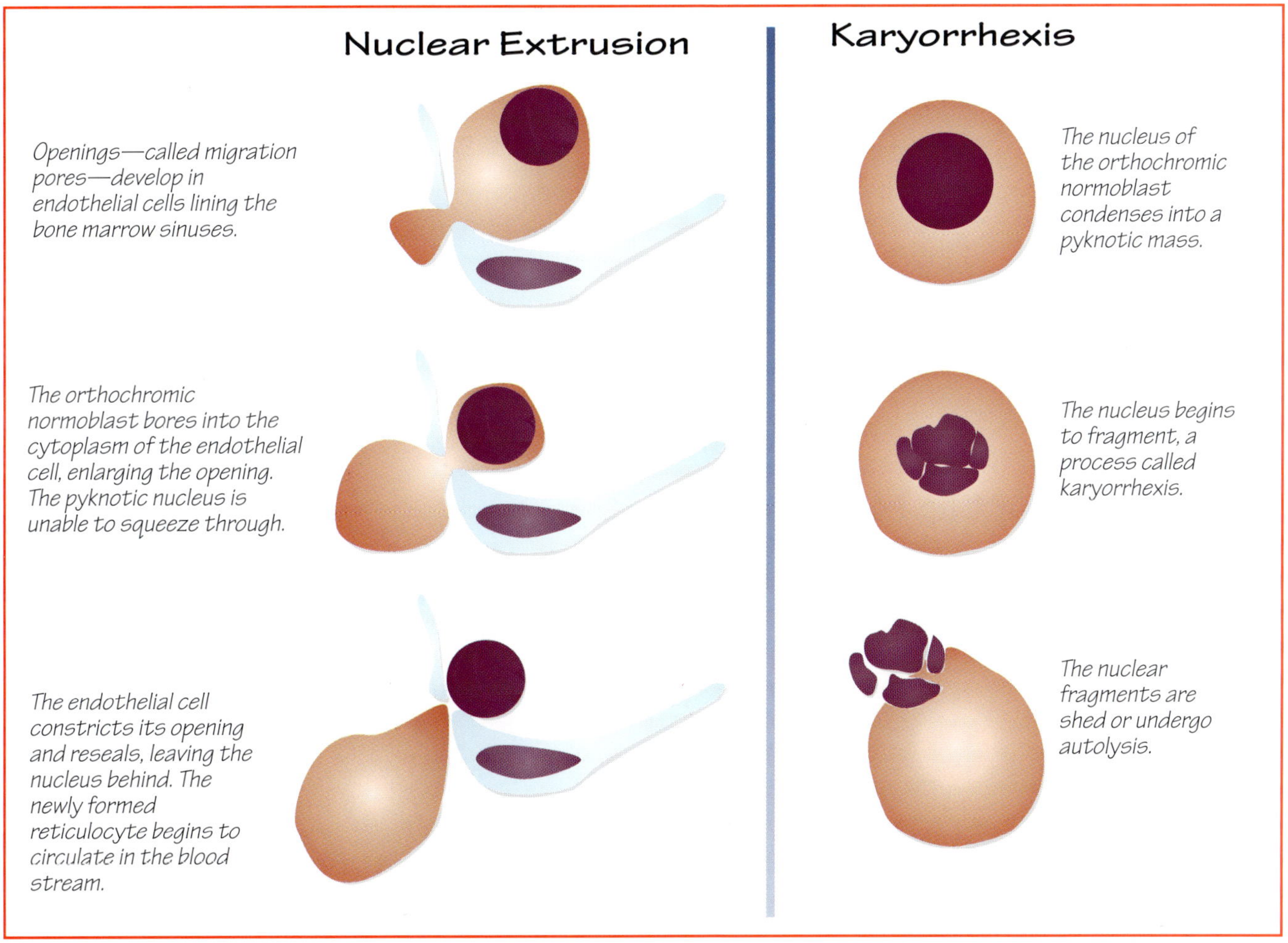

Nuclear Extrusion

Openings—called migration pores—develop in endothelial cells lining the bone marrow sinuses.

The orthochromic normoblast bores into the cytoplasm of the endothelial cell, enlarging the opening. The pyknotic nucleus is unable to squeeze through.

The endothelial cell constricts its opening and reseals, leaving the nucleus behind. The newly formed reticulocyte begins to circulate in the blood stream.

Karyorrhexis

The nucleus of the orthochromic normoblast condenses into a pyknotic mass.

The nucleus begins to fragment, a process called karyorrhexis.

The nuclear fragments are shed or undergo autolysis.

Nucleated Red Cell, Megaloblastic (Bone Marrow)

SYNONYMS
  megaloblast

VITAL STATISTICS
  size .... larger than normal counterpart
  N:C ratio .... less than normal counterpart
  chromatin .... more immature than normal counterpart
  nucleoli .... may persist in more mature stages and be more prominent when compared to normal counterpart
  cytoplasm .... for a given degree of nuclear immaturity may demonstrate more orangeophilic cytoplasm representing increased hemoglobin synthesis

KEY DIFFERENTIATING FEATURES
  compared to their normoblastic counterparts, megaloblastic cells are larger in size, have slightly decreased N:C ratios, and have immature nuclear chromatin from the degree of cytoplasmic maturation

OTHER FINDINGS
  cytoplasmic basophilic stippling
  multiple Howell-Jolly bodies

POTENTIAL LOOK ALIKES
  dysplastic maturing granulocyte (in cases with severe megaloblastic change and dyserythropoiesis reflected by abnormal nuclear lobation and multinuclearity)

ASSOCIATED DISEASE STATES AND CONDITIONS
  vitamin B_{12} deficiency
  folate deficiency
  veganism
  gastric malabsorption due to pernicious anemia or gastrectomy
  severe ileal disease as seen in tropical sprue, ileal resection, Crohn's disease, fish tapeworm
  gluten induced enteropathy
  increased rate of cell turnover
  drugs (anticonvulsants, hydroxyurea)
  myelodysplasia
  acute leukemias

Each of the nucleated erythroid cells can demonstrate megalobastic changes. These changes are the result of defective DNA synthesis and are associated with a variety of disorders. Overall, megaloblastic cells are larger for each stage of maturation than normal and demonstrate nuclear and cytoplasmic maturation asynchrony. The degree of cytoplasmic maturation is ahead of the degree of nuclear maturation. This results in the cells continuing to undergo normal hemoglobinization of the cytoplasm while maintaining a more immature nuclear chromatin pattern. Co-existing features of dyserythropoiesis, such as multinucleate cells, abnormal nuclear configurations, and Howell-Jolly bodies, are often seen.

The cytoplasm of megaloblastic erythroid cells should be opaque and devoid of granules. This may aid in appropriate classification of a cell as belonging to the erythroid series in cases of severe dysplasia. In pathologic states associated with dyserythropoiesis, cytoplasmic basophilic stippling may be present. These abnormal cytoplasmic aggregates consist of condensed areas of RNA.

Megaloblastic anemia is often associated with a macrocytosis of the mature red cells present in the peripheral blood. Often these macrocytes are oval in shape. They have an increased MCV but contain normal amounts of hemoglobin (increased MCH and normal MCHC). In addition, marked anisocytosis and poikilocytosis may be present. The reticulocyte count can be either decreased, normal, or increased. Leukopenia, primarily due to a neutropenia as well as thrombocytopenia, is usually present. Hypersegmented neutrophils (1 PMN with 6 lobes or 6 PMNs with 5 lobes/100 WBCs) are often sited as the hallmark of megaloblastic anemia due to B_{12} or folate deficiency.

Megaloblastic Nucleated RBCs

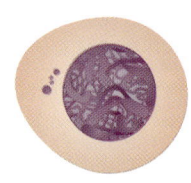
Orthochromatophilic

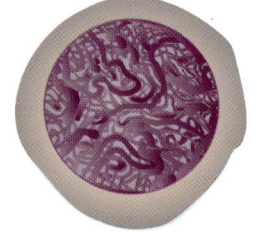
Polychromatophilic

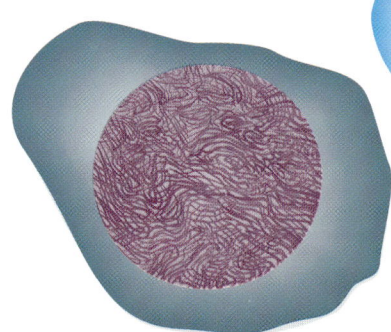
Basophilic, Late

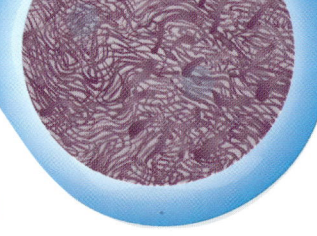
Basophilic, Early

H-6, 1982 (Bone Marrow, Wright-Giemsa, X400)

Identification	Referee %	Participant %
Pronormoblast, megaloblastic	88.9	65.1
Pronormoblast	11.1	7.6

The arrowed cell is a megaloblastic pronormoblast. It has a high N:C ratio with immature chromatin with several nucleoli present. The cytoplasm is for the most part deep blue but has a hint of blue-gray discoloration. Other erythroid precursors in the field also demonstrate megaloblastic changes. As discussed in the following *A Closer Look At...*, it is not possible to reliably separate normoblastic and megaloblastic pronormoblasts for a given single cell. The clue is the surrounding nucleated red cells, which clearly show nuclear-cytoplasmic dyssynchrony.

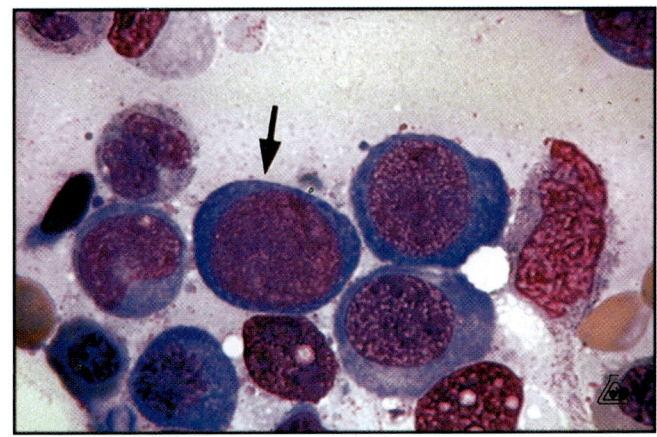

H1-33, 1984 (Bone Marrow, Wright-Giemsa, X400)

Identification	Referee %	Participant %
Basophilic megaloblast	63	55
Polychromatophilic megaloblast	16	16

The arrowed cell is a megaloblastic nucleated red cell. It has a moderately high N:C ratio and very immature chromatin. Distinct nucleoli are not present. The gray-basophilic cytoplasm would place this cell in the late basophilic or early polychromatophilic stage of erythroid maturation. The fine and delicate chromatin pattern is suggestive of a cell more immature than the cytoplasm would dictate. The megaloblastic cell below the arrow contains multiple Howell-Jolly bodies. These represent aberrant chromosomes that become separated from the nucleus during mitotic division. This is a feature of the dyserythropoiesis often seen in cases with megaloblastic changes. (See *A Closer Look At...* page 168).

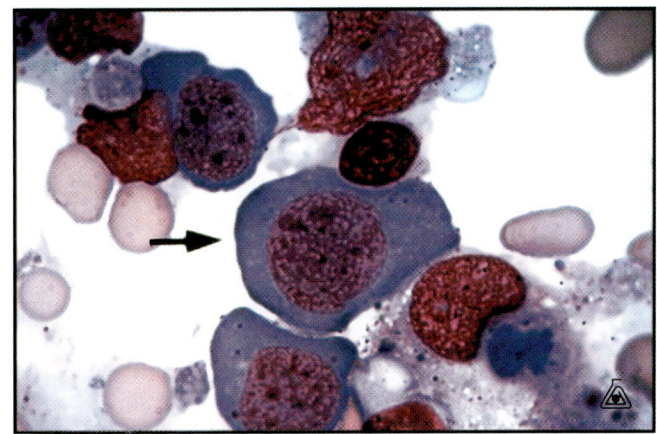

H1-47, 1989 (Bone Marrow, Wright-Giemsa, X375)

Identification	Referee %	Participant %
Polychromatophilic megaloblast	85	69
Orthochromatophilic megaloblast	10	11
Basophilic megaloblast	5	11

The arrowed cell is a polychromatophilic megaloblast. The cell is larger than its normoblastic counterpart. The cytoplasm is gray-pink (dishwater gray), indicative of active hemoglobin formation. However, the nucleus is markedly immature with fine, delicate chromatin for this stage consistent with megaloblastic change. The degree of cytoplasmic hemoglobinization present is more than is seen in a basophilic megaloblast. Several other polychromatophilic megaloblasts are present in the field. To the left of the arrowed cell is an orthochromatophilic megaloblast. The degree of cytoplasmic maturation (hemoglobinization) is more pronounced in this cell than in the arrowed cell while the nucleus is too immature for an orthochromatophilic normoblast. Above the arrowed cell is a giant band that may also be seen in megaloblastic processes.

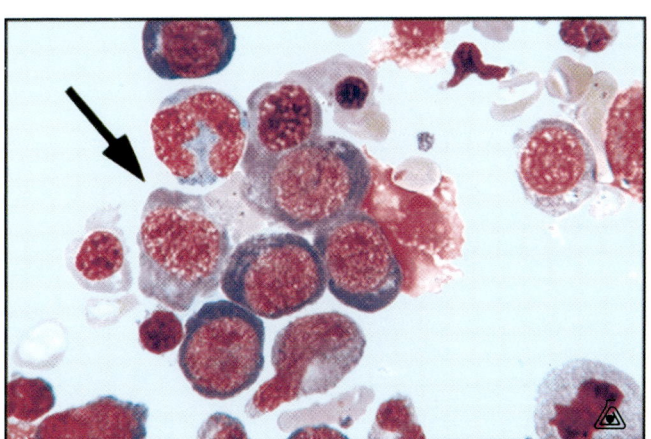

A Closer Look At...

Megaloblastic Morphology

In pathologic states abnormal maturation of the nucleus and cytoplasm may occur. The normal reduction in cell size and condensation of nuclear chromatin associated with cell maturation may not occur. In megaloblastic erythropoiesis the nuclear maturation lags behind the cytoplasmic maturation. This nuclear to cytoplasmic dyssynchrony, a result of impaired DNA synthesis, is the classic feature of megaloblastic change. In addition, due to the conservation of DNA production and impaired DNA synthesis, fewer cell divisions occur at each stage resulting in an overall increase in cell size. It is often difficult to accurately classify these cells as an immature appearing erythroid precursor nucleus may be associated with mature, hemoglobinized cytoplasm. The assumption is that cytoplasmic maturation is appropriate and nuclear maturation is delayed or impaired, resulting in cell identification based on cytoplasmic characteristics.

Megaloblastic morphologic change is very difficult to appreciate in the pronormoblast and is best appreciated in basophilic, polychromatophilic, and orthochromatophilic cells. Megaloblastic pronormoblasts have a similar chromatin pattern to normal pronormoblasts with a slightly decreased N:C ratio secondary to increased cytoplasm.

Basophilic megaloblasts have immature nuclear features similar to the megaloblastic pronormoblast, but have a greater amount of deep blue cytoplasm. The overall size is somewhat larger compared with its normal counterpart.

The nuclear chromatin of the polychromatophilic megaloblast begins to demonstrate coarse condensation, with the parachromatin remaining abundant and distinct. The cytoplasm ranges from basophilic to orange, varying with the hemoglobin concentration.

The nucleus of the normoblastic orthochromatophilic cell is dense and pyknotic. The nucleus of the megaloblastic orthochromatophilic cell may have retained some degree of open parachromatin. The cytoplasm ranges from orange to pink and is often abundant compared to its normal counterpart.

The net result of the megaloblastic change of erythroid precursors is for the mature red cell in the peripheral blood to be larger in size (oval macrocytes with increased MCV) due to decreased cell divisions.

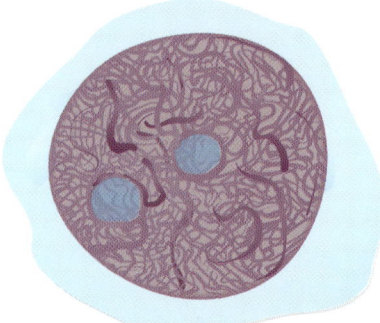

Pronormoblast, normoblastic

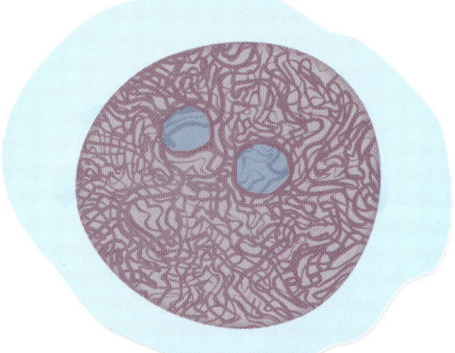

Pronormoblast, megaloblastic

There is little morphologic difference between normoblastic and megaloblastic pronormoblasts. They cannot be reliably distinguished. Early basophilic normoblasts and megaloblasts are similarly difficult to differentiate. Diagnosis relies on evaluation of surrounding more mature cells. Nuclear-cytoplasmic dyssynchrony is better seen in polychromatophilic and orthochromatophilic cells.

Comparison of Normal and Megaloblastic Erythroid Cells

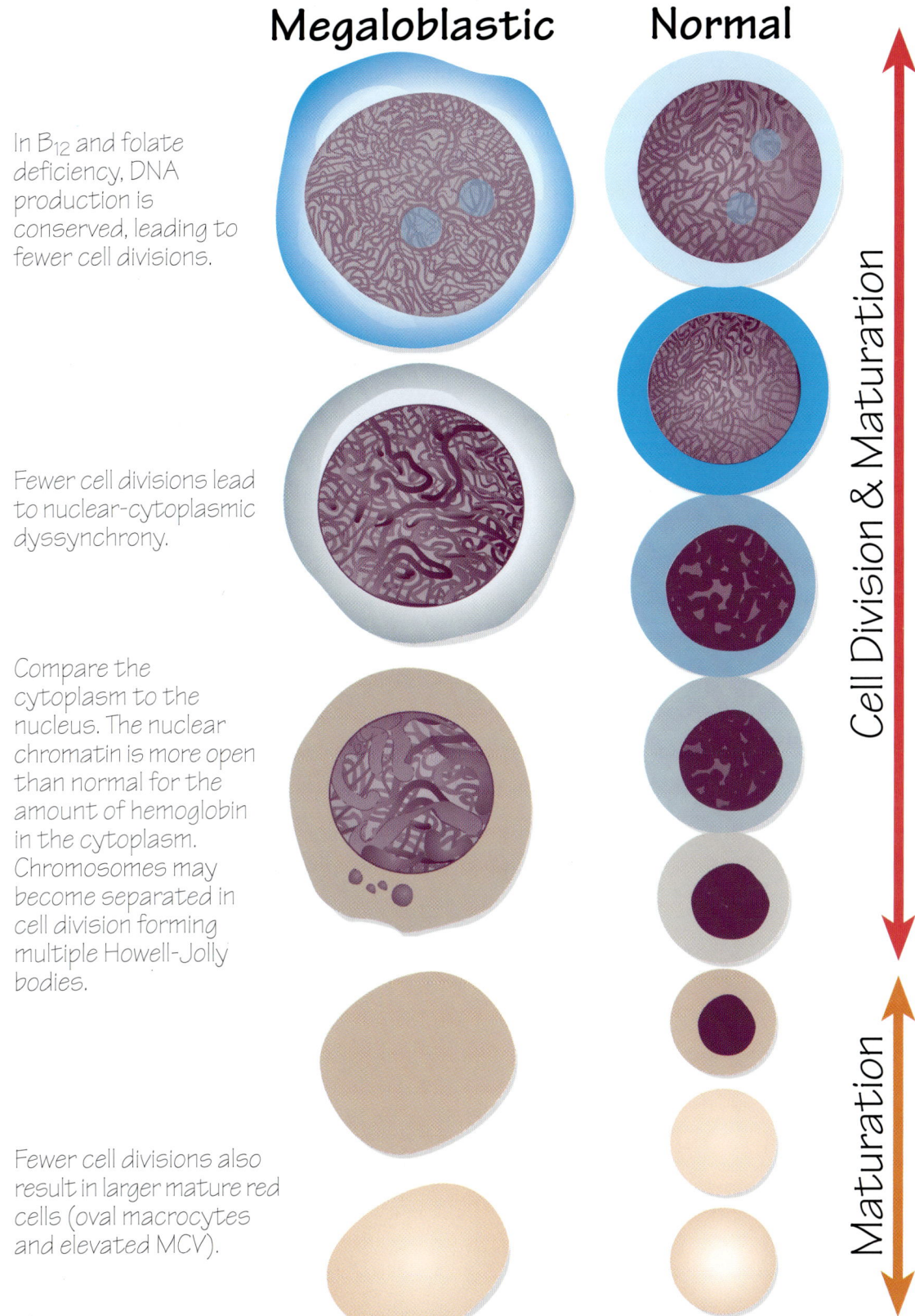

In B₁₂ and folate deficiency, DNA production is conserved, leading to fewer cell divisions.

Fewer cell divisions lead to nuclear-cytoplasmic dyssynchrony.

Compare the cytoplasm to the nucleus. The nuclear chromatin is more open than normal for the amount of hemoglobin in the cytoplasm. Chromosomes may become separated in cell division forming multiple Howell-Jolly bodies.

Fewer cell divisions also result in larger mature red cells (oval macrocytes and elevated MCV).

Nucleated Red Cells

Nucleated Red Cell, Normal or Abnormal (Blood)

SYNONYMS
NRBC, dyplastic, megalobastic, and megaloblastoid nucleated red cell

VITAL STATISTICS
- size .... varies with the stage of maturation
- N:C ratio .... varies with the stage of maturation
- cell shape .... round to oval
- nuclear shape .... round to oval if normal or megaloblastic; multinucleate, cloverleaf or abnormal due to nuclear budding if dysplastic
- chromatin .... varies with the stage of maturation
- nucleoli .... usually absent
- cytoplasm .... varies with the stage of maturation; may show coarse basophilic stippling or multiple Howell-Jolly bodies if dysplastic

KEY DIFFERENTIATING FEATURES
- normal nucleated red cell morphology matching bone marrow morphology
- if dysplastic, may exhibit abnormalities in cell size and nuclear configuration or maturation

OTHER FINDINGS
- multiple Howell-Jolly bodies
- basophilic stippling

POTENTIAL LOOK-ALIKES
- necrobiotic polymorphonuclear leukocytes
- lymphocytes

ASSOCIATED DISEASE STATES AND CONDITIONS
- severe stress reaction
- myelofibrosis (myelophthisic processes)
- thalassemias
- hemolytic anemias
- other severe anemias
- acute leukemias
- myeloproliferative disorders

The term nucleated red cell is used to state the presence of normoblasts in the peripheral blood and includes all normoblasts regardless of the stage of maturation. Typically, the circulating nucleated red cell is at the orthochromatophilic stage of differentiation. Both megaloblastic (nuclear and cytoplasmic dyssynchrony) and dysplastic changes (abnormal nuclear shapes, nuclear budding, and nuclear fragmentation) can be seen in these circulating red cells reflecting simultaneous erythroid maturation abnormalities present in the bone marrow. Caution should be used in classifying a circulating nucleated red cell as dysplastic on the basis of abnormal nuclear shape (lobated or fragmented) as these changes may occur during their egress from the marrow space and may not be present in the maturing erythroids present in the marrow. For the purposes of CAP proficiency testing it is adequate to identify a cell as a nucleated red cell when it is present in the peripheral blood, be it normal or abnormal (i.e., exhibiting megaloblastic or dysplastic changes). For bone marrow photographs, "nucleated red cell" is insufficient identification; staging and assessment of dyserythropoietic changes are necessary.

Normal Nucleated Red Blood Cells in Peripheral Blood

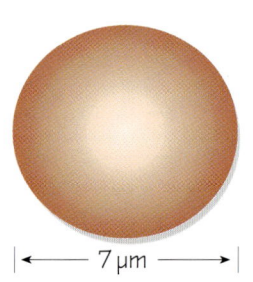

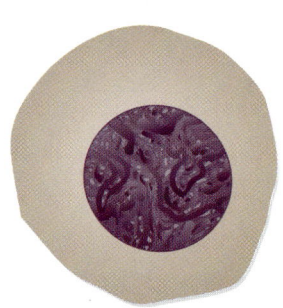

|← 7 μm →|
size of normal red blood cell

XH-14, 1990 (Blood, Wright-Giemsa, X400)

Identification	Referee %	Participant %
Nucleated red cell, blood	95	94

The arrowed cells are nucleated red blood cells present in the peripheral blood and have small nuclei with clumped chromatin and pink to slightly chromatophilic cytoplasm. A small amount of parachromatin is still present suggestive of late polychromatophilic maturation. The mature red cells in the background demonstrate moderate anisocytosis and poikilocytosis. Microcytes and a teardrop cell are also present.

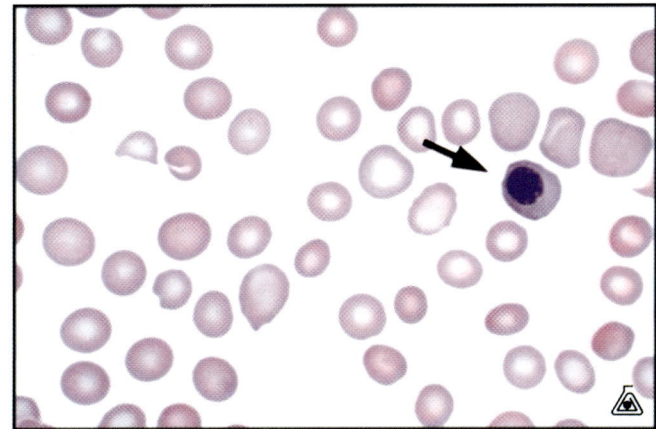

XL-33, 1989 (Blood, Wright-Giemsa, X400)

Identification	Referee %	Participant %
Nucleated red cell, blood	100	96

The arrowed cells represent circulating nucleated red cells with normal morphology corresponding to the orthochromatophilic stage of maturation. The nucleus is condensed and parachromatin is not appreciated. Also present are spherocytes, red cell fragments, and polychromatophilic cells—changes seen in hemolytic anemia. This specimen was taken from a newborn with ABO hemolytic disease.

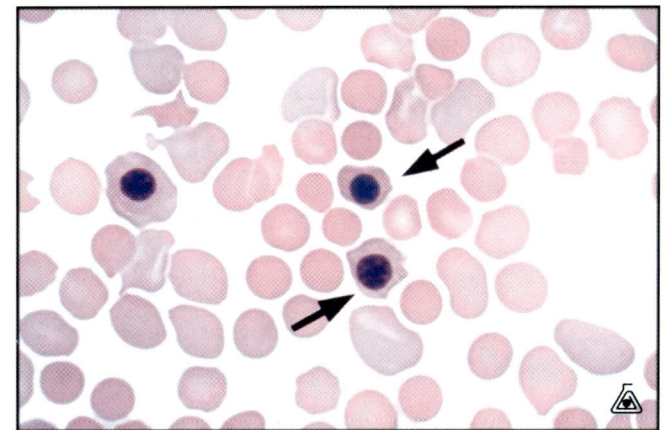

Dysplastic Nucleated Red Blood Cells in Peripheral Blood

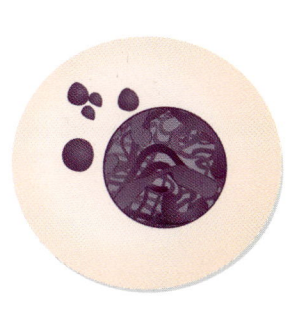
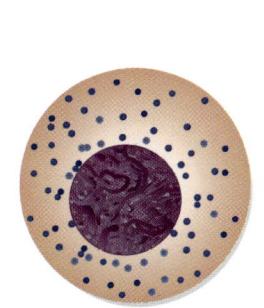
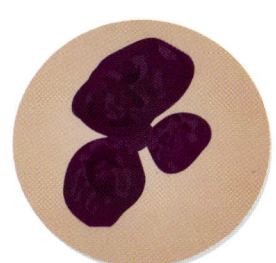

Nucleated Red Cell, Dysplastic (Bone Marrow)

SYNONYMS
none

VITAL STATISTICS
- size .... similar normal counterpart
- N:C ratio .... may be normal or increased
- cell shape .... usually round or oval
- nuclear shape .... strikingly abnormal; lobated, fragmented, multinucleated
- chromatin .... often coarsely clumped "megaloblastoid"
- nucleoli .... usually not present
- cytoplasm .... may contain vacuoles (PAS positive), DNA fragments (Howell-Jolly bodies), or coarse basophilic stippling

KEY DIFFERENTIATING FEATURES
- abnormal nuclear and cytoplasmic features corresponding to a state of dyserythropoiesis
- dysplastic erthroid cells demonstrate PAS cytoplasmic positivity; normal erythroid cells are PAS negative

OTHER FINDINGS
- may have associated megaloblastic, dysplastic changes in the granulocytic megakaryocytic series

POTENTIAL LOOK-ALIKES
- normal or necrobiotic polymorphonuclear leukocytes
- lymphocytes
- metastatic tumor cells

ASSOCIATED DISEASE STATES AND CONDITIONS
- vitamin B_{12} deficiency
- folate deficiency
- DiGuglielmo's syndrome (FAB M6, erythroleukemia)
- acute myeloid leukemias
- myelodysplasia
- chronic myeloproliferative disorders
- congenital dyserythropoietic anemia
- heavy metal poisoning
- ethanol
- antimetabolites

The term dyserythropoiesis is used to encompass abnormal erythroid development of both megaloblastic and dysplastic types. Megaloblastic abnormalities involve nuclear and cytoplasmic dyssynchrony most classically occurring in cases of folate and or B_{12} deficiency. Dysplastic nucleated red cells exhibit strikingly abnormal nuclear features. The nucleus may be grossly misshapen due to "nuclear budding" (lobation or rosette formation), fragmentation, or multinucleation. The cytoplasm may demonstrate vacuoles, contain multiple Howell-Jolly bodies, or exhibit coarse basophilic stippling. Some of the cytoplasmic abnormalities may also be seen in severe cases of megaloblastic change. Megaloblastoid change is a more subtle type of dysplasia. Megaloblastoid findings are present when the nuclear chromatin is more clumped and the chromatin strands are much coarser than in a corresponding normoblastic cell, and the clear spaces between the dense chromatin strands, called parachromatin, are more prominent. These changes are most easily detected in the later stages of red cell maturation. (See *A Closer Look At…* page 174).

Dysplastic Nucleated Red Cells in Bone Marrow

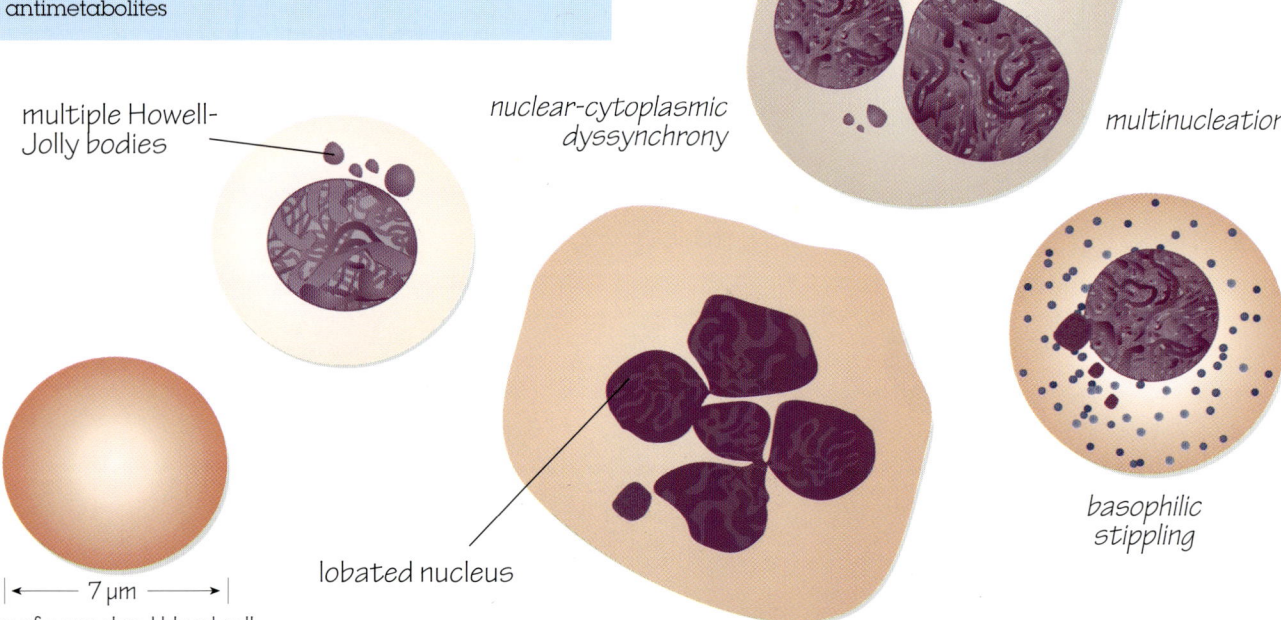

- multiple Howell-Jolly bodies
- nuclear-cytoplasmic dyssynchrony
- multinucleation
- lobated nucleus
- basophilic stippling
- 7 μm — size of normal red blood cell

HE-47, 1996 (Bone Marrow, Wright-Giemsa, X400)

Identification	Referee %	Participant %
Nucleated red cell, dysplastic	88	71.9
Nucleated red cell, normal or abnormal (blood)	8.0	7.9
Orthochromic normoblast	-	4.7

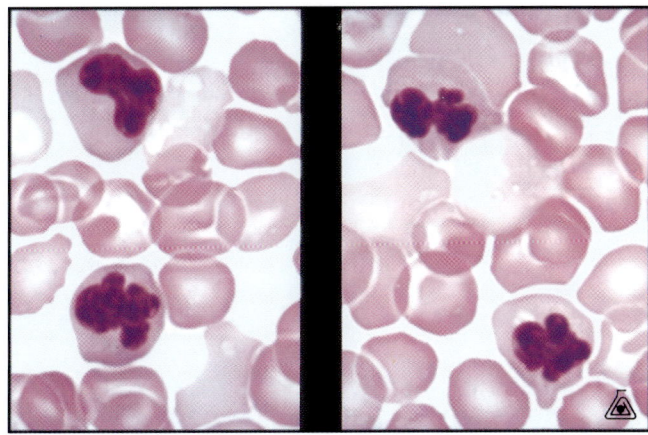

The split panel photograph demonstrates several dysplastic nucleated red cells. The nuclei are abnormal with irregularly lobated and multilobulated forms present. The nuclear shape is so distorted as to resemble the nuclei of bands or polymorphonuclear leukocytes. These cells can be distinguished from dysplastic myeloid cells by noting the hemoglobinized cytoplasm.

HE-14, 1996 (Bone Marrow, Wright-Giemsa, X400)

Identification	Referee %	Participant %
Nucleated red cell, dysplastic	83	60
Nucleated red cell, megaloblastic	4	18

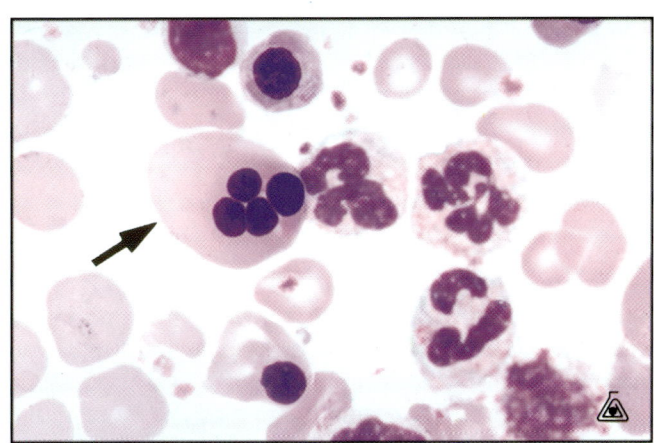

The arrowed cell is a dysplastic nucleated red cell that contains four, dark, hyperchromatic nuclei and has abundant pink, agranular cytoplasm. Dysplastic erythroid cells contain abnormal nuclei that may be lobated, multilobulated, fragmented or multinucleated. Occasionally a thin filament may connect the multinucleated forms. Dysplastic changes include the range of abnormalities seen in megaloblastoid cells as well as abnormally large and multinucleated forms. Megaloblastic change refers specifically to nuclear-cytoplasmic dyssynchrony. These changes are most evident in the latter stages of erythroid maturation and demonstrate an immature nucleus compared to the degree of cytoplasmic maturation. The chromatin is more open and immature than one would expect for the degree of cytoplasmic hemoglobinization. The arrowed cell is not a dysplastic or degenerating myeloid cell due to the dense, homogeneous orangeophilic cytoplasm. Compare this cytoplasm to the cytoplasm of the two orthochromic normoblasts in the same field.

PAS Staining of Dysplastic NRBCs

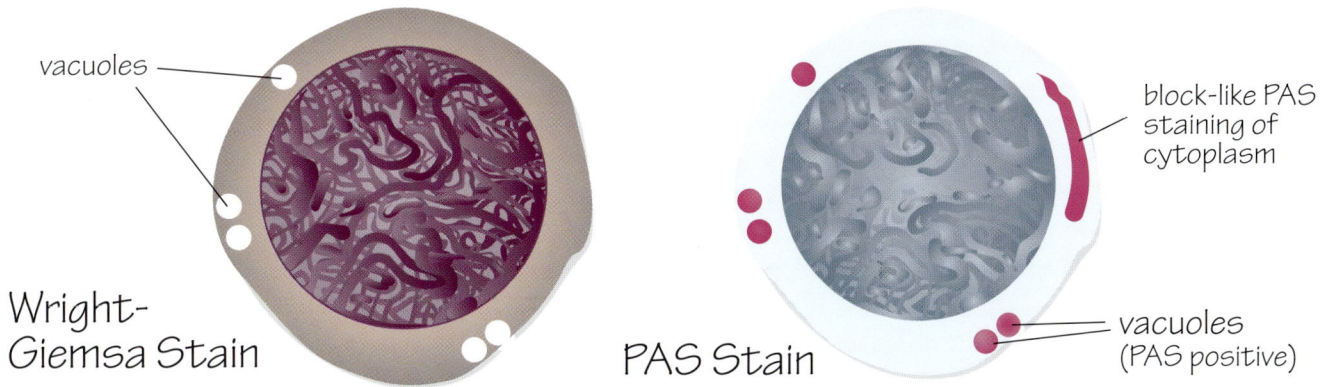

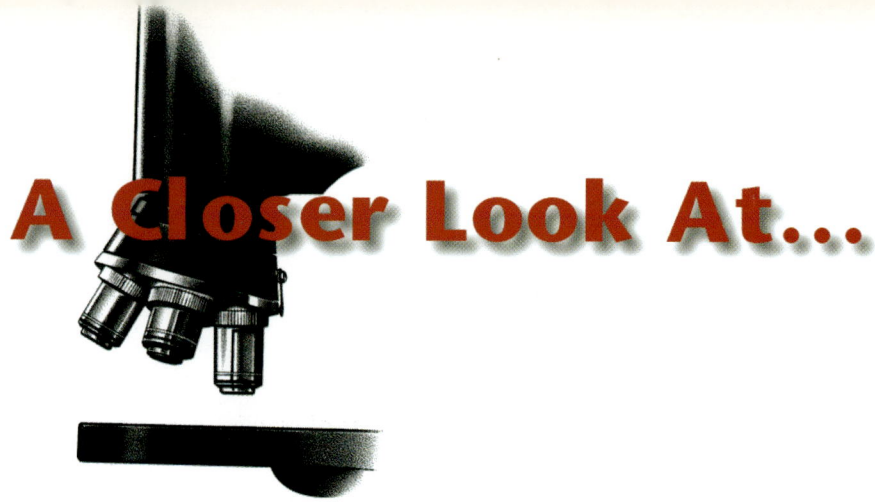

A Closer Look At...

Megaloblastic vs. Megaloblastoid Erythroid Maturation

Megaloblastic and megaloblastoid erythroid maturation are subdivisions under the general term dyserythropoiesis. Abnormal erythroid maturation of the megaloblastic type is characterized by nuclear-cytoplasmic dyssynchrony. The nuclear maturation present lags behind the cytoplasmic maturation resulting in a cell which has an immature nucleus with more open chromatin compared to the degree of cytoplasmic maturation, which is represented by the degree of hemoglobinization (orangeophilia) present. In addition, the megaloblastic forms of erythroid cells are larger than their normoblastic counterparts.

Megaloblastoid erythroid maturation is a more subtle form of dyserythropoiesis and is felt to be an intermediate type of abnormal erythroid maturation. The most prominent feature of megaloblastoid maturation is the presence of an abnormal chromatin pattern which is more condensed and clumped when compared to the normoblastic counterpart. This results in more prominent parachromatin spaces. Hyperclumping of the chromatin is somewhat similar to that which is sometimes seem in the atypical lymphocytes of chronic lymphocytic leukemia. Megaloblastoid maturation is also characterized by cells which are somewhat larger than their normoblastic counterparts and demonstrate a mild degree of nuclear-cytoplasmic dyssynchrony. Neither of these last two features are as prominent as in their megaloblastic counterpart. The etiology of these changes is unclear, but is thought to be related to abnormal DNA synthesis. Megaloblastoid maturation is most commonly seen in DiGuglielmo's syndrome (FAB M6), other acute myelogenous leukemia, myelodysplastic conditions and following exposure to various toxic agents such as organic phosphates, ethanol, and antimetabolites.

Comparison of Normal, Megaloblastoid, and Megaloblastic Red Blood Cell Maturation

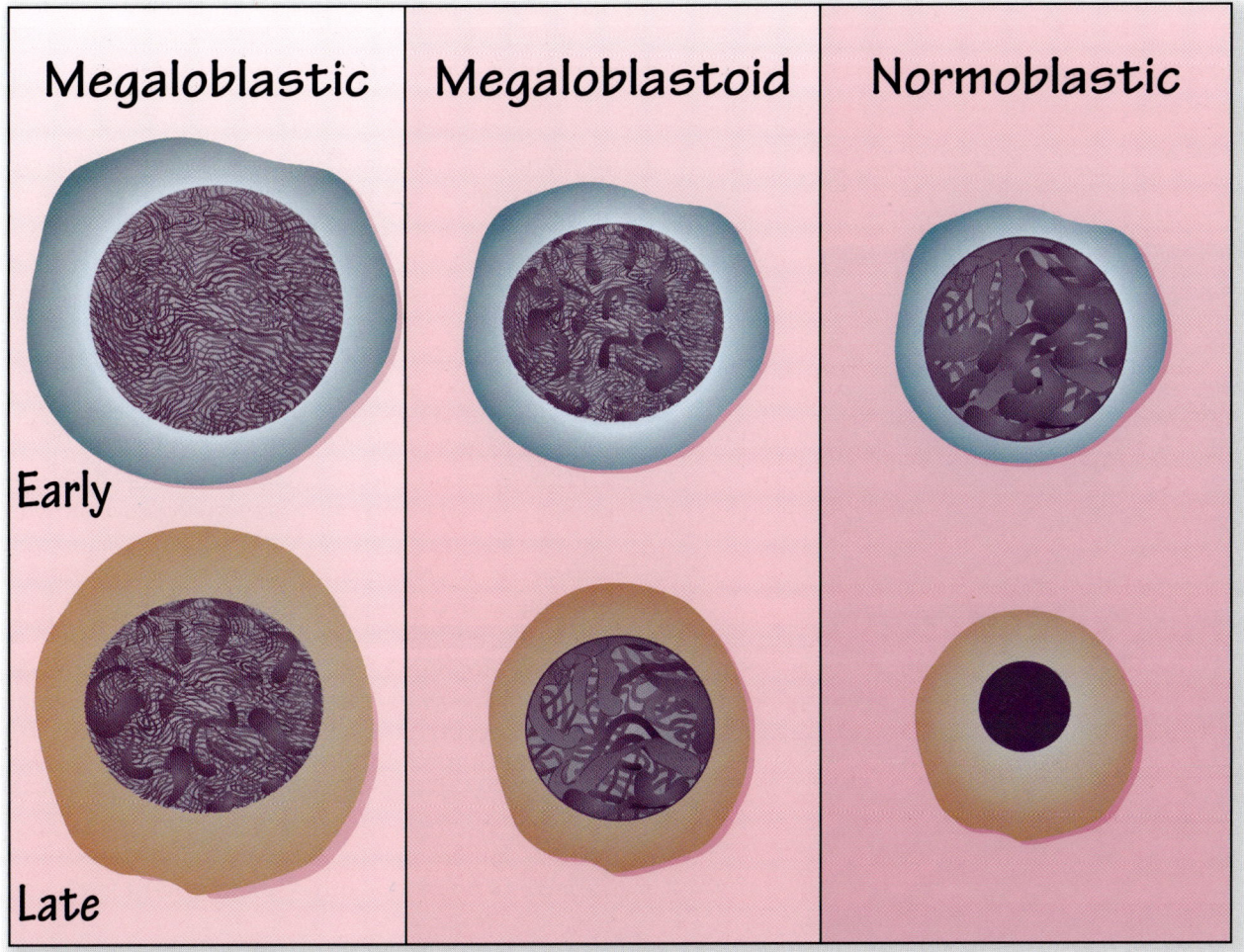

Megaloblastoid change is characterized by the following:
1. cells usually larger than corresponding normoblastic erythrons
2. dissociation of nuclear-cytoplasmic maturation, but less than in megaloblastic maturation
3. chromatin pattern is clumped and more coarse than in megaloblastic maturation but more open than in normoblastic maturation

Sideroblast (Iron Stain)

SYNONYMS
none

VITAL STATISTICS
- size .... varies with stage of maturation
- N:C ratio .... varies with disease state, usually normal or decreased
- cell shape .... round or oval
- nuclear shape .... may be round or abnormal
- chromatin .... varies with disease state
- nucleoli .... usually not present
- cytoplasm .... may contain Pappenheimer bodies on Wright-Giemsa stained material; blue granules seen after iron staining (Perls' reaction)

KEY DIFFERENTIATING FEATURES
cytoplasmic granules must demonstrate a positive reaction with an iron stain

POTENTIAL LOOK-ALIKES
- Howell-Jolly bodies (iron negative)
- Heinz bodies (iron negative; not visible on Wright-Giemsa stained smears)
- hemoglobin H inclusions (iron negative; supravital stain only)
- RNA bodies

ASSOCIATED DISEASE STATES AND CONDITIONS
normal finding in bone marrow
increased in:
- dyserythropoiesis
- iron overload
- intramedullary hemolysis

Normoblasts can contain cytoplasmic inclusions that stain positively with Prussian blue or Perls' stain for iron. In the bone marrow the red cell is usually at the polychromatophilic or orthochromatophilic stage of normoblastic maturation. The inclusions are called *siderosomes*. Siderosomes consist of ferritin molecules wrapped in a lysosomal membrane. Under normal conditions, no more than 5 siderosomes are present per cell.

On peripheral smears, siderosomes may be present in mature red cells and are termed *Pappenheimer bodies*. Non-nucleated red blood cells that contain Pappenheimer bodies are referred to as *siderocytes*. Nucleated red cells containing siderosomes are designated *sideroblasts*. Siderocytes and sideroblasts are present in normal bone marrow samples. Up to 50% of erythrocyte precursors may be sideroblasts. The three types of sideroblasts are discussed on pages 178 and 179. Siderocytes and sideroblasts are not normally found in peripheral blood.

The figure on the next page illustrates the life cycle of iron in a red blood cell. Iron is absorbed from intestinal villi and transported in the plasma by transferrin. Transferrin is composed of the protein apotransferrin and one or two atoms of iron. Receptors on the red cell bind transferrin. The membrane invaginates forming an intracytoplasmic vesicle called an *endosome*. Acid-containing vesicles fuse with the endosome creating an acid environment which liberates iron from transferrin. Most of the iron (80-90%) is transported to mitochondria for production of heme. The rest is stored in the protein *ferritin*. Ferritin is a complex of iron and the protein apoferritin. The protein subunits form a sphere capable of holding about 4,500 atoms of ferric iron.

Sideroblast (Prussian Blue Stain)

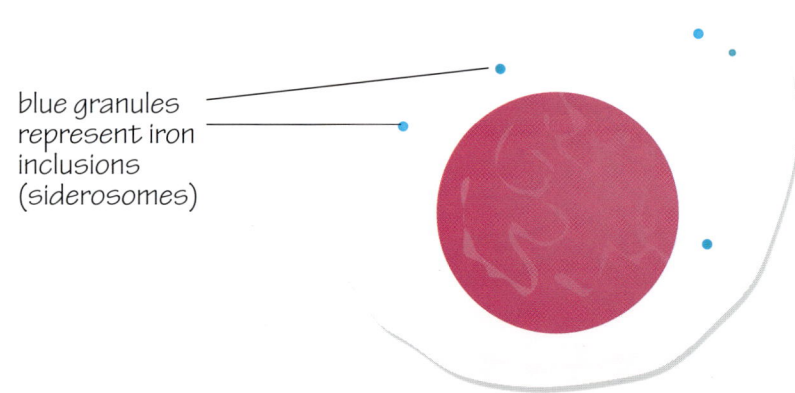

blue granules represent iron inclusions (siderosomes)

the granules are randomly located in the cytoplasm (not primarily peri-nuclear)

no more than 5 granules are normally present (type I sideroblast)

if iron is not effectively utilized, 6 or more granules may be found (type II sideroblast)

H-51, 1979 (Bone Marrow, Prussian Blue, X400)

Identification	Referee %	Participant %
Sideroblast (iron stain)	85.7	79.4
Polychromatophilic normoblast	14.3	4.2
Pappenheimer bodies (iron stain)	-	6.8

Nucleated red blood cells normally contain iron inclusions (siderosomes). They are distributed within the cytoplasm and do not concentrate around the nucleus. This distinguishes normal sideroblasts from ring sideroblasts. Participants were asked to identify the cell, not the inclusions; therefore, Pappenheimer bodies is not a correct choice. Pappenheimer bodies may be found in sideroblasts and siderocytes. They are visible on Wright-Giemsa smears and an iron stain is used to confirm them. Normal siderosomes are invisible on Wright-Giemsa stains.

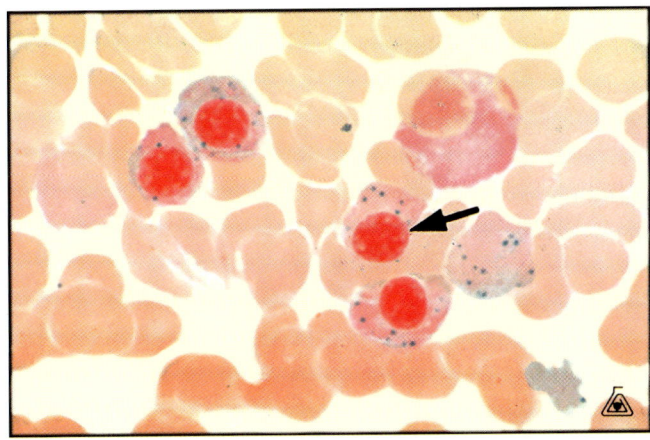

Iron Uptake, Storage, and Utilization in Red Cells

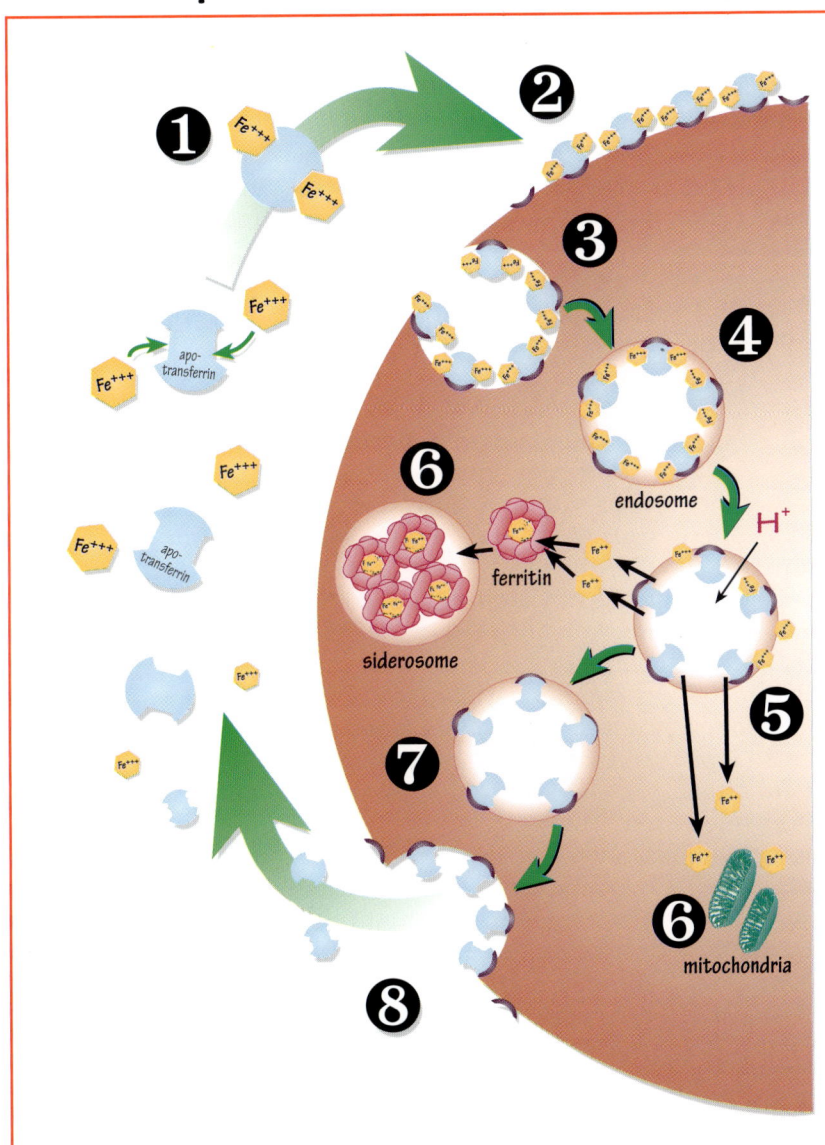

❶ Whenever molecules of iron enter the plasma (e.g., from intestinal villi), they attach to apotransferrin. The resulting complex is called *transferrin*.

❷ Transferrin attaches to receptors on the surface of a red cell.

❸ The cell membrane invaginates.

❹ The vesicle that forms is called an *endosome*. It contains transferrin molecules bound to receptors.

❺ Acid enters the siderosome, triggering release of iron from apotransferrin.

❻ Iron can be used by mitochondria to form heme (see page 178) or may be stored in ferritin molecules. Aggregates of ferritin may be enclosed in a lysosomal organelle, called a *siderosome*.

❼ The vesicle containing the receptors and apotransferrin is transported to the surface of the cell.

❽ The vesicle fuses with the cell membrane and opens, releasing apotransferrin back into the plasma.

A Closer Look At...

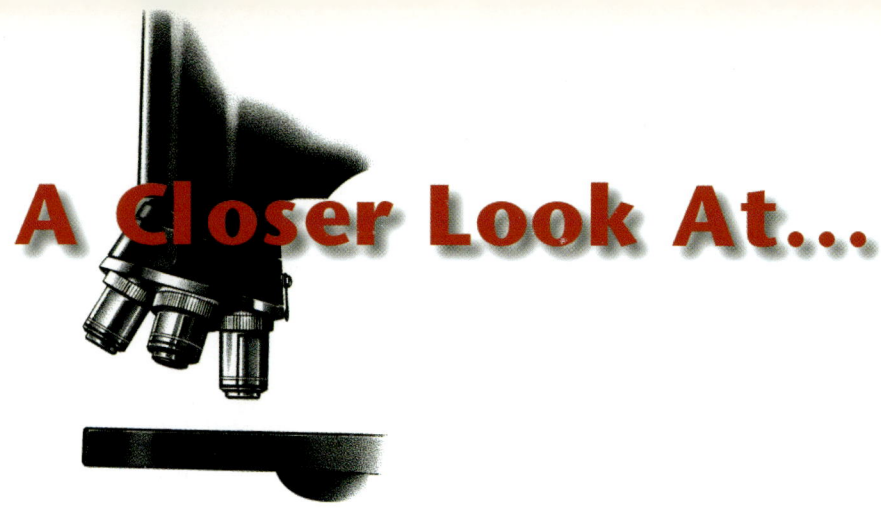

Sideroblasts and Siderocytes

The vast majority of iron that enters the maturing red cell is incorporated into heme. The rest is stored as ferritin. Prussian blue staining of the bone marrow allows for a qualitative assessment of iron stores (hemosiderin and ferritin). Under normal physiologic conditions, hemosiderin and ferritin will be deposited in the bone marrow macrophages and maturing erythroid cells. Nucleated red cells that contain Prussian blue positive cytoplasmic granules are termed sideroblasts (types I, II, and III).

Ferritin molecules may be dispersed throughout the cytoplasm of the cell or clustered together and surrounded by a lysosomal organelle to form a *siderosome*. Siderosomes concentrate enough iron to be visible by light microscopy and iron stains.

Type I sideroblasts contain up to 5 siderosomes that are faintly positive by the Prussian blue reaction. They normally represent up to 50% of marrow normoblasts. In the normal physiologic state, these granules decrease in number as the normoblast matures. Occasionally the stored iron is not effectively utilized and Type II sideroblasts are present. They contain greater than 6 siderosomes that are scattered randomly throughout the cytoplasm. Ringed sideroblasts (Type III sideroblasts) are always pathologic. They are often thought to be the result of insufficient heme formation secondary to impaired or defective protoporphyrin production (usually related to decreased d-aminolevulinic acid synthase activity such as in lead poisoning and ethanol abuse). Uncommonly, the formation of ringed sideroblasts may be due to impaired globin production (thalassemias). See *A Closer Look At...* on page 184 for a discussion of how ringed sideroblasts form.

Anucleate cells with Prussian blue positive cytoplasmic granules are termed siderocytes. When the siderotic granules are identifiable on Wright-Giemsa stained peripheral blood smears they are referred to as Pappenheimer bodies. These may be particularly prominent in cases of functional hyposplenia or asplenia. Reticulocytes that demonstrate positive iron staining have been termed sidero-reticulocytes. Circulating siderocytes are found in many hematopoietic disorders, particularly sideroblastic anemias. They are much less prevalent than Pappenheimer bodies and are abundant only after splenectomy.

Although individuals with ringed sideroblasts often appear to have adequate marrow iron stores, they are usually anemic. The ringed sideroblastic anemias are categorized as either acquired or hereditary. Acquired causes include the myelodysplastic syndromes, acute myelogenous leukemia (FAB M6), ethanol toxicity, lead poisoning, zinc toxicity, copper deficiency, as well as chloramphenicol and isoniazid therapy. Hereditary causes include the congenital sideroblastic anemias and some hemoglobinopathies. Bone marrow findings are characterized by erythroid hyperplasia and dysplasia. The reticulocyte count is usually normal or only slightly increased. The circulating red cells are usually hypochromic and microcytic. Occasionally a dimorphic red cell population consisting of a hypochromic/microcytic population in conjunction with a normochromic/normocytic population (or rarely a macrocytic population) may also be present.

Sideroblasts | Siderocytes

Iron Stain   Wright-Giemsa Stain   Iron Stain   Wright-Giemsa Stain

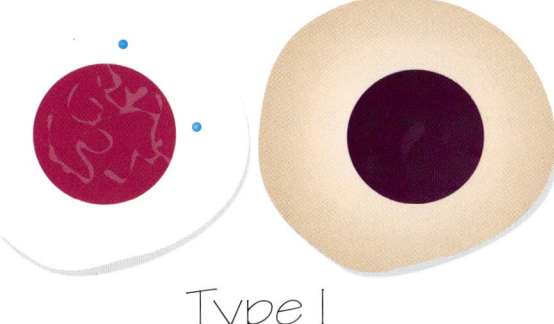

Type I

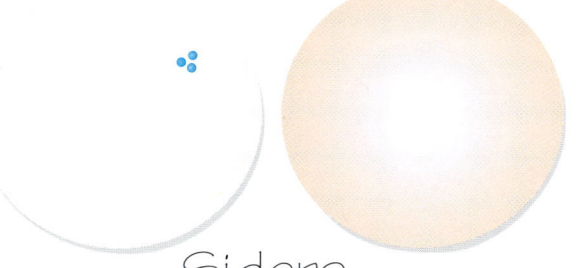

Sidero-Reticulocyte

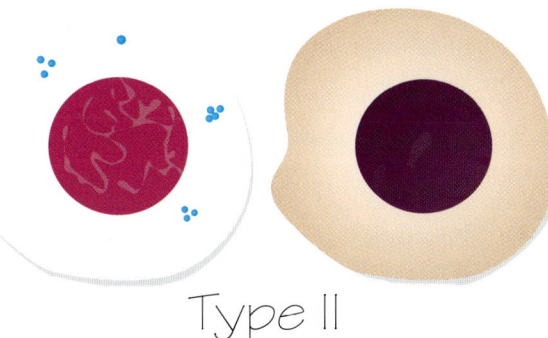

Type II

Siderocyte

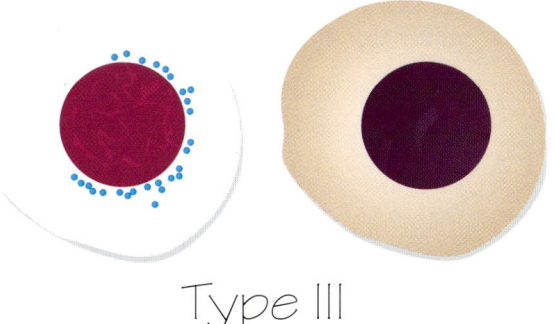

Type III

Siderocyte with Pappenheimer Bodies

Sideroblast, Ringed (Iron Stain)

SYNONYMS
ring sideroblast

VITAL STATISTICS
- size .... varies with stage of maturation
- N:C ratio .... varies with disease state, usually normal or decreased
- cell shape .... round or oval
- nuclear shape ... may be round or abnormal
- chromatin .... varies with disease state
- nucleoli .... usually not present
- cytoplasm .... may contain Pappenheimer bodies on Wright-Giemsa stained material; blue granules encircling the nucleus after iron staining

KEY DIFFERENTIATING FEATURES
a ringed sideroblast must have at least 5 granules that cover at least one half of the nuclear circumference
abnormal sideroblasts may have multiple, larger than normal granules, or granules that are polarized at one end of the cell

OTHER FINDINGS
nuclear to cytoplasmic dyssynchrony and abnormal nuclear morphology may also be present
increased iron stores

POTENTIAL LOOK-ALIKES
Howell-Jolly bodies (iron negative)
Heinz bodies (iron negative; not visible on Wright-Giemsa-stained smears)
hemoglobin H inclusions (iron negative; supravital stain only)
RNA bodies

ASSOCIATED DISEASE STATES AND CONDITIONS
myelodysplasia
hemosiderosis
hemoglobinopathies
sideroblastic anemia
alcoholism
hyposplenism
lead poisoning
drugs (isoniazid, chloramphenicol)
copper deficiency
zinc intoxication

Nucleated red cells that stain positive for iron granules are termed sideroblasts. If the granules appear as a full or partial ring around the nucleus, the term *ringed sideroblast* is used. This perinuclear location corresponds to mitochondrial deposition of iron. The deposition of iron within the mitochondria is associated with changes in heme synthesis resulting in ineffective erythropoiesis.

Sideroblasts are divided into three types, as described on pages 178 and 179. Ringed sideroblasts are type III sideroblasts. They must have more than 5 iron-containing granules covering at least 50% of the nuclear circumference. The individual granules are often larger than normal siderosomes. Background iron stores are usually increased as well. The Wright-Giemsa stained erythroblasts may show dysplastic features such as nuclear-cytoplasmic dyssynchrony and/or abnormal nuclear morphology.

Ringed sideroblasts are seen in the blood and/or bone marrow in sideroblastic anemias, myelodysplasias, and other dyserythropoietic states. Sideroblastic anemias are a heterogeneous group of disorders that all share the unique finding of iron deposits in erythroblast mitochondria. Impaired production of protoporphyrin or defective insertion of iron into protoporphyrin results in decreased heme production leading to accumulation of iron within mitochondria. The delivery of iron to the red cell (detailed on page 178) does not stop; iron is transported normally to mitochondria where it continues to accumulate. Defective globin synthesis, such as in thalassemia, can also lead to iron accumulation in mitochondria. Since mitochondria are preferentially located near the nucleus, a circumferential iron staining pattern results. These events are detailed on pages 184 and 185 in *A Closer Look At...Formation of Ringed Sideroblasts*.

Ringed Sideroblast (Prussian Blue Stain)

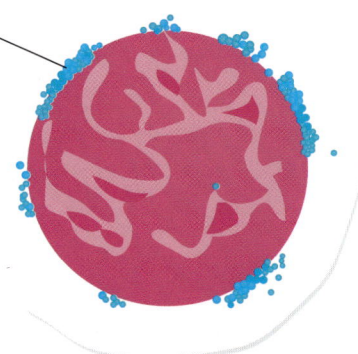

iron-containing mitochondria

ringed sideroblasts must have more than 5 iron-containing granules covering at least 50% of the nuclear circumference

ringed sideroblasts are also known as type III sideroblasts

H-26, 1981 (Bone Marrow, Prussian Blue, X400)

Identification	Referee %	Participant %
Ringed sideroblast	83.3	81.9
Sideroblast	16.7	11.4

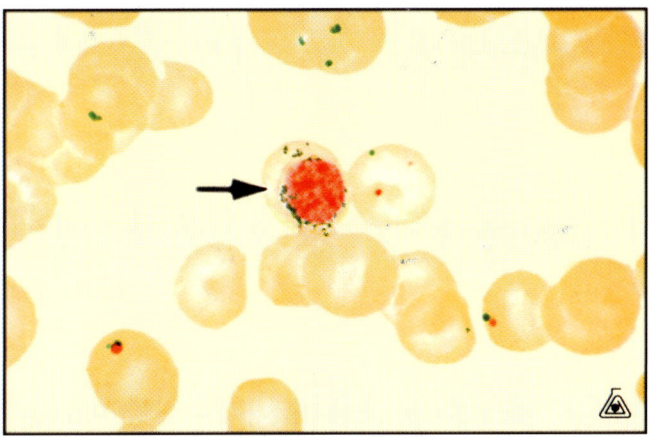

The photomicrograph is a Prussian Blue-stained bone marrow aspirate. The arrowed cell is a ringed sideroblast. Blue granules partially surround the nucleus. The granules represent iron deposition within mitochondria. Notice the coarse nature of the siderotic particles and their perinuclear location. More than 5 granules are present and these are more than half way around the nucleus, fulfilling the definition of ringed sideroblast. Many of the non-nucleated red cells in the same field contain iron-positive granules. These are *siderocytes*, not sideroblasts, because they do not contain a nucleus. If the inclusions are found on Wright-Giemsa staining as well, they are termed Pappenheimer bodies.

H-50, 1979 (Bone Marrow, Prussian Blue, X400)

Identification	Referee %	Participant %
Ringed sideroblast	93.3	85.7
Pappenheimer bodies (iron stain)	3.0	14.3
Sideroblast	1.5	-

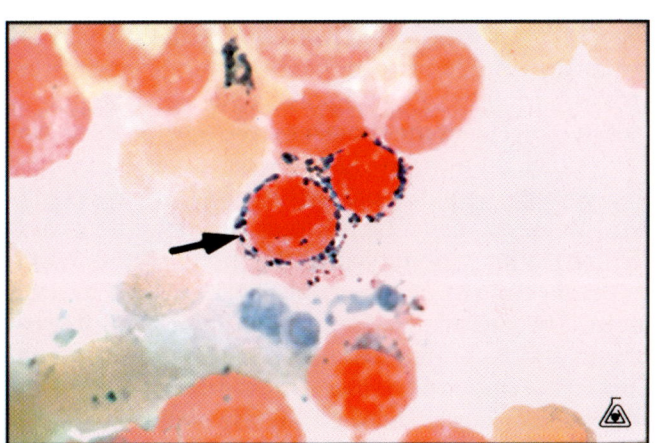

The two arrowed cells are ringed sideroblasts. Once again, the Prussian blue-stained bone marrow aspirate clearly shows iron granules surrounding the nucleus. Iron accumulates within mitochondria due to abnormalities in heme or globin production. Since the mitochondria are preferentially located near the nucleus, iron deposition produces the characteristic ringed pattern.

H1-44, 1987 (Bone Marrow, Prussian Blue, X375)

Identification	Referee %	Participant %
Ringed sideroblast	100	95.7

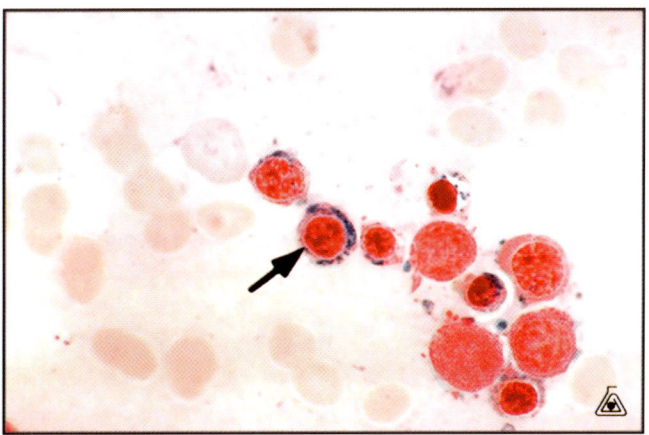

The arrowed cell is a ringed sideroblast. The Prussian blue-positive granules within the cytoplasm form a partial ring around the nucleus. Sometimes the staining is so intense it almost forms a solid band, as in this cell, rather than the punctate staining present in the ringed sideroblasts in the previous two photomicrographs (H-26, 1981 and H-50, 1979). Iron inclusions can be seen in non-nucleated red cells in the same field. These are *siderocytes*. Some of the inclusions may represent Pappenheimer bodies, if they can be seen by Wright-Giemsa stain as well.

A Closer Look At...

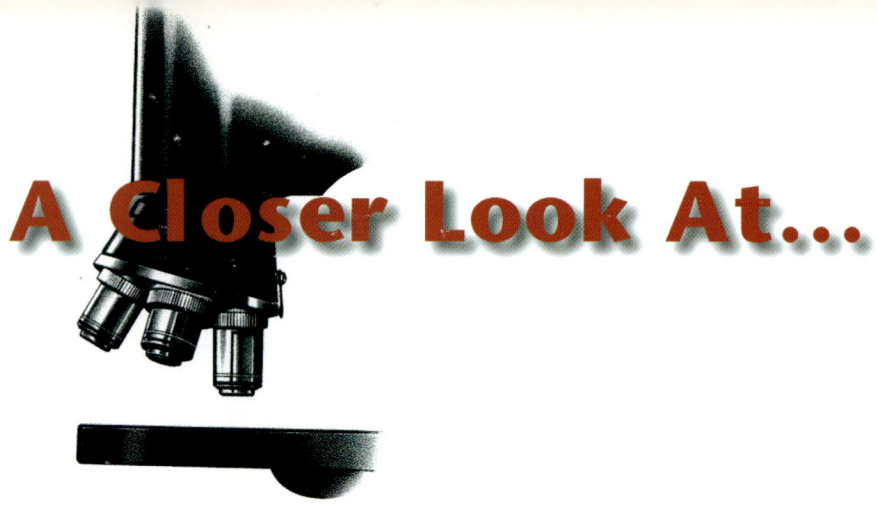

Hemoglobin Formation and Iron Utilization

The change in Wright-Giemsa staining of the erythroid precursor cytoplasm from blue to orange reflects increased amounts of hemoglobin synthesis. The hemoglobin molecule is the protein in the red blood cell that carries oxygen from the lung to the tissues. Hemoglobin synthesis begins in proerythroblasts. The hemoglobin molecule consists of four polypeptide chains (globin) and a nonpolypeptide (heme). The heme molecule consists of an organic molecule and an iron atom. The organic component of heme is protoporphyrin and is formed from succinyl CoA and glycine. Succinyl CoA and glycine, in the presence of d-aminolevulinic acid (ALA) synthetase and pyridoxal 5'-phosphate form ALA. This initial step is the rate limiting step of heme synthesis. Two of the ALA molecules combine to form porphobilinogen. Four of the porphobilinogen molecules then form uroporphyrinogen III. Uroporphyrinogen undergoes decarboxylation to form coproporphyrinogen III and oxidation to form protoporphyrin IX. Within the cytoplasmic mitochondria, protoporphyrin IX combines with ferrous iron (Fe^{++}) to form heme.

The iron that is incorporated into the heme molecule can be derived from heme and non-heme sources. Heme iron is derived from exogenous or endogenous hemoglobin, myoglobin, and other heme proteins. Non-heme iron is exogenously acquired through the diet and absorbed in the duodenum and upper jejunum. Under normal circumstances only 5-10% of ingested iron is absorbed. Once absorbed, iron is complexed to transferrin, a carrier protein in the plasma. The transferrin-iron complex is then routed to transferrin receptors of various cells within the body that require iron. The complex is internalized and the iron is liberated from transferrin which returns to the plasma. As erythrocytes mature, iron is incorporated into the heme molecule. A small amount of iron remains in the erythroid cytoplasm as ferritin. The ferritin may be concentrated in membrane-bound packets called *siderosomes*. When stained with Prussian blue, ferritin granules dispersed in the cytoplasm are too small to be visible. Siderosomes, however, are large enough to be seen. Maturing nucleated erythroid cells with iron-staining siderosomes are referred to as *sideroblasts*. They can be seen in the cytoplasm of 20-60% of normoblasts.

Globin chain synthesis involves chromosome 16 which contains 2 genes for the alpha globin chain, and chromosome 11 which contains one gene for the beta globin chain. Each gene contains exons and introns that undergo RNA transcription and translation to form an amino acid polypeptide chain.

Each final hemoglobin molecule then contains four polypeptide chains, four heme groups and four oxygen molecules. The four polypeptide chains are held together by non-covalent bonds. The four chains are arranged as a tetrahedral structure with the heme groups located near the exterior of the molecule. The amino acid sequence of each of the four polypeptides is critical because it determines the hemoglobin molecule's tertiary structure.

Heme and Globin Formation

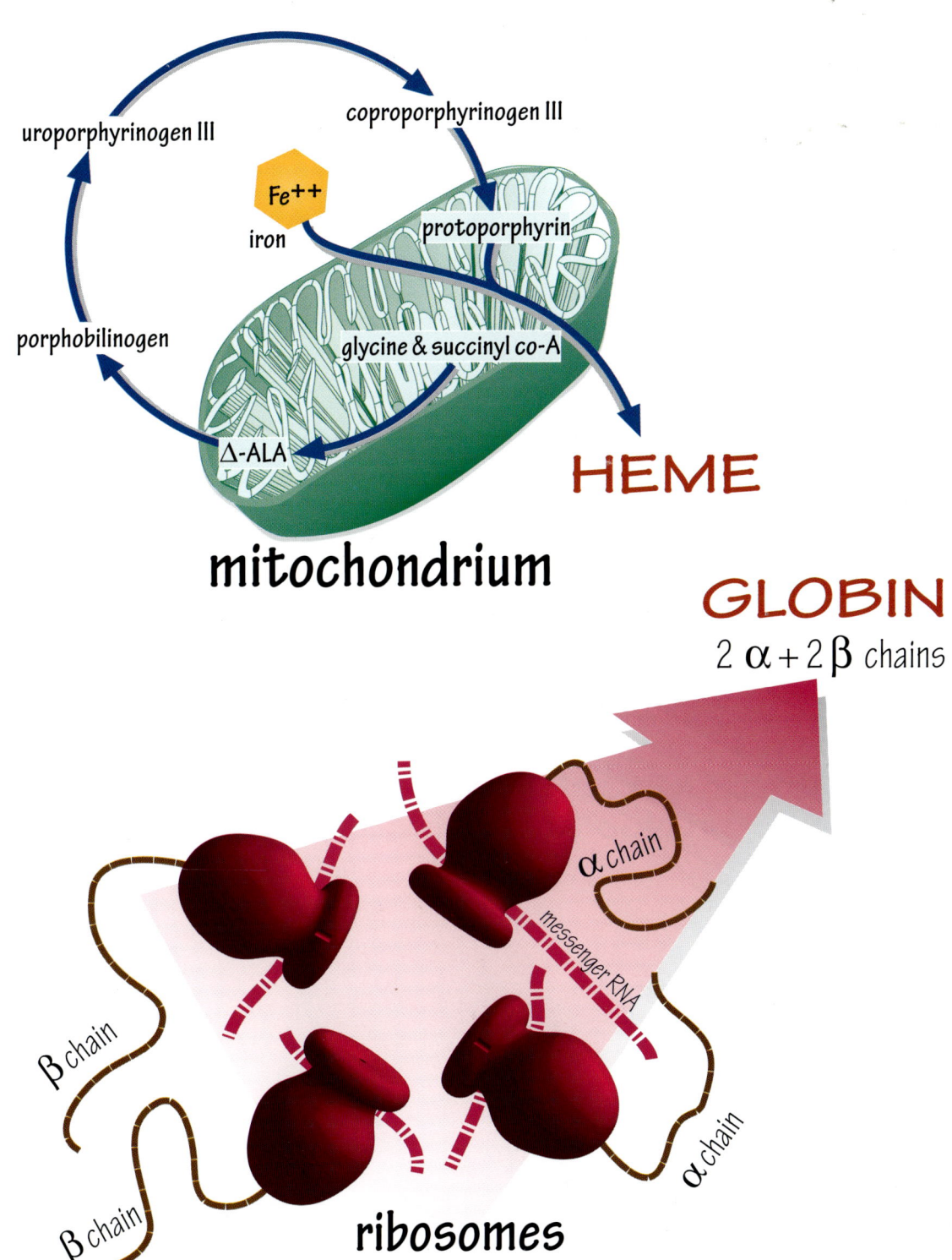

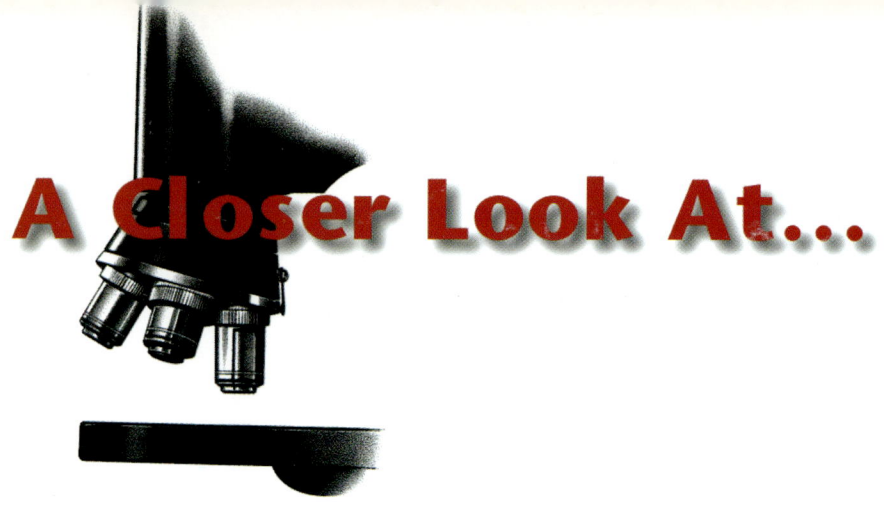

A Closer Look At...

Formation of Ringed Sideroblasts

Ringed sideroblasts are formed by the deposit of iron in the mitochondria of erythroid precursors. The iron is deposited in the form of ferric phosphate and ferric oxide. The mitochondria are preferentially located close to the nucleus, giving rise to the ringed staining pattern seen with iron stains. Ultrastructurally the iron is deposited within the thin, delicate cristae of the mitochondria resulting in mitochondrial dysfunction. Ringed sideroblasts are always pathologic and can be found in a variety of disease states, the most common being sideroblastic anemia. The unifying pathologic process in the sideroblastic anemias is thus thought to be a defect in heme synthesis.

The sideroblastic anemias can be classified as congenital or acquired. The acquired form is either primary or secondary. The primary acquired sideroblastic anemias are the most common and are part of the spectrum of myelodysplastic disorders (refractory anemia with ringed sideroblasts). Other causes of primary acquired sideroblastic anemia include those cases associated with previous chemotherapy or irradiation. Secondarily acquired sideroblastic anemias are most often due to drugs including alcohol, isoniazid, and chloramphenicol.

Location of Mitochondria and Siderosomes in Nucleated Red Cells

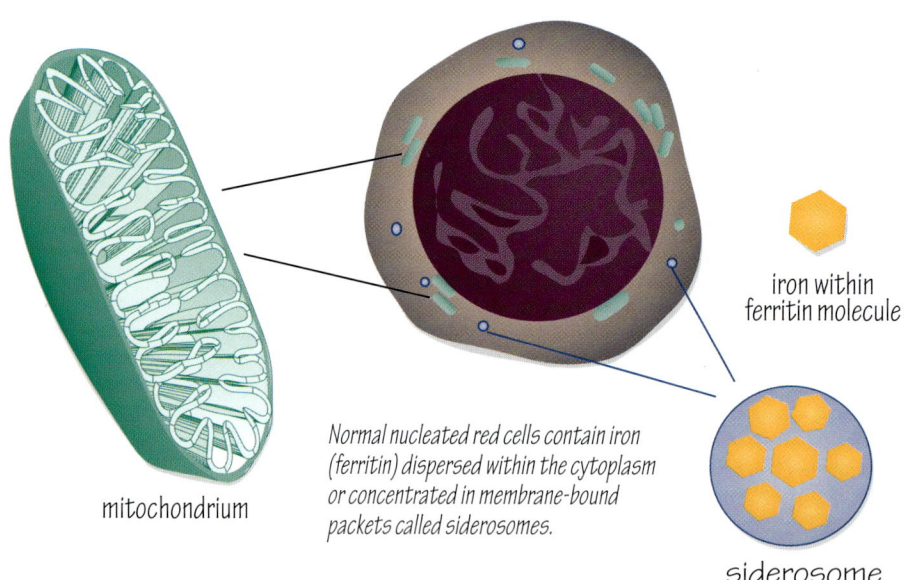

mitochondrium

Normal nucleated red cells contain iron (ferritin) dispersed within the cytoplasm or concentrated in membrane-bound packets called siderosomes.

iron within ferritin molecule

siderosome

Examples of Heme & Globin Synthesis Abnormalities Leading to Mitochondrial Iron Deposition

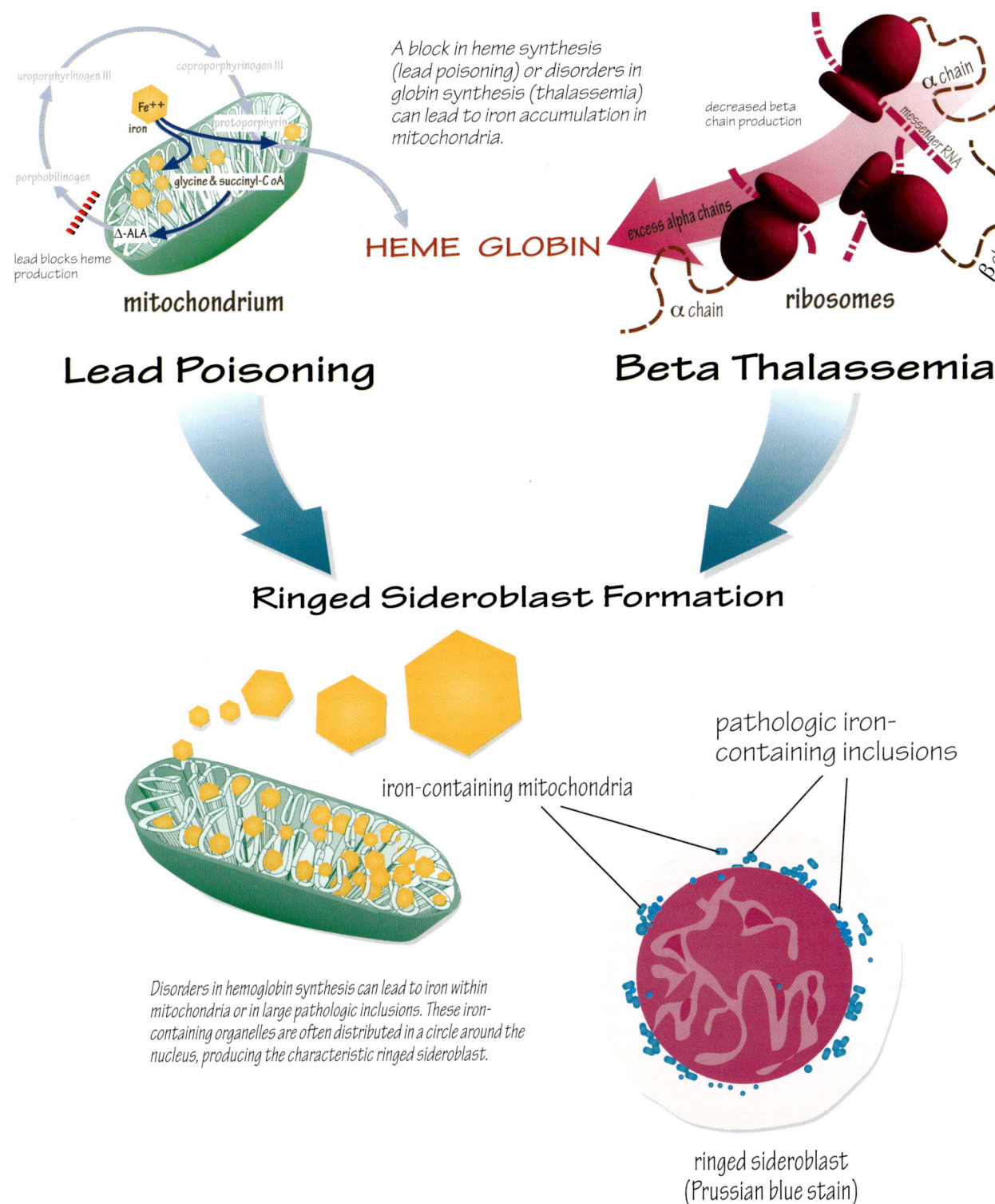

Megakaryocytic Cells and Thrombocytes

Introduction 187
Megakaryocyte or Precursor, Normal 188
    A Closer Look At…Megakaryocyte Maturation 190
Megakaryocyte or Precursor, Abnormal 192
    A Closer Look At…Dysplastic Megakaryocytes 194
Megakaryocyte Nucleus 196
Platelet, Normal 198
    A Closer Look At…Platelet Formation 200
Platelet, Giant 202
Platelet, Hypogranular 204
Platelet Satellitism 206
    A Closer Look At…Platelet Satellitism 208

Introduction

Megakaryocytes are the largest cell in the bone marrow. They develop through a complex process involving proliferation of committed stem cells, nuclear duplication without cell division, and maturation. The final step is cytoplasmic fragmentation, releasing a shower of platelets into the blood stream.

The same stem cell responsible for producing granulocytes and nucleated red cells gives rise to the committed stem cells that eventuate in mature megakaryocytes. The sequence of events is unique because it involves endoreduplication (also known as endomitosis). Here, chromosomes double in number but the cell does not divide.

At some point, polyploid megakaryocytes begin to mature. The trigger for this is unknown. Some start the process after only a few cycles of endomitosis while others delay until they have reached 32 or 64N ploidy. The cytoplasm becomes granulated as a complex of tubules and membrane invaginations subdivide the cytoplasm into small packets. These cytoplasmic territories are future platelets.

Mature megakaryocytes are usually located next to bone marrow sinuosoids. The cell cytoplasm penetrates endothelial cells and forms long strands dangling in the blood stream. These eventually break into small platelet fragments. Residual megakaryocyte nuclei are phagocytized by bone marrow macrophages. Some nuclear fragments and lobes, often surrounded by wisps of cytoplasm, enter the blood stream. These megakaryocyte fragments are usually seen in myeloproliferative and myelodysplastic states.

It takes approximately five days for a megakaryoblast to mature and release platelets. These small disc-shaped cytoplasmic fragments become activated after injury and participate in several aspects of hemostasis.

Like all the other hematopoietic elements, megakaryocytes and their progeny may display abnormal morphology. Most cases are associated with the myeloproliferative and myelodysplastic disorders. Dysplastic megakaryocytes may be abnormally small or large with hypo or hyperlobation. Nuclei may be abnormallly lobated. Unusual forms of platelet morphology include cells that are larger than red cells or exhibit hypogranulation.

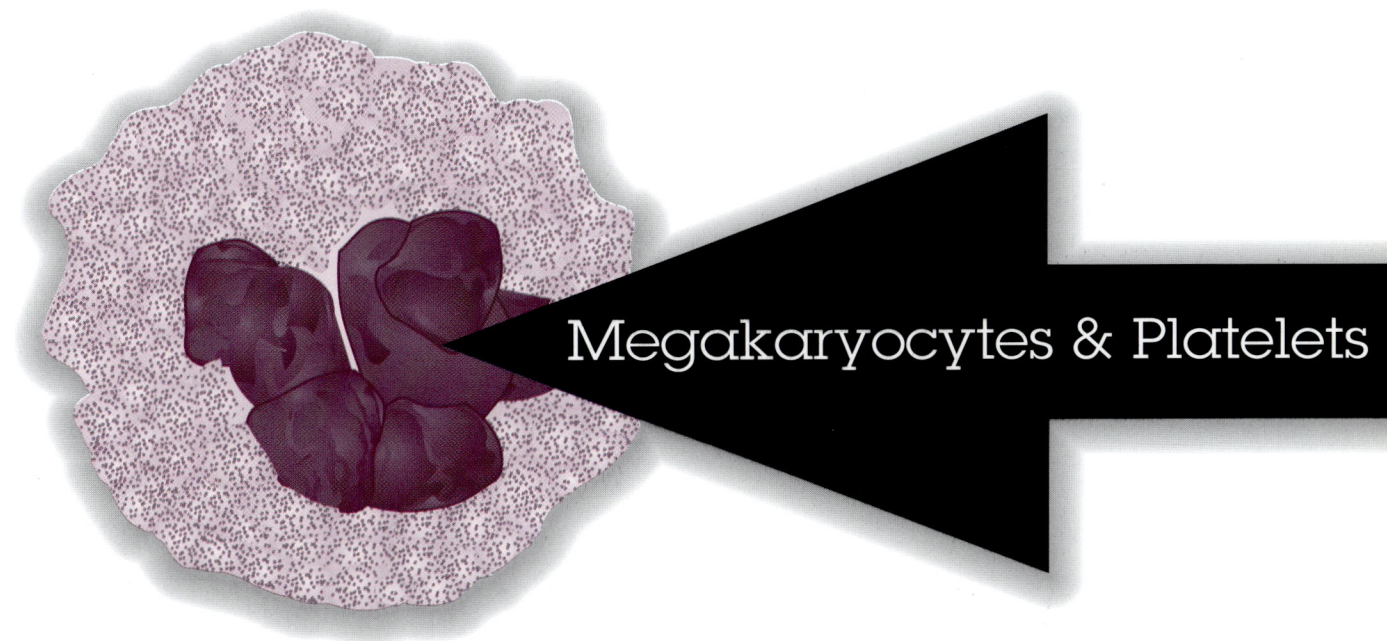

Megakaryocyte or Precursor, Normal

SYNONYMS
none

VITAL STATISTICS
- size .... 20-160 μm in diameter
- N:C ratio .... varible, depending on maturation of cell; early forms have a high N:C rato which decreases as cell matures and acquires cytoplasm; at the end of cell lifespan, the cytoplasm is discharged as platelets and the N:C ratio increases again
- cell shape .... variable; may be round or have irregular cytoplasmic contours; platelets may form at the periphery producing a fragmented sillouette
- nuclear shape .... young cells: round or horseshoe shaped; mature cells: irregularly lobed, ring-shaped or doughnut-shaped; lobes are connected; not multinucleated
- chromatin .... dense; stains dark purple-blue; less clumped in young cells
- nucleoli .... immature cells only
- cytoplasm .... young cells: basophilic and agranular or a few granules; mature cells: abundant light blue and packed with fine azurophilic granules that cluster producing a checkerboard pattern

KEY DIFFERENTIATING FEATURES
- mature cells: low N:C ratio, large cell size, highly lobed nucleus, light blue cytoplasm packed with pink granules, platelets sometimes at periphery
- young cells: moderate N:C ratio, moderately clumped chromatin, basophilic cytoplasm with irregular boarder, para-nuclear early granule formation
- blasts: high N:C ratio, round nucleus, evenly distributed chromatin, nucleoli, basophilic cytoplasm

POTENTIAL LOOK-ALIKES
- histiocytes and macrophages (Langerhans and Touton giant cells, Gaucher's and other storage disease cells)
- osteoclast and osteoblast
- lymphoma (hyperlobated cell, Reed-Sternberg cell)
- granulocytic precursors (mimic micromegakaryocytes)
- metastatic tumor cells

ASSOCIATED DISEASE STATES AND CONDITIONS
normal finding in bone marrow

Megakaryocytes develop from a series of committed stem cells, the last one designated CFU-MK. The committed cell goes through a sequence of nuclear duplication without cell division called *endomitosis* or *endoreduplication*. The result is a large cell with abundant cytoplasm and a hyperdiploid nucleus. The cytoplasm then matures, dividing into territories which eventually become mature platelets. The entire maturation sequence is detailed in the following *A Closer Look At...Megakaryocyte Maturation* discussion on page 190.

The CFU-MK stem cell is a mononuclear lymphoid-like cell with megakaryocyte-specific cell markers but no morphologic distinguishing features. As the cell develops, three stages are recognized:
- Stage I: megakaryoblast
- Stage II: promegakaryocyte
- Stage III: granular or mature megakaryocyte

The mononuclear megakaryoblast is at least 15 μm in size. The nucleus is round or a slightly indented with evenly distributed chromatin. Nucleoli are generally visible and may be prominent. The nucleus is surrounded by a small rim of basophilic cytoplasm.

The promegakaryocyte, also knows as basophilic megakaryocyte, is at least 20 μm in size and has a lobated or horseshoe-shaped nucleus. Chromatin starts to show significant clumping. There is a moderate amount of intensely basophilic cytoplasm that may be irregular in shape with blebs and extensions. The earliest site of platelet production occurs next to the

Mature Megakaryocyte

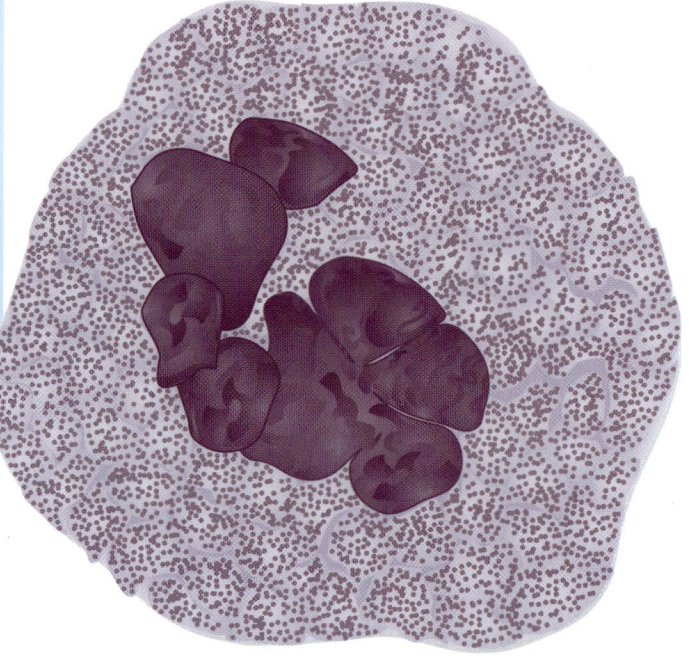

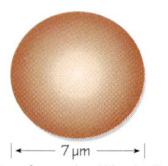

|← 7μm →|
size of normal red blood cell

nucleus. Here, azurophilic granules form. Later stages may have a patchy eosinophilic cytoplasm. This stage marks the end of DNA duplication.

Granular megakaryocytes are capable of platelet production. They are the largest bone marrow hematopoietic cell, meauring at least 25-50 μm. They are normally pleomorphic and a spectrum of cell shapes and sizes is typical. The numerous nuclear lobes are of various sizes, connected by large bands or fine chromatin threads. The chromatin is initially coarse and clumped and later pyknotic in the fully mature megakaryocyte. The abundant cytoplasm stains pink or wine-red and contains fine azurophilic granules which may be clustered due to formation of demarcation lines. This produces a checkered pattern.

Increased numbers of megakaryocytes are seen in chronic myeloproliferative disorders, myelodysplastic syndromes, acute megakaryoblastic leukemia (M7), ITP, hypersplenism, infections, blood loss (intra or extravascular), and some malignancies.

Decreased numbers of megakaryocytes are seen in acute leukemia, infiltration of the marrow by neoplastic cells (histiocytes, lymphoma, carcinoma, etc.), occasional myelodysplastic syndromes, amegakaryocytic thrombocytopenia, viral infections, aplastic anemia, and radiation or toxic-drug treatments.

HE-44, 1992 (Bone Marrow, Wright-Giemsa, X300)

Identification	Referee %	Participant %
Megakaryocyte or precursor, normal	47.4	39.7
Megakaryocyte or precursor, abnormal	52.6	48.0

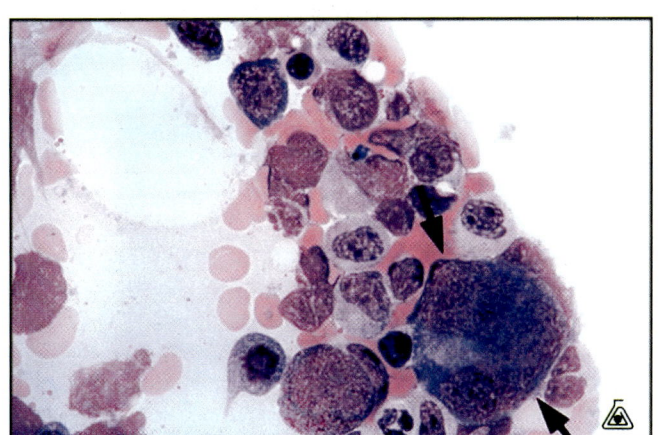

The arrowed cell is a normal megakaryocyte precursor (promegakaryocyte). The nucleus is lobated and the chromatin is coarse but relatively evenly distributed. No nucleoli are visible. The cytoplasm is basophilic and lacks the marked granularity associated with mature megakaryocytes. Early granule production is seen near the golgi region. Many of the participants and referees incorrectly identified this cell as an abnormal megakaryocyte. Such cells are generally too small (micromegakaryocytes), gigantic, or have too few or too many nuclear lobations. None of these dysplastic features are seen in the arrowed cell. Its only "aberration" is immaturity.

HE-43, 1992 (Bone Marrow, Wright-Giemsa, X300)

Identification	Referee %	Participant %
Megakaryocyte or precursor, normal	100	83.5
Megakaryocyte or precursor, abnormal	-	11.4

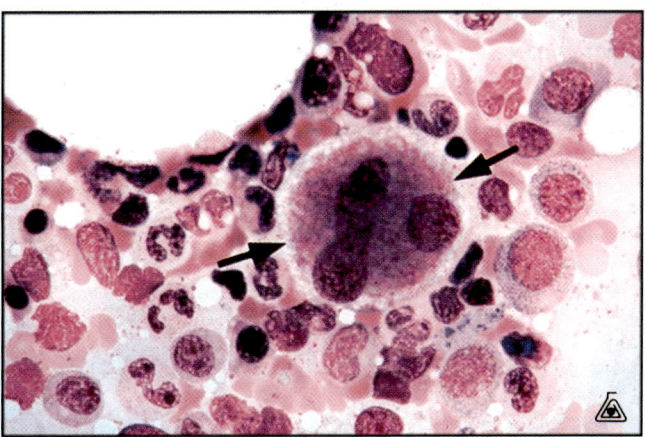

The arrowed cell is a normal mature megakaryocyte. The large cell has multiple, overlapping nuclear lobes and abundant granulated cytoplasm. Three nuclear lobes are visible; one appears separate from the other two which are overlapping. The chromatin is clumped. No nucleoli are visible. Notice how the cytoplasm is divided into smaller platelet territories. Soon it will fragment into thousands of small platelets. The remaining nucleus will condense and be digested by bone marrow macrophages.

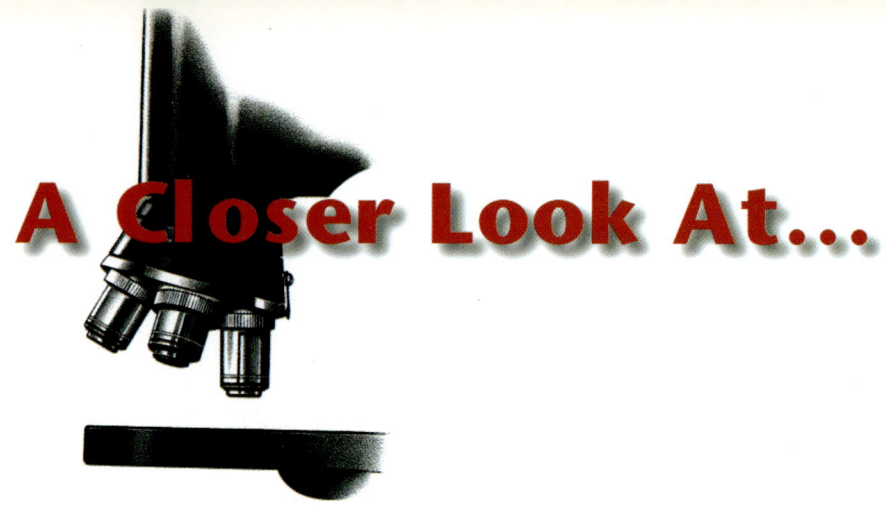

A Closer Look At...

Megakaryocyte Maturation

Megakaryopoiesis is a complex process that involves maturation, nuclear development, and platelet production. The illustrations below and on the next page portray these events in a stylized fashion.

Bone marrow stem cells undergo normal cell division and sequence through several stages, eventuating in the CFU-MK cell. This committed stem cell (called a promegakaryoblast) develops into morphologically-recognizable megakaryocytes in a three-stage process.

In stage I, megakaryoblasts form. These cells measure 15 µm or more in size and have a round nucleus with a small to moderate amount of slightly basophilic cytoplasm. Nuclear chromatin is coarse, without much clumping. This cell has a normal amount of DNA (2N).

Stage II begins after a series of amplification steps. The megakaryoblast becomes a promegakaryocyte. The cell stops dividing and instead DNA doubles in amount, forming cells with 4, 8, 16, 32, and rarely 64 sets of chromosomes. This unusual process of polyploidization goes by either the term *endomitosis* or nuclear *endoreduplication*.

In stage III, granular megakaryocytes form. Sometime during endoreduplication, the cell stops doubling the DNA content and instead focuses on cytoplasmic maturation. There is no direct associaton between the amount of DNA in the cell and when maturation is trig-

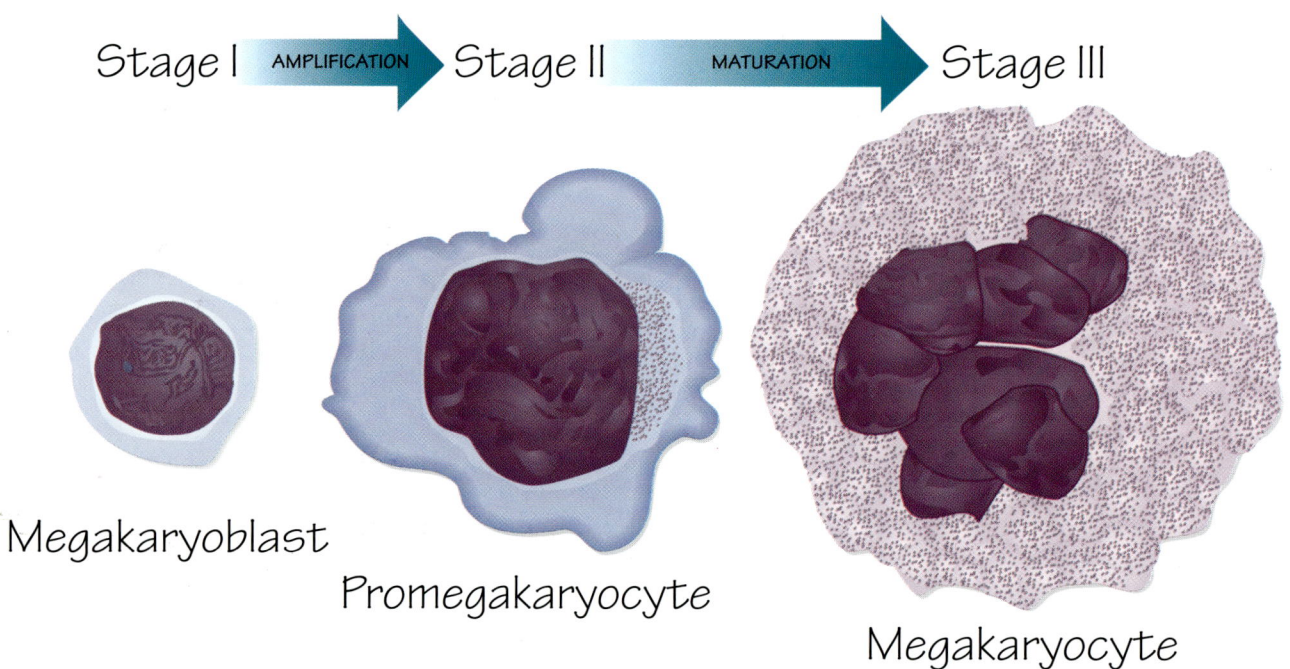

Megakaryocytic Cells and Thrombocytes

gered. Some cells with 8N begin to mature, while others do not start the process until the 32N stage. This is illustrated in the drawing below. The nucleus develops lobes, with each lobe roughly containing a single complement of chromosomes. Cells with 16N nuclei are the most common and these have 8 lobes. The cytoplasm, which has approximately doubled in amount with each nuclear multiplication, also begins to mature. Proteins and other biochemical constituents of platelets are produced giving the cytoplasm a pink granular appearance. Demarcation membranes develop, dividing the cell into territories that will eventually become platelets. Cells with increased ploidy—and therefore increased cytoplasm— produce platelets that are smaller and less dense. Lower ploidy cells produce fewer numbers of platelets that are larger, denser and more functionaly active. The process of platelet release is illustrated on page 201. The pyknotic nucleus is left behind to be phagocytized by marrow histiocytes.

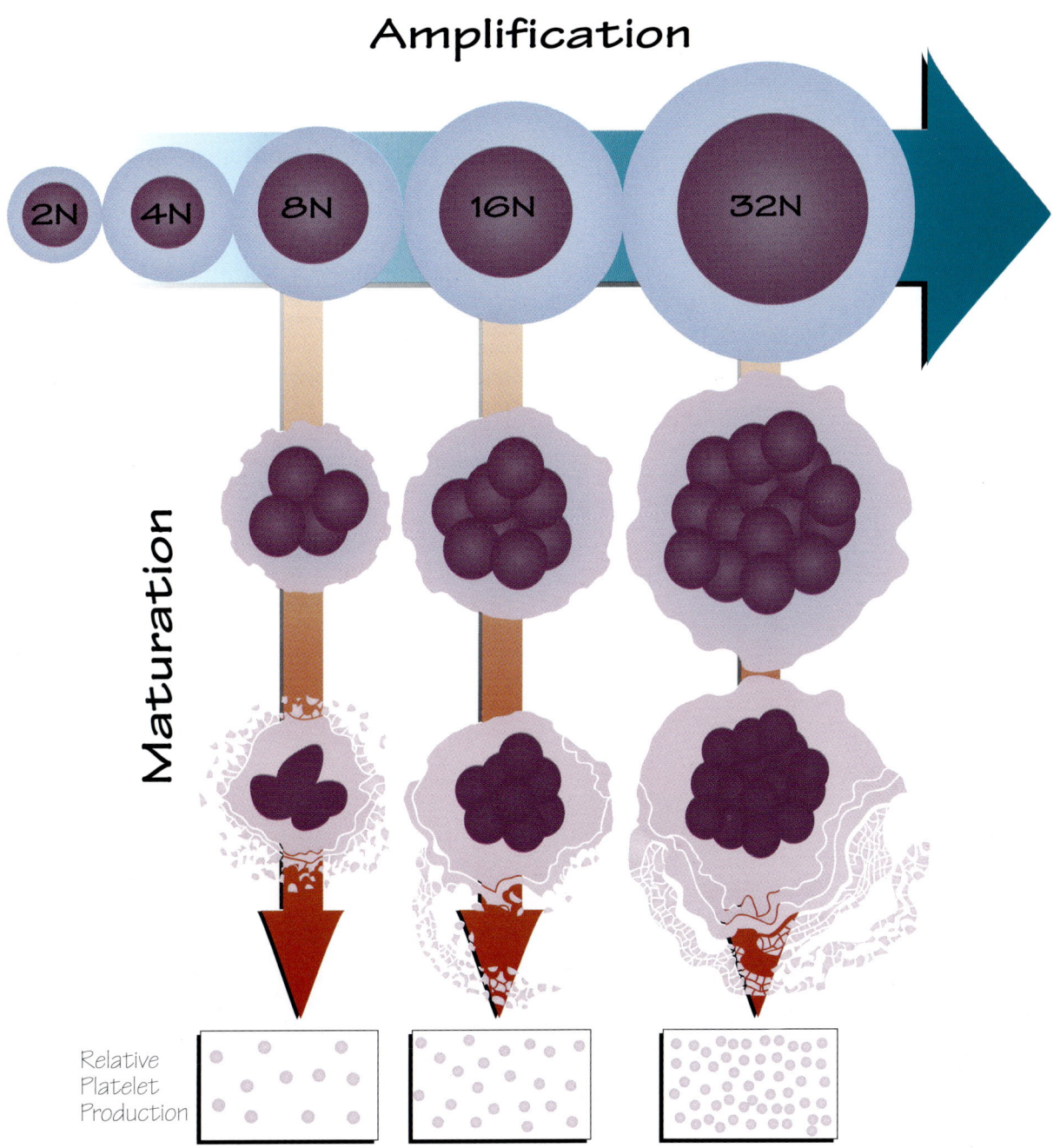

Megakaryocyte or Precursor, Abnormal

SYNONYMS
dysplastic or atypical megakaryocyte

VITAL STATISTICS
- size .... micromegs 15-39 μm (most <20 μm); very large megs 160 μm or more
- N:C ratio .... highly variable; micromegs 1:1 to 1:2; larger cells lower ratio
- cell shape .... micromegs irregular with cytoplasmic budding or blebs common; large cells highly pleomorphic
- nuclear shape .... micromegs round, oval, bilobed or trilobed; large cells are hyper- or hypolobated
- chromatin .... dense or puddled; naked nuclei may be pyknotic (apoptosis)
- nucleoli .... usually none; micromegs may have small nucleoli
- cytoplasm .... pale blue or pink with minimal or very abundant granularity; platelet production may be visible

KEY DIFFERENTIATING FEATURES
clustering
paratrabecular location (visible on bone biopsies only)
small size (micromegakaryocytes) or markedly enlarged mononuclear and hyperlobated forms
cytoplasmic hypogranularity
dyspoiesis present in other cells lines (granulocytes and nucleated red blood cells)
striking variability from cell to cell and field to field

POTENTIAL LOOK-ALIKES
histiocytes and macrophages (Langerhans and Touton giant cells, Gaucher's and other storage disease cells)
osteoclast and osteoblast
lymphomas (large cell types, Reed-Sternberg cells)
granulocytic precursors (micromegakaryocytes)
metastatic tumor cells

ASSOCIATED DISEASE STATES AND CONDITIONS
newborns (micromegs a normal finding in cord blood)
chronic myeloproliferative disorders (CML, PRV, AMM, ET)
myelodysplastic sydromes
5q- syndrome
acute megakaryocytic leukemia (M7)
other variants of AML
B_{12} and folate deficiency

Dysplasia in bone marrow megakaryocytes may manifest as abnormalities in cell size, nuclear shape, and cell location. *Micromegakaryocytes* are the most common example. These cells, also known as dwarf megakaryocytes, are abnormally small megakaryocytes that usually measure 15 to 39 μm in diameter (most are <20 μm). The N:C ratio is 1:1 or 1:2. They are morphologically mature but have impaired polyploidization. The nucleus may be hypolobated or may have multiple small lobes reminiscent of the pmn's in megaloblastic anemia. The cytoplasm is pale blue and may contain pink granules. Micromegakaryocytes are usually found in the marrow in myelodysplastic syndromes. They may also circulate in the blood. When they lack any significant cytoplasm, they are best termed *megakaryocyte nuclei* or fragments.

Larger abnormal megakaryocytes are highly variable in morphology. Some show marked nuclear lobation while others are hypolobated or mononuclear. Normal megakaryocyte nuclei are connected in series. Dysplastic nuclei may be separated. The finding of triple nuclei forming a pawn-ball pattern is a particularly useful marker of dysplasia.

Normally, megakaryocytes are single cells, well separated from each other and from the bony trabeculae. Dyspoiesis may be manifested by cell clustering and a paratrabecular location. Large sheets of highly pleomorphic cells may be found. This feature is best seen on bone marrow biopsies and clot specimens rather than aspirate smears.

Uniform hypolobated megakaryocytes are a feature of 5q- syndrome. This subtype of myelodysplasia occurs most commonly in elderly females. Patients have a macrocytic anemia with normal or elevated platelets. The prognosis is better than other subtypes of myelodysplasia.

Circulating micromegakaryocytes in adults are abnormal; they are seen most commonly in myeloproliferative conditions, especially agnogenic myeloid metapalsia. They are a normal finding in cord blood.

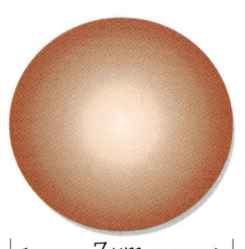

|← 7μm →|
size of normal red blood cell

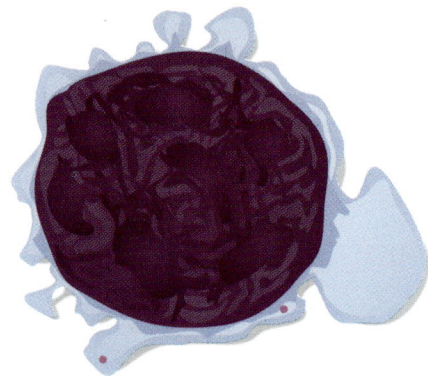

Micromegakaryocytes

HE-45, 1995 (Bone Marrow, Wright-Giemsa, X313)

Identification	Referee %	Participant %
Megakaryocyte or precursor, abnormal	73.9	58.8
Megakaryocyte or precursor, normal	21.7	24.6
Megakaryocyte nucleus	4.2	0.3
Osteoblast	-	2.6
Plasma cell, immature	-	2.7

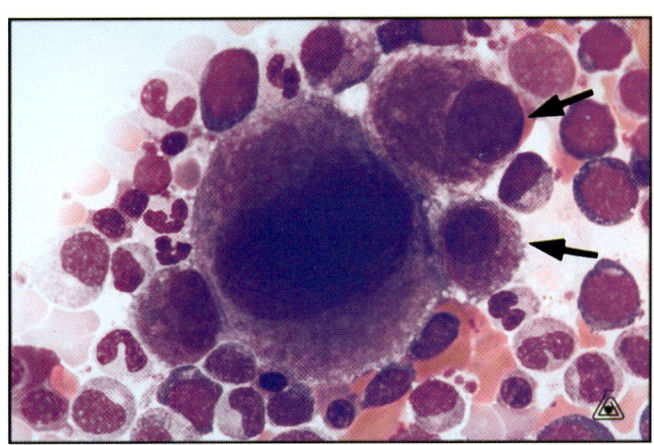

The bone marrow is from a patient with myelodysplasia. The large central cell and the surrounding three smaller cells, two of which are arrowed, are all dysplastic megakaryocytes. The cytoplasm is heavily granulated but the nucleus is round or minimally lobated. The small cells are best designated micromegakaryocytes. Megakaryocyte nuclei are stripped of most of their cytoplasm, unlike these cells. Osteoblasts have blue cytoplasm and a prominent clear zone (Golgi) a short distance away from the nucleus. Plasma cells have blue cytoplasm and a clear zone adjacent to the nucleus.

H1-31, 1988 (Bone Marrow, Wright-Giemsa, X330)

Identification	Referee %	Participant %
Megakaryocyte or precursor, abnormal	70	49
Megakaryocyte or precursor, normal	20	11.3
Myelocyte	10	24.7

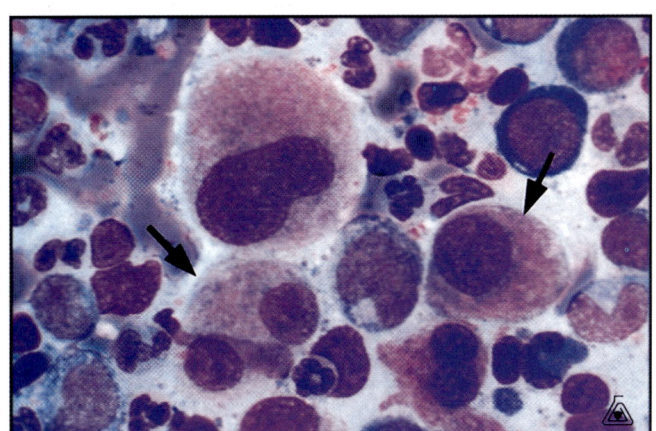

This is a case of chronic myelogenous leukemia. The bone marrow is hypercellular with markedly increased megakaryopoiesis. In this field, there are four recognizable abnormal megakaryocytes, two of which are arrowed. The arrowed cells are abnormally small (micromegakaryocytes) and have a single round nucleus. The cytoplasm exhibits varying degrees of granularity. The small bilobed cell beneath them is a heavily granulated megakaryocyte beginning to shed platelets. The larger megakaryocyte above them is hypolobated for the degree of cytoplasmic maturity. The size of the arrowed cells far exceeds that of myelocytes; in addition, no cytoplasmic granules suggestive of myelocytes are seen.

HE-11, 1994 (Blood, Wright-Giemsa, X400)

Identification	Referee %	Participant %
Megakaryocyte or precursor, abnormal	48.1	28.3
Megakaryocyte or precursor, normal	18.5	16.8
Megakaryocyte nucleus	11.1	10.8

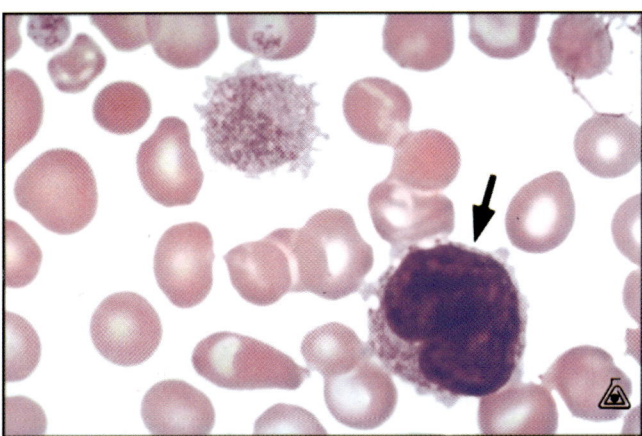

The arrowed cell is a micromegakaryocyte circulating in the peripheral blood of an adult. The N:C ratio is high. The nucleus is attempting to lobate. Chromatin is smudged. The pink granular cytoplasm forms small projections from the cell that are similar in appearance to the giant platelet above it. Circulating micromegakaryocytes are abnormal in adults but they are a normal finding in cord blood. For CAP proficiency testing purposes, the term *megakaryocyte nucleus* refers to cells that have very little or no cytoplasm. This cell has too much cytoplasm for that designation. (See page 196 for a discussion of megakaryocyte nuclei).

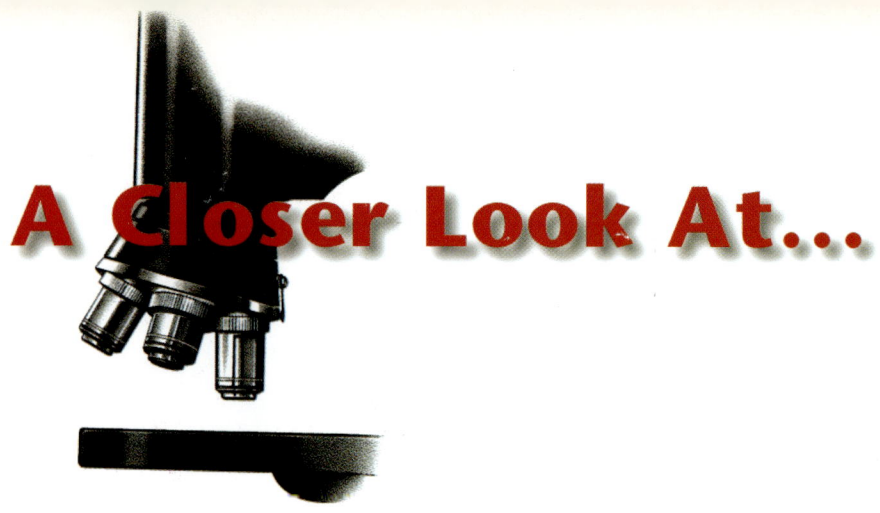

A Closer Look At...

Dysplastic Megakaryocytes

Normal megakaryocytes display considerable pleomorphism which may seem to render the term "abnormal" moot at times. Nevertheless, there are distinctive morphologic changes that are indicative of dysplasia. The illustrations below and to the right highlight some of these features.

Unusual cell changes in shape, size, and nuclear configuration are seen in the montage on the next page. Dysplastic megakaryocytes may be abnormally large or abnormally small. The nucleus may be hypo- or hyperlobated.

Tri-polar nuclei giving a pawn-ball appearance are uncommon but clear markers of dysplasia. Likewise, nuclei with two distinct and separated lobes (so called *Marty Feldman cells*, named after the comedian with prominent bulging eyes) are also indicators of myelodysplasia.

The schematic below emphasizes that nuclear shape and cell size are not the only factors indicative of dysplasia. Nuclear chromatin in dysplastic megakaryocytes typically demonstrates abnormal clumping. Sometimes this takes the form of large clumps that exhibit periodicity reminiscent of the markings on the back of a turtle. A large dark swath of clumped chromatin is also abnormal.

Although leukemic megakaryoblasts are abnormal, for the purposes of CAP proficiency testing the master list item *abnormal megakaryocyte* refers to more mature cells, rather than blasts.

Schematic of Micromegakaryocyte Nuclei

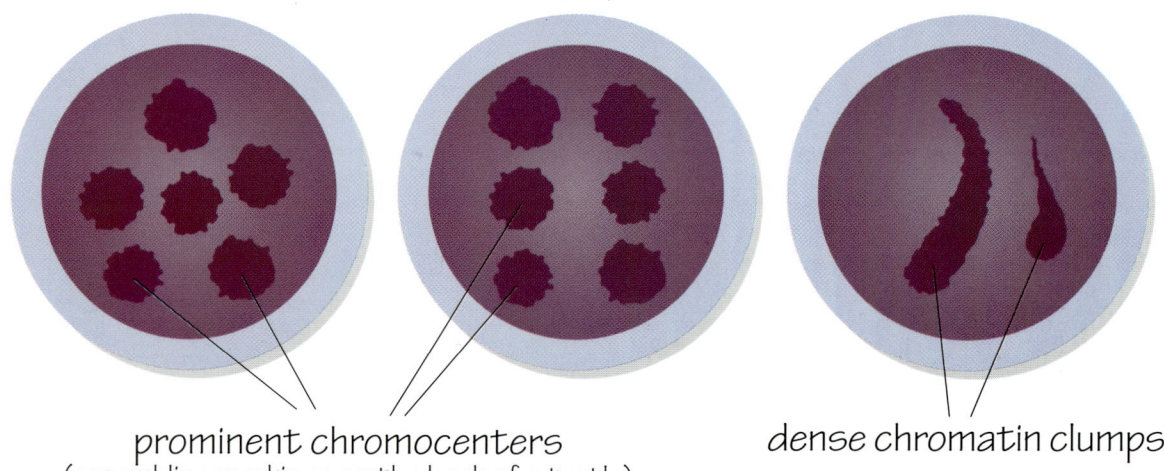

prominent chromocenters
(resembling markings on the back of a turtle)

dense chromatin clumps

Dysplastic Megakaryocytes

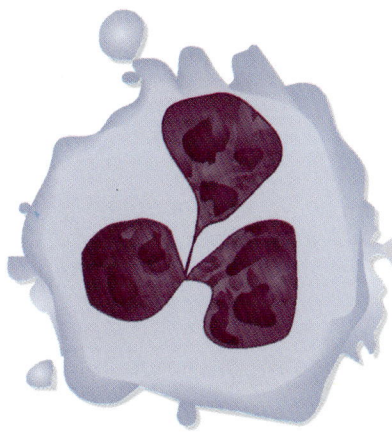

Abnormal Nuclear Shape
(Pawnball)

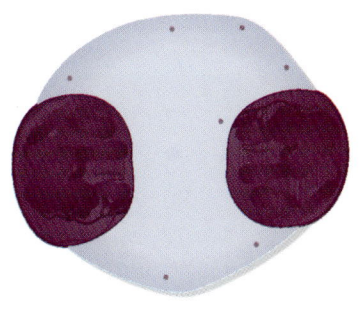

Abnormal Nuclear Shape
("Marty Feldman Cell")

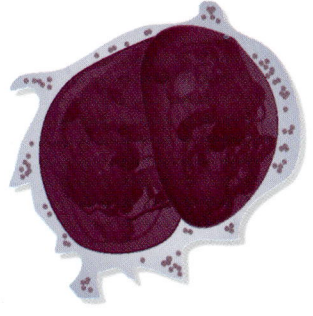

Micromegakaryocyte

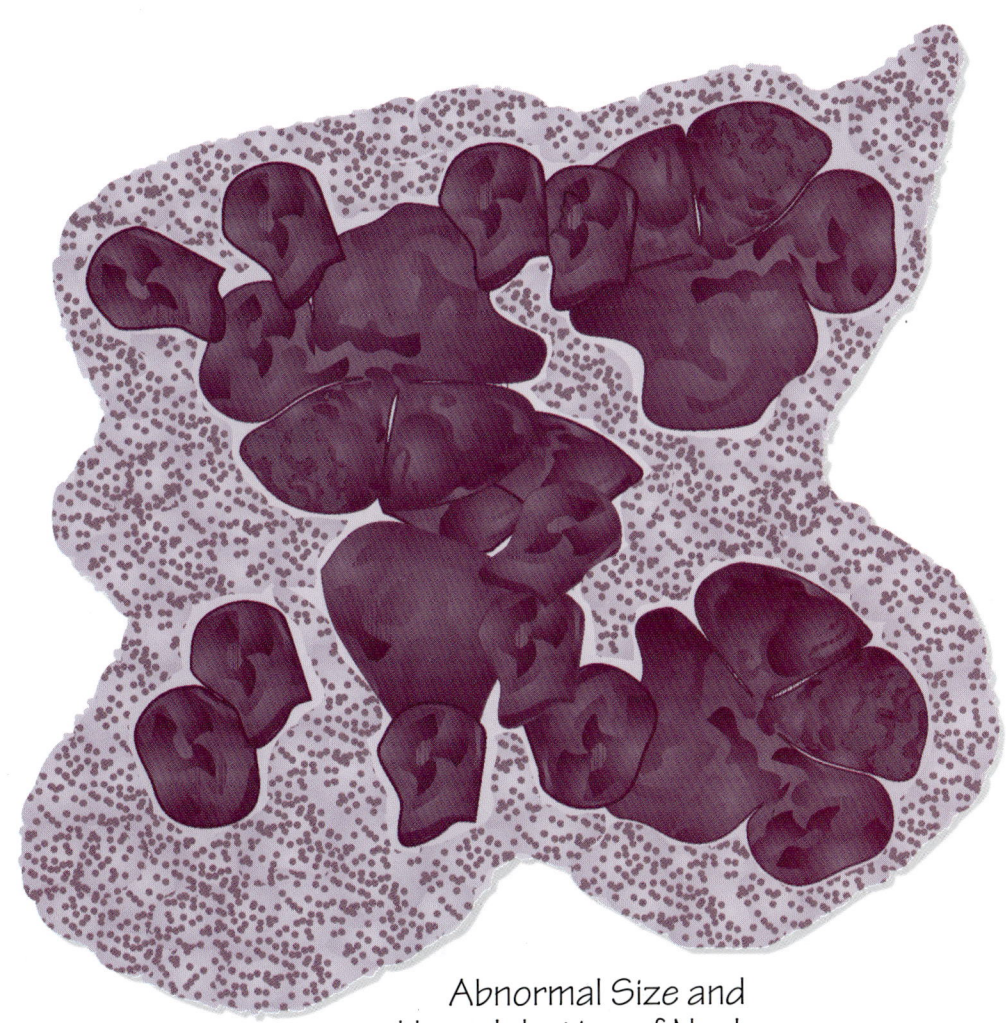

Abnormal Size and
Hyperlobation of Nucleus

Megakaryocyte Nucleus

SYNONYMS
megakaryocyte fragment

VITAL STATISTICS
- size .... highly variable; generally 15 to 30 μm
- N:C ratio .... very high
- cell shape .... irregular or round, depending on contour of cytoplasmic remnants
- nuclear shape .... round or oval; may be binucleate or bilobed
- chromatin .... deep purple; variably smudged, "puddled" or in discreet clumps
- nucleoli .... absent
- cytoplasm .... basophilic, dappled pink, or peppered blue-pink; forms a thin rim around nucleus; may show characteristic pseudopods or ear-like cytoplasmic projections

KEY DIFFERENTIATING FEATURES
nuclear morphology (smudged or "puddled" chromatin)
thin rim of cytoplasm with projections
cytoplasm may have staining characteristics of platelets

POTENTIAL LOOK-ALIKES
micromegakaryocyte
micromyeloblast
lymphocyte
granulocytic precursors
smudge cell or necrobiotic nucleus
plasma cell
monocyte and precursors
macrophage

ASSOCIATED DISEASE STATES AND CONDITIONS
rarely found in normal adults
newborns
pregnancy
myeloproliferative disorders
myelodysplastic syndromes
refractory anemia and preleukemia
acute leukemia
thrombotic thrombocytopenic purpura
B_{12} and folate deficiency (pernicious anemia)
lead poisoning
Hodgkin's disease
cancer
after surgical procedures, chest injury, cardiac massage
in association with severe leukemoid reactions

Having discharged their cytoplasm to form platelets, megakaryocyte fragments may occasionally enter the circulation. This may happen normally but is accelerated in disorders associated with myelofibrosis. Marrow fibrosis scars and distorts the normal marrow: blood sinusoid exit sites and as a result, immature cells and spent megakaryocyte fragments escape into the circulation. The megkaryocyte fragments are composed of a nucleus (or rarely two nuclei) and they have little or no cytoplasm.

Although the cell size may vary considerably and some cells may be binucleated, most have quite distinctive morphology. The N:C ratio is very high. The nucleus has smudged or "puddled" chromatin and is either totally naked or surrounded by a very scant amount of basophilic cytoplasm. If cytoplasmic remnants are present, they create a wispy, frilly, or fragmented rim. There may be small cytoplasmic blebs or a few adherent platelets.

When the cytoplasm is completely missing, the cell can be recognized as a megakaryocyte by the distinctive clumped nuclear chromatin pattern that forms deep purple masses reminiscent of a turtles' back. (See

Megakaryocyte Nuclei

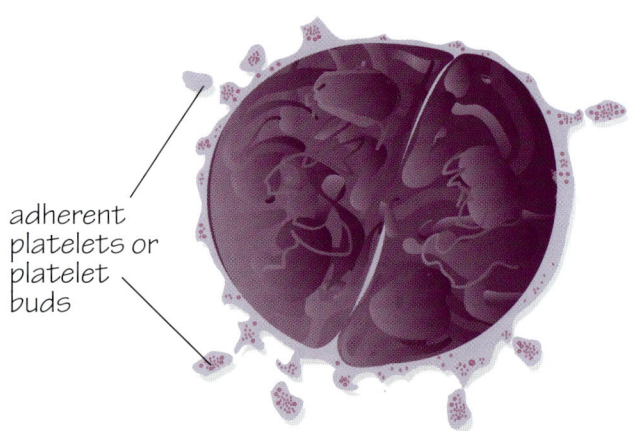

adherent platelets or platelet buds

very thin rim of cytoplasm

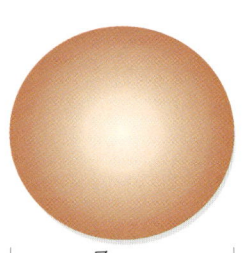

7 μm
size of normal red blood cell

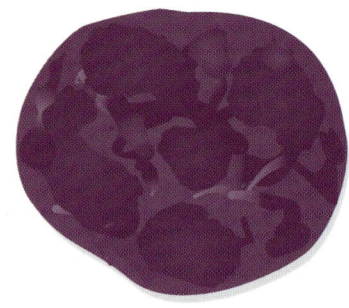

naked nucleus with "turtle-back" chromatin

A Closer Look At... Dysplastic Megakaryocytes on page 194).

If the cytoplasmic characteristics are not appreciated, megakaryocyte nuclei may be mistakenly identified as lymphocytes. Sometimes the rim of cytoplasm is only a small "fringe" and the nucleus is nondescript. Finding megakaryocyte cytoplasmic fragments and giant platelets in the field are helpful clues to the origin of the nucleus. It is important to remember that these cells are not mechanically distorted or degenerating cells; therefore the chromatin pattern does not have the characteristics of basket cells.

Pyknotic megakaryocytes in the marrow are sometimes seen in HIV infection. The naked or near-naked nuclei are composed of dark masses of chromatin. The cells reflect apoptosis (programmed cell death).

Megakaryocyte nuclei are easily confused with circulating micromegakaryocytes. Megakaryocyte nuclei have been stripped of their cytoplasm; only a few torn fragments may remain. Micromegakaryocytes are dysplastic cells that have a moderate amount of intact cytoplasm; the N:C ratio is high, but a rim of clearly delineated cytoplasm is evident.

For CAP proficiency testing purposes, megakaryocyte nuclei are almost always confined to the blood whereas micromegakaryocytes can be found either in the bone marrow or circulating. If the cells have small remnants or wisps of cytoplasm and perhaps a few attached platelets, the term *megakaryocyte nucleus* is appropriate. If the cell has more abundant, clearly defined cytoplasm, the term *abnormal megakaryocyte* (micromegakaryocyte) is preferred.

H1-30, 1988 (Blood, Wright-Giemsa, X350)

Identification	Referee %	Participant %
Megakaryocyte nucleus	95	77.3
Megakaryocyte, abnormal	-	3.5
Basket cell/smudge cell	-	7.9

The case is from a patient with chronic myelogenous leukemia. Platelet count was unusually elevated, exceeding 3 million. The red blood cells show non-specific aniso- and poikilocytosis. Platelets are generally well granulated and not overtly dysplastic. The arrowed cell is a megakaryocyte nucleus. The chromatin is clumped and "smudgy." There is a suggestion of lobation. The cytoplasm is nearly completely gone; only a few projections and whisps remain. Megakaryocyte nuclei have a very high N:C ratio. The chromatin is too clumped for the cell to be a blast and too well defined to represent a smudge cell. Also, basket/smudge cells do not have any rim of cytoplasm. The term *abnormal megakaryocyte* is best reserved for dysplastic megakaryocytes that have more than just a few wisps of cytoplasm.

HE-44, 1995 (Blood, Wright-Giemsa, X373)

Identification	Referee %	Participant %
Megakaryocyte nucleus	31.8	33.1
Blast cell	27.3	22.2
Myeloblast	-	17.5
Megkaryocyte or precursor (abnormal)	-	4.3

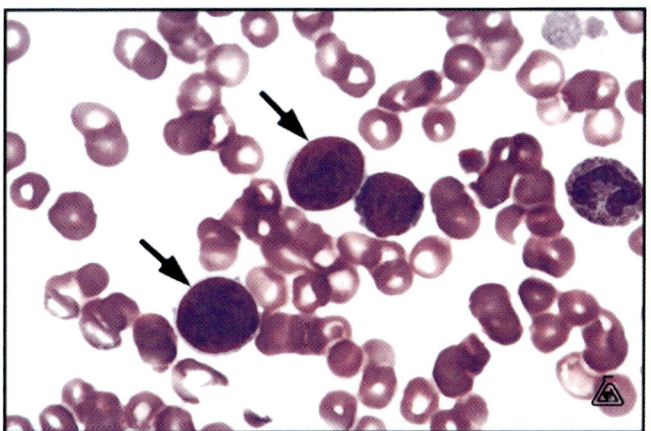

The arrowed cells are megakaryocyte nuclei. They can be recognized by their small size, dark staining clumped, or "puddled" chromatin, and scant or absent cytoplasm. Chromocenters are abnormally prominent, resembling the markings on the back of a turtle (see page 194). The upper nucleus is surrounded by buds of cytoplasm that are morphologically similar to platelets. Although these cells resemble blasts, the nuclei are too mature for them to be blasts. Also, the cytoplasm shows platelet maturation which does not occur in the blast stage. A large hypogranular platelet is also in the upper right corner of the field. A lymphocyte and band are also present.

Platelet, Normal

SYNONYMS
thrombocyte, amebocyte

VITAL STATISTICS
- size .... 1-5 µm in diameter; majority 1.5-2.5 µm in diameter (one quarter to one third the diameter of a normal red cell)
- cell shape .... wide variation; typically round, or elliptical; sometimes long or veil-like cytoplasmic extensions
- cytoplasm .... clear or slightly blue-gray containing purple or red granules; the granules are dispersed or form a central aggregate

KEY DIFFERENTIATING FEATURES
pale cytoplasm with centrally located purple-red granules
small size

POTENTIAL LOOK-ALIKES
extracellular babesia
stain precipitate
fragments of non-megakaryocytic cell cytoplasm

ASSOCIATED DISEASE STATES AND CONDITIONS
normal finding
increased in
 essential thrombocythemia
 myeloproliferative disorders
 malignancy
 acute or chronic inflammation
 anemias (acute blood loss, iron deficiency, hemolytic)
 surgery (especially splenectomy)
 drug reaction
 exercise
 premature infants
decreased in
 aplastic anemia
 marrow infiltration (malignancy, fibrosis, etc.)
 drugs and radiation
 megakaryocytic aplasia
 viral infections
 nutritional deficiencies (B_{12}, folate, or iron)
 non-immune and immune destruction (various causes)
 sequestration due to hypersplenism or hypothermia
 massive transfusion
 hereditary conditions (including Fanconi's syndrome, thrombocytopenia with absent radii, Bernard-Soulier syndrome, gray platelet syndrome, May-Hegglin anomaly, Alport syndrome variants, and Wiskott-Aldrich syndrome)

Platelets are small round or oval blue-gray fragments of megakaryocyte cytoplasm. They are typically 1.5 to 3 µm in diameter. Platelets are usually single but may form aggregates. Platelets larger than 7 µm (larger than a normal red blood cell) are termed *giant platelets*. Abnormally small platelets are seen in Wiskott-Aldrich syndrome.

The cell shape is variable but most platelets are round or elliptical. They may also be comma shaped, cigar shaped, or appear as stars with three or more points. Some have long cytoplasmic extensions or irregular ruffled margins. Shape and size variation increases when platelet production is accelerated. If too large a drop of blood is used when preparing smears, platelets may be artifactually dark due to excessive shrinkage during the prolonged drying period.

Normal platelets contain at least some azurophilic granules. The granules are dispersed or more frequently either form a crown around a central clear area or are tightly packed in the center of the platelet, giving the appearance of a nucleus.

Platelet granules are of three types. *Delta (dense) granules* contain seratonin, ADP, and calcium. *Alpha granules* contain platelet factor 4, platelet-derived growth factor, fibrinogen, and other clotting factors. Lysozomes are the third type of granule. When the platelet is activated, the contents of alpha and delta granules are released; this is important in the control of bleeding. Besides their key role in coagulation, platelets are also involved in inflammatory reactions.

The concentration of platelets can be estimated by scanning the smear. If the platelet count is normal, you should see 8 to 15 platelets per each 100x oil-immersion field or about one platelet for every 10 to 20 RBCs. The screened box to the left details the clinical conditions associated with increased and decreased counts.

Most platelets circulate for 7-10 days and then are removed by the spleen. See *A Closer Look At... Platelet Formation* for a more complete discussion of the life cycle (page 200).

Normal Platelets

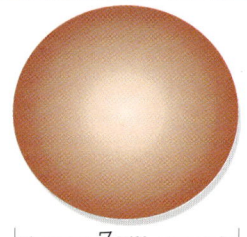

|←— 7 µm —→|
size of normal red blood cell

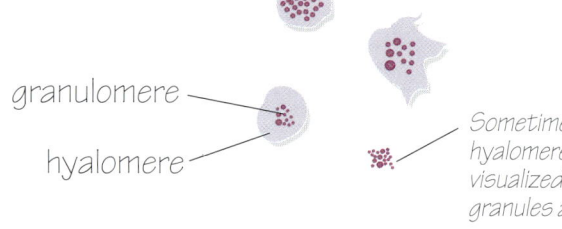

H-41, 1982 (Blood, Wright-Giemsa, X360)

Identification	Referee %	Participant %
Platelet, normal	100	92.3
Platelet, abnormal	-	5.9

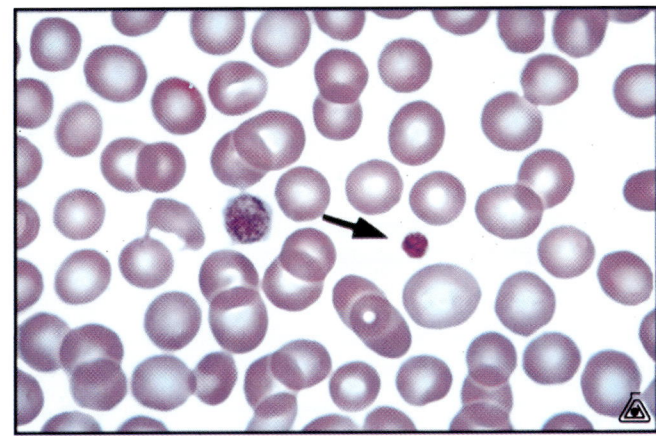

The arrowed cell is a normal platelet. The center, called the granulomere, contains azurophilic granules. It is surrounded by a blue rim devoid of granules, called the hyalomere. Normal platelets may be quite variable in size and shape, but they must be smaller than a normal red blood cell. The other platelet in the field located to the left of the arrow is a large platelet, also with unremarkable morphology. The granulomere and hyalomere are sharply demarcated. The erythrocytes are not remarkable.

HE-21, 1994 (Blood, Wright-Giemsa, X330)

Identification	Referee %	Participant %
Platelet, normal	100	94.8
Platelet, giant	-	4.7

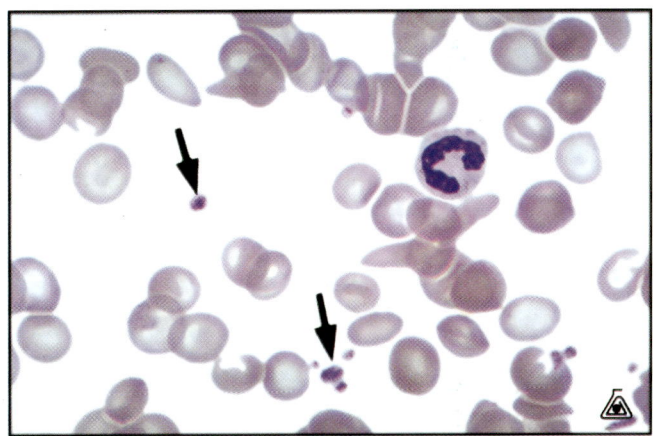

The arrowed cell is a normal platelet. It is larger than the surrounding platelets but still smaller than a normal red blood cell and thus is not a giant platelet. The centrally located granules are azurophilic and abundant. The surrounding hyalomere is barely visible. Sometimes it cannot be seen at all. The red blood cells are slightly hypochromic and microcytic. The lone leukocyte in the field is a band.

A-68, 1984 (Blood, Wright-Giemsa, X330)

Cell	Referees	Participants
Platelet, normal	94.7	94.4

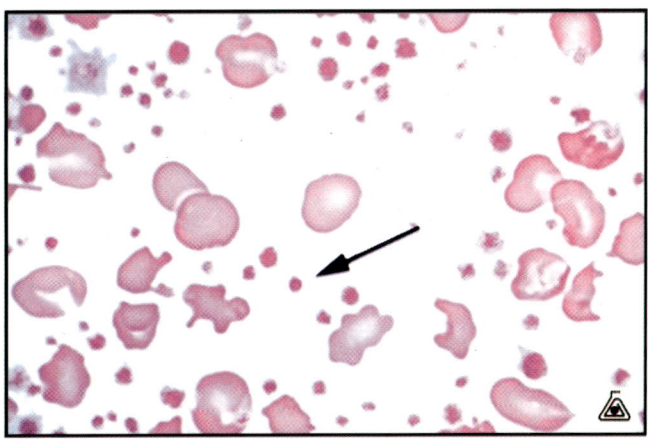

The field is dominated by platelets in this patient with marked thrombocytosis (count >1,000,000/µL). Most are small and well granulated. None are overtly dysplastic. The arrowed cell is a normal platelet. The size is about 2 µm. Azurophlic granules fill the center of the cell. Notice the morphologic variation in platelet size and shape. The large platelet in the left upper corner shows a well-demarcated hyalomere and granulomere. The red cells show moderate non-specific aniso- and poikilocytosis.

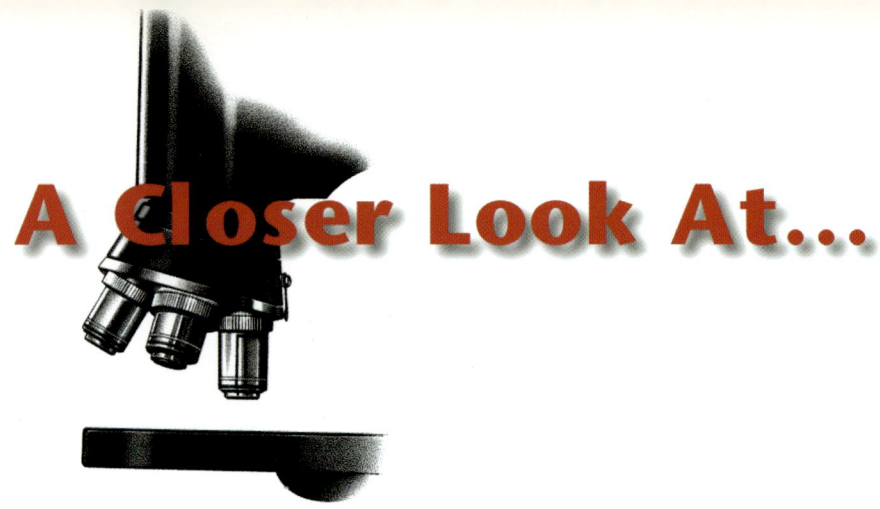

A Closer Look At...

Platelet Formation

During megakaryocyte maturation, microvesicles form in the cytoplasm, dividing the cell into subdomains that become platelet territories. Dense core granules, lysosomes, and other proteins are synthesized within the territories. Eventually, the cytoplasm resembles one large jigsaw puzzle, composed of thousands of pieces that will eventually break off and become circulating platelets.

Platelet release occurs either by rapid fragmentation of the megakaryocyte cytoplasm or by controlled release into the bone marrow sinusoids. In the later method, the megakaryocyte extends its cytoplasm through or between endothelial cells lining the sinuses. Long strands of cytoplasm dangle in the bloodstream. Each megakaryocyte produces seven to eight such tentacles called *proplatelets*. The long strands constrict at demarcation points and rupture, releasing individual platelets into the marrow sinuses. The naked megakaryocyte nucleus, now shorn of platelets, condenses and is phagocytized by bone marrow macrophages. The entire process is illustrated on the next page.

Megakaryocyte maturation and platelet production are under control of the hormone *thrombopoietin*, which is made in the liver. Other regulatory cytokines may also be involved. Each megakaryocyte makes about 4,000 platelets. About 35,000 platelets per microliter of blood are produced each day. Platelet production can increase 8 fold during times of increased demand. Normal platelet life span is 8 to 10 days.

Megakaryocyte size, DNA ploidy, and degree of maturation determine the size and number of platelets released. DNA ploidy directly correlates with the number of demarcation membranes formed. Cells with 64n nuclei are larger and release numerous small, less granulated platelets. If platelet formation is suppressed, a greater proportion of megakaryocytes are in the 4n or 8n ploidy stage; these cells release fewer platelets which are larger and denser. See *A Closer Look At...Megakaryocyte Maturation* on page 190.

Megakaryocytes are also normally found in the lung. Intact megakaryocytes escape the bone marrow and become lodged in the pulmonary microvasculature. Rapid blood flow causes the megakaryocyte cytoplasm to fragment into variably sized platelets that enter the circulation. Pulmonary sources make up about 10% of the total platelet mass.

How Platelets Form

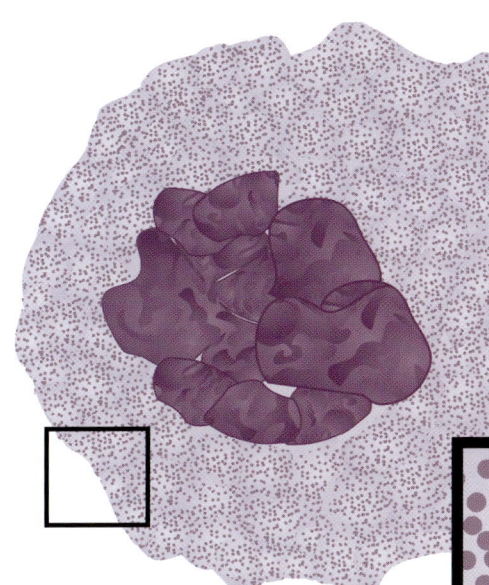

platelet-forming megakaryocyte

As the megakaryocyte matures, numerous cytoplasmic invaginations form a meshwork of tubules extending throughout the cell. These **demarcation membranes** surround territories that are destined to become platelets when the cytoplasm fragments.

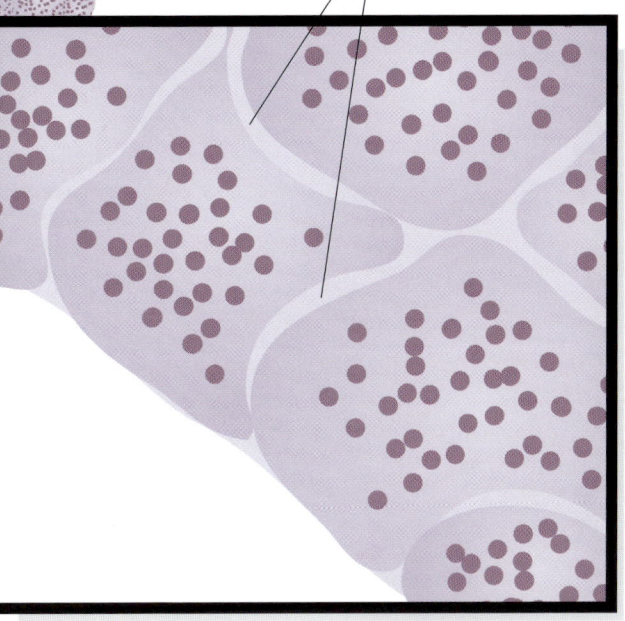

demarcation membranes separating future platelets

Some megakaryocytes quickly fragment, releasing a shower of platelets. Others have a parasinusoidal location and reel out a chain of platelets through perforations in the bone marrow sinus walls. The chains develop constrictions and rupture. The remaining condensed nucleus, devoid of cytoplasm, is phagocytized by macrophages.

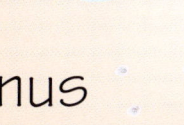

Sinus

proplatelets

parasinusoidal megakaryocyte

endothelial cell

Chains of platelets are carried away in the bloodstream. They normally break into small platelets but may persist in thrombopathies, TTP, and thrombocythemias.

Megakaryocytic Cells and Thrombocytes

Platelet, Giant

SYNONYMS
giant thrombocyte, giant amebocyte

VITAL STATISTICS
size .... 10-20 μm in diameter; larger than a normal-sized red cell
cell shape .... wide variation; periphery may be rounded, scalloped, or stellate
cytoplasm .... clear or slightly blue-gray containing purple or red granules that are dispersed or form a central aggregate; granules may fuse into giant granules

KEY DIFFERENTIATING FEATURES
size larger than normal red cell

POTENTIAL LOOK-ALIKES
large platelet (smaller than normal-size red cell)
cytoplasmic debris of non-megakaryocyte (pseudothrombocyte)
red cell with polychromasia

ASSOCIATED DISEASE STATES AND CONDITIONS
myeloproliferative disorders
myelodysplastic syndromes
preleukemia
acute leukemia
autoimmune thrombocytopenia (recovering phase of drug-induced platelet destruction)
following severe blood loss
splenectomy
severe leukemoid reactions
monoclonal gammopathies
rare inherited conditions
   May-Hegglin anomaly
   Bernard-Soulier syndrome
   "thrombopathic" thrombocytopenia
   "Montreal" platelet syndrome
   familial macrothrombocytopenia
   Mediterranean macrothrombocytopenia
   Alport's syndrome variants
     Alport's syndome
     Epstein's syndrome
     Fechtner's syndrome
   mucopolysaccharidoses
   disorders of connective tissue
     Marfan syndrome
     Ehlers-Danlos syndrome

Platelets may be quite variable in size and shape. Normal platelets are usually 1-4 μm in diameter. So called large platelets are 4 to 7 μm in diameter. Giant platelets are usually 10 to 20 μm in diameter. Because a micrometer is often not available, the term *giant platelet* is used if the size is greater than that of a normal red cell. For CAP proficiency testing purposes, if the MCV is in the normal range, you may assume that the average red cell size in the photographic field reflects that MCV. Any platelet larger than the average red cell is appropriately labeled *giant*.

The cell shape may be smooth and round or irregular with a ruffled or scalloped periphery. The cytoplasm may be agranular or contain a normal number of centrally located azurophilic granules. The granules may occasionally fuse to form giant granules.

Mechanical disruption of non-megakaryocytes can produce so-called *pseudothrombocytes*. These cytoplasmic fragments are usually basophilic and round. Most are agranular or contain a few granules that are distributed throughout the cytoplasm and not aggregated in the center. True platelets exhibit *zoning*—rings of dark and light coloration of the cytoplasm. See *Platelet, Hypogranular* discussion and illustration on page 204.

In non-stem cell disorders, large platelets are young platelets. They are increased in diseases associated with increased platelet loss or destruction with compensatory platelet production. This can be viewed as a stress-induced "shift to the left" in megakaryopoiesis in which the megakaryocytes exhibit smaller size and less nuclear lobation. The platelets produced by these cells are larger than normal. Stem cell abnormalities such as the myeloproliferative disorders and myelodysplastic syndromes often exhibit giant platelets. These are reflective of disordered megakaryopoiesis.

Giant Platelets

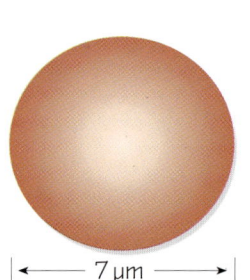
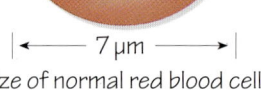
size of normal red blood cell

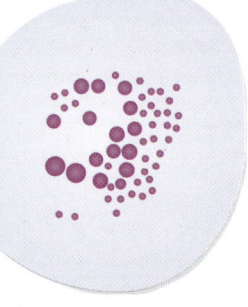

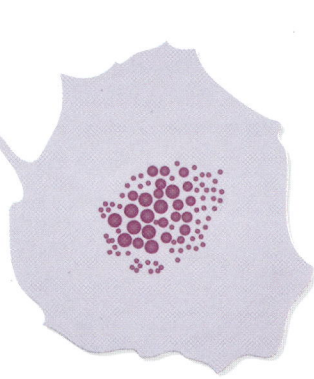

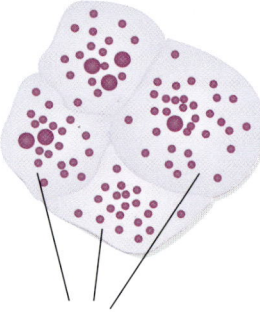
Giant platelets are typically formed from fragments of megakaryocyte cytoplasm containing multiple demarcation zones.

HE-06, 1994 (Blood, Wright-Giemsa, X400)

Identification	Referee %	Participant %
Platelet, giant	92.6	97.7
Platelet, abnormal	7.4	1

The blood film is from a patient with agnogenic myeloid metaplasia. The platelet is larger than the surrounding red blood cells. The normal central placement of the granules is present. The cell shape may be round or irregular with a ruffled or scalloped periphery. Giant platelets are one type of abnormal platelet. They are typically found in myeloproliferative and myelodysplastic states. They are reflective of disordered megakaryopoiesis. The cell in the left upper part of the field is a micromegakaryocyte. There is a small rim of granular cytoplasm which has a "frilly" boarder. The nucleus is partially lobated and has dark, clumped, and smudged chromatin. The cytoplasm is a little too abundant to refer to the cell as a megakaryocyte nucleus.

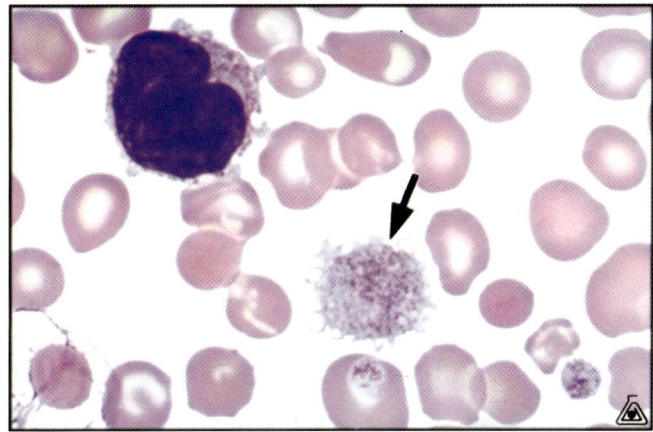

XL-71, 1987 (Blood, Wright-Giemsa, X360)

Identification	Referee %	Participant %
Platelet, giant	94.4	77.5
Basket cell, smudge cell	-	5.1
Leukocyte (various types)	5.6	5.1
Megakaryocyte	-	3.5
Platelet, abnormal	-	2.9

The large arrowed cell is a giant platelet. The central collection of azurophilic granules creates the illusion of a nucleus, but it lacks a membrane and the staining is too azurophilic for DNA. The surrounding pale blue hyalomere is free of granules. Giant platelets should not be confused with smudge cells which lack any definable granularity or structure. Cytoplasm stripped from other cells may also resemble giant platelets. These structures do not exhibit zoning, rings of dark and light coloration of the cytoplasm which are typical of platelets, even when they do not contain any granules.

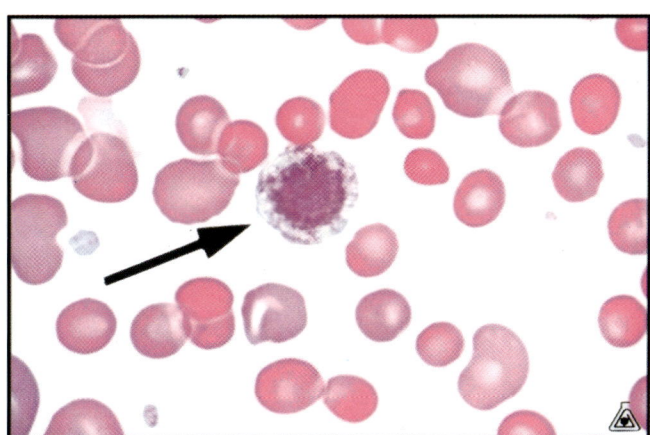

H-47, 1978 (Blood, Wright-Giemsa, X330)

Identification	Referee %	Participant %
Platelet, abnormal (giant)	87.5	80.5

This is a case of May-Hegglin anomaly. The segmented neutrophil contains a prominent Döhle body. The arrowed cell is a giant platelet. Only *normal platelet* and *abnormal platelet* were choices on the CAP proficiency testing master list in 1978, so we do not have statistics for a choice of giant platelet. Nevertheless, the cell is larger (in its long axis) than the average red cell in the field. Granules are heavily concentrated and there is little surrounding hyalomere. The other platelet in the field is large but not giant. Its granulomere and hyalomere are easily distinguished. May-Hegglin anomaly is a rare autosomal dominant disorder characterized by Döhle bodies, giant platelets, and variable thrombocytopenia. Unlike the cell photographed here, many giant platelets in this condition are poorly granulated. Premature megakaryocyte fragmentation probably accounts for the large platelet size and thrombocytopenia. See page 46 for a more complete discussion.

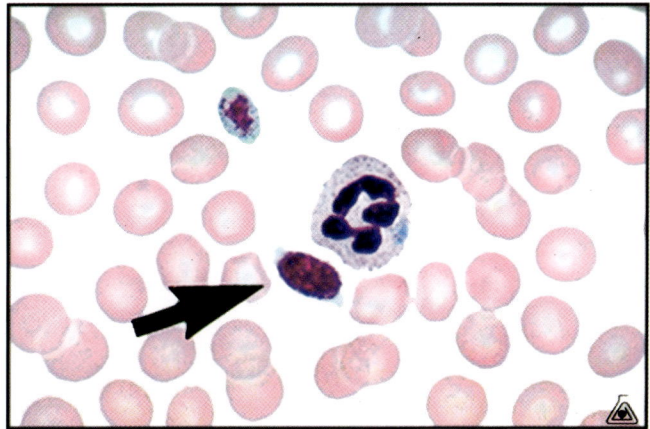

Platelet, Hypogranular

SYNONYMS
dysplastic platelet

VITAL STATISTICS
- size .... normal to giant platelet size (4 to 6 μm)
- cell shape .... round, oval or irregular; larger forms usually have small surface projections
- cytoplasm .... light gray or pale blue; absent or very faint pink-purple granularity; distinct dark and light staining zones

KEY DIFFERENTIATING FEATURES
- lack of granules
- zoning

POTENTIAL LOOK-ALIKES
- non-megakaryocyte cell fragment (pseudothrombocyte)
- parasites
- poorly stained normal well-granulated platelets (note: abnormal size, shape, and granule appearance may be an artifact of poorly collected specimens or after storage of anticoagulated blood)
- red cell with polychromasia

ASSOCIATED DISEASE STATES AND CONDITIONS
- acute leukemia
- chronic myeloproliferative disorders
- myelodysplastic syndromes
- gray platelet syndrome (alpha storage pool disease)

A hypogranular platelet is one type of abnormal platelet. As the name implies, they have reduced or absent granularity. Normal platelets are composed of a hyalomere and a granulomere. The hyalomere is the platelet cytoplasm which exhibits darker and lighter staining zones. The granulomere is composed of moderate numbers of azurophilic granules which are dispersed or centrally located. If the granules are dramatically reduced in number or absent altogether, the terms *hypogranular* and *agranular* are used respectively. Hypogranular platelets may be normal in size, shape, and configuration or they may be enlarged and misshapen. The cytoplasm stains pale blue or blue-gray.

Cytoplasmic fragments from cells other than megakaryocytes may resemble hypogranular or agranular platelets. The cytoplasm does not display the characteristic zones of the platelet hyalomere. These amorphous cytoplasmic fragments are variously known as *pseudothrombocytes*, *lymphoglandular bodies*, and *hyaline bodies*.

Morphologically abnormal platelets are usually found in association with myeloproliferative disorders (acute myelogeneous leukemia, chronic myelogenous leukemia, polychthemia rubra vera, essential thromb-

Hypogranular and Agranular Platelets

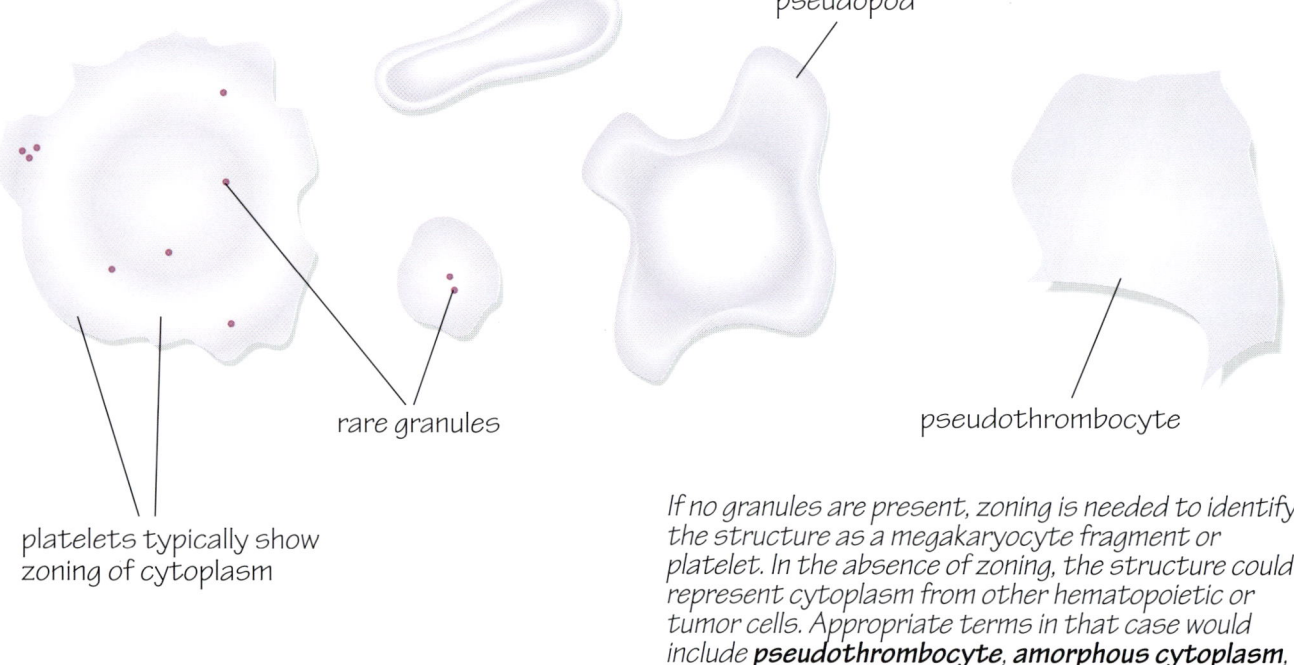

*If no granules are present, zoning is needed to identify the structure as a megakaryocyte fragment or platelet. In the absence of zoning, the structure could represent cytoplasm from other hematopoietic or tumor cells. Appropriate terms in that case would include **pseudothrombocyte**, **amorphous cytoplasm**, **hyaline body**, and **lymphoglandular body**.*

ocythemia, and agnogenic myeloid metaplasia) or myelodysplastic syndromes. Hypogranular platelets are one form of abnormal platelet morphology. Other morphologic abnormalities include irregular shape, unusual pseudopod projections, giant size, increased basophilia of cytoplasm, vacuolization of cytoplasmic membrane, abnormal aggregation of granules, and hypergranularity. Some diseases display a fairly characteristic morphology. The platelets in essential thrombocythemia, for example, are usually uniform but markedly enlarged. Extreme platelet pleomorphism is uncommon in reactive thrombocytic conditions.

Alpha storage pool disease—also known as gray platelet syndrome—is a rare autosomal trait characterized by moderate thrombocytopenia and abnormal platelets. The thrombocytes are moderately enlarged and stain gray or blue. They have a washed-out or ghost-like appearance.

HE-43, 1995 (Blood, Wright-Giemsa, X400)

Identification	Referee %	Participant %
Platelet, hypogranular	62.5	23.3
Platelet, giant	29.2	66.9
Platelet, normal	8.3	8.6

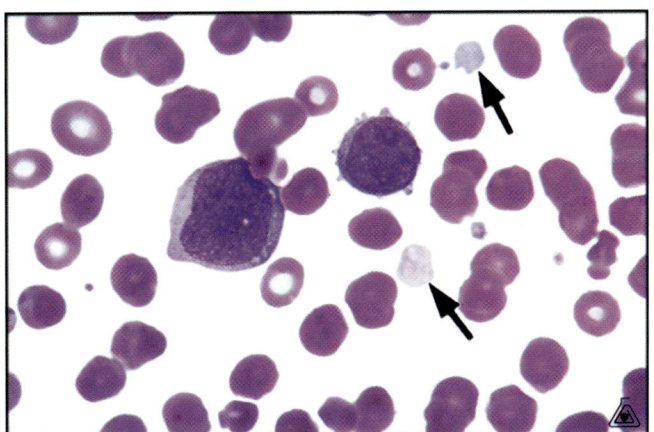

The case is from a patient with chronic myelogenous leukemia in blast crisis. The two leukocytes are blasts. One has small cytoplasmic blebs, raising the possibility that the cell is a megakaryoblast. The arrowed objects are large hypogranular platelets. This is a form of atypia. Smaller, granulated platelets are also in the field and they can be compared to the arrowed dysplastic forms. Hypogranular platelets have just a few granules, while agranular platelets lack any granularity at all. They may be mistaken for cytoplasmic fragments from non-megakaryocytes. Platelets are recognized by the presence of *zoning*—concentric light and dark regions of the cytoplasm which are not seen in other cell types. The two arrowed cells are not giant platelets because they are not as large as the surrounding red cells.

Platelet Satellitism

SYNONYMS
platelet rosette, platelet satellitosis

VITAL STATISTICS
size .... variable, depending on the number of platelets attached to the leukocyte
cell shape .... the central leukocyte (usually a neutrophil but may be a monocyte) is round or slightly irregular; the surrounding platelets are single or form small clumps which may impart an irregular shape

KEY DIFFERENTIATING FEATURES
adherence of 4 or more platelets to the surface of a segmented neutrophil, band or monocyte
morphology of leukocyte and platelet is normal
may produce false thrombocytopenia with automated cell counters
in vitro phenomenon requiring EDTA-anticoagulated blood

POTENTIAL LOOK-ALIKES
circulating megakaryocyte
macrophage

ASSOCIATED DISEASE STATES AND CONDITIONS
not associated with any specific disease, but more readily found in the following conditions (according to some authors):
 ill, hospitalized patients
 autoimmune disorders
 pregnancy
 Behçet's disease

Platelet satellitosis, also known as *platelet rosettes,* is a rare peripheral blood finding that was first reported by Field in 1963. Kjeldsberg was the first to point out that it may be a cause of thrombocytopenia. The phenomenon is transient and not related to any medication, clinical disease, or other hematologic finding.

Patients reported in the literature have ranged in age from 14 to 85 years of age. Although some patients may be totally asymptomatic, platelet satellitosis has been reported in a variety of clinical conditions including Behçet's disease. It appears to be associated with a high incidence of thromboembolism. The amount of satellitosis has no association with the severity of clinical disease.

The spurious low platelet count is due to the clumping and adherence of platelets to neutrophils. These large masses are counted as white cells. The photomicrographs illustrate this phenomenon well. Segmented neutrophils and bands are almost exclusively involved. There may be a small amount of platelet phagocytosis. Rare monocytes may demonstrate a few peripheral or phagocytized platelets but other white cells—lymphocytes, eosinophils, basophils, myelocytes, and metamyelocytes—are not involved. The platelets and neutrophils are normal in morphology and function. Platelet satellitosis may be found in conjunction with other causes of true thrombocytopenia. It is not an artifact of staining and occurs in wet unstained preparation as well.

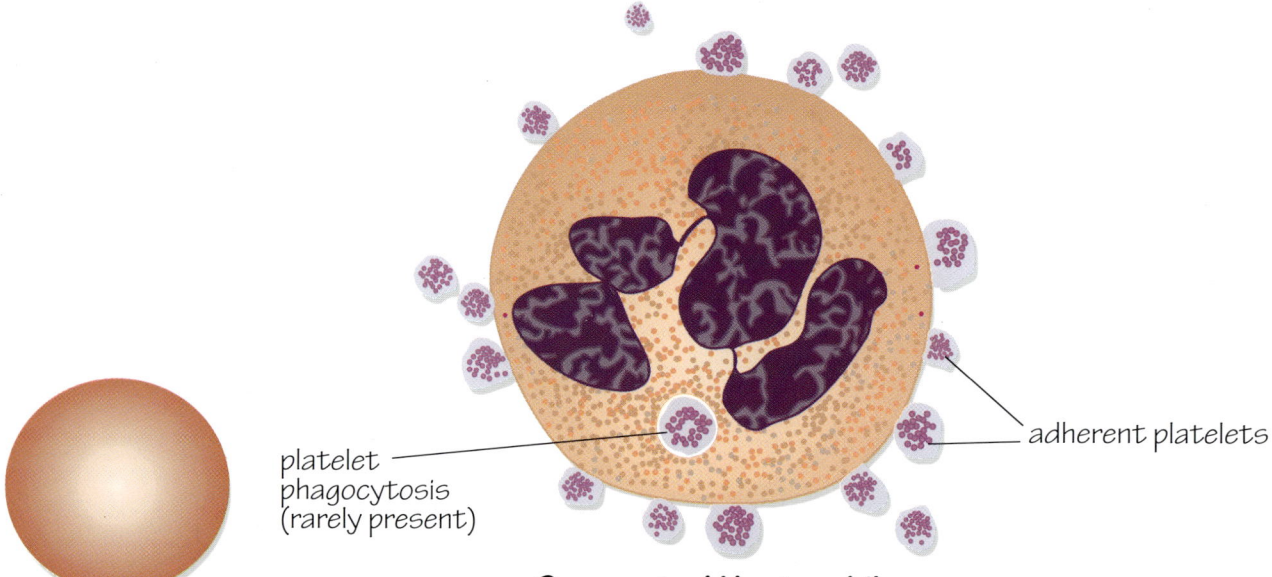

HE-26, 1993 (Blood, Wright-Giemsa, X370)

Identification	Referee %	Participant %
Platelet satellitism	100	96.6

The peripheral blood phenomenon illustrated here is *platelet satellitism*. All the leukocytes are segmented neutrophils. They are surrounded by platelet wreaths. The platelets themselves exhibit normal size and granularity. Platelets may adhere to neutrophils or rarely monocytes in the presence of EDTA. This may result in spurious thrombocytopenia. In this patient, the automated platelet count was 163,000/μl and the true count 275,000/μl. Pseudothrombocytopenia may be much more marked in some patients. If not recognized on the peripheral blood smear, it may result in undue diagnostic testing, cancellation of surgery, or even unnecessary surgery (splenectomy). See HE-22, 1993 on page 91 and HE-25, 1993 on page 287 for other examples of platelet satellitism.

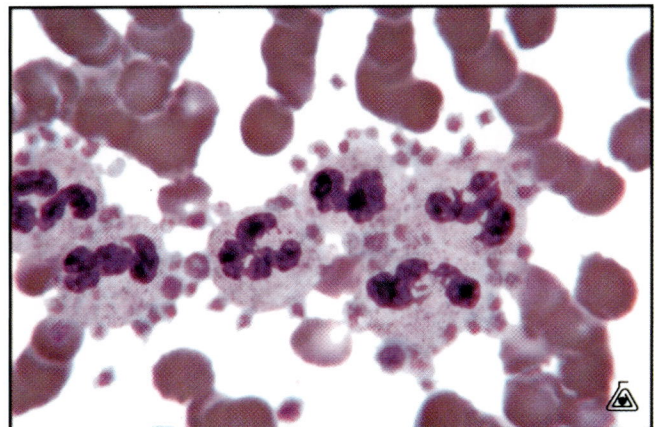

Platelet Satellitism

Band Neutrophil

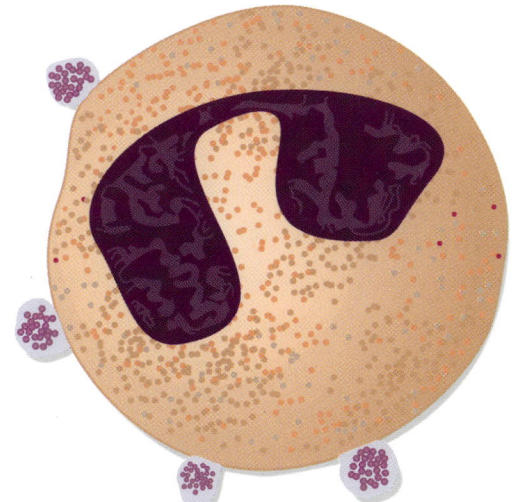

bands and segmented neutrophils are almost exclusively involved in the phenomenon

diagnosis requires 4 or more adherent platelets

Monocyte

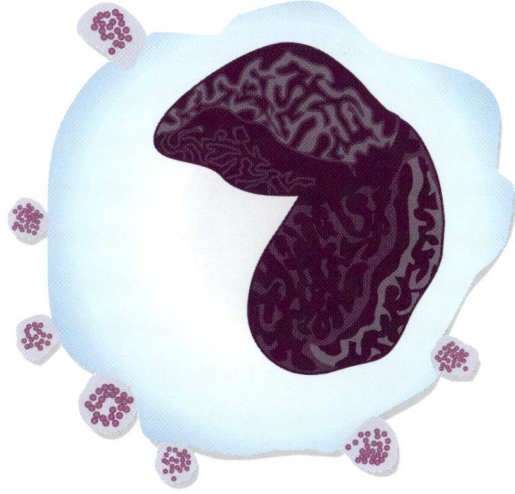

very rarely, monocytes may show platelet satellitosis

Megakaryocytic Cells and Thrombocytes

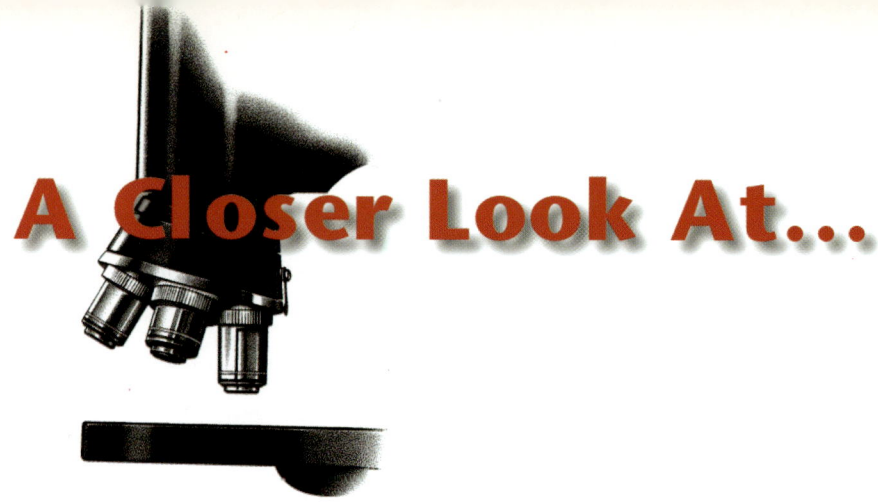

A Closer Look At...

Platelet Satellitism

The illustration on the facing page diagrams the test tube interactions that result in platelet satellitosis. The phenomenon is important because it is a cause of pseudo-thrombocytopenia. Finding a low platelet count should initiate a peripheral smear review for clumps or satellitosis.

Platelet satellitism is found almost exclusively in peripheral blood collected in EDTA. EDTA (ethylene diaminetetracetic acid) is a heavy metal chelator. It is used instead of oxalate or other anticoagulants in automated instruments because EDTA has a greater ability to prevent platelet clumping (another cause of pseudothrombocytopenia). A small amount of satellitosis has been observed, however, with other anticoagulants and in non-anticoagulated blood.

Satellitosis occurs best at room temperature and is time dependent, maximizing at 60 minutes. Only a small amount of satellitosis is found in blood incubated at 37°C. EDTA alters the conformation of the GPIIb/IIIa complex on the surface of the platelet. This facilitates IgG antibody attachment. The coated platelets then non-specifically attach to the surface of the leukocytes.

Platelet Satellitism

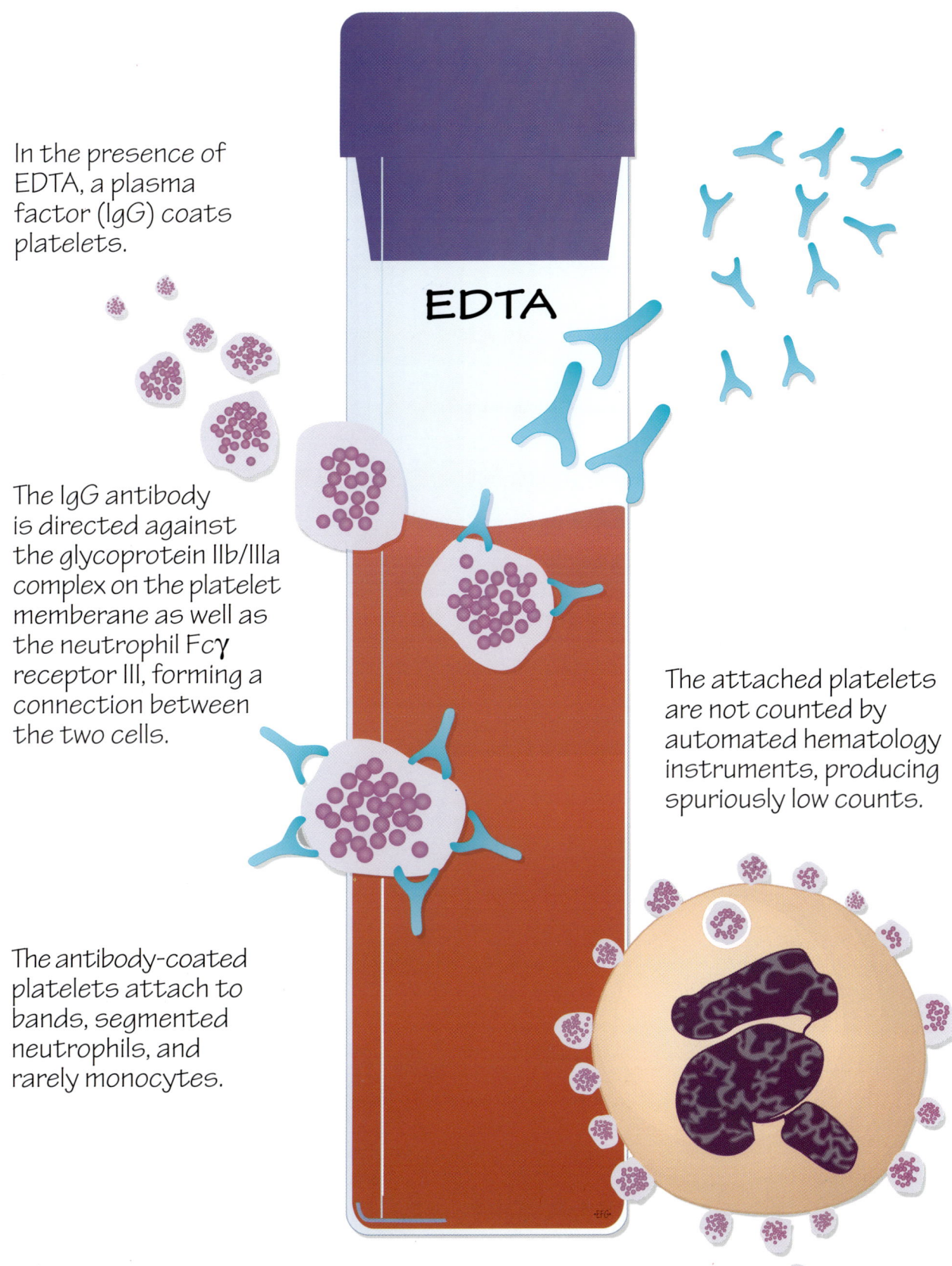

In the presence of EDTA, a plasma factor (IgG) coats platelets.

The IgG antibody is directed against the glycoprotein IIb/IIIa complex on the platelet memberane as well as the neutrophil Fcγ receptor III, forming a connection between the two cells.

The attached platelets are not counted by automated hematology instruments, producing spuriously low counts.

The antibody-coated platelets attach to bands, segmented neutrophils, and rarely monocytes.

Lymphocytic and Plasmacytic Cells

Introduction 211
Hairy Cell 212
   *A Closer Look At…*Hairy Cell Leukemia 214
Lymphoblast 216
Lymphocyte, Mature 218
   *A Closer Look At…*Normal vs. Reactive Lymphocytes 220
Lymphocyte, Reactive 222
   *A Closer Look At…*Reactive vs. Neoplastic Lymphocytes 226
Lymphoma Cell 228
   *A Closer Look At…*Normal Lymphocyte Maturation and Malignant Transformation 230
   *A Closer Look At…*B Cell Neoplasms 232
   *A Closer Look At…*T Cell and Putative NK Cell Neoplasms 236
Plasma Cell, Mature 238
   *A Closer Look At…*Plasma Cell Maturation 240
Plasma Cell, Immature or Abnormal (Myeloma Cell) 242
Plasma Cell or Precursor with Inclusion Body 244
Prolymphocyte 246
   *A Closer Look At…*Prolymphocytes 248
Sézary Cell 250

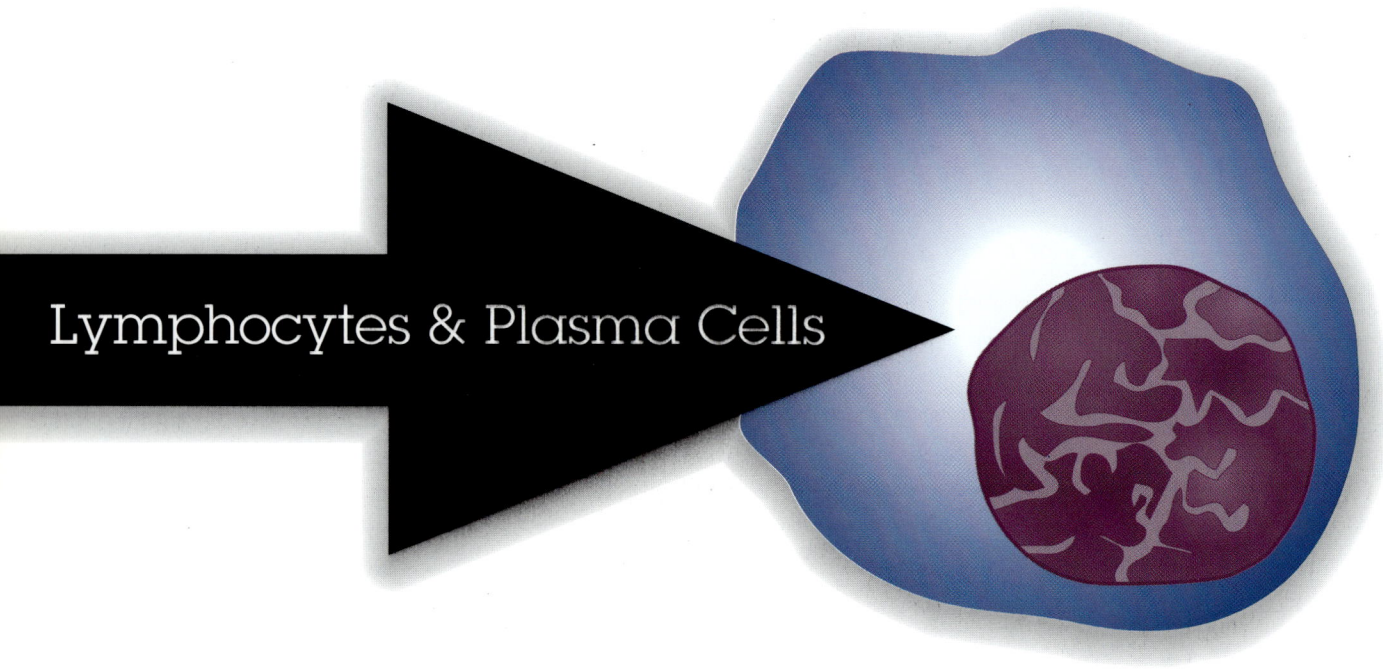

Introduction

Lymphoid cells are involved in many immunologic reactions such as the recognition of self from non-self, generation of antibody responses to infectious organisms, and are responsible for the development of immunity. Most lymphoid cells are found within the lymphatic system, which is made up of lymph nodes, spleen, lymphatic ducts, thymus, and bone marrow. These cells circulate in the blood, comprising one third to one half of all white blood cells. Infants and children have higher numbers of circulating lymphocytes which decrease to adult levels by adolescence.

The major types of lymphoid cells are T, B, natural killer (NK), and null cells. These cells can be identified by the presence of characteristic proteins and receptors on their cell surface using methods such as flow cytometry. The majority of circulating lymphocytes are T cells, which are mainly composed of CD4 cells (helper/inducer) and CD8 cells (suppressor/cytotoxic). B cells and NK cells make up most of the remaining blood lymphocytes with a small number of null cells.

T cells mature in the fetal thymus in response to the hormone thymosin, which is released by the epithelial cells of this organ. Here, they differentiate (mature) and acquire the ability to perform their various immunologic functions. As these cells differentiate, they change the types of cell surface receptors and proteins. The stage of development can be identified by using flow cytometry to characterize these surface markers.

Once T cells leave the thymus, they circulate in the blood and migrate in and out of various lymphoid tissues. When these cells encounter a foreign antigen, such as a protein from the cell wall of a bacteria, they increase in size and divide. These large transformed lymphoid cells correspond to the atypical or reactive lymphocytes seen in various infections such as infectious mononucleosis (Epstein-Barr virus infection). T cells can recognize antigens using a family of molecules called T cell receptors. These receptors resemble immunoglobulins found on B cells.

The specific actions of an activated T cell depend on how it was "programmed" in the thymus. Cytotoxic T cells can directly kill facultative intracellular organisms by killing the cells in which these organisms are living. T cells also generate substances called lymphokines that act on other cells. The lymphokine gamma interferon can activate macrophages and enable them to kill various organisms. Interleukin 2 (IL-2), another lymphokine, aids the growth and maturation of B cells. It is released by helper T cells. Suppressor T cells help control the production of antibodies so that uncontrolled or inappropriate antibody responses are prevented. T cells are also able to recognize two classes of histocompatibility antigens allowing differentiation of self from non-self.

B cells are conditioned and differentiate in the bone marrow of mammals and in the bursa of Fabricius in birds. These cells also acquire and lose various cell surface proteins and receptors as they differentiate. Flow cytometry is useful for identifying the stage of maturation of B cells, since morphologically B and T cells are indistinguishable. Mature B cells circulate in the blood and lymphatics, but most are found in the germinal centers of lymph nodes and in the white pulp of the spleen. The most mature form of a B cell is the plasma cell, which can secrete immunoglobulins.

Once a mature B cell encounters an antigen or is stimulated by IL-2, it proliferates and differentiates into a plasma cell. Some agents can directly induce B cells to differentiate. Other agents need to have the cooperation of T cells and macrophages. The first type of immunoglobulin made by B cells is IgM. The production of these antibodies are usually short lived and soon followed by production of other immunoglobulins such as IgD, IgG, IgA, or IgE. Each plasma cell can make only one type of immunoglobulin.

Natural Killer (NK) lymphocytes have the ability to kill various abnormal cells such as those damaged by trauma, aging, viruses, and possibly cancer cells. NK cells do not need to be stimulated or "primed" by previous recognition of the cell, antibodies, or lymphokines. These cells are stimulated by interferon. NK lymphocytes exhibit a characteristic pattern of cell surface markers and can be identified by flow cytometry.

Null cells are very immature lymphocytes which have not differentiated into T or B cells. Some may even be stem cells which have the potential to divide and differentiate into various types of mature lymphocytes.

Hairy Cell

SYNONYMS
leukemic reticuloendotheliosis

VITAL STATISTICS
- size .... 12 to 20 μm
- N:C ratio .... 4:1 to 2:1
- cell shape .... round or ovoid
- nuclear shape .... ovoid to indented to "kidney bean" shaped; may be folded or dumbbell-shaped; usually central, can be eccentric
- chromatin .... homogeneous, fine to slightly coarse; parachromatin is scant and evenly dispersed
- nucleoli .... one or more, small; rarely single and prominent
- cytoplasm .... moderate to abundant; pale blue to gray-blue and agranular; fine (hairy), irregular, filamentous projections; the projections can be thick, blunted, smudged, or serrated; some cases lack projections and have a smooth cytoplasmic border; occasional cells may contain a few, fine, azurophilic granules; small vacuoles may be present

KEY DIFFERENTIATING FEATURES
- medium to larger lymphoid cells with oval to indented nuclei, fine chromatin, moderate amount of cytoplasm, and fine, filamentous projections
- positive staining with tartrate resistant acid phosphatase (TRAP)

OTHER FINDINGS
- commonly associated with massive splenomegaly and pancytopenia (including monocytopenia)
- some cases may have lymphocytosis, rarely greater than 25 X 10^9/L
- bone marrow aspiration often results in a "dry tap" due to reticulin fibrosis

POTENTIAL LOOK-ALIKES
- reactive lymphocytes
- prolymphocytes
- lymphoma cells
- Sézary cells
- monocytes
- immature monocytes (promonocytes)

ASSOCIATED DISEASE STATES AND CONDITIONS
- hairy cell leukemia

Hairy cell leukemia is a chronic lymphoproliferative disease of B cell origin. It occurs most commonly in middle-aged to elderly males. Classic hairy cells are round to ovoid lymphoid cells that measure 12-20 μm and are larger than normal, mature lymphocytes. The N:C ratio ranges from 4:1 to 2:1 and they contain moderate to abundant pale blue to grayish blue cytoplasm. The cell borders are often indistinct secondary to the presence of characteristic elongated, fine (hairy), cytoplasmic projections. These projections are frequently irregular and may be thick, blunted, smudged, serrated, or short. Occasional cases lack these projections and have a smooth cytoplasmic border. The majority of cells lack granules; however, occasional fine azurophilic granules may be seen in some cases. Small vacuoles can be present and often give a mottled appearance to the cytoplasm.

The nuclei of hairy cells are usually oval to indented. They can be folded, bean-shaped, angulated, or dumbbell-shaped and are either centrally or eccentrically located. The chromatin is finer than in normal lymphocytes or chronic lymphocytic leukemia cells. It is evenly distributed with intervening parachromatin and may be slightly to moderately coarse. A small single nucleolus is often visible. Some cells have multiple small nucleoli or a single larger nucleolus.

Hairy Cells

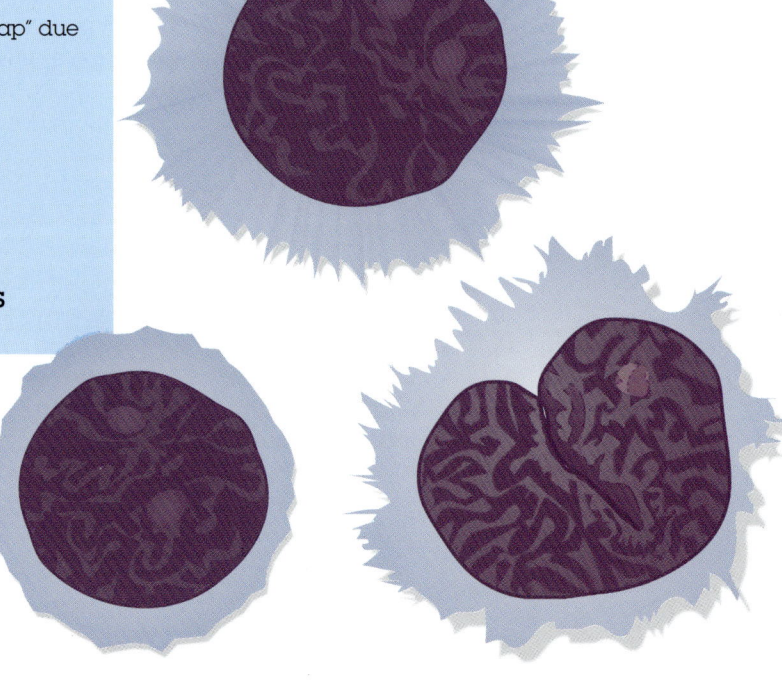

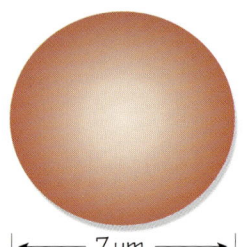

|← 7 μm →|
size of normal red blood cell

H-26, 1980 (Blood, Wright-Giemsa, X400)

Identification	Referee %	Participant %
Hairy cell	100	86.5
Lymphocyte, normal	-	3.6

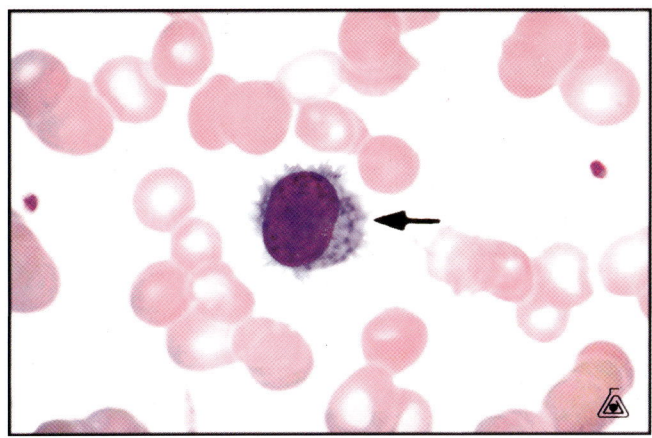

The red blood cells are normochromic and normocytic with slight clumping that resembles rouleaux formation. This effect is probably secondary to the photomicrograph being taken in a thick area of the blood film. Two normal appearing platelets are present. Dirt and/or stain precipitate is also seen. The arrowed cell is a hairy cell. It is slightly larger than a normal lymphocyte and has an oval nucleus with moderately coarse chromatin and visible parachromatin. A definite nucleolus is not seen. The cytoplasm is blue/gray with indistinct borders and fine, barely visible, projections.

H1-42, 1984 (Blood, Wright-Giemsa, X400)

Identification	Referee %	Participant %
Hairy cell	100	80.7
Lymphocyte, reactive	-	9.5

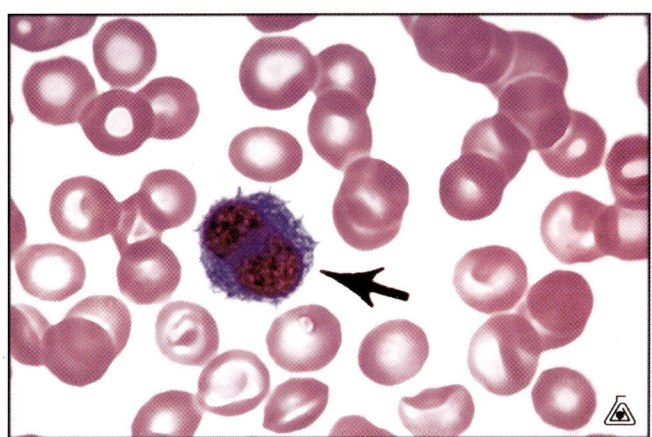

This photomicrograph is from a 68-year-old white male who presented with an elevated white count and thrombocytopenia. The single arrowed cell is a hairy cell. It is slightly larger than a normal mature lymphocyte. The nucleus is ovoid and indented giving it a bean-shaped appearance. The chromatin is moderately coarse and a nucleolus is not visible. There is a moderate amount of blue/gray cytoplasm with indistinct borders showing a few fine projections. The red blood cells are normocytic with scattered target cells and stomatocytes. No platelets are present.

H1-44, 1984 (Blood, Wright-Giemsa, X400)

Identification	Referee %	Participant %
Hairy cell	100	83.6
Lymphocyte, reactive	-	7.0

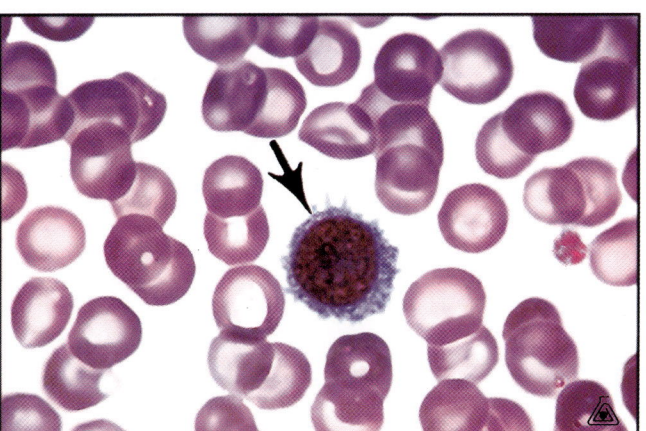

This blood film shows another hairy cell from the same case as slide H1-42, 1984. A single normal platelet is present. The red blood cells are normocytic with a few target cells. The arrowed cell is larger than a normal lymphocyte with a round nucleus containing moderately coarse chromatin. No nucleoli are visible. The moderate amount of blue/gray cytoplasm has irregular margins and fine projections.

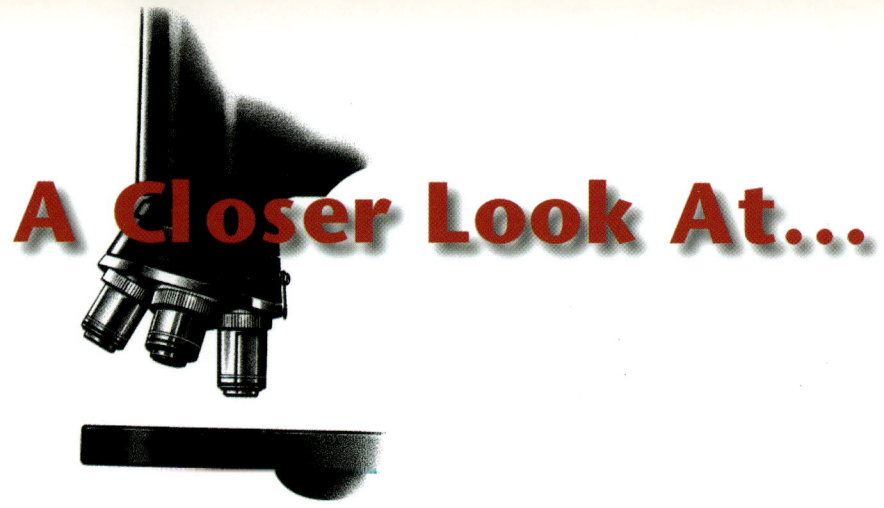

Hairy Cell Leukemia

Hairy cell leukemia accounts for about 2-5% of all cases of leukemia and is a chronic lymphoproliferative disorder. It occurs more commonly in males (3-5 times more frequently than females). The median age at diagnosis is 52 and about half the cases occur between 40 and 60 years of age. Splenomegaly, often massive, is present in over 50% of patients and is associated with variable degrees of pancytopenia (anemia, neutropenia, monocytopenia, and thrombocytopenia). The majority of patients have normal or low absolute lymphocyte counts with hairy cells comprising from 5-50% of leukocytes. Some cases exhibit lymphocytosis that rarely exceeds 25×10^9/L and is predominantly composed of hairy cells.

The malignant cells infiltrate the spleen, bone marrow, and liver. Lymph node involvement is less common. Bone marrow involvement is associated with an increase in reticulin fibrosis that often results in unsuccessful attempts at bone marrow aspiration (dry tap).

Hairy cells show positive staining for acid phosphatase that is resistant to preincubation with tartrate (so called tartrate resistant acid phosphatase stain or *TRAP*). Most hairy cells show a diffuse or finely granular staining pattern. Other neoplastic lymphoid cells may be TRAP positive, but the pattern is focal.

Flow cytometry reveals a characteristic mature B cell phenotype and a monoclonal staining pattern for surface immunoglobulin light chain. Dual positive staining for both CD22 (mature B cell antigen) and CD11c (a membrane adhesion molecule) is an important diagnostic finding. Hairy cells also show positive staining for CD25 (IL-2 receptor) and CD103 (α E integrin).

Various types of lymphoid cells may be confused with hairy cells. Generally, these cells lack the characteristic cytoplasmic projections seen on hairy cells and the clinical situation differs. Some of the lymphoid cell types that must be distinguished from hairy cells are reactive lymphocytes, lymphoma cells (such as splenic marginal zone lymphoma), prolymphocytes, large granular lymphocytes, and Sézary cells. Occasionally, hairy cells can be confused with monocytes and immature monocytes (promonocytes). These cells are slightly larger, contain more abundant cytoplasm, frequent vacuoles, fine azurophilic granules, and often exhibit more irregular nuclear shapes. Comparison with other cells seen in the blood film, correlation with the clinical history, and confirmation with special stains or flow cytometry may be necessary to arrive at the correct diagnosis. The table on the right highlights the key findings used to differentiate various lymphocytic leukemias. It is important to recognize hairy cell leukemia because these patients have a good prognosis when treated with newer chemotherapeutic regimens.

Comparison of Lymphocytes Resembling Hairy Cells

	Leukocyte Count	Morphology	TRAP Stain	Immunophenotype
Hairy Cell Leukemia	low; often pancytopenia	>2 RBCs in size; round or dumbell-shaped nuclei with spongy chromatin; small nucleoli; pale cytoplasm with numerous projections	strong diffuse staining in most cells	positive: CD19, CD20, CD22, CD11c, CD25, CD103, FMC7 variable: CD23 negative: CD5
Prolymphocytic Leukemia	markedly elevated (>100,000/μL)	>2 RBCs in size; round nuclei with clumped chromatin; single prominent central nucleolus; moderate basophilic cytoplasm	weak to moderate focal or granular staining in many cases	positive: CD19, CD20, CD22, CD23, FMC7 variable: CD5, CD11c, CD25 negative: CD103
Splenic Lymphoma with Villous Lymphocytes	variable; usually not markedly increased (<40,000/μL)	1-2 RBCs in size; round nuclei with clumped blocky chromatin; nucleoli indistinct; scant to moderate cytoplasm; thin short eccentric projections (villi may be concentrated at one pole or bipolar)	variable; weak to moderate focal or granular staining in some cases	positive: CD19, CD20, CD21, CD22 variable: CD11c, CD25, CD5 negative: CD23, CD103
Large Granular Lymphocytic Leukemia	mildly elevated (<20,000/μL); high counts in aggressive variants	>2 RBCs in size; round to oval nuclei with clumped chromatin; absent or small indistinct nucleoli; moderate pale cytoplasm; multiple fine or coarse azurophilc granules	variable; weak to moderate focal or granular staining in some cases	positive: CD2, CD8, CD11c, CD56, variable: CD7, CD3, CD57, CD11c, CD5 negative: CD4, CD25

TRAP= tartrate resistant acid phosphatase

Lymphoblast

SYNONYMS
none

VITAL STATISTICS
- size .... 10 to 20 μm
- N:C ratio .... 7:1 to 4:1
- cell shape .... round to oval
- nuclear shape ..... usually round to oval; occasionally clefted, folded, convoluted, oblong, or angular
- chromatin .... fine and lacy, but more granular than in myeloblasts; can be moderately granular; parachromatin is abundant to moderate
- nucleoli .... one or more; may be indistinct; if multiple, are usually small to medium size; can be single, large, and centrally located.
- cytoplasm .... scant to moderate; moderately to deeply basophilic; usually agranular; vacuoles may be present and sometimes prominent; can appear pulled to one side and give a "hand mirror" appearance

KEY DIFFERENTIATING FEATURES
- medium to larger size cells with high nuclear to cytoplasmic ratio, immature chromatin pattern, one or more nucleoli, and scant, agranular, basophilic cytoplasm
- in the absence of data concerning cell surface markers or cytochemistry, individual blast cells cannot reliably be distinguished from each other

OTHER FINDINGS
- often associated with markedly increased white blood cell count, anemia, thrombocytopenia, hepatosplenomegaly; pancytopenia in some cases

POTENTIAL LOOK-ALIKES
- blasts (myeloblasts, monoblasts, megakaryoblasts)
- lymphoma cells
- reactive lymphocytes
- prolymphocytes

ASSOCIATED DISEASE STATES AND CONDITIONS
- acute lymphoblastic leukemia (ALL)
- lymphoid blast crisis of chronic myelogenous leukemia and other chronic myeloproliferative disorders

Lymphoblasts are the most immature cell of the lymphoid series. They are most commonly seen in acute lymphoblastic leukemia (ALL), but they can also occur in the lymphoid blast crisis of chronic myelogenous leukemia (CML) and other chronic myeloproliferative disorders. Morphologically, lymphoblasts have been separated into three subtypes by the French-American-British (FAB) cooperative group. These types are designated L-1, L-2, and L-3. Using cell surface markers, ALL can be divided into B-cell ALL, T-cell ALL, and undifferentiated (null cell) ALL. Both T- and B-cell ALL can be further subdivided based on the pattern of various cell surface markers.

The L-1 type of ALL is characterized by a homogeneous population of lymphoblasts. These cells are relatively small with regular, round nuclei. Scattered larger cells can be present. The nuclear contour is smooth; however, occasional clefts or indentations may be seen. The chromatin pattern is homogeneous, but coarser and more compact than in other leukemic blasts. Nucleoli are inconspicuous due to the denser chromatin pattern. If seen, they are small and single. The cytoplasm is scant and slightly to moderately basophilic. A few vacuoles may be present and the cytoplasm is agranular. The nuclear to cytoplasmic ratio is very high.

L-2 lymphoblasts exhibit marked heterogeneity in cell size with larger blasts predominating. The nuclei are variable and range from round or oval to irregular with prominent indentations, folding, and clefting. They may appear monocytoid and be confused with monoblasts. When the nuclei are more regular in appearance, these cells resemble myeloblasts. The chromatin pattern is also variable, even within the same

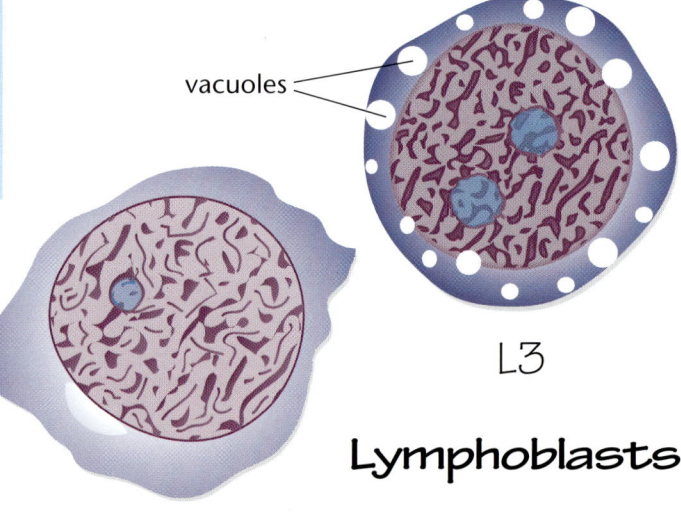

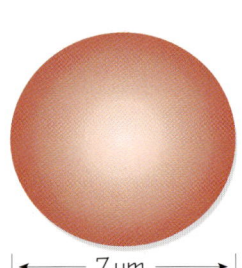
size of normal red blood cell — 7 μm

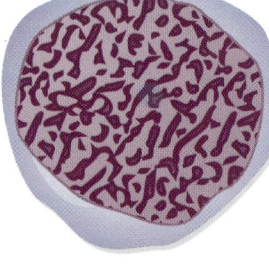

L1 L2 L3

Lymphoblasts

case. It can range from finely dispersed to coarsely condensed. One or more large, basophilic nucleoli may be seen. They can vary considerably in size and number. The cytoplasm ranges from scant to moderate and the staining intensity varies from light to deeply basophilic. Granules and Auer rods are absent. Vacuoles may be found, but they are not prominent.

In contrast, the lymphoblasts seen in L-3 ALL exhibit a characteristic appearance. These cells are large and uniform in size and shape. The nuclei are round to oval with a smooth contour. While the chromatin pattern is dense, it is homogeneous and finely stippled. Most cells demonstrate one or more prominent vesicular nucleoli. These have a moderate amount of deeply basophilic cytoplasm containing frequent, similar sized, round vacuoles that surround the nucleus. Vacuoles may even be noted to lie over the nucleus.

Since lymphoblasts are quite variable in appearance, it is often impossible to correctly classify an individual cell based on the morphology alone. Lymphoblasts can be indistinguishable from other types of blasts (myeloblasts, monoblasts, and megakaryoblasts), lymphoma cells, prolymphocytes, and some reactive lymphocytes. Additional information from cytochemical stains or cell surface markers is necessary to make the correct diagnosis. For identification purposes, one should classify individual cells exhibiting this type of morphology as blast cells when additional confirmatory information is unavailable.

H-23, 1982 (Blood, Wright-Giemsa, X350)

Identification	Referee %	Participant %
Lymphoblast	77.8	46.5
Blast	22.2	29.7
Prolymphocyte	-	7.0
Myeloblast	-	5.7

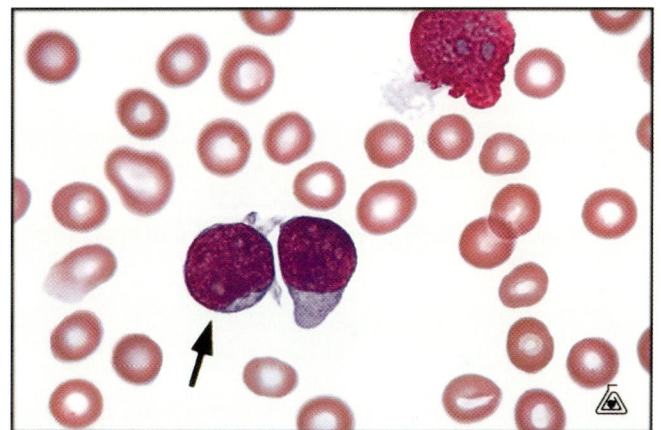

This blood film shows two lymphoblasts and a smudge cell in a field of normochromic-normocytic red cells. No platelets are present. The arrowed cell is over two times larger than a red blood cell with a very high N:C ratio. The slightly ovoid nucleus contains finely dispersed chromatin and 2 to 3 nucleoli. The cytoplasm is scant, agranular, and blue-gray. The adjacent cell is another lymphoblast which contains slightly more cytoplasm and exhibits a similar chromatin pattern. The case is from a 14-year-old male with T-cell ALL.

H-25, 1982 (Blood, Wright-Giemsa, X350)

Identification	Referee %	Participant %
Lymphoblast	55.6	29.3
Blast	33.3	23.7
Monoblast	11.1	18.0
Monocyte or precursor	-	9.9
Myelomonoblast	-	6.7

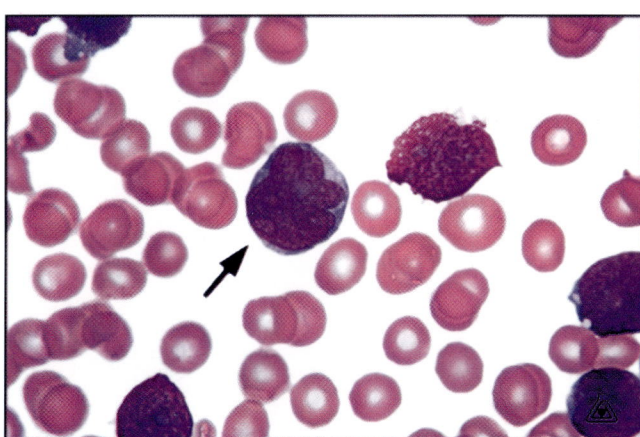

This photomicrograph exhibits another lymphoblast from the same case as H-23 1982. The red blood cells are normochromic-normocytic and show rouleaux formation, since this view is from a thicker area of the blood film. No platelets are visible. The arrowed cell is large with a high N:C ratio and an irregular nuclear membrane with deep indentations and folds. The chromatin is homogeneous and fine. Multiple nucleoli are visible. The cytoplasm is agranular and blue-gray. The other leukocytes are also lymphoblasts which exhibit similar morphology. A basket or smudge cell is to the right of the arrowed cell.

Lymphocyte, Mature

SYNONYMS
none

VITAL STATISTICS
- size .... 7 to 15 µm
- N:C ratio .... 5:1 to 2:1
- cell shape .... round to ovoid
- nuclear shape .... generally round to oval; occasionally notched or slightly indented
- chromatin .... diffusely dense or coarse with clumpy masses; minimal or absent parachromatin
- nucleoli .... not visible; sometimes a small, pale chromocenter is present
- cytoplasm .... scant to moderately abundant; pale blue to moderately basophilic; may have a perinuclear clear zone; sometimes a paranuclear hof; granules are absent in small lymphocytes; larger lymphocytes with more cytoplasm often contain a few coarse azurophilic granules

KEY DIFFERENTIATING FEATURES
- small cells with compact, coarse chromatin and scant cytoplasm
- nucleoli are lacking
- cells with more cytoplasm may exhibit a few azurophilic granules

POTENTIAL LOOK-ALIKES
- lymphoma cells (i.e. chronic lymphocytic leukemia or peripheralized low-grade lymphomas)
- some reactive lymphocytes
- nucleated red blood cells
- orthochromic normoblasts in the bone marrow

ASSOCIATED DISEASE STATES AND CONDITIONS
- acute infections (pertussis, typhoid fever, *Mycoplasma pneumonia*, etc.)
- chronic infectious or inflammatory disorders
- viral illnesses
- drug reactions
- endocrine disorders (i.e. thyrotoxicosis)

Mature lymphocytes are a normal constituent of blood and bone marrow. While the majority of lymphocytes seen in a blood film are fairly homogeneous, these cells normally exhibit a range of morphology. Most lymphocytes are small cells with round to oval nuclei that may be slightly indented or notched. Some normal lymphocytes are medium sized due to an increased amount of cytoplasm. The chromatin is diffusely dense or coarse and clumped. Nucleoli are not visible. Some cells may exhibit a small, pale chromocenter that may be mistaken for a nucleolus.

The majority of lymphocytes have a scant amount of pale blue to moderately basophilic, agranular cytoplasm. Occasionally, the edges may be slightly frayed or pointed due to artifacts induced during smear preparation. Some cells show a perinuclear clear zone or halo that surrounds the nucleus. Occasional lymphocytes will have a small clear zone or hof adjacent to one side of the nucleus.

Lymphocytes with more abundant cytoplasm often contain a few, coarse, unevenly distributed, azurophilic granules. These are referred to as large granular lymphocytes. These cells are found in blood smears from normal individuals and may also be increased in association with reactive lymphocytes. Cell surface marker studies show that these cells are generally either natural killer lymphocytes or CD8 positive suppressor/cytotoxic T lymphocytes.

Mature lymphocytes must be distinguished from reactive lymphocytes. See *Lymphocyte, Reactive* (page 222) and *A Closer Look at…Normal vs. Reactive Lymphocytes* (page 220) for more information. In cases of diffuse small lymphocytic lymphoma and/or chronic lymphocytic leukemia (CLL) the malignant cells can be morphologically indistinguishable from normal, mature lymphocytes. This difficulty is more apparent in cases of early disease or with low numbers of malignant cells. Additional information, such as from cell surface marker studies, is often necessary to make the correct identification. See *A Closer Look At…Reactive vs. Neoplastic Lymphocytes* on page 226.

Mature, Non-Reactive Lymphocytes

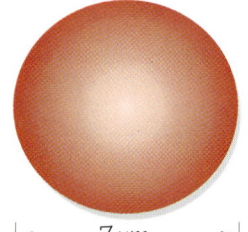

|← 7 µm →|
size of normal red blood cell

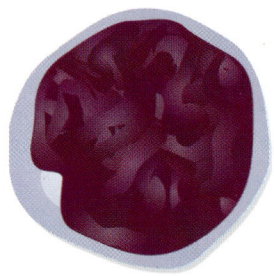

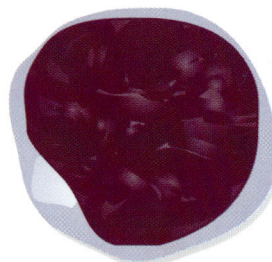

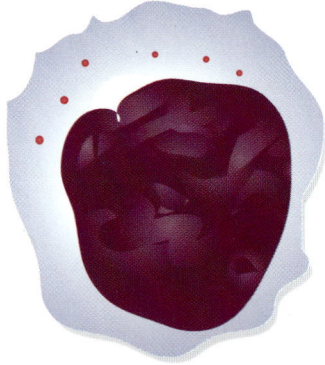

large granular lymphocyte

A-66, 1983 (Blood, Wright-Giemsa, X400)

Identification	Referee %	Participant %
Lymphocyte	91.7	92.3

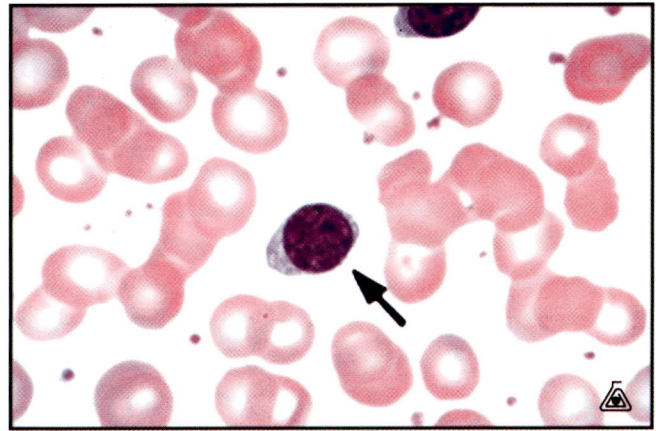

This blood film shows a high power view of a normal lymphocyte. The platelets appear unremarkable and small. Red blood cells exhibit rouleaux formation, but are otherwise unremarkable. The arrowed cell has a small round nucleus with darkly clumped, coarse chromatin. No nucleoli are present, but a small, dark chromocenter is seen. The cytoplasm is eccentric, scant, and pale blue without granules. The non-arrowed cell at the top of the field is another mature lymphocyte.

HE-21, 1995 (Blood Wright-Giemsa, X400)

Identification	Referee %	Participant %
Lymphocyte	85.7	79.3
Lymphocyte, reactive	14.3	17.6

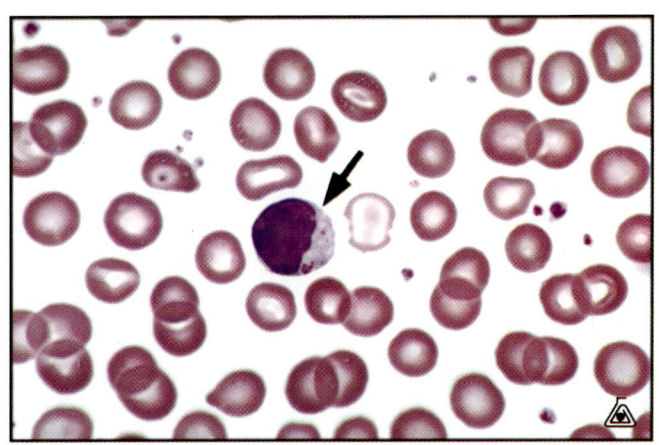

The arrowed cell is a normal lymphocyte. The red blood cells are normocytic with slight poikilocytosis. Frequent platelets are present. The lymphocyte has an eccentric nucleus with clumped chromatin. It has a moderate amount of pale blue cytoplasm containing scattered, unevenly distributed azurophilic granules. This cell is a granulated lymphocyte.

HE-25, 1995 (Blood, Wright-Giemsa X400)

Identification	Referee %	Participant %
Lymphocyte	82.1	81.4
Lymphocyte, reactive	17.9	15.5

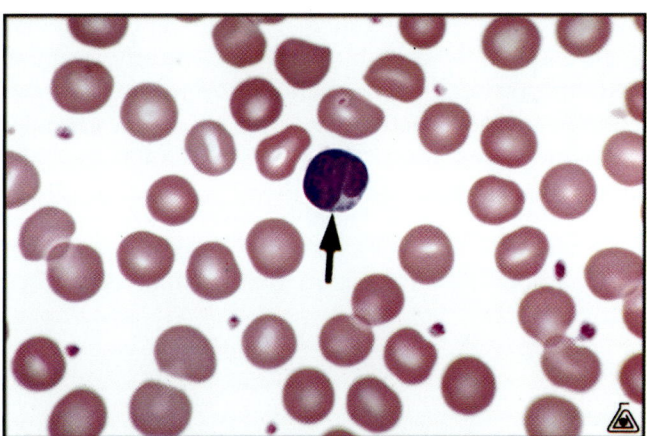

The cell in this blood film is another type of normal lymphocyte. Red blood cells are normocytic with mild poikilocytosis. Platelets are unremarkable. This lymphocyte has an indented or reniform nucleus with clumped, dark chromatin. The cytoplasm is scant and pale blue. Lymphocytes exhibiting this morphologic appearance are normal and are more frequently seen in infants and small children.

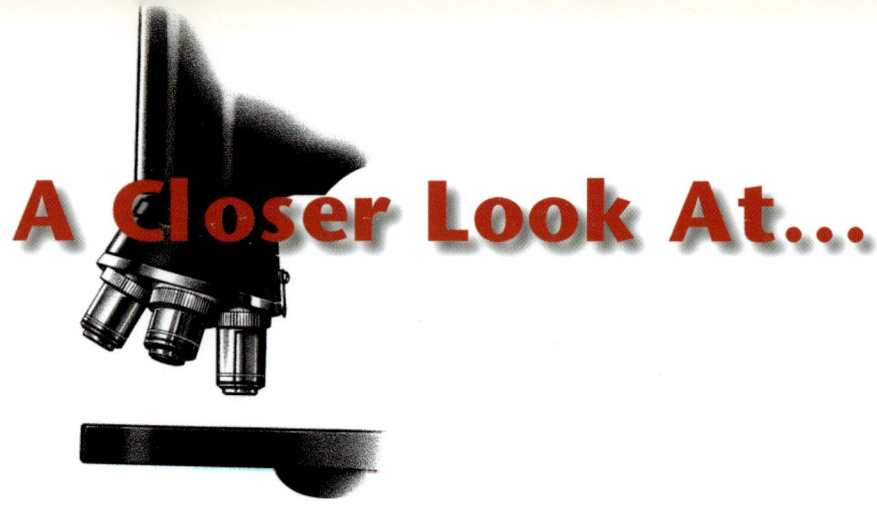

A Closer Look At...

Normal vs. Reactive Lymphocytes

Blood and bone marrow lymphocytes are generally homogeneous; however, they do show a range of morphologic appearances. Well stained Wright-Giemsa smears reveal that most normal lymphocytes have small round to ovoid nuclei with dense, compact or clumped chromatin and scant, pale blue cytoplasm. But, if one is observant, other types of lymphocytes are found. Lymphocytes having a small nuclear indentation or notch are frequent. Some lymphocytes are medium size and contain a moderate amount of agranular cytoplasm. A paranuclear hof next to the nucleus or a clear zone surrounding the nucleus is apparent in other cells. Then, there are large granular lymphocytes that have moderate to abundant pale cytoplasm containing scattered fine to coarse azurophilic granules. All these types of lymphocytes are normal cells and their presence does not signify any abnormality.

In contrast, reactive lymphocytes are characterized by their even greater range of morphologic appearance within the same blood film. Generally, reactive lymphocytes have more abundant cytoplasm that frequently contains vacuoles, a lower N:C ratio, irregular nuclei, a more open chromatin pattern, and nucleoli. These cell types include the Downey type I, II, and III cells and plasmacytoid lymphocytes.

Downey type I cells are small lymphocytes with small amounts of cytoplasm that contain occasional azurophilic granules and numerous small vacuoles. The nuclei are frequently indented or lobulated. Downey type II cells exhibit a smeared nuclear chromatin pattern and have abundant, agranular cytoplasm that stains darker at the edges and often partially surrounds adjacent red blood cells. Immunoblasts are another name for Downey type III cells. These large cells have fine to moderately coarse chromatin, one or more prominent nucleoli, and moderate to abundant cytoplasm that stains deeply basophilic. Plasmacytoid reactive lymphocytes are medium size with round nuclei. Their chromatin pattern resembles that of plasma cells and they have abundant blue cytoplasm with a prominent perinuclear hof.

When attempting to distinguish a normal, mature lymphocyte from a reactive lymphocyte on a photomicrograph, care should be taken. First, examine the clinical history and CBC results. Next, review all the photomicrographs pertaining to the case. The other slides will frequently show additional lymphoid cells for comparison and contrast. By referring to this atlas one can review the pertinent points necessary for identification of a mature lymphocyte versus a reactive lymphocyte. Finally, correlate the features of the illustrated cell with all the information available and arrive at the correct diagnosis.

Comparison of Mature and Reactive Lymphocytes

	Mature	Reactive
Size	7-15 μm	10-25 μm
N:C Ratio	5:1-2:1	3:1-1:2
Shape	round to oval	round, oval, irregular
Nucleus	round to oval	variable
Chromatin	dense, clumped	variable
Parachromatin	none to scant	variable
Nucleoli	none	none to multiple
Cytoplasm	scant to moderate; pale to moderately basophilic	moderate to abundant; pale to deeply basophilic
Vacuoles	none	occasional
Granules	few, some cells	some cells
Other Findings	normal cells	viral infections, etc.

Normal Lymphocytes

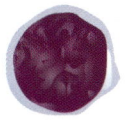 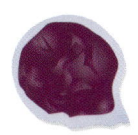 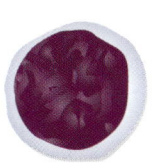 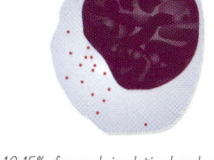

Chromatin is dense and clumped. Nucleoli should not be visible. Cytoplasm is usually scant but can be moderate in amount. Some cells may have a tadpole shape.

10-15% of normal circulating lymphocytes are large granular lymphocytes (NK cells). They have abundant pale cytoplasm and distinct azurophilic granules.

CLL Lymphocytes

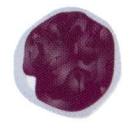 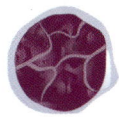

Nuclei are round or slightly indented. The chromatin is heavily clumped and may have distinctive chunky, block-like chromatin. No nucleoli are visible. Typical cases have <10% prolymphocytes. Mixed cell types of CLL have 10% to 55% prolymphocytes or variable numbers of large lymphoid cells.

Reactive Lymphocytes

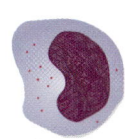

Downey Type I

Nucleus is kidney-bean shaped or lobated. Nucleoli may be visible. Cytoplasm is basophilic, foamy or vacuolated. Azurophilic granules may rarely be seen.

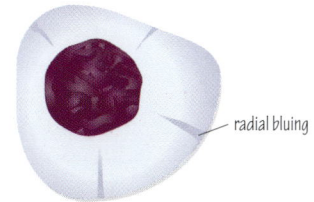

radial bluing

Downey Type II

Nucleus has loosely clumped chromatin. It may be eccentrically located. Cytoplasm is pale and abundant; radial bluing may be present. The periphery is scalloped, often producing a "ballerina skirt" appearance. Surrounding red blood cells may indent the cytoplasm.

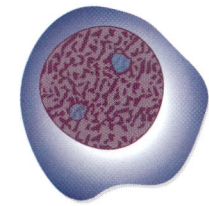

Downey Type III

These are the least common Downey cell. They resemble immunoblasts. The chromatin is fine and diffuse or moderately coarse. There may be one or two nucleoli. The cytoplasm is moderate to abundant and deeply basophilic.

Lymphocyte, Reactive

SYNONYMS
atypical lymphocyte, plasmacytoid lymphocyte, immunoblast, stimulated lymphocyte, variant lymphocyte, virocytes

VITAL STATISTICS
- size .... 10 to 25 μm
- N:C ratio .... 3:1 to 1:2
- cell shape .... variable; round, oval, irregular
- nuclear shape .... variable; round, oval, notched, indented, folded, cleaved, or lobulated
- chromatin .... may be fine, medium, or coarse; parachromatin is scant or abundant and distinct
- nucleoli .... none to multiple; vary in size and staining characteristics
- cytoplasm .... generally moderate to abundant; staining ranges from gray through pale blue to deeply basophilic; may be darker at the periphery and lighter near the nucleus; plasmacytoid lymphocytes often have a paranuclear clear zone or hof; fine azurophilic granules are sometimes seen; occasional cells contain vacuoles; the cytoplasm may be indented by adjacent red cells

KEY DIFFERENTIATING FEATURES
- marked variability in cell size and shape, nuclear chromatin characteristics, and amount of cytoplasm
- nucleoli are often present
- cytoplasm may be indented by adjacent red cells

OTHER FINDINGS
- total lymphocyte count may be normal or increased
- rarely seen in bone marrow smears

POTENTIAL LOOK-ALIKES
- lymphoma cells
- normal lymphocytes
- blasts (including lymphoblasts, myeloblasts, monoblasts, and megakaryoblasts)
- prolymphocytes
- monocytes
- immature monocytes (promonocytes)
- plasma cells
- Sézary cells

ASSOCIATED DISEASE STATES AND CONDITIONS
- Epstein-Barr virus infection (infectious mononucleosis)
- CMV infection
- viral hepatitis
- other viral infections
- drug reactions
- chronic inflammatory disorders (systemic lupus erythematosis, rheumatoid arthritis, etc.)

The key distinguishing feature of reactive lymphocytes is their wide range of morphologic appearance within the same blood film. These cells are reacting to an abnormal stimulus and are frequently increased in viral illnesses. The classic example is Epstein-Barr virus infection (infectious mononucleosis). Reactive or atypical lymphocytes can also be found in a variety of other viral infections (CMV, herpes viruses, HIV, mumps, measles, rubella, etc.); protozoal infections such as toxoplasmosis; some drug reactions (Dilantin); connective tissue diseases and other chronic inflammatory disorders such as SLE and rheumatoid arthritis; and after a major stress to the body's immune system such as sickle-cell anemia with vasoocclusive crisis or after radiation exposure.

A variety of reactive lymphocyte forms have been described and they are often seen concurrently in the same blood film. A classification scheme proposed by Downey lists five major types of cells. The Wood and Frenkel classification scheme has also been used. Many individuals prefer more of a descriptive classification that includes plasmacytoid lymphocytes, immunoblasts, monocyte-like lymphocytes, etc.

Downey type I cells are small and have indented or lobulated nuclei. Their chromatin is clumped. Nucleoli, if visible, are small. The cytoplasm is small in amount and basophilic. Numerous small vacuoles may be present. Occasional azurophilic granules may be seen.

Another type of reactive lymphocyte resembles a large lymphocyte and corresponds to a Downey type II cell. These cells have a round to oval nucleus, moderately clumped chromatin giving it a "smeared" appearance, and absent or indistinct nucleoli. They contain abundant pale gray-blue cytoplasm. Frequently, these reactive lymphocytes have an amoeboid cytoplasm that partially surrounds adjacent red cells and has a darker staining, furled margin. Occasionally basophilia radiating out from the nucleus is present, so called "radial bluing."

Immunoblasts and immunoblastic-like reactive lymphocytes are larger (15-20 μm) cells with round to oval nuclei. They have moderately dispersed chromatin with abundant parachromatin and one or more prominent nucleoli. These transformed cells may resemble lymphoma cells or blasts. Their cytoplasm is moderately abundant and stains deeply basophilic. The N:C ratio is high (3:1 to 2:1). These reactive lymphocytes correspond to Downey type III cells.

Plasmacytoid reactive lymphocytes resemble plasma cells and are intermediate in size (10 to 20 μm) and round to oblong in shape. They have round nuclei that are centrally placed or slightly eccentric. The chromatin is slightly to moderately coarse and forms small dense masses or a mesh of strands, resembling that of plasma cells. Nucleoli are generally not visible, but some cells may have one or two small irregular nucleoli. The cytoplasm is moderately abundant, homogeneous, light blue to deep slate-blue, and shows a paranuclear clear zone or hof.

The Spectrum of Reactive Lymphocytes

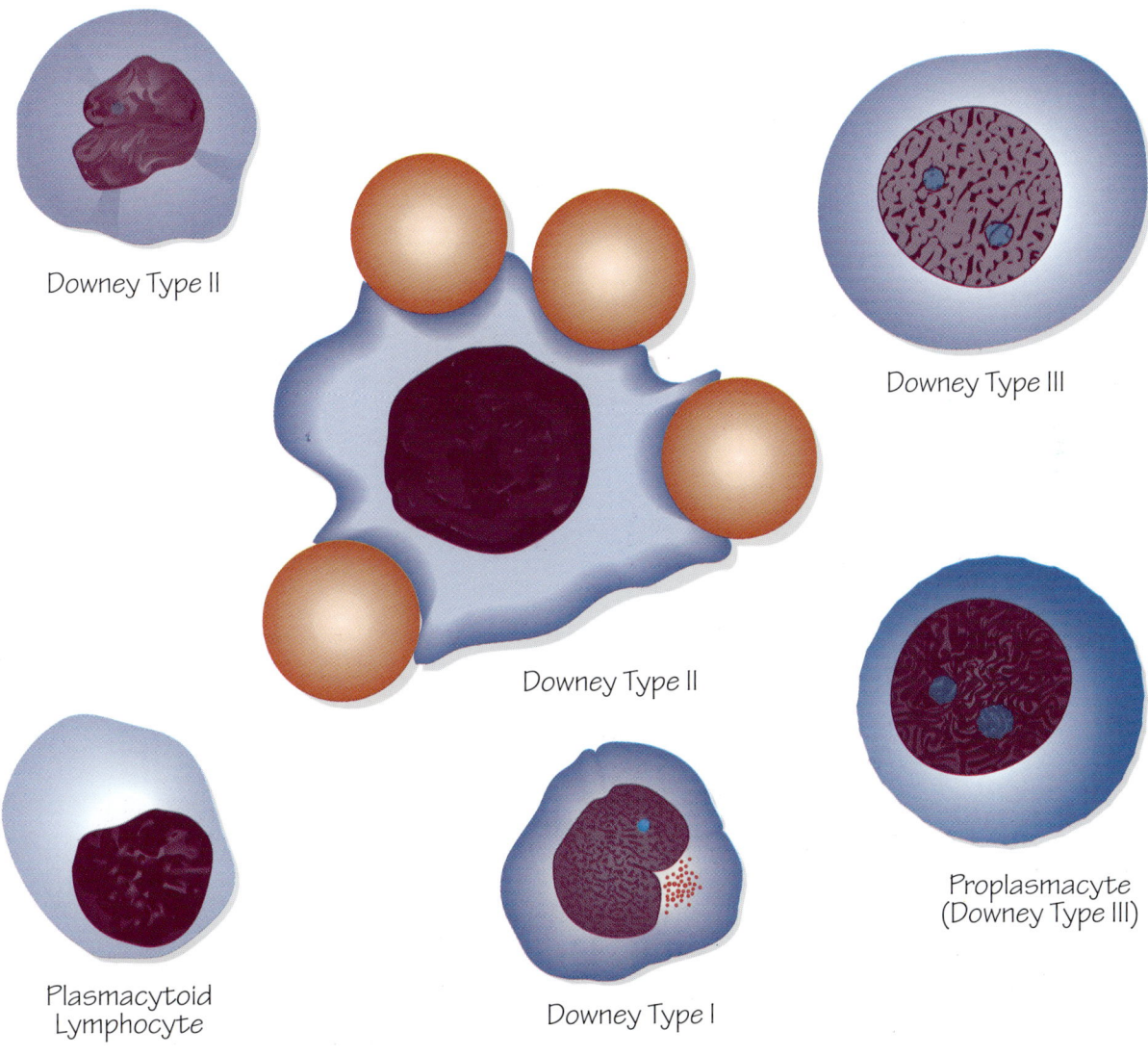

Lymphocytic and Plasmacytic Cells

H-22, 1980 (Blood, Wright-Giemsa, X375)

Identification	Referee %	Participant %
Lymphocyte, reactive	85.7	92.9
Monocyte	14.3	5.4

A reactive lymphocyte is present in this blood film. Three normal platelets are seen. Red blood cells are normochromic and normocytic. The arrowed cell is large with an irregular, slightly indented, ovoid nucleus. Its chromatin is fine to moderately coarse with some areas showing more clumping. No nucleoli are visible. The abundant, moderately basophilic cytoplasm contains a few, small azurophilic granules and surrounds adjacent red cells, appearing darker at the edges.

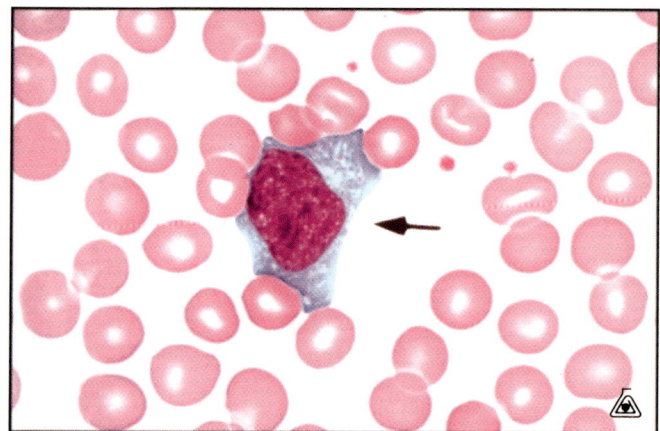

A-27, 1984 (Blood, Wright-Giemsa, X375)

Identification	Referee %	Participant %
Lymphocyte, reactive	100	91.4

This blood film shows a reactive lymphocyte. No platelets are present. Red cells are unremarkable. The arrowed cell is large with an angulated, indented nucleus. The chromatin is moderately coarse with a few more condensed areas and some open areas of parachromatin that resemble nucleoli. The cytoplasm is abundant, moderately basophilic, agranular, and contains a few small vacuoles. It appears darker at the margins.

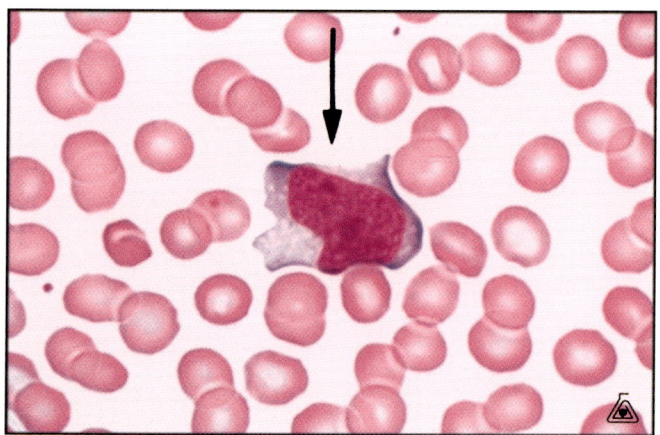

XL-88, 1989 (Blood, Wright-Giemsa, X350)

Identification	Referee %	Participant %
Lymphocyte, reactive	95	86.8
Monocyte	-	6.7

A reactive lymphocyte is present in this blood film. A few normal appearing platelets are visible. Red blood cells are normochromic and normocytic. The arrowed cell has a round nucleus with coarsely condensed chromatin. No nucleoli are visible. The abundant cytoplasm is light blue/gray with a pinkish tint. It is agranular and appears darker at the margins. The morphology of this cell corresponds to a Downey type II cell. The nonarrowed cell in the field is a basket/smudge cell. This case is from a 19-year-old white female with infectious mononucleosis.

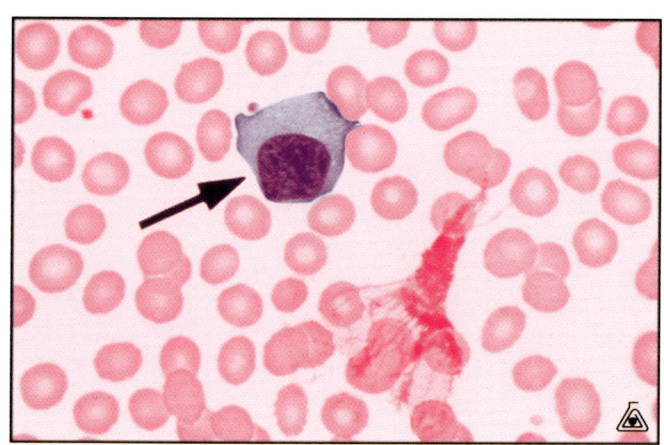

A-67, 1983 (Blood, Wright-Giemsa, X375)

Identification	Referee %	Participant %
Lymphocyte, reactive	100	91.4

Two reactive lymphocytes are seen in this blood film. A single normal platelet is adjacent to the arrowed cell. Red cells show artifactual changes secondary to being photographed in the thick area of the blood film. The arrowed cell is much larger than a normal lymphocyte and has an ovoid to angulated nucleus. The chromatin is fairly homogeneous and moderately to finely condensed. A distinct, single nucleolus is present. The abundant cytoplasm is blue with darkening at the edges. It is agranular and surrounds adjacent red cells. The non-arrowed cell in the field is another reactive lymphocyte which exhibits similar morphology.

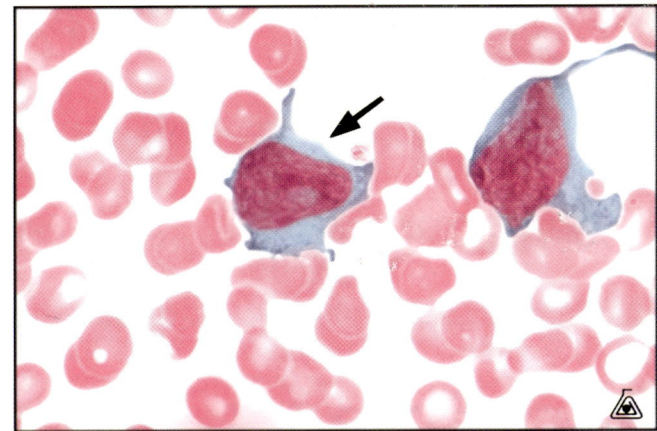

H1-18, 1983 (Blood, Wright-Giemsa, X350)

Identification	Referee %	Participant %
Lymphocyte, reactive	100	95.2

This blood film shows another type of reactive lymphocyte. Scattered, normal platelets are present. Red blood cells are unremarkable. The arrowed cell is larger than a mature lymphocyte with an irregular, indented nuclear membrane. The chromatin is moderately coarse with a small, indistinct nucleolus. There is a moderate amount of blue/gray, agranular cytoplasm which appears darker at the edges and surrounds adjacent red cells. This case is from a patient with infectious mononucleosis and was used to illustrate the types of reactive lymphocytes seen in this condition.

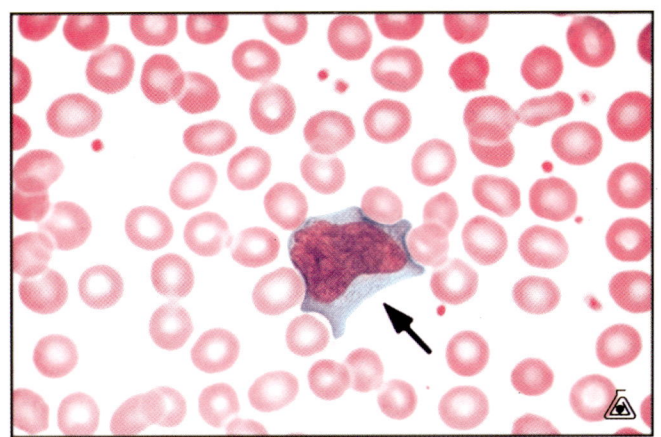

H1-20, 1983 (Blood, Wright-Giemsa, X350)

Identification	Referee %	Participant %
Lymphocyte, reactive	100	96.3

Another reactive lymphocyte from the same case as slide H1-18, 1983 is illustrated in this blood film. Red blood cells are normochromic and normocytic. The platelets appear normal. The large arrowed cell has an angulated nucleus with moderately clumped chromatin and open areas of parachromatin that resemble small nucleoli. The abundant cytoplasm surrounds adjacent red cells, is gray/blue without obvious granules, and appears darker at the margins. A few small vacuoles are present.

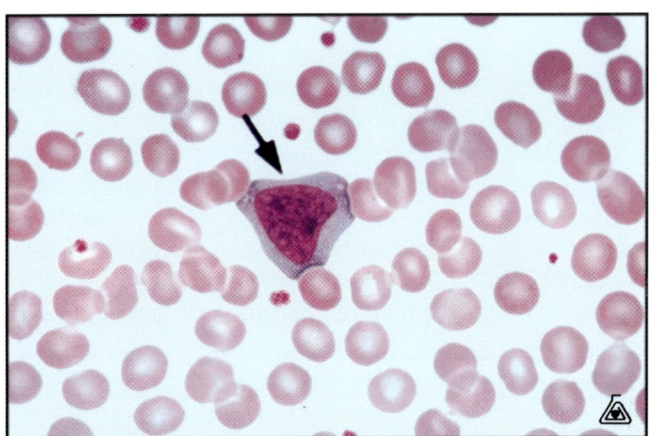

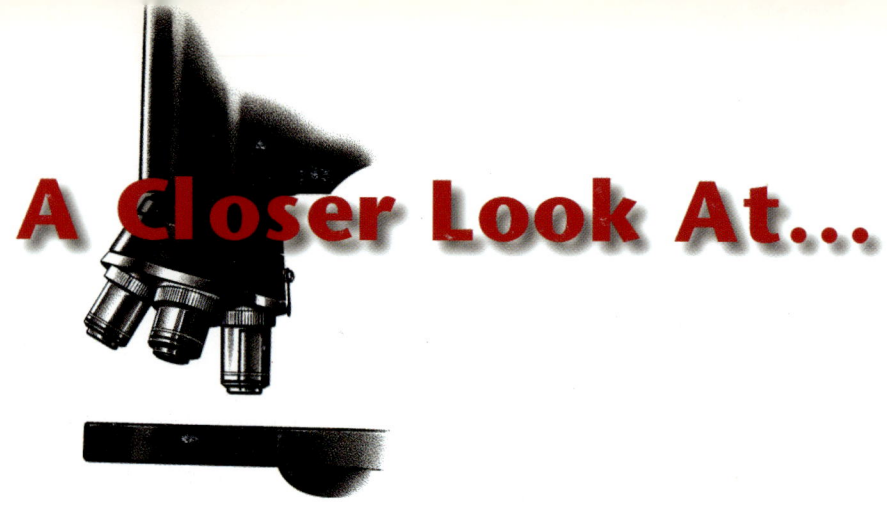

A Closer Look At...

Reactive vs. Neoplastic Lymphocytes

It is often difficult to distinguish reactive lymphocytes from lymphoma cells, lymphoblasts, and prolymphocytes. This problem is more apparent when photomicrographs of single cells are used to make a diagnosis. Therefore, one must rely on the clinical history and CBC findings that are supplied, along with any additional photomicrographs from the same case. If given, immunophenotype information is invaluable.

Of these cell types, reactive lymphocytes and lymphoma cells exhibit the most similarities. However, this apparent similarity is somewhat deceiving. Reactive lymphocytes are characterized by their wide range of morphologic appearance within the same blood film. In contrast, while lymphoma cells can exhibit a wide variety of appearances, any individual case tends to show a monotonous population of the abnormal cells. The most important distinction between reactive lymphocytes and lymphoma cells is the difference in their N:C ratios. The N:C ratio tends to be low in atypical lymphocytes, while it is high in lymphoma cells. The table on the next page compares features of reactive lymphocytes to various malignant lymphocytes.

Reactive lymphocytes are seen in cases of viral infection, protozoal infections, some drug reactions, connective tissue diseases, and some stress reactions. Cases due to viral infections are more common in children and young adults. Lymphoma cells are often seen in patients with a previous diagnosis of lymphoma at some other site. These disorders are more common in middle age to elderly adults.

Other cells that can be confused with reactive lymphocytes are lymphoblasts and prolymphocytes. Lymphoblasts are immature cells with fine chromatin and one or more nucleoli. Prolymphocytes have a central nucleus with moderately coarse chromatin (between that of a lymphoblast and a mature lymphocyte), a single prominent nucleolus, and moderate blue cytoplasm. Lymphoblasts are seen in patients with acute lymphoblastic leukemia, which occurs more commonly in the pediatric population. In contrast, prolymphocytes are seen in adults with chronic lymphocytic leukemia (CLL), CLL with prolymphocytic transformation, and prolymphocytic leukemia.

While these features will frequently allow one to make a diagnosis based on morphology alone, supplemental studies are often necessary. Flow cytometric analysis is the most reliable means of separating these cell types. Reactive lymphocytes are most commonly activated CD8+ T cells. Lymphoma cells of B cell origin show clonality with a single light chain type. Cases of T cell lymphoma are less common and they may show loss of normal pan-T-cell markers. Lymphoblasts are most commonly immature B cells, but immature T cells are also seen. Prolymphocytes are B cells in CLL but may be either of B or T cell origin in prolymphocytic leukemia.

Comparison of Reactive and Neoplastic Lymphocytes

	Reactive	Lymphoma	Lymphoblast	Prolymphocyte
Size	10-25 µm	8-30 µm	10-20 µm	10-18 µm
N:C Ratio	3:1-1:2	7:1-3:1	7:1-4:1	5:1-3:1
Shape	round, oval, irregular	variable	round to oval	round to oval
Nucleus	variable	variable	round to oval	round to oval
Chromatin	variable	variable	fine	clumped
Parachromatin	none to scant	variable	none to abundant	indistinct
Nucleolus	none to multiple	none to multiple	one to multiple	one; prominent
Cytoplasm	moderate to abundant; pale to deeply basophilic	scant to moderate; pale to deeply basophilic	scant to moderate; moderate to deeply basophilic	moderate; moderately basophilic
Vacuoles	occasional	occasional	sometimes	none
Granules	some cells	none	none	rare
Associated Disease States	viral infection, etc.	lymphoma	acute lymphoblastic leukemia	chronic lymphocytic or prolymphocytic leukemia

Lymphocytic and Plasmacytic Cells

Lymphoma Cell

SYNONYMS
none

VITAL STATISTICS
- Size .... 8 to 30 μm
- N:C ratio .... 7:1 to 3:1
- cell shape .... round or oval, can be irregular
- nuclear shape .... variable; usually clefted, folded, convoluted, or lobulated; can be round, oval, or angulated; dependent on type of lymphoma
- chromatin .... variable, depending on type of lymphoma; ranges from compact and clumped to fine and open; parachromatin is variable
- nucleoli .... variable number and size
- cytoplasm .... variable; ranges from scant and pale blue to moderate and deeply basophilic; vacuoles may be present; agranular

KEY DIFFERENTIATING FEATURES
- presence of a monotonous population of lymphoid cells with a similar appearance
- atypical features such as prominent nucleoli, vacuoles, prominent lobulation or clefting

OTHER FINDINGS
- anemia, thrombocytopenia, and lymphocytosis
- rouleaux formation in some cases
- may have history of lymphoma at other site

POTENTIAL LOOK-ALIKES
- blasts (myeloblasts, lymphoblasts, monoblasts, megakaryoblasts, erythroblasts)
- prolymphocytes, atypical, or reactive lymphocytes
- immature plasma cells

ASSOCIATED DISEASE STATES AND CONDITIONS
- any type of malignant lymphoma including:
  - diffuse small lymphocytic lymphoma/CLL
  - follicular center cell lymphomas (small, large and mixed cell types)
  - mantle cell lymphoma
  - marginal zone lymphoma
  - large cell lymphomas and immunoblastic lymphoma
  - small noncleaved cell lymphoma (Burkitt's and Burkitt's-like)
  - lymphoblastic lymphoma
  - cutaneous T cell lymphoma or Sézary's syndrome
  - adult T cell lymphoma/leukemia

Lymphoma cells can exhibit a variety of appearances. The cellular morphology is variable and dependent on the underlying type of lymphoma. While lymphoma cells are usually round to oval, they can be irregular. Cell size varies from 8 to 30 μm and the N:C ratio varies from 7:1 to 3:1. It is critical to obtain an accurate clinical history, since knowledge of any previous diagnosis of lymphoma greatly aids in the identification of these cells. Supplemental studies such as cytochemical stains and immunophenotyping are often necessary to arrive at a diagnosis.

Lymphoma cells are more frequently seen in the bone marrow, since many patients with low-grade lymphomas will have bone marrow involvement. Morphological identification of circulating lymphoma cells is less common. However, some studies have found that more than 80% of patients presenting with non-Hodgkin's malignant lymphomas have circulating malignant cells when sensitive techniques such as flow cytometry are used.

In diffuse small lymphocytic lymphoma (the tissue equivalent of chronic lymphocytic leukemia), the cells are generally small with round to oval nuclei, compact and coarse chromatin, and have a scant amount of basophilic cytoplasm. They may be the same size as normal lymphocytes or slightly larger. Occasionally, the nuclei exhibit an angulated appearance with slightly more open chromatin. A small nuclear indentation may be present. Nucleoli are not seen. Scattered prolymphocytes are often present which are larger cells with a centrally placed nucleus, a prominent single nucleolus, and moderate basophilic cytoplasm.

In the small cell follicular center cell lymphomas, the cells are slightly larger than normal lymphocytes and have an angulated appearance. The majority of nuclei have clefts, indentations, folds, convolutions, and may

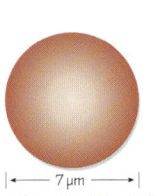
7 μm
size of normal red blood cell

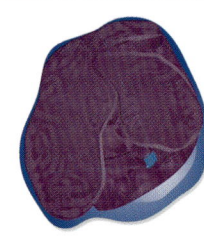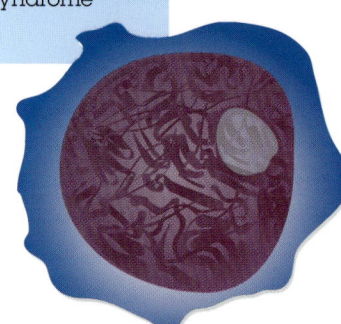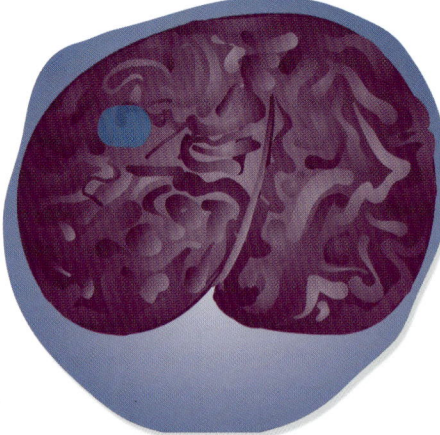

Various Lymphoma Cells

even be lobulated. The chromatin is moderately coarse and one or more nucleoli may be visible. The cytoplasm is scant to moderate and basophilic.

The cells in small noncleaved cell lymphomas (Burkitt's and Burkitt's-like lymphomas) are morphologically similar to FAB L3 lymphoblasts (See *Lymphoblast*, page 216). These cells are generally moderate size (10-25 µm) and have a round to oval nucleus with moderately coarse chromatin and one or more prominent nucleoli. The cytoplasm is moderate, stains dark blue, and may contain numerous small vacuoles.

Large cell lymphomas and immunoblastic lymphomas may exhibit some of the most blast-like and abnormal morphology. These cells are large, varying from 20 to 30 µm and have a scant to moderate amount of deeply basophilic cytoplasm. The nuclei are generally round to oval, but may be angulated, folded, indented, or convoluted. Nucleoli are prominent and may be single or multiple. Vacuoles can occasionally be seen in the cytoplasm. These cells can be easily confused with blasts and additional studies such as immunophenotyping may be necessary to make the correct diagnosis.

T cell lymphomas can exhibit similar morphology to any of the above types of lymphoma. The typical appearance of a Sézary cell is a variably sized cell with a markedly convoluted nucleus having a cerebriform or grooved pattern. The chromatin is moderately coarse and nucleoli are not apparent. The cytoplasm is generally scant and blue.

H1-30, 1987 (Blood, Wright-Giemsa, X325)

Identification	Referee %	Participant %
Lymphoma cell	84.2	74.8
Lymphoblast	10.5	11.3

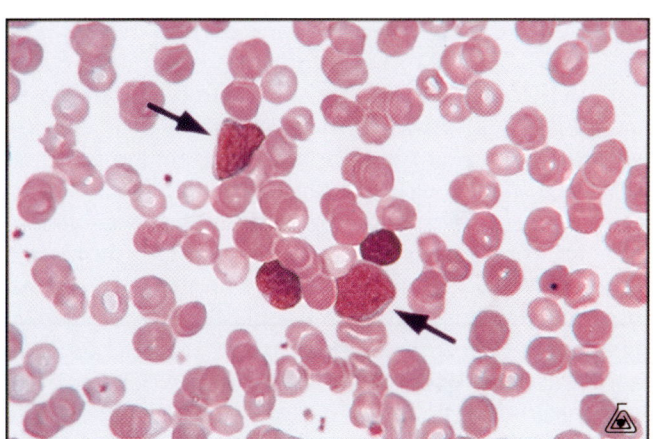

This blood film shows normochromic normocytic red cells. Rouleaux formation appears to be present, although this photomicrograph may be in a thicker portion of the slide. The platelets appear normal. The two arrowed cells are medium size, angulated, have a high N:C ratio, and contain scant cytoplasm. Both cells display folding or clefting of the nucleus. Their chromatin is moderately coarse and the lower arrowed cell appears to have two small peripheral nucleoli. The two nonarrowed cells in the center of the field are normal lymphocytes for comparison. One has a round nucleus with very dark clumped chromatin and the other is similar, but has a small nuclear indentation. This case is from a patient with peripheralized small cleaved cell lymphoma.

H1-42, 1987 (Bone Marrow, Wright-Giemsa, X350)

Identification	Referee %	Participant %
Lymphoma cell	89.4	91.3

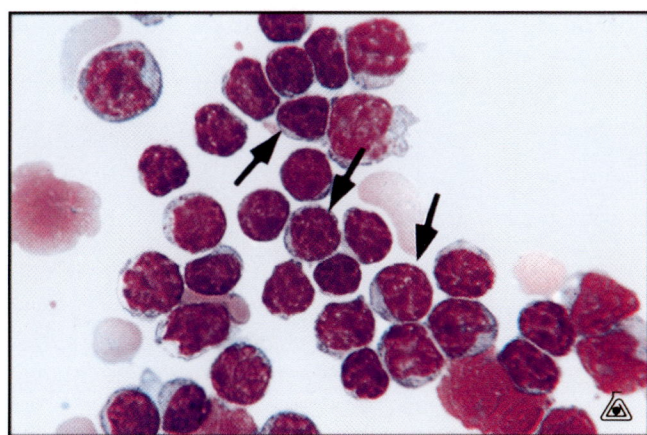

This bone marrow aspirate shows a field of monotonous appearing small lymphoid cells of which the three arrowed cells are representative. These cells have a round to oval nucleus, coarsely clumped chromatin, and a scant amount of pale basophilic cytoplasm. A few of the small cells display slight nuclear indentations. Two larger cells with a moderate amount of cytoplasm are present. They have more open chromatin and the one at about 10 o'clock has a central nucleolus. Two smudge cells are also visible. This case is from a bone marrow with involvement by diffuse small lymphocytic lymphoma. The small cells are the major component of this malignancy and the larger cells are prolymphocytes, which are also seen in this disorder.

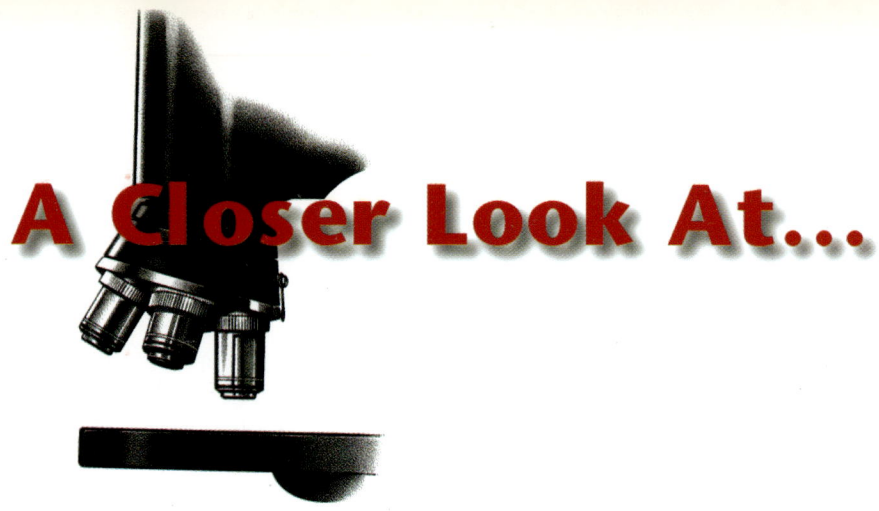

A Closer Look At...

Normal Lymphocyte Maturation and Malignant Transformation

Knowledge about the normal process of differentiation of T and B cells is important for the recognition of the various lymphoid malignancies. Acute lymphoblastic leukemia (ALL) arises from immature T or B cells. In contrast, malignant lymphomas, chronic lymphocytic leukemia, hairy cell leukemia, and multiple myeloma arise from more mature lymphoid cells. These malignancies are composed of transformed lymphoid cells that exhibit uncontrolled growth and invade normal tissues. The cause of these neoplastic proliferations is unknown. Exposure to ionizing radiation, chemicals, and viruses are possible etiologies for the development of genetic alterations and mutations that could lead to growth of a malignant clone of cells.

The classification of malignant lymphoid disorders is often complex. Past attempts to organize these malignancies have been based on the histological appearance of these neoplastic cells in lymph nodes, blood, and bone marrow. Recent advances regarding cell surface markers and the biology of these diseases has led to the recognition of new disease categories and reclassification of other disorders.

The schematic illustration on the next page follows lymphoid maturation and transformation. All the details of this sequence have not been ellucidated. The chart highlights some of the leukemias and lymphomas that can develop when this sequence is disrupted. Notice that the same cell type can result in either a leukemia (starting in the bone marrow) or a lymphoma (starting in lymph nodes or extra-nodal tissue).

Recent reviews of lymphomas have attempted to clarify the organization and define the various types of lymphoid malignancies (see *References* section page 343). Please refer to these papers for a detailed discussion. The following pages are not intended to be all inclusive, but rather to give an overview of common lymphoid neoplasms involving the blood and bone marrow.

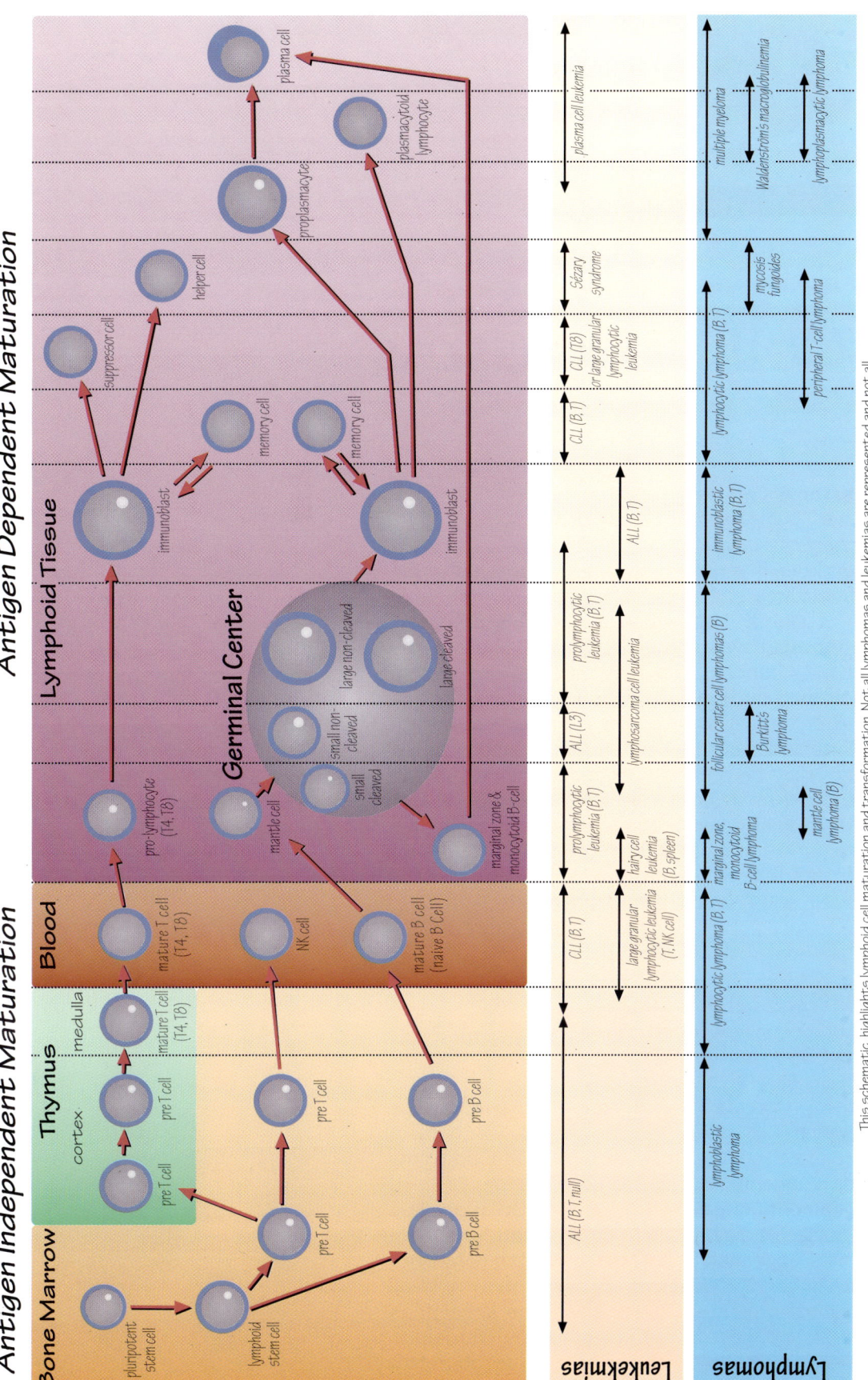

A Closer Look At...

B Cell Neoplasms

Precursor B Cell Neoplasms
Precursor B Lymphoblastic Leukemia/Lymphoma (Lymphoblastic Lymphoma and B Cell ALL)

This disorder is regarded as a high-grade malignant lymphoid disease. The primary cell is a lymphoblast which is slightly larger than a normal lymphocyte. Lymphoblasts have round to oval nuclei, fine and lacy chromatin, abundant parachromatin, and one or more nucleoli that can range from small and indistinct to large and centrally located. The cytoplasm is scant to moderate and stains moderately to deeply basophilic. Vacuoles may be present. Cell surface marker studies are required to determine whether these are B or T cells. This disease occurs most commonly in children and accounts for about 80% of cases of ALL. Flow cytometry studies show that these cells mark as immature B cells and characteristically are positive for CD19, CD10, HLA-DR, and TdT. They may also express other B cell antigens such as CD20 and CD22.

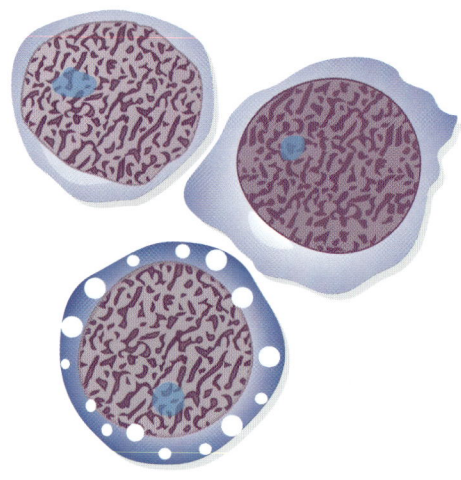

Precursor B Lymphoblasts

Peripheral B Cell Neoplasms
B Cell Chronic Lymphocytic Leukemia (CLL)
Prolymphocytic Leukemia (PLL)
Small Lymphocytic Lymphoma

Synonyms include well-differentiated lymphocytic lymphoma. CLL cells resemble normal lymphocytes but are often slightly larger. They have a round to occasionally indented nucleus, clumped chromatin, and a scant amount of pale blue cytoplasm. Occasionally, a small nucleolus may be seen. Some variants have more angulated appearing nuclei and more abundant cytoplasm. Frequently, serum studies may show a small monoclonal protein. Prolymphocytes are larger than CLL cells and have a prominent central nucleolus, clumped chromatin, and a moderate to abundant amount of basophilic cytoplasm. PLL is characterized

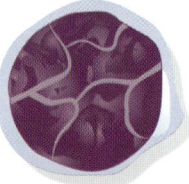

B-cell CLL

by greater than 50% of these cells in the blood or bone marrow. The majority of these cases occur in older adults and most individuals have blood and bone marrow involvement at the time of diagnosis. Sometimes, the lymph node involvement predominates. Clinically, cases of CLL display an indolent course, but they are incurable with current chemotherapy regimens. Transformation to prolymphocytic leukemia or large cell lymphoma (Richter's syndrome) can occur. De novo PLL usually presents with a markedly elevated white blood count and splenomegaly. The prognosis is poor. CLL typically expresses the B cell markers CD19, CD20, and CD23. They also exhibit CD5, weak surface light chain, and may be negative or weak for CD22, CD11c, and FMC-7. PLL may be negative for CD5 and have stronger expression of surface light chain, CD22, and FMC-7.

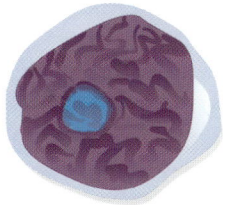

B cell Prolymphocyte

Lymphoplasmacytoid Lymphoma
Immunocytoma

These tumors are composed of small lymphocytes, plasmacytoid lymphocytes, and plasma cells. Cell marker studies show a different pattern than in CLL. Cases with this morphology, monoclonal IgM protein spikes, and the proper clinical criteria correspond to Waldenström's macroglobulinemia. This disorder also occurs in older adults and has an indolent clinical course. The lymph nodes, spleen, and bone marrow are frequently involved while blood involvement is less common. Some patients may have hyperviscosity syndrome due to high levels of serum IgM. These cells exhibit positivity by flow cytometry for CD19, CD20, and CD22; they lack CD5 and CD10. The cells show strong surface light chain expression in contrast to CLL, which is weak or negative for surface light chain.

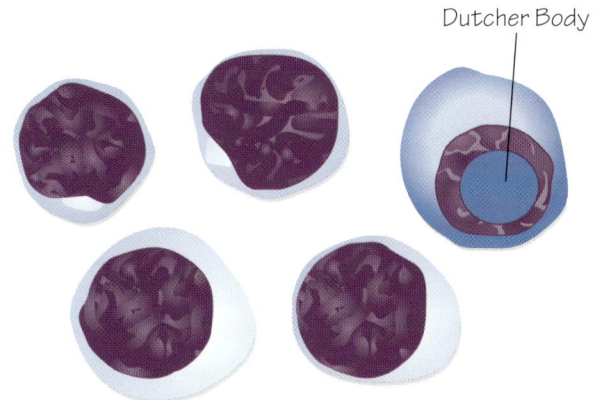

Waldenström's Macroglobulinemia

Mantle Cell Lymphoma

These cells are small to medium size, have moderately clumped chromatin, irregular nuclei that may be indented, folded or "cleaved," and a scant amount of pale blue cytoplasm. In some cases the nuclear contour is even and round, making these cells indistinguishable from CLL cells. Occasional cases can transform into a "blastic" or "lymphoblastoid" variant that has a very aggressive clinical course. These tumors occur in older adults and involve lymph nodes, spleen, bone marrow and blood. Gastrointestinal tract involvement is frequent. Their clinical course is moderately aggressive and survival is shorter than in CLL or small lymphocytic lymphoma. Flow cytometry is often necessary to aid in diagnosis. These cells exhibit positive staining for CD5, CD19, CD20, CD22, and FMC-7. Surface light chain expression is strong. They are negative to weak for CD23 and negative for CD11c.

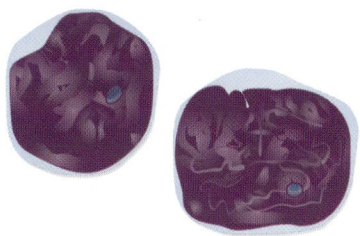

Mantle Zone Lymphoma Cells

Follicular Center Cell Lymphomas

Follicular center cell lymphomas include diffuse and follicular variants of small cell, mixed small and large cell and large cell B cell lymphomas. Synonyms are the variations of cleaved cell lymphomas and poorly differentiated lymphoma. The small cells in these tumors are slightly larger than normal lymphocytes, have a irregular nuclear outline with frequent indentations, foldings, angulations, and "cleaving," moderately clumped chromatin with an occasional small nucleolus, and a scant amount of basophilic cytoplasm. The larger cells have more abundant blue cytoplasm, oval to angulated and folded nuclei, more open chromatin, and may have more distinct nucleoli. These tumors occur in adults and account for about 40% of non-Hodgkin's lymphomas in the United States. The clinical course is generally indolent, but varies depending on the grade and subtype. Lymph node, splenic, and bone marrow involvement are common. Circulating cells can be found in some cases. Flow cytometry is somewhat variable, but most cases are positive for CD19, CD20, and CD22 with strong surface light chain expression. CD5 and CD11c are negative. CD10, CD23, and FMC-7 may be weakly positive or negative.

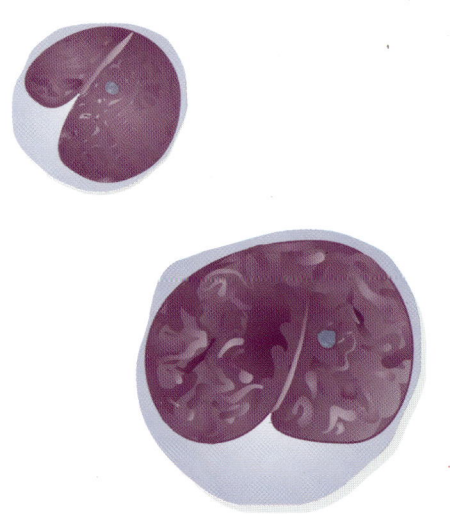

Follicular Center Cell Lymphoma Cells

Splenic Marginal Zone Lymphoma with or without Villous Lymphocytes

This disease is also known as splenic lymphoma with circulating villous lymphocytes and is only recently recognized. These cells range from small, unremarkable appearing lymphocytes to medium size cells with round to irregular nuclei, moderately coarse chromatin, an occasional nucleolus, and an abundant amount of pale basophilic cytoplasm that may exhibit eccentric fine projections. Since these cells can mimic hairy cells, and cases often present in a similar manner with lymphocytosis and splenomegaly, confirmation of the diagnosis by other methods is necessary. Typically, patients will have splenic, bone marrow, and blood involvement. Lymphadenopathy is uncommon. Many patients will have a small monoclonal protein spike in the serum. These patients tend to have a long, indolent clinical course and splenectomy often results in prolonged remissions. By flow cytometry, these cells are positive for CD19, CD20, CD22, FMC-7, and show strong surface light chain expression. CD5 is variable. CD10 and CD103 are negative. CD23 is negative to weak. CD11c and CD25 may be either positive or negative. These cells are usually negative for tartrate resistant acid phosphatase. (A few cases may show weak focal staining in contrast to the strong diffuse staining in hairy cell leukemia.)

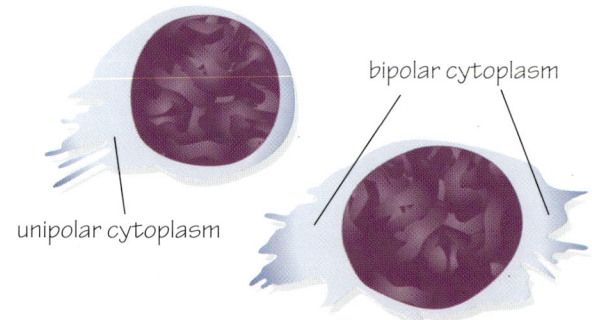

Splenic Lymphoma with Villous Lymphocytes

Hairy Cell Leukemia

These cells are slightly larger than normal lymphocytes and have an oval to indented nucleus which may be folded, bean-shaped, angulated or dumbbell-shaped. The chromatin is finer than normal lymphocytes and small nucleoli may be present. They contain moderate to abundant pale blue cytoplasm that classically exhibits numerous fine, hairlike projections. This disorder involves the spleen, bone marrow, and blood. Lymphadenopathy is rare. Patients are adults who often present with pancytopenia and may only have a few hairy cells circulating. Occasionally, there is a prominent lymphocytosis. The clinical course is indolent. Treatment with newer chemotherapeutic agents such as interferon, 2-chlorodeoxyadenosine (2-CDA), and deoxycoformycin have produced long-term remissions. Hairy cells display strong and diffuse staining for tartrate resistant acid phosphatase (TRAP). Flow cytometry shows a classic immunophenotype with positive staining for CD19, CD20, CD22, CD25, CD103, FMC-7, and strong surface light chain expression. CD23 is negative to weak. CD5 and CD10 are negative. The cells also show strong expression of CD11c.

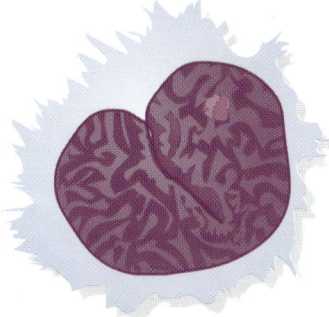

Hairy Cell

Plasmacytoma
Plasma Cell Myeloma, Multiple Myeloma

This neoplasm is composed of either mature or immature plasma cells. Plasma cells are medium size and have an eccentric round nucleus with coarse chromatin that is often arranged in a cartwheel-like or clock-face pattern. Cytoplasm is abundant and ranges from pale gray-blue to deeply basophilic and often shows an area of paranuclear clearing or "hof." Immature plasma cells exhibit a finer chromatin pattern, increased nuclear to cytoplasmic ratio, and may have one or more nucleoli. These tumors occur in older adults and most often involve the bone marrow. Patients may present with pathologic fractures, back pain, amyloidosis, or renal failure. Most patients will have a monoclonal immunoglobulin or light chain in either the serum or urine. These cells contain large amounts of cytoplasmic immunoglobulins, but lack surface light chain expression. Flow cytometry is less useful, since they lack most B-cell markers. The cells are positive for CD38 and may have CD56 on their surface.

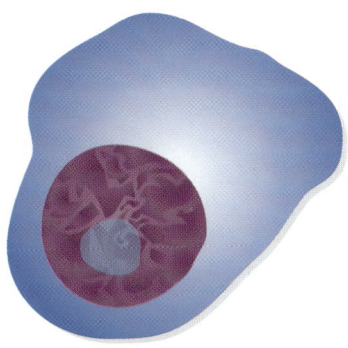

Myeloma Cell

A Closer Look At...

T Cell and Putative NK Cell Neoplasms

Precursor T Cell Neoplasms
Precursor T Lymphoblastic Lymphoma/Leukemia (T Cell ALL and Lymphoblastic Lymphoma)
These cells are morphologically identical to the cells of B cell ALL. Patients are usually adolescents or young adults. They often present with rapidly enlarging symptomatic mediastinal masses and/or lymphadenopathy. Cases of ALL may present with anemia, thrombocytopenia, pancytopenia, or leukocytosis with circulating blasts. Immunophenotyping by flow cytometry is necessary to establish the diagnosis. These cells frequently express CD2, CD3, and CD7. CD5 staining may be negative or positive. Some cases are positive for both CD4 and CD8, but both may be negative. Typically, these cases are positive for TdT.

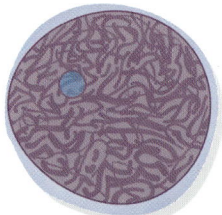
T Lymphoblast

Peripheral T Cell and NK Cell Neoplasms
T Cell Chronic Lymphocytic Leukemia
Prolymphocytic Leukemia
Most cases of chronic T cell leukemia have cells that look identical to B cell prolymphocytic leukemia. Cases of T cell CLL are rare. These neoplasms comprise less than 1% of all cases of CLL and about 20% of cases of prolymphocytic leukemia. Patients are adults and usually present with white blood counts greater than 100,000 and often have mucosal and/or skin involvement. The bone marrow, spleen, liver, and lymph nodes may be involved. These diseases are more aggressive than their B cell counterparts and are incurable with current therapies. Flow cytometry shows positive staining for CD2, CD3, CD5, and CD7. Most cases are CD4 positive, but cases with both CD4 and CD8 are found. These cells are CD25 negative.

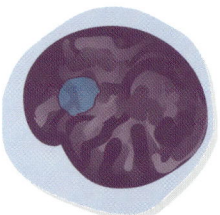
T Prolymphocyte

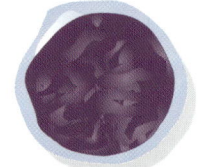
T4-CLL

Large Granular Lymphocyte Leukemia (LGL)

Both T and NK cell types of this disorder are known. These cells are identical to normal large granular lymphocytes. They have round to oval nuclei, moderately coarse chromatin, rare nucleoli, and an abundant amount of pale blue cytoplasm that contains scattered fine to coarse azurophilic granules. These neoplasms occur in adults who often present with neutropenia, mild anemia, and a mild to moderate, stable lymphocytosis. Most patients have splenomegaly, but bone marrow involvement is sparse. Lymphadenopathy is uncommon. The clinical course is usually indolent, but some patients have more rapidly progressive disease. Flow cytometry reveals that the T cell type is positive for CD2, CD3, CD8, and CD16. CD4, CD5, and CD25 are negative. Some cases that lack both CD4 and CD8 (gamma-delta T cells) have been described. The NK cell type is positive for CD2, CD16, and may have CD56 and/or CD57.

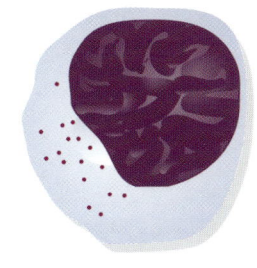
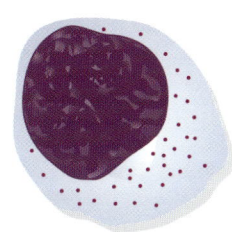

Large Granular Lymphocytes
(T8-CLL, NK cell leukemia, gamma-delta T-Cell Leukemia)

Mycosis Fungoides
Sézary Syndrome

These tumor cells are usually small with markedly convoluted nuclei, giving them a "cerebriform" appearance. Larger cells can be found with a similar nuclear morphology. This disease primary affects the skin, but can involve lymph nodes, bone marrow, and the blood. Patients are adults who present with multiple skin plaques or nodules. Sometimes they may have generalized erythroderma. Flow cytometry reveals that these cells are usually positive for CD2, CD3, CD5, and CD4. CD7 is positive in about one third of cases. Rare cases of CD8 positive mycosis fungoides have been reported.

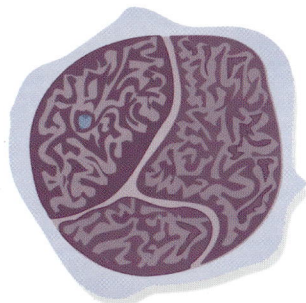

Sézary Cell

Plasma Cell, Mature

SYNONYMS
  plasmacyte

VITAL STATISTICS
  size .... 10 to 20 μm
  N:C ratio 1:2
  cell shape .... round to oval
  nuclear shape .... round to ovoid; usually eccentric; may be binucleated; rarely multinucleated
  chromatin .... coarse and clumped with dense masses often arranged in a clock-face or wheel-like pattern; parachromatin absent or scant
  nucleoli .... absent
  cytoplasm .... moderate to abundant; staining ranges from blue-gray to medium blue to deeply basophilic; occasionally may be pink-red (flame color); prominent, pale or lightly stained hof touching one side of nucleus; agranular; may have vacuoles of varying size

KEY DIFFERENTIATING FEATURES
  round nucleus with clock-face chromatin pattern
  paranuclear hof
  abundant dark blue cytoplasm

OTHER FINDINGS
  normal cell seen in bone marrow; rarely seen in normal blood films

POTENTIAL LOOK-ALIKES
  immature plasma cells
  osteoclasts
  reactive lymphocytes (plasmacytoid forms)
  lymphoma cells
  polychromatophilic normoblasts

ASSOCIATED DISEASE STATES AND CONDITIONS
  chronic infectious or inflammatory conditions
    bacterial (streptococcal sepsis, typhoid, endocarditis)
    viral (Epstein-Barr, HIV, mumps, rubella)
    parasites (malaria)
  malignancies including lymphomas
  autoimmune disorders
  alcoholic liver disease and cirrhosis
  drug reactions and hypersensitivity reactions
  sarcoidosis
  granulomatous disease
  monoclonal gammopathy of undetermined significance

Plasma cells are a normal constituent of the bone marrow, lymph nodes, spleen, gastrointestinal tract, and connective tissues. They are rarely seen in a normal blood film. Increased numbers in the blood or bone marrow are associated with a variety of chronic infectious and inflammatory disorders that result in increased antibody production. Plasmacytosis in the blood can be found in bacterial infections (streptococcus, syphilis, tuberculosis), viral infections (Epstein-Barr, HIV, mumps, rubella, rubeola), protozoal infections (malaria, trichinosis), chronic liver disease, autoimmune and collagen vascular disorders, various malignancies, drug and toxin exposure, hypersensitivity reactions, and serum sickness. Bone marrow plasmacytosis can be found in similar circumstances and also in Hodgkin's disease, non-Hodgkin's lymphoma, various anemias, myeloproliferative and myelodysplastic disorders, aplastic anemia, granulomatous diseases, diabetes mellitus, amyloidosis, and monoclonal gammopathy of undetermined significance (benign monoclonal gammopathy).

Plasma cells are generally easy to recognize. They are medium size, round to oval cells with moderate to abundant cytoplasm and eccentric nuclei. Their nuclei are generally round to ovoid and have prominently coarse and clumped chromatin that is often arranged in a cartwheel-like or clock-face pattern. Nucleoli are absent. The cytoplasm stains gray-blue to deeply basophilic. A prominent hof or paranuclear zone of pale or lighter staining cytoplasm is seen towards one side of the nucleus. This area corresponds to the Golgi zone, which is prominent in cells which produce large

Normal Plasma Cell

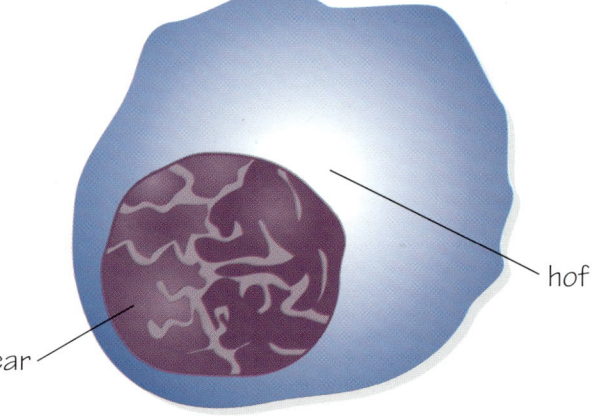

hof
clumped nuclear chromatin

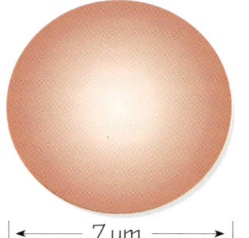

|← 7 μm →|
size of normal red blood cell

Lymphocytic and Plasmacytic Cells

amounts of protein (immunoglobulins in the case of plasma cells). Granules are absent and scattered vacuoles of varying size may be seen. In some cases of malignancy, plasma cells may show a pink-red cytoplasm. These cells are called *flame cells.*

While mature plasma cells have a distinctive appearance, they may be confused with morphologically immature plasma cells, plasma cells, or precursors with inclusion bodies, some reactive lymphocytes (plasmacytoid forms), some lymphoma cells, and normoblastic or megaloblastic polychromatophilic normoblasts in the bone marrow. Generally, these cell types show a different, often immature, nuclear chromatin pattern and may have distinct nucleoli. Also, the cytoplasmic hof will be absent or smaller and less prominent than in mature plasma cells. These cells have less abundant cytoplasm and a higher nuclear to cytoplasmic ratio. When cytoplasmic inclusions are noted within an otherwise mature appearing plasma cell, the preferred identification is plasma cell or precursor with inclusion body. Osteoclasts may also closely resemble plasma cells, but these cells have a cytoplasmic clear zone away from the nucleus (See *Osteoclast* page 340 and *A Closer Look At...Osteoblast vs. Plasma Cell*, page 338).

HE-28, 1995 (Blood, Wright-Giemsa, X375)

Identification	Referee %	Participant %
Plasma cell, mature	96.4	85.4
Nucleated red cell, megaloblastoid or dysplastic	3.6	3.7
Plasma cell, immature	-	3.7

A normal mature plasma cell is seen in this blood film. The red cells show mild artifactual changes. A few platelets are present. The plasma cell has an eccentric round nucleus with clumped masses of chromatin. No nucleoli are visible. A prominent perinuclear hof is seen within the abundant, deeply basophilic cytoplasm. A smudge/basket cell is located in the upper right side of the photomicrograph.

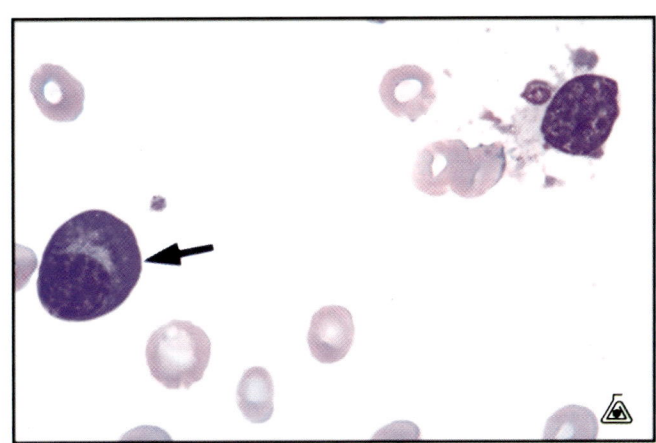

Variations of Normal Plasma Cells

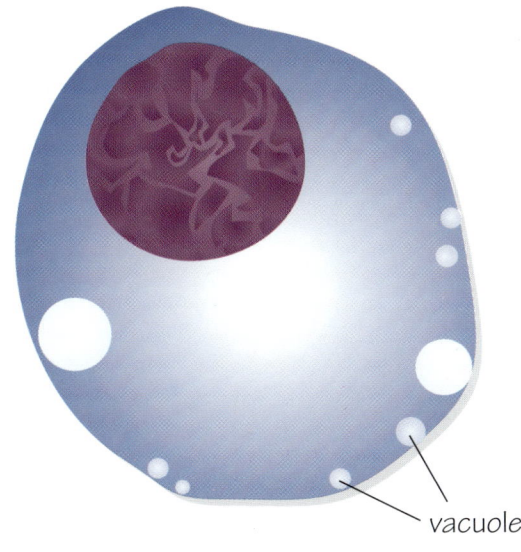

vacuoles

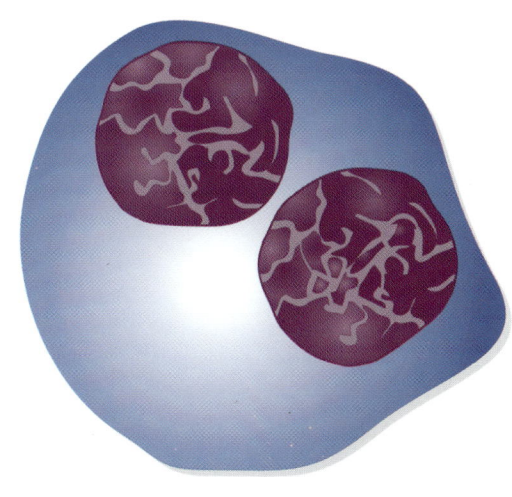

binucleation

Lymphocytic and Plasmacytic Cells

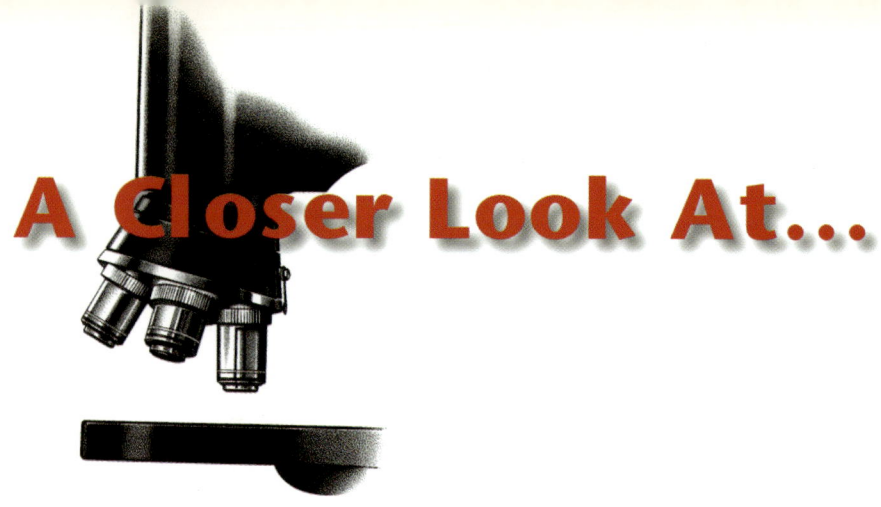

A Closer Look At...

Plasma Cell Maturation

Plasma cells are the most mature form of B-lymphocytes. Three recognizable stages of maturation have been described. The most immature form is the immunoblast or plasmablast. While some investigators feel that plasmablasts are derived from immunoblasts and they are two different stages of maturation, others feel that since these cells are difficult if not impossible to distinguish morphologically, they should be considered the same cell. The next recognizable stage is the proplasmacyte that then develops into a mature plasma cell.

Immunoblasts/plasmablasts are the largest and least mature form in the maturation sequence. These round to oval cells are moderate to large in size (25-40 µm) and may have a smooth cytoplasmic surface. Frequently, the cytoplasmic edges are ragged with bleb and bud formation. The nuclei are round to oval and may be eccentric or centrally placed. The N:C ratio is high at 2:1 to 1:1. The chromatin is finely dispersed with distinct parachromatin and one or more prominent nucleoli are present. A scant to moderate amount of pale to deep blue cytoplasm is present and a small, poorly demarcated, paranuclear area of clearing called a *hof* is often present. Occasional small vacuoles may be seen and sometimes immunoglobulin inclusions (Russell bodies) are present.

Proplasmacytes are intermediate between plasmablasts and mature plasma cells. These cells are moderate to large (15-30 µm) and generally contain a single, round or oval, often eccentric nucleus. The N:C ratio ranges from 1.5:1 to 1:1. The chromatin is fine to moderately coarse and tends to form small aggregates that are more notable adjacent to the nuclear membrane. Therefore, smaller areas of visible parachromatin are present. One to two small nucleoli are often seen. The cytoplasm stains pale to deep blue and a hof is easily identified. Granules are absent and scattered vacuoles of varying size may be seen. Immunoglobulin inclusions (Russell bodies) can be found in some cases.

Immature plasma cells have a variety of appearances and may be confused with morphologically mature plasma cells, plasma cells, or precursors with inclusion bodies, some reactive lymphocytes (plasmacytoid forms), some lymphoma cells, and polychromatophilic and basophilic nucleated red blood cells (both normoblastic and megaloblastic) in the bone marrow. The most atypical forms can sometimes be difficult to distinguish from blasts (myeloblasts and lymphoblasts) and pronormoblasts. Mature plasma cells display coarsely clumped chromatin, a lower nuclear to cytoplasmic ratio, and a prominent cytoplasmic hof. In the majority of these other cell types, the cytoplasmic hof will be absent or smaller than in immature plasma cells.

Plasma Cell Maturation

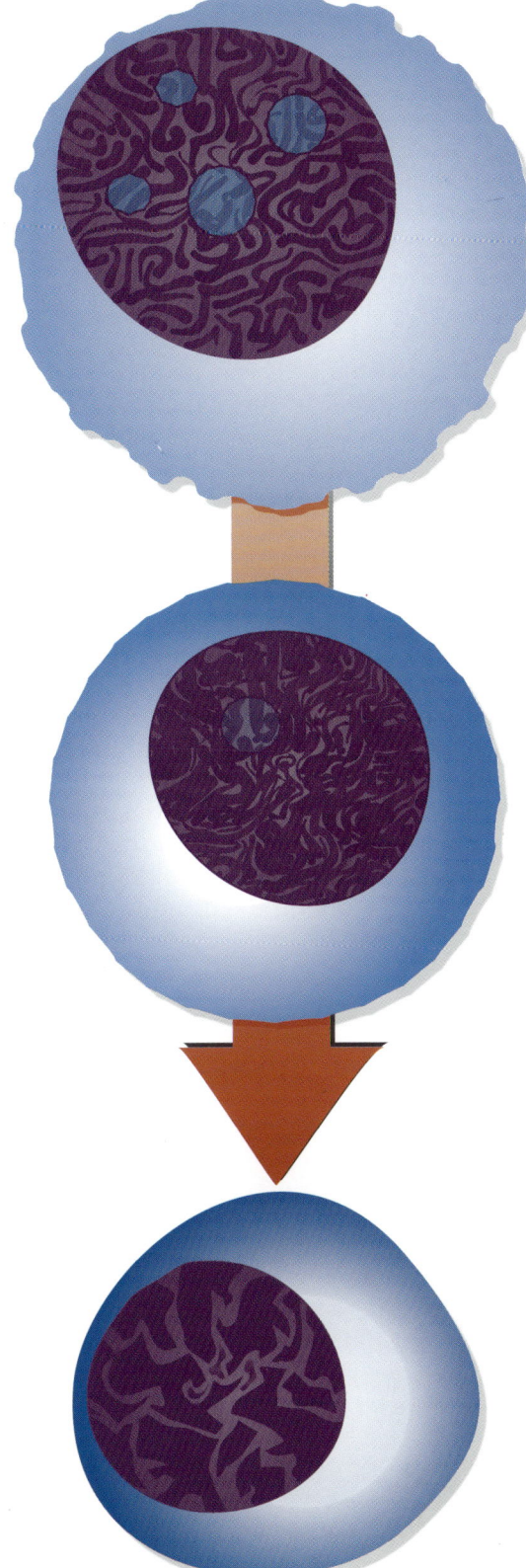

Plasmablast

- 25-40 μm
- cytoplasm
    - light or moderately blue cytoplasm
    - indistinct hof
- nucleus
    - eccentrically located
    - round or oval
    - fine chromatin
- nucleoli
    - 0 to 6, well demarcated

Proplasmacyte

- 15-30 μm
- cytoplasm
    - moderate to dark blue
    - distinct paranuclear hof
- nucleus
    - eccentrically located
    - round or oval
    - thick nuclear membrane
    - moderately clumped chromatin
- nucleoli
    - 1 to 2, partially masked by chromatin

Plasma Cell

- 7-25 μm
- cytoplasm
    - very dark blue
    - distinct paranuclear hof
- nucleus
    - eccentrically located
    - round
    - thick nuclear membrane
    - significantly clumped chromatin
- nucleoli
    - none

Plasma Cell, Immature or Abnormal (Myeloma Cell)

SYNONYMS
plasmablast, proplasmablast, myeloma cell, atypical plasma cell, immature plasma cell

VITAL STATISTICS
- size .... 15 to 25 µm
- N:C ratio .... 2:1 to 1:1
- cell shape .... round to oval
- nuclear shape ... round to oval; central or eccentric; can be binucleated or multinucleated
- chromatin .... ranges from moderately coarse to finely reticulated; parachromatin scant to abundant and distinct
- nucleoli .... often present; may be multiple; range from small to large and prominent
- cytoplasm .... scant to moderate; pale to dark blue; small to variably-sized perinuclear clear zone (hof); agranular; may be vacuolated

KEY DIFFERENTIATING FEATURES
eccentrically located round nucleus; immature chromatin
single or multiple nucleoli
moderate blue cytoplasm with paranuclear hof

OTHER FINDINGS
seldom found in normal bone marrow and in nonmalignant conditions
rarely seen in blood films except in plasma cell leukemia
associated with plasma cell dyscrasias, amyloidosis, lytic bone lesions, pathologic fractures, and renal failure
rouleaux formation may be prominent on the blood film

POTENTIAL LOOK-ALIKES
morphologically mature plasma cells
plasma cells or precursors with inclusion bodies
osteoclasts
reactive lymphocytes (plasmacytoid forms)
lymphoma cells
normoblastic and megaloblastic polychromatophilic and basophilic normoblasts in the bone marrow
blasts (myeloblasts, lymphoblasts, pronormoblasts)

ASSOCIATED DISEASE STATES AND CONDITIONS
multiple myeloma
monoclonal gammopathy of undetermined significance
plasmacytoma
amyloidosis
plasma cell leukemia (large numbers of circulating cells)

Immature plasma cells (immunoblasts/plasmablasts and proplasmacytes) are a normal constituent of the bone marrow; however, these cells are present in very low numbers and are rarely identified in nonmalignant conditions. Increased numbers of these immature or atypical plasma cells in the bone marrow are associated with a variety of plasma cell dyscrasias including multiple myeloma, monoclonal gammopathy of undetermined significance, plasmacytoma, and amyloidosis. Large numbers (2000 X 10^9/L or 20% plasma cells in the differential) of circulating immature plasma cells are present in plasma cell leukemia. Lower numbers of circulating immature plasma cells can be seen in multiple myeloma and other plasma cell dyscrasias.

Immature plasma cells can range from those that are easily recognized to those that are almost impossible to classify without supplemental stains or special techniques like flow cytometry or electron microscopy. See *A Closer Look At... Plasma Cell Maturation* on page 240 for a more detailed description.

Malignant plasma cells, as seen in multiple myeloma, may show a variety of morphologic features and may include some or all forms of immunoblasts/plasmablasts, proplasmacytes, and mature plasma cells. Binucleated and multinucleated forms may be frequent and, when present, often display immature nuclear characteristics. Atypical mitotic figures may also be found.

The diagnosis of multiple myeloma can be difficult. Bone marrow plasma cells may be increased in a number of benign conditions. The following criteria are generally used to confirm the diagnosis.

Abnormal Plasma Cell

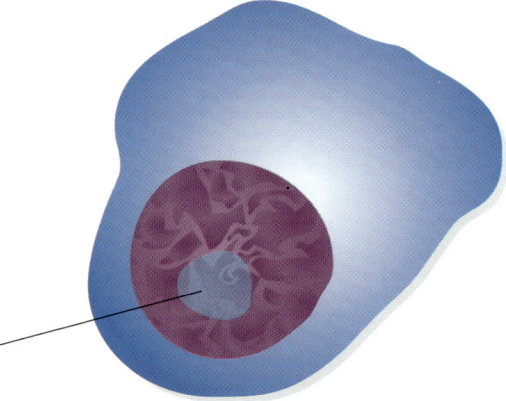

prominent nucleolus

the larger the nucleolus, the more likely the cell is malignant

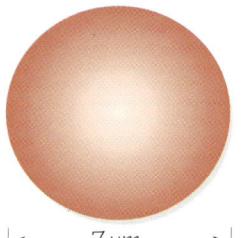

|← 7 µm →|
size of normal red blood cell

Major Criteria
  I. Plasmacytoma on tissue biopsy
  II. Marrow plasmacytosis with >30% plasma cells
  III. Monoclonal globulin spike on serum protein electrophoresis >3.5 g/dL for IgG or >2.0 g/dL for IgA, or 1.0 g/24 hr of kappa or lambda light chain excretion on urine protein electrophoresis in the absence of amyloidosis

Minor Criteria
  a. Marrow plasmacytosis with 10-30% plasma cells
  b. Monoclonal globulin spike present, but less than the levels defined above
  c. Lytic bone lesions
  d. Normal IgM <50 mg/dL, IgA <100 mg/dL, or IgG <600 mg/dL

Multiple myeloma can be diagnosed when specific combinations of major and minor criteria are present in symptomatic patients with clearly progressive disease. The diagnosis requires a minimum of one major plus one minor criterion or three minor criteria that must include a and b. Possible combinations are listed below. Of note, the finding of plasmacytoma on tissue biopsy and a bone marrow plasmacytosis of 30% or less is not sufficient for a diagnosis of multiple myeloma.

1. I + b, I + c, I + d (I + a is not sufficient)
2. II + b, II + c, II + d
3. III + a, III + c, III + d
4. a + b + c, a + b + d

H1-4, 1983 (Bone Marrow, Wright-Giemsa, X350)

Identification	Referee %	Participant %
Plasma cell, immature	92.8	85.8

This bone marrow smear shows a plasmablast. The other cells present in the field are difficult to identify due to artifacts and the thickness of the smear in this area. The nucleus of either a band or segmented neutrophil is present in the upper right. The arrowed cell is very large with a round nucleus, moderately coarse and homogeneous chromatin, and a single, prominent central nucleolus. It has an abundant amount of eccentric, deeply basophilic cytoplasm. The paranuclear hof is not visible. No granules are present in the cytoplasm. This case is from a 72-year-old white male with multiple myeloma.

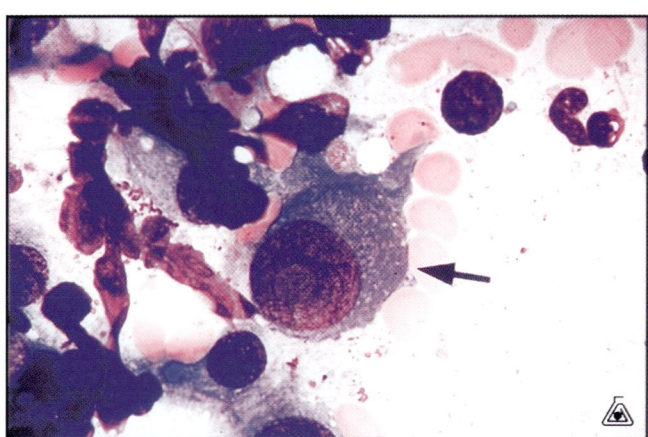

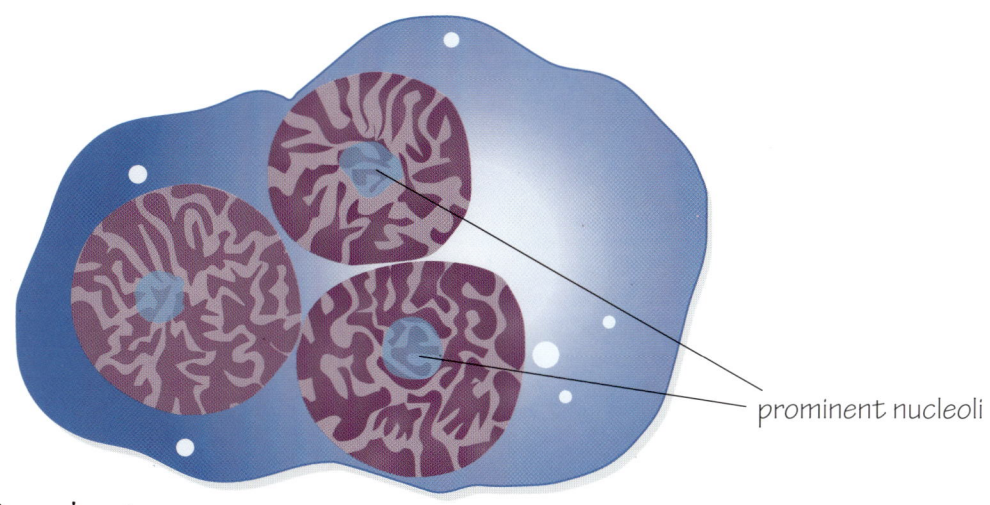

Abnormal Plasma Cell

trinucleate — prominent nucleoli

Plasma Cell or Precursor with Inclusion Body

SYNONYMS
flame cells, Mott cells, grape cells, morula cells

VITAL STATISTICS

size	10 to 25 µm
N:C ratio	1:2 to 1:3
cell shape	round to oval
nuclear shape	round to oval; usually eccentric; sometimes binucleated and rarely multinucleated
chromatin	coarse and clumped with dense masses often arranged in a clock-face or wheel-like pattern; parachromatin absent or scant
nucleoli	absent
cytoplasm	moderate to abundant; staining ranges from blue-gray to medium blue to deeply basophilic; may be pink-red (flame cells); contains single or multiple large, eosinophilic inclusions (Russell bodies), intranuclear inclusions (Dutcher bodies), or crystals that are granular, elongated or diamond-shaped; the crystals are colorless or stain blue, purple, or bright red

KEY DIFFERENTIATING FEATURES
cells exhibit nuclear characteristics of plasma cell with either unusual colored cytoplasm (flame cell) or presence of single or multiple cytoplasmic inclusions (Russell bodies), intranuclear inclusions (Dutcher bodies), or crystalline inclusions
presence of cytoplasmic hof may be helpful

POTENTIAL LOOK-ALIKES
mature and immature plasma cells
reactive lymphocytes (plasmacytoid forms)
some lymphoma cells
macrophages (lipophage, Niemann-Pick cell, phagocytized organisms)

ASSOCIATED DISEASE STATES AND CONDITIONS
normal finding (a few cells may be present)
increased numbers seen in any condition associated with bone marrow plasmacytosis (see listing under *Plasma Cell, Mature*, page 238 or *Plasma Cell, Immature or Abnormal*, page 242)

Plasma cells are the most mature form of B lymphocytes and normally produce and secrete immunoglobulins. This protein product may appear in different forms within the cytoplasm of the cell. When production within a particular plasma cell is increased or secretion is blocked, immunoglobulins accumulate. This finding can occur in mature, immature, or malignant plasma cells.

These immunoglobulin accumulations often appear as large eosinophilic cytoplasmic globules called Russell bodies. Sometimes intranuclear inclusions called Dutcher bodies are seen. While Dutcher bodies appear to be within the nucleus, they are actually pseudoinclusions that occur when a cytoplasmic globule invaginates through the nucleus or is surrounded by the nucleus. The nuclear membrane remains intact and, therefore, Dutcher bodies are actually within the cytoplasm, not the nucleus.

When multiple Russell bodies are present, these cells are called "Mott cells." If the Russell bodies are numerous and form a cluster or occupy the entire cytoplasm, the cell is called a "grape cell" or a "morula cell." These cells are often confused with macrophages containing lipid or ingested microorganisms. However, grape cells contain multiple, often refractile globules of similar size. Frequently, these globules stain red or eosinophilic, but they may appear pale pink or be colorless. The nucleus remains visible and exhibits the character-

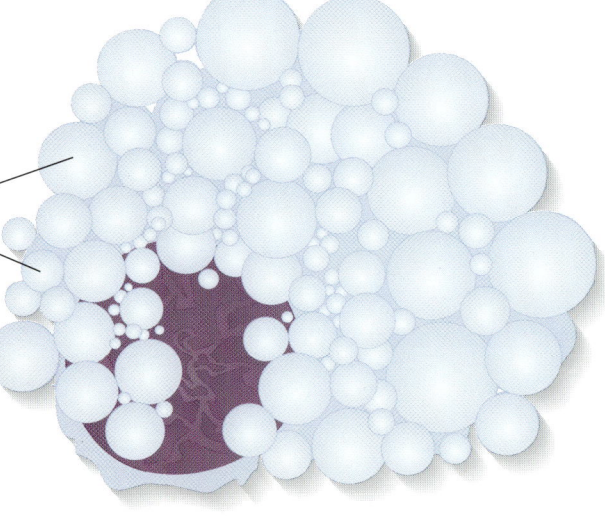

Mott Cell

Russell Bodies

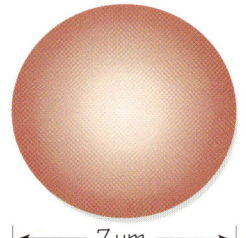

|← 7 µm →|
size of normal red blood cell

istic clumped chromatin pattern of plasma cells. A hof may often be seen, despite the presence of numerous Russell bodies.

Occasionally, the immunoglobulin can crystallize or combine with other compounds and form elongated or diamond-shaped cytoplasmic crystals. These crystals can be colorless or stain blue, purple, or bright red. Sometimes proteins will form small granules within plasma cells. In all these cases, the nuclear morphology of the plasma cell is similar with clumped chromatin that often forms a cartwheel or spoke-like pattern. The cytoplasmic hof is frequently present and often prominent and the cytoplasm stains pale to deep blue.

Flame cells are plasma cells with bright red to pink cytoplasm. They can be found in normal individuals, in cases associated with chronic infections or inflammation, and in cases of malignancy including various plasma cell dyscrasias such as multiple myeloma, amyloidosis, and monoclonal gammopathy of undetermined significance.

HE-29, 1995 (Bone Marrow, Wright-Giemsa, X250)

Identification	Referee %	Participant %
Plasma cell with inclusion body	70.4	52.1
Macrophage	11.1	16.2
Lipophage	7.4	11.4
Niemann-Pick cell	-	6.1

This split screen photomicrograph exhibits two different plasma cells with inclusion bodies. Both views are from bone marrow smears. The arrowed cell on the left is very large with two ovoid nuclei. The chromatin pattern is clumped, forming dense masses. The abundant dark blue cytoplasm is filled with uniform round, colorless inclusions (Russell bodies). The arrowed cell on the right is very large and has an eccentric round nucleus with dark compact chromatin. The cytoplasm contains multiple ovoid blue-green inclusions (Russell bodies). Two orthochromic normoblasts are also present.

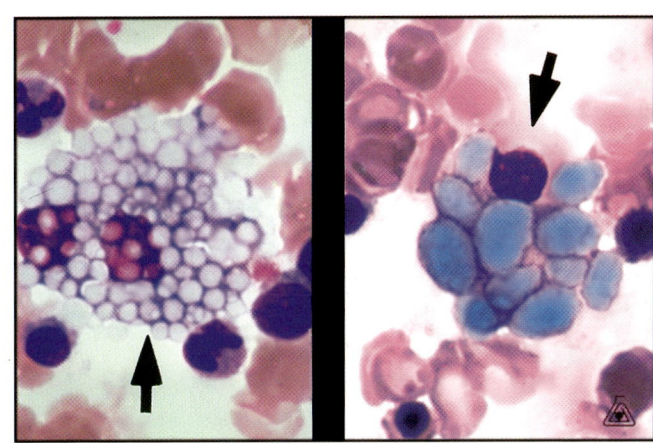

Plasma Cells with Cytoplasmic Inclusions

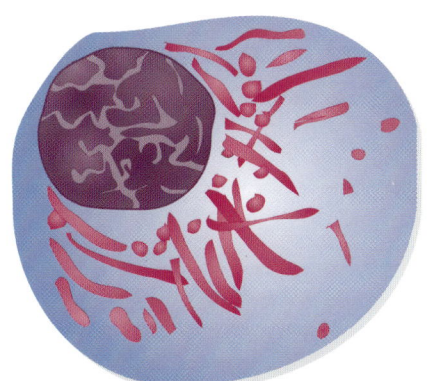

crystaline-like inclusions

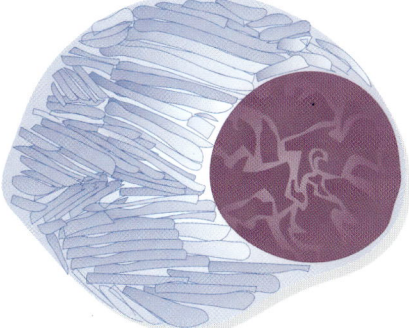

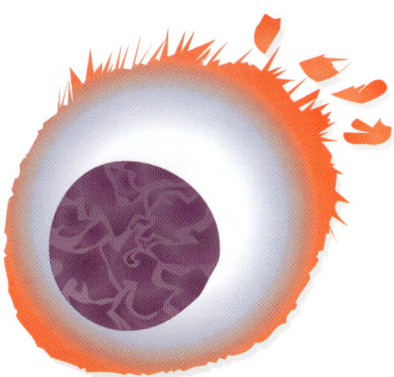

flame cell

flame cells are due to plugging of peripheral secretory channels by precipitated immunoglobulin; peripheral cytoplasm may fragment away

Prolymphocyte

SYNONYMS
none

VITAL STATISTICS
- size .... 10 to 18 µm
- N:C ratio .... 5:1 to 3:1
- cell shape .... round to ovoid
- nuclear shape .... round to oval; may be slightly indented; centrally placed
- chromatin .... somewhat condensed; coarser than in lymphoblasts and more open than in lymphocytes; parachromatin is indistinct
- nucleoli .... typically single and prominent; rarely may have two nucleoli
- cytoplasm .... moderate amount; stains homogeneously blue and may contain a few azurophilic granules

KEY DIFFERENTIATING FEATURES
- similar size to lymphoblasts and larger than mature lymphocytes
- centrally placed nucleus with high N:C ratio
- larger amount of cytoplasm than blasts or lymphocytes
- chromatin is moderately condensed
- single, prominent nucleolus
- cytoplasm stains homogeneous blue

OTHER FINDINGS
- lymphocytosis, often marked
- splenomegaly, anemia, and thrombocytopenia are frequent
- small numbers seen in chronic lymphocytic leukemia
- increased numbers found in prolymphocytic leukemia

POTENTIAL LOOK-ALIKES
- blasts (myeloblasts, monoblasts, lymphoblasts)
- malignant lymphoma cells
- reactive lymphocytes

ASSOCIATED DISEASE STATES AND CONDITIONS
- chronic lymphocytic leukemia
- prolymphocytoid transformation of chronic lymphocytic leukemia
- prolymphocytic leukemia

Prolymphocytes are not detected in normal blood films or bone marrow smears. These abnormal cells are most commonly seen in cases of chronic lymphocytic leukemia (CLL) where they typically comprise less than 10 percent of lymphoid cells. They can also be found in prolymphocytoid transformation of CLL and pro-lymphocytic leukemia (PLL).

These round to ovoid cells range from 10 to 18 µm and their N:C ratio varies from 5:1 to 3:1. Prolymphocytes are larger than normal lymphocytes and the typical lymphoid cells in CLL and are similar in size to lymphoblasts. A centrally placed, oval to round nucleus and a moderate amount of homogeneously staining blue cytoplasm is typical. The cytoplasm is more abundant than in normal lymphocytes and blasts. It may rarely contain a few, small azurophilic granules. The nucleus shows condensed chromatin (coarser than in lymphoblasts and more open than in mature lymphocytes) with indistinct parachromatin and, typically, a single, prominent nucleolus. Rarely, these cells may exhibit more than one nucleolus. See *A Closer Look At... Prolymphocytes* on page 248 for a more detailed discussion.

Prolymphocytes

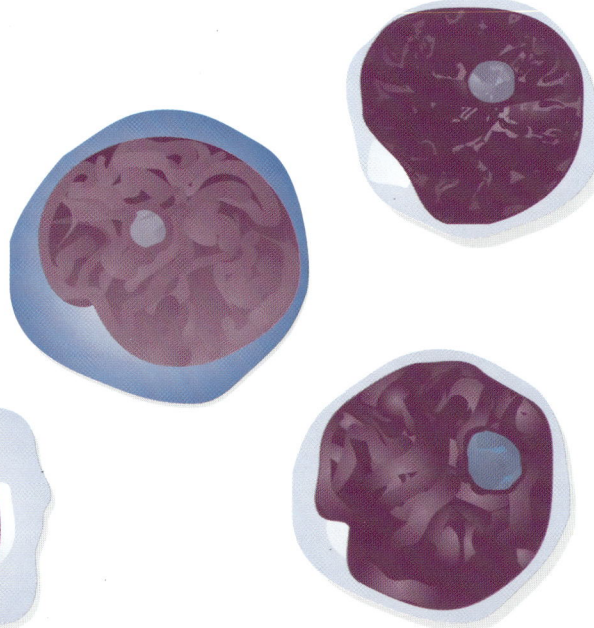

all have clumped chromatin and a single prominent nucleolus

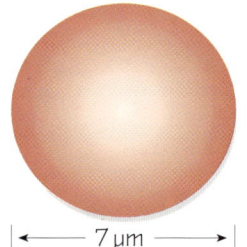

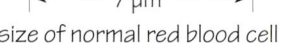

size of normal red blood cell

HE-28, 1996 (Blood, Wright-Giemsa, X380)

Identification	Referee %	Participant %
Prolymphocyte	84.6	56.6
Lymphocyte, mature	7.7	8.1
Lymphoycte, reactive	3.8	6.5
Lymphoblast	3.8	20.3

Four prolymphocytes are present in this blood film. The red blood cells are normocytic. A few platelets are visible. The lymphocytes are large cells with oval to slightly angulated nuclei containing moderately coarse chromatin. Each has a single, prominent nucleolus. There is a moderate amount of pale blue, agranular cytoplasm. This photomicrograph is from a patient with CLL that has undergone prolymphocytoid transformation.

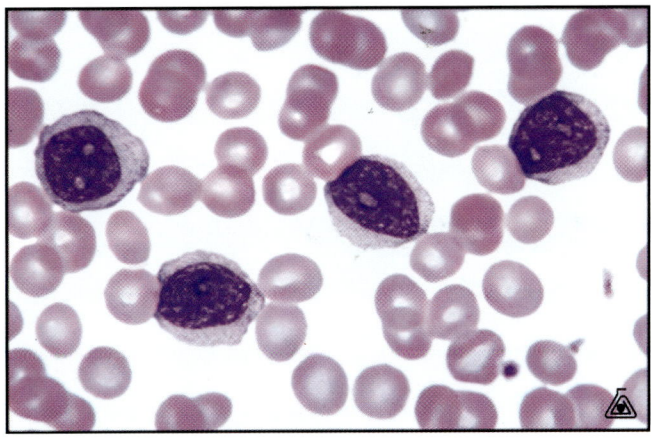

H-23, 1980 (Blood, Wright-Giemsa, X400)

Identification	Referee %	Participant %
Prolymphocyte	28.6	54.2
Lymphoblast	42.9	29.4
Lymphocyte, reactive	14.3	7.2
Blast cell	14.3	3.2

This blood film shows a prolymphocyte in a field of smaller lymphocytes. One normal appearing platelet is present. Red blood cells are normochromic and normocytic. Some have some dirt lying on top of them. The arrowed cell is slightly larger than the other lymphocytes. It has moderately coarse chromatin which appears slightly more open than the other cells. A single, prominent, central nucleolus is present. The cytoplasm is moderately basophilic and agranular. This cell has slightly more cytoplasm than the other lymphoid cells in the field. While some of the non-arrowed lymphoid cells have one or two of these characteristics, they lack a prominent nucleolus and, thus, are not prolymphocytes. Rather, these cells are the typical lymphocytes seen in chronic lymphocytic leukemia.

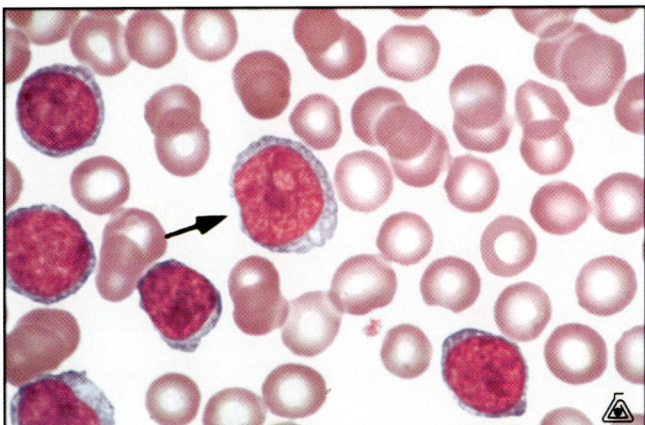

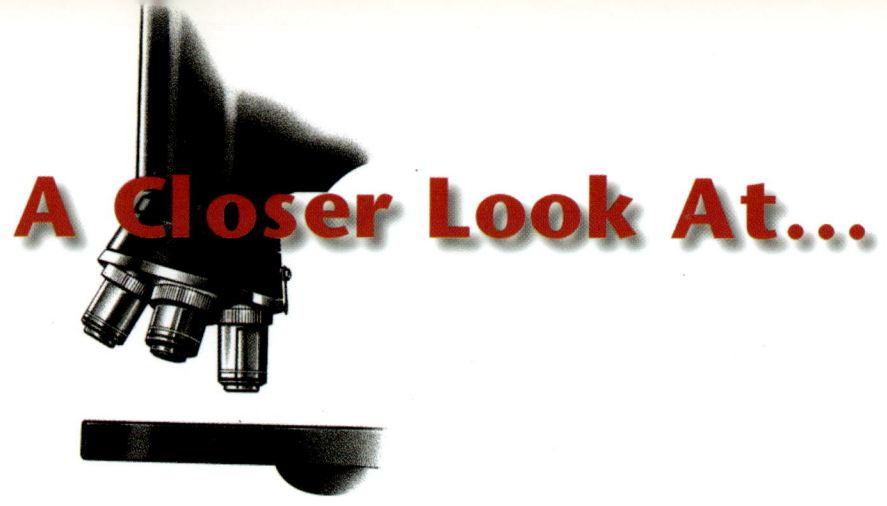

A Closer Look At...

Prolymphocytes

Prolymphocytes are abnormal cells that can be confused with lymphoblasts, reactive lymphocytes, and lymphoma cells. While these cells are lymphoma cells, they exhibit a characteristic morphologic appearance that usually allows their specific identification. Most commonly, prolymphocytes are seen in cases of chronic lymphocytic leukemia (CLL). However, they are also found in patients with prolymphocytoid transformation of CLL and prolymphocytic leukemia. When present in classic CLL, prolymphocytes usually comprise less than 10% of the lymphoid cells. In these cases, prolymphocytes are generally fairly easily recognized when contrasted to the remainder of the mature appearing small lymphocytes.

While only a small percentage of lymphocytes in most cases of CLL are prolymphocytes, one subgroup of CLL has been described that shows a dimorphic population of lymphoid cells. These cases of "mixed cell type" CLL have between 10 and 55% prolymphocytes and appear to have a worse prognosis than classic B cell CLL. In contrast, a second kind of mixed cell type CLL has been recognized. Patients with this disorder have a spectrum of lymphoid cells ranging from small to large. However, prolymphocytes comprise less than 10% of the lymphoid cells. The prognosis of this subtype of CLL appears similar to classic CLL.

Transformation of CLL into a more aggressive disease can occur when the proportion of prolymphocytes increases (prolymphocytoid transformation). These cases often have an insidious onset and are associated with an increasing white blood count, enlarging spleen and lymph nodes, and increased proportion of prolymphocytes from the patient's baseline. Unfortunately, there is no consensus in the literature regarding the proportion of prolymphocytes necessary to classify a case of prolymphocytoid transformation in CLL and numbers have ranged from 10 to 55%.

In contrast, prolymphocytic leukemia (PLL) is a more aggressive disease and defined by the presence of greater than 55% prolymphocytes in the blood. Some of these cases can arise de novo; however, many result from transformation of CLL. Cases of PLL typically have a white blood count greater than $100 \times 10^9/L$, massive splenomegaly, and no adenopathy except in the terminal stages. About 50% of patients are over 70 years old at diagnosis. In contrast to the lymphocytes of CLL, prolymphocytes are reported to show a slightly different immunophenotype by flow cytometry. Cases of PLL typically are negative or weak for CD5, show stronger expression of surface immunoglobulin, and may have stronger expression of CD20 and CD22 than cases of classic CLL.

The table and illustrations on the next page compare important features of various subtypes of CLL and PLL as well as the small cell type of follicular center cell lymphoma.

Morphology of Small Cell Lymphocytic Neoplastic Disorders

	Size	Nuclear Outline	Chromatin	Nucleolus	Cytoplasm	Azurophilic Granules
B CLL	<2 RBCs	usually regular; 15% of cases are reniform (Rieder cells)	clumped in block-like pattern	absent	scant	none
T CLL (CD4+)	<2 RBCs	irregular, notched, convoluted	clumped	absent	moderate	none
T CLL (CD8+) (large granular lymphocytes)	>2 RBCs	reniform or oblong; smoothly indented	clumped	absent or inconspicuous	moderate	numerous
CLL mixed with large cells	>2 RBCs	usually regular	clumped	small or inconspicuous	variable; may be abundant	none
CLL mixed with prolymphocytes	>2 RBCs	usually regular	clumped	single, central, prominent	moderate	none
B PLL	>2 RBCs	65% regular; 20% clefted	clumped	prominent, single	moderate	rare
T PLL	>2 RBCs	50% very irregular	clumped	prominent, single	abundant	often numerous
Follicular lymphoma (small cell type)	1-2 RBCs	reniform, clefted (buttock cells)	coarse; evenly distributed	absent or 1-2 inconspicuous	scant	none

Prolymphocytes in Chronic Leukemias

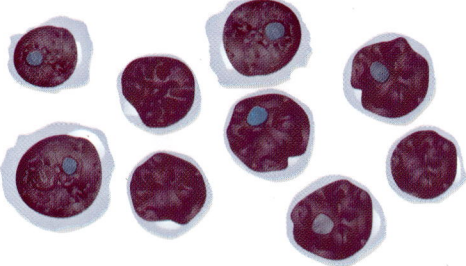

Prolymphocytic Leukemia
(>55% prolymphocytes)

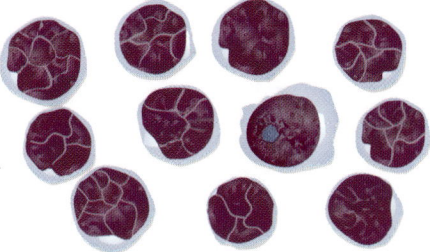

CLL (B cell type)
(<10% prolymphocytes)

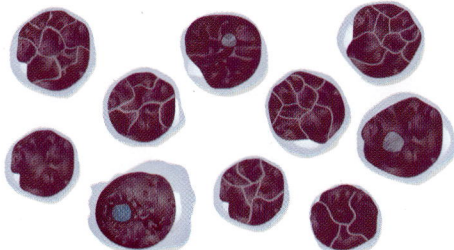

Mixed CLL
(10-55% prolymphocytes)

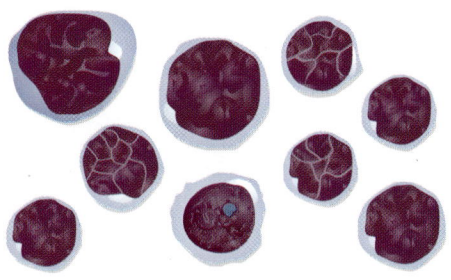

Mixed CLL
(variable numbers of large cells with <10% prolymphocytes)

Sézary Cell

SYNONYMS
cutaneous T cell lymphoma, mycosis fungoides

VITAL STATISTICS
- size .... 8 to 20 μm
- N:C ratio .... 7:1 to 3:1
- cell shape .... round or oval, can be irregular
- nuclear shape .... irregular with varying degrees of folding, grooving, and convolutions (cerebriform or snake-like)
- chromatin .... hyperchromatic with dense clumping in smaller cells; larger cells may show more open, dispersed chromatin; parachromatin is absent or scant
- nucleoli .... inconspicuous or not seen; rarely, larger cells may have a single, small, nucleolus
- cytoplasm .... scant, pale, and basophilic; agranular; occasional cells may have multiple, small, clear vacuoles that closely surround the nucleus

KEY DIFFERENTIATING FEATURES
lymphoid cells with prominently folded, convoluted, often cerebriform nuclei
the chromatin is hyperchromatic and cytoplasm scant
cells may be slightly larger to twice the size of normal lymphocytes

OTHER FINDINGS
some cases have lymphocytosis
patients generally have widespread, erythematous skin lesions of mycosis fungoides, lymphadenopathy, splenomegaly, and bone marrow involvement
anemia and thrombocytopenia may be found with extensive disease

POTENTIAL LOOK-ALIKES
atypical or reactive lymphocytes
malignant lymphoma (both B and T cell types, often with cleaved cell morphology)
normal lymphocytes (generally T cells)

ASSOCIATED DISEASE STATES AND CONDITIONS
mycosis fungoides
Sézary syndrome
benign dermatoses including eczema, psoriasis, and lichen planus
HIV infection and other viral illnesses

Sézary cells are classically found in patients with mycosis fungoides, which is a cutaneous T cell lymphoma. Sézary syndrome refers to the stage of this disease characterized by diffuse, extensive skin involvement that gives it a red, scalded appearance called erythroderma, extreme pruritus, lymphadenopathy, splenomegaly, and a leukemic blood picture. These individuals frequently have increased white blood counts that can reach greater than 200×10^9/L composed predominantly of abnormal, atypical lymphoid cells. Sézary cells can also be found in patients with earlier stages of mycosis fungoides, but are present in lower numbers.

Sézary cells are usually round to oval but can be irregular. They range in size from 8 to 20 μm and the N:C ratio varies from 7:1 to 3:1. Smaller Sézary cells are slightly bigger than normal lymphocytes and have folded, grooved, or convoluted nuclear membranes that may give them a cerebriform appearance. The chromatin is dark and hyperchromatic without visible

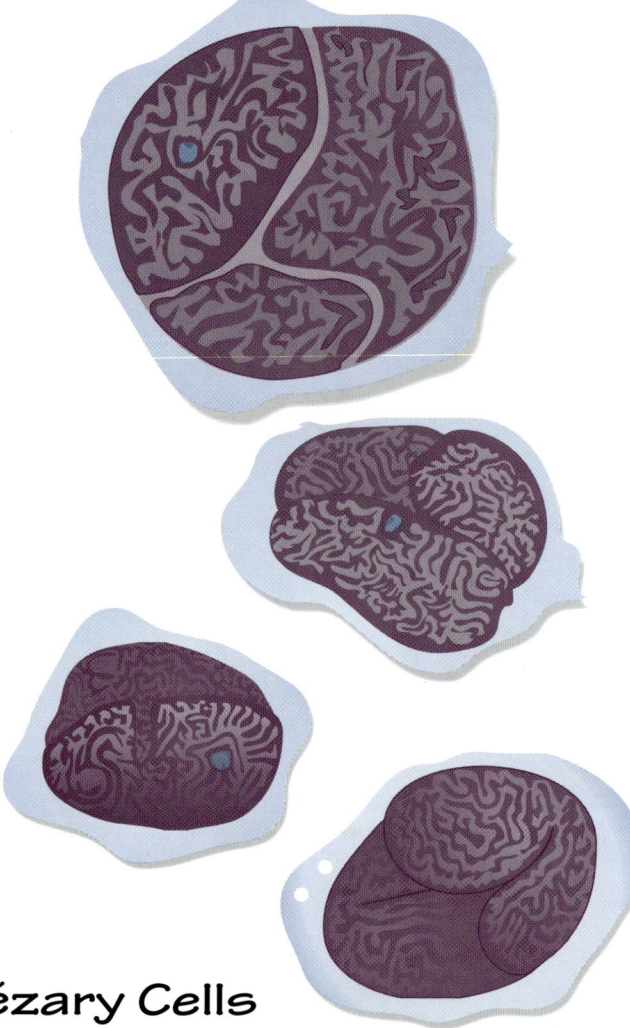

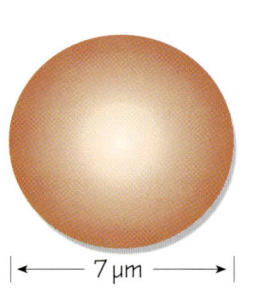
7 μm
size of normal red blood cell

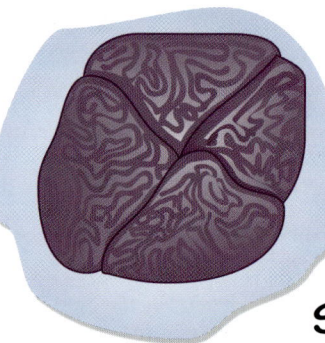

Sézary Cells

nucleoli. The pale, blue to gray cytoplasm is scant and may contain from one to two dozen small, vacuoles that lie adjacent to the nucleus. Larger Sézary cells can be more than twice the size of normal lymphocytes. The nucleus is also convoluted and cerebriform with hyperchromatic chromatin. Often the nuclear membrane is so tortuous and folded that the nucleus may appear lobulated or even like a cluster of berries. Some cells may exhibit a small nucleolus; this finding is not a prominent feature. The larger cells also have a scant amount of pale blue, agranular cytoplasm.

While the appearance of Sézary cells is distinctive, occasionally other cells may exhibit similar morphology. Some reactive lymphocytes can be indistinguishable. Other kinds of T cell lymphomas, such as HTLV-associated adult T cell lymphoma/leukemia, may have similar appearing cells. Some cases of follicular center B cell lymphoma can mimic Sézary cells and require special studies such as immunophenotyping to obtain the correct diagnosis. Also, many authors have described low proportions of Sézary-like cells, comprising up to 6% of lymphocytes, in normal healthy individuals.

Immunophenotyping by flow cytometry has demonstrated that Sézary cells are helper-inducer (CD4 positive) T cells in the majority of cases. In contrast, the Sézary-like cells described in other, non-malignant conditions are typically CD8 positive T cells.

HE-11, 1996 (Blood, Wright-Giemsa, X400)

Identification	Referee %	Participant %
Sézary cell	68	39.5
Lymphoma cell	12	5.3
Monocyte, immature	12	34.1
Monocyte	4	11.3

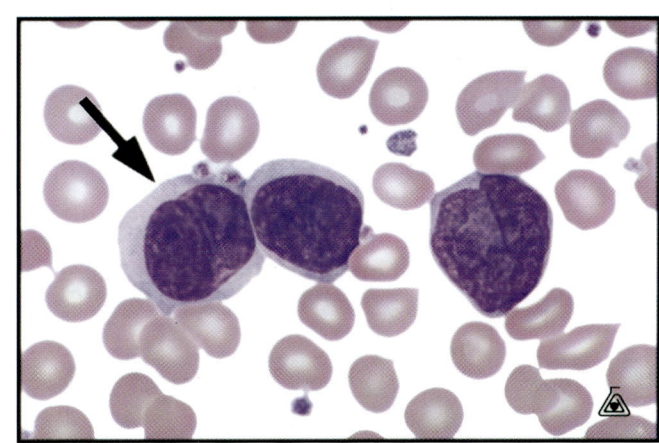

Three Sézary cells are featured in this photomicrograph. The red blood cells display mild poikilocytosis and a spherocyte is on the left side. Scattered normal platelets are visible. The arrowed cell is large with an ovoid, folded nucleus containing fine to moderately coarse chromatin. No nucleoli are seen. The moderate amount of pale blue cytoplasm is agranular. The other two cells are also Sézary cells. The cell in the center has an oval nucleus without folds, while the one on the left shows a prominent nuclear cleft with scant cytoplasm.

HE-12, 1996 (Blood, Wright-Giemsa, X400)

Identification	Referee %	Participant %
Sézary cell	75	38.4
Lymphoma cell	7.1	35.9
Monocyte, immature	3.6	8.4
Monocyte	3.6	7.3

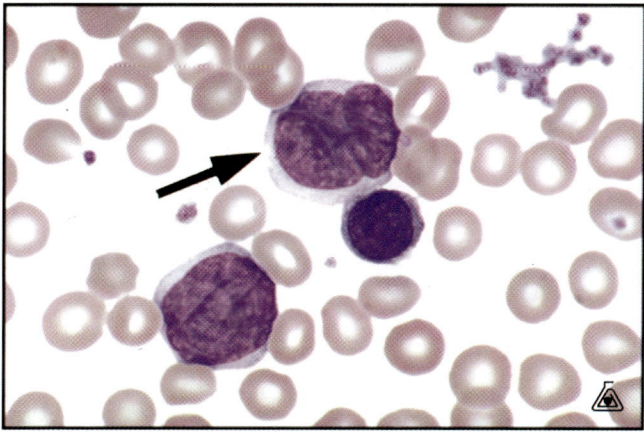

This blood film exhibits two Sézary cells with a round lymphocyte for comparison. The red blood cells appear unremarkable. Scattered platelets are seen with a clump in the upper right. The arrowed cell is 2-3 times the size of a normal lymphocyte. The folded nucleus contains fine to moderately coarse chromatin without nucleoli. A moderate amount of pale blue, agranular cytoplasm is present. The other large cell exhibits similar features and is another Sézary cell. The normal lymphocyte in the center has a round nucleus, clumped nuclear chromatin, and scant blue cytoplasm.

Microorganisms

Introduction 253
Babesia 254
   A Closer Look At...Babesiosis vs. Malaria 256
Bacteria (Cocci or Rod), Extracellular 258
Bacteria (Spirochete) 260
Fungi, Extracellular 262
Leukocyte (Blood) with Phagocytized Bacteria 264
Leukocyte (Blood) with Phagocytized Fungi 266
Macrophage with *Histoplasma*, *Leishmania*, or *Toxoplasma* 268
Macrophage with Phagocytized Mycobacteria 270
Malaria (Intracellular and Extracellular) 272
   A Closer Look At...Species Differences Among Malarial Parasites 274
Microfilaria 276
   A Closer Look At...Species Differences Among Microfilariae 278
Protozoan (Non-Malarial) 280
   A Closer Look At...African Trypanosomiasis 282

Introduction

A variety of microorganisms can be seen in the blood and bone marrow, including bacteria, fungi, and parasites. Although they are not commonly seen, their identification in the blood or bone marrow can be key to the proper and timely treatment of the patient. In some cases, such as infections with malaria, babesia, microfilariae, borrelia, and trypanosomes, visual identification is the only or best method available for diagnosis. In other instances, such as infections with bacteria, some fungi and mycobacteria, culture will be more sensitive and reliable. In addition, serology and special stains, such as AFB, GMS, gram stain, and acridine orange under fluorescence, can be useful adjuncts to diagnosis. Therefore one must be alert at all times to the unusual possibility of infectious organisms in blood and bone marrow, and when they are encountered, one must then be aware of their morphologic manifestations for accurate diagnosis.

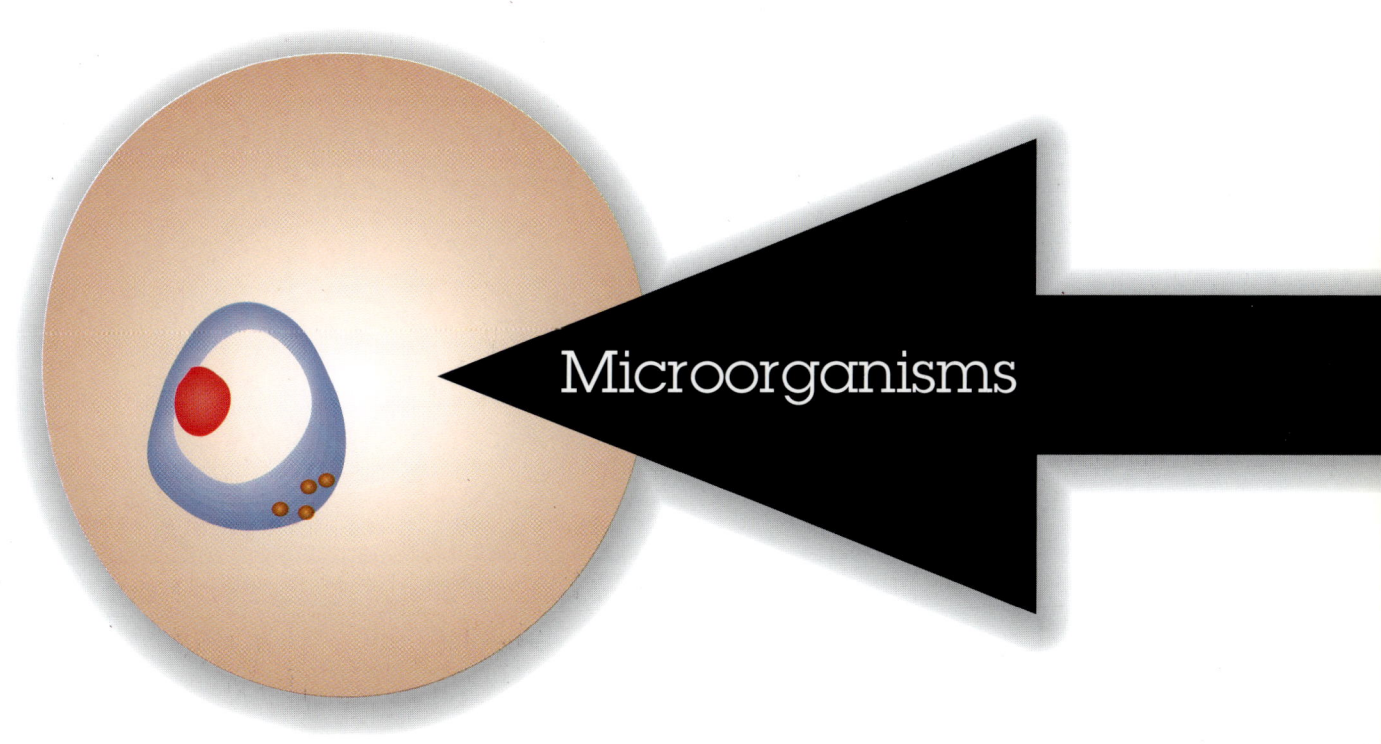

Babesia

SYNONYMS
  babesiosis, piroplasmosis

VITAL STATISTICS
  size .... range from 1-5 µm, mimicking the ring forms of malaria
  shape .... may be round, oval, elongate, ameboid or pyriform; pyriform organisms form a "Maltese cross" after division into four organisms

OTHER FINDINGS
  tetrad arrangement of the merozoites and the lack of other findings on the peripheral blood smear are most helpful in distinguishing these organisms from malaria
  Schüffner's granules are absent, as are the schizont and gametocyte forms of malaria
  extracellular organisms are seen only with *Babesia* (note: plasmodium organisms surrounded by a thin sheath of red blood cell membrane can mimic extracellular organisms; malarial merozoites may also be released if red cells are mechanically ruptured when making smears or if blood is old; when in doubt about the presence of extraerythrocytic organisms, draw a fresh sample)

POTENTIAL LOOK-ALIKES
  ring forms of malaria
  platelets overlying erythrocytes
  stain precipitate overlying erythrocytes

ASSOCIATED DISEASE STATES AND CONDITIONS
  babesiosis; severe disease is more common in splenectomized or immunosuppressed patients; bovine species more virulent than rodent species

Babesia microti is the main cause of babesiosis in non-splenectomized patients in the United States. It is endemic in parts of Massachusetts and the east coast and has been reported in Indiana and Wisconsin. It is transmitted by ticks, which serve as an intermediate host. Mammals such as deer and mice serve as the reservoir, and humans are only incidentally infected. Most patients have subclinical or mild undiagnosed disease, although fatal infections with severe hemolysis can occur, typically in splenectomized or immunocompromised patients. In California and other parts of the world, the disease is more common in splenectomized patients and follows a more fulminant course; the organisms involved may represent *B. bovis*, *B. divergens*, or as yet unrecognized species of *Babesia*. Rare cases of transfusion-associated disease have also been described. These usually are associated with severe parasitemia necessitating exchange transfusion.

If symptoms develop, they occur 10-14 days after the tick bite and include malaise with chills, fever, diaphoresis, weakness, headache, myalgia, and arthralgia. Hemolysis may be present, as well as hepatosplenomegaly. Detectable levels of parasitemia are usually

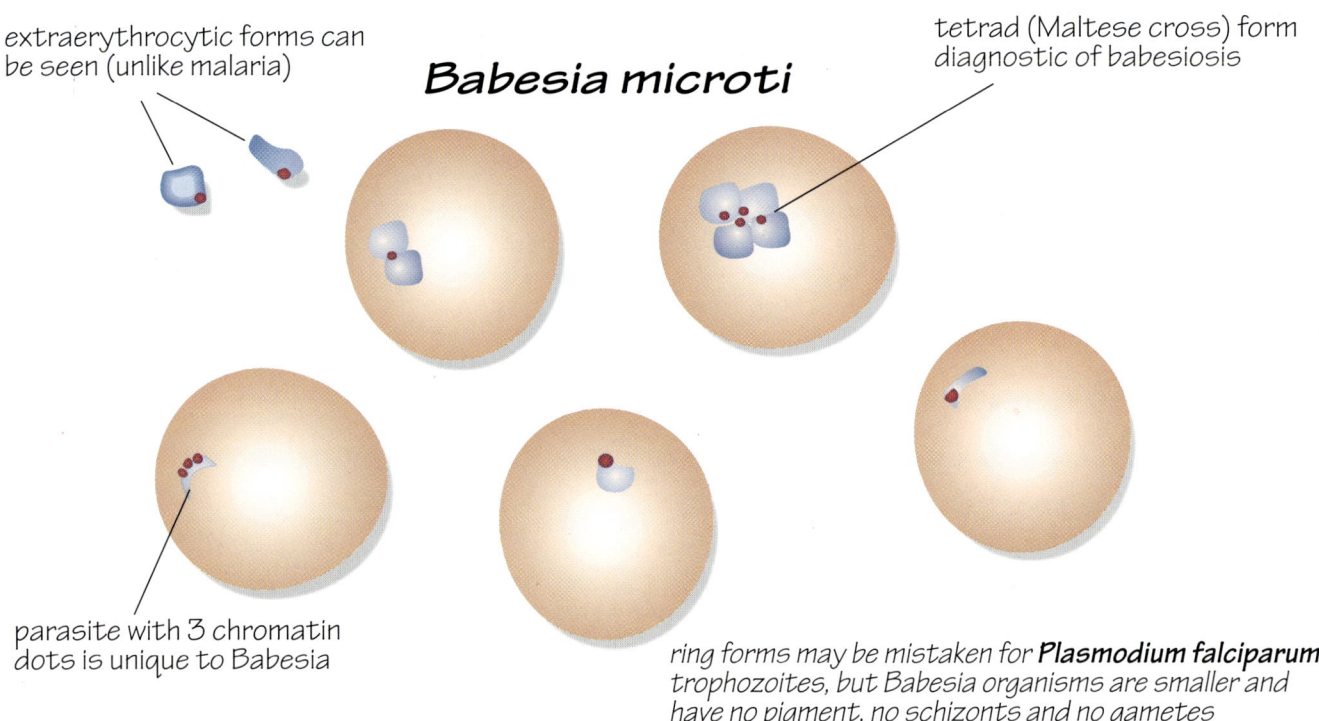

Babesia microti

extraerythrocytic forms can be seen (unlike malaria)

tetrad (Maltese cross) form diagnostic of babesiosis

parasite with 3 chromatin dots is unique to Babesia

ring forms may be mistaken for **Plasmodium falciparum** trophozoites, but Babesia organisms are smaller and have no pigment, no schizonts and no gametes limited to patients with severe infections. The parasite invades red blood cells and undergoes asexual reproduction, forming the tetrad or binary arrangement of the merozoites.

Thick blood films are preferred for diagnosis, where one sees tiny chromatin dots and wispy cytoplasm. These organisms can easily be confused with malaria, but are smaller and gametocytes are not seen. As noted above, patients with subacute or chronic disease typically have very low levels of parasitemia, and blood film evaluations are often negative. However, serologic tests can be very useful in these patients, for although three to four weeks must pass before antibody levels rise, many of these patients do not seek medical treatment until several months have passed. Unfortunately, interpretation of serologic results is limited by some degree of cross-reactivity with malaria. Therefore, since both morphologic and serologic methods do not always clearly separate these two diseases, careful clinical history is required to recognize babesiosis, particularly as the treatment differs for these two blood-borne parasitic pathogens.

H-15, 1996 (Blood, Wright-Giemsa, X400)

Identification	Referee %	Participant %
Malaria	65.4	67.3
Babesia	30.8	29.7

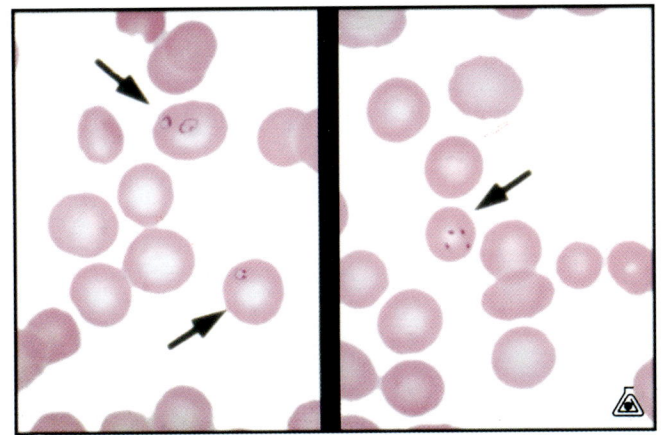

The panel on the left side shows two arrowed red blood cells containing ring forms of *Babesia microti*. The right panel shows a red blood cell containing four small, red-purple dots, also representing *Babesia* organisms. This is a tetrad of merozoites. Note the small size of the organisms compared to malarial ring forms. Although they can be easily confused with malaria, the merozoites are smaller and tetrads are diagnostic.

A Closer Look At...

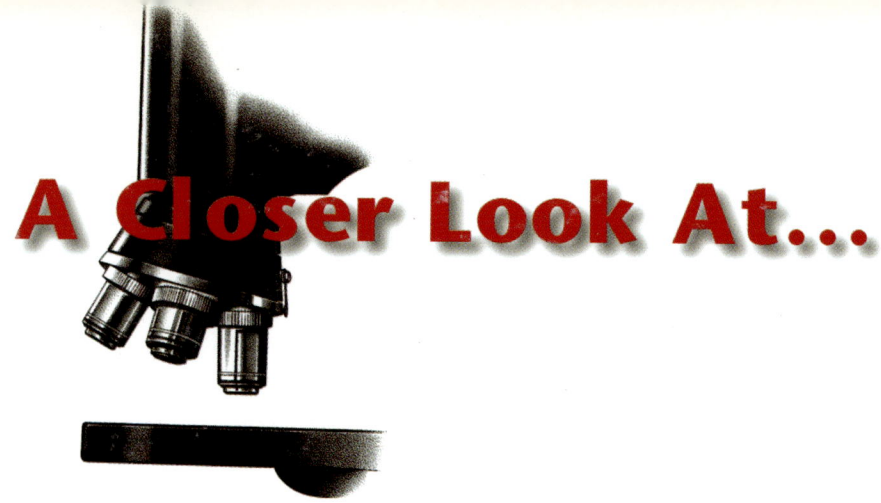

Babesiosis vs. Malaria

The differences between *Babesia* species and *Plasmodium* species are listed in the table below and the illustration on the opposite page. The major diagnostic feature of *Babesia* is the presence of four small merozoites forming a tetrad. The occasional presence of three chromatin dots is another unique feature. The infected red blood cells also do not contain pigment. In heavily infected patients, extraerthyrocytic merozoites can be detected in the peripheral blood.

Serologic tests can help to confirm the diagnosis of Babesiosis when parasitemia is not readily detected. Indirect immunofluorescence is the most sensitive test. Cross reactivity with *Plasmodium* species occurs but the titer is not as high as in *Babesia* infections. A significant increase in titer is diagnostic of acute infection. Another option that has proven to be a sensitive technique for recovering the parasite is to inject patient's blood into a hamster or gerbil.

Comparison of Malaria and Babesiosis

	Malaria	Babesiosis
Insect vector	mosquito	tick
Parasites per red cell	1 to 3	1 to 12
Trophozoite	small rings (*P. falciparum*) or ameboid cytoplasm with size >1/3 of RBC	round, ovoid, or pear-shaped; tetrads distinctive; multiple ring forms in single RBC
Pigment in trophozoite (Schüffner's pigment)	present	absent
Chromatin dots per parasite	1 or 2	1 to 3
Schizont	rare in *P. falciparum*; commonly present in other species	absent
Gametocyte	round or banana-shaped	absent
Extra-erythrocytic forms	absent	present
Serologic testing	+ *Plasmodium* antigen	+ *Babesia* antigen

Comparison of Babesia and Plasmodium Species

The small ring forms of *Babesia* may be difficult to distinguish from the ring forms of malarial parasites, especially *Plasmodium falciparum*. Other morphologic clues may help to separate the two parasites.

Babesia species | | Plasmodium species

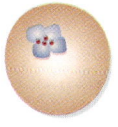 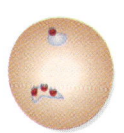

small ring forms, some with multiple chromatin dots (3 dots seen only in *Babesia*); tetrads—although not numerous—are diagnostic of babesiosis

Size & Number
Ring forms of *Babesia* are smaller (1.2 to 2.0 µm) in diameter than *Plasmodium*. Both species may have one or two chromatin dots per parasite but three dots are unique to *Babesia*. Up to 12 parasites may be found per red cell in *Babesia*. Up to 3 are found in *Plasmodium*.

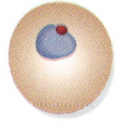 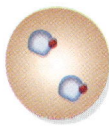

delicate ring forms of *P. falciparum* are very similar to *Babesia* trophozoites; multiple rings may be seen, especially in *P. falciparum* but no tetrads

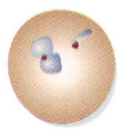

small ring forms only; no pigment

Shape & Pigment
Babesia are always found as small ring forms. The trophozoites of *P. falciparum* are small rings while other species are large and ameboid. Pigment is always absent in *Babesia*, even in red cells infected with mature parasites.

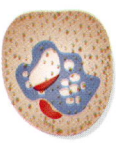 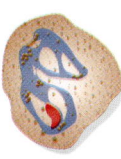

ameboid cytoplasm of *P. vivax* trophozoites; Schüffner's dots present

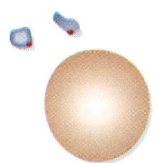

merozoites outside of red cell membrane

Extraerythrocytic Forms
Babesia merozoites may be found outside of the red cell in heavily infected patients (usually those without a spleen). Malarial parasites are always located inside the red cell. (Note: only fresh blood samples should be examined; old blood or mechanical pressure may rupture red cells, releasing malarial merozoites. Also, RBC membrane may be quite thin and nearly invisible).

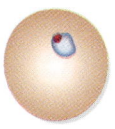

malarial parasites are confined to the red cell if blood is fresh and smears are properly prepared

Schizonts & Gametocytes
Schizonts and gametocytes are not found in babesiosis.

not found

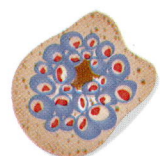 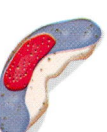

schizonts and gametocytes from *P. vivax* and *P. falciparum*

Bacteria (Cocci or Rod), Extracellular

SYNONYMS
none

VITAL STATISTICS
size .... individual organisms are typically around 1 µm in size, although there is considerable variation
shape .... range from cocci to bacilli, can occur singly, in clusters, or in chains

OTHER FINDINGS
gram stain is useful in separating organisms into Gram positive and negative groups

POTENTIAL LOOK-ALIKES
stain precipitate
platelets

ASSOCIATED DISEASE STATES AND CONDITIONS
traumatic or surgical wounds
burns
injuries to bones and joints
brain abscess
skin infections
meningitis
pneumonia
lung abscess
empyema
mycotic aneurysm
cardiac anomalies
peritonitis
intestinal or biliary obstruction
cholangitis
carcinoma
urinary obstruction
nephropathies
post-partum endometritis
septic abortion
immunosuppressive states

Although bacteremia is relatively common, it is quite unusual to identify bacteria on a random blood film, and in most cases, this finding represents an overwhelming infection. Blood cultures are much more likely to detect bacteremia, as large volumes of blood are collected and incubated for at least one week to encourage bacterial growth. A peripheral blood film should therefore never be used as a diagnostic modality. In the vast majority of circumstances, recognizing bacteria on the peripheral blood film will be a fortuitous event. The most likely error in interpretation is to misidentify stain precipitate as microorganisms. This error can be avoided by remembering that bacteria tend to be relatively uniform in size and shape, while stain precipitate is often irregular in shape and individual grains vary considerably in size. The morphology of stain precipitate is further discussed on pages 294–295. Differences between extracellular bacteria and stain precipitate are illustrated on the bottom of the next page.

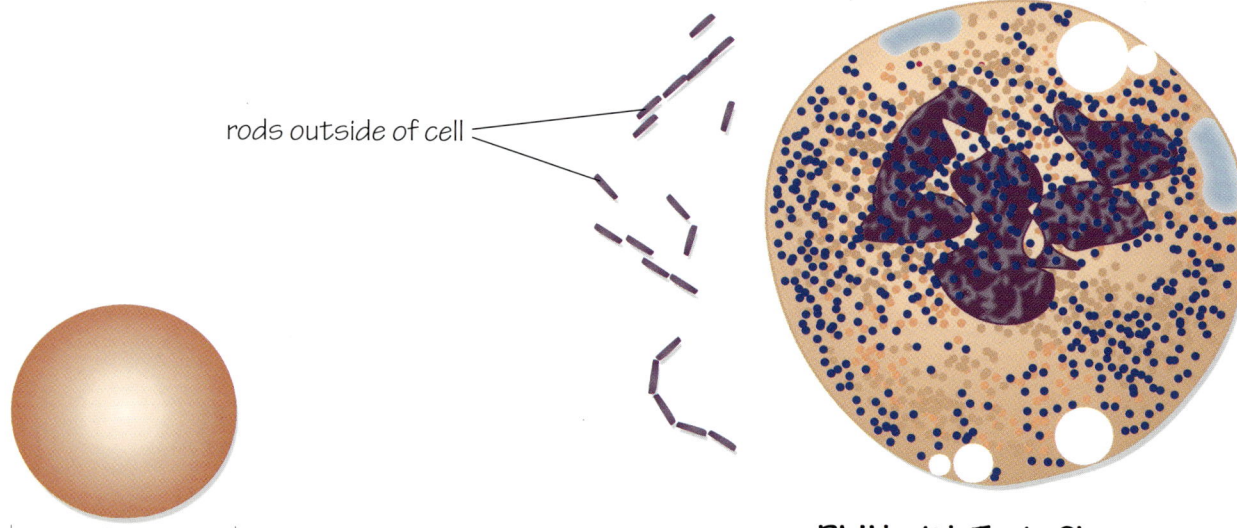

Extracellular Bacteria

rods outside of cell

PMN with Toxic Changes

7 µm
size of normal red blood cell

H1-42, 1985 (Blood, Wright-Giemsa, X450)

Identification	Referee %	Participant %
Bacteria (cocci/rod), extracellular	100	98.9

The bacteria in this photomicrograph exhibit a definite bacillary shape and are arranged in chains, end to end. This clearly represents a thick area of the blood film, as the red blood cells are overlapping and exhibit some slow drying artifact. A poorly-preserved monocyte is also present to the right of the field.

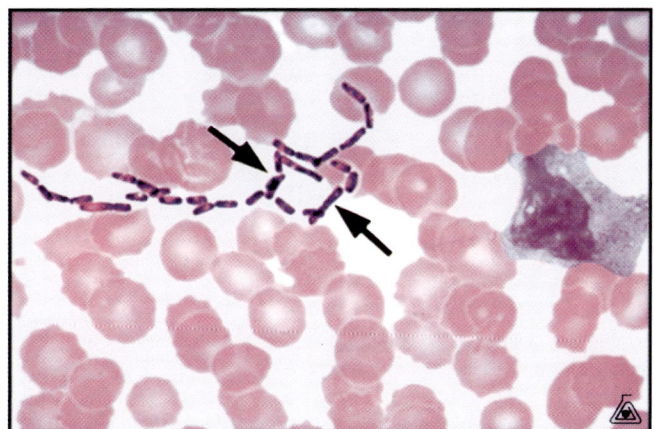

Differences Between Extracellular Bacteria and Stain Precipitate

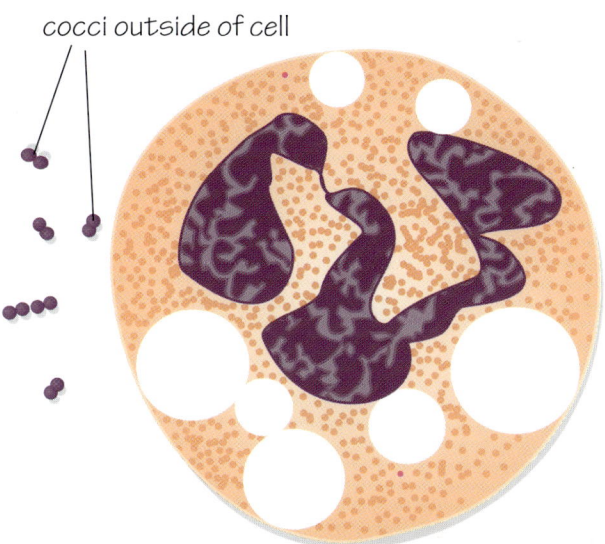

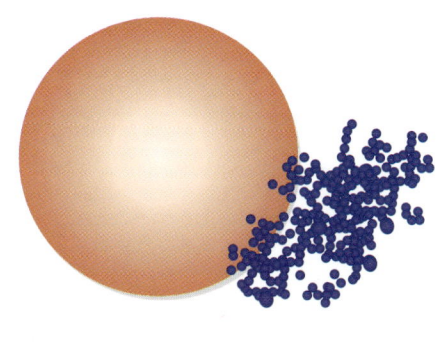

PMN with Toxic Vacuoles and Extracellular Bacteria

RBC with Stain Precipitate

Stain precipitate may resemble extracellular or intracellular bacteria. If the precipitate appears intracellular, check the plane of focus; stain will be in a different focal plane than the cell. Bacteria are not as dark as stain precipitate and are more regular in size and shape. Individual particles of precipitated stain vary considerably in size and sometimes shape. Bacteria in peripheral blood are usually few in number and found randomly on the slide. Precipitated stain, on the other hand, is not so dispersed and tends to form clumps in a selected area. Gram stain may be helpful in difficult cases.

Bacteria (Spirochete)

SYNONYMS
none

VITAL STATISTICS
- size .... *Borrelia* species vary from 5-25 μm in length and 0.2-0.5 μm in width
- shape .... *Borrelia* species demonstrate from 4-30 helical coils

OTHER FINDINGS
organisms can be seen in fresh wet mount preparations, on thin Giemsa stained blood films, or on thick Giemsa stained blood preparations
concentration technique can be used in mildly infected persons

POTENTIAL LOOK-ALIKES
fiber, thread or hair contamination may mimic spirochetes, but should be easily distinguished as an artifact, given their lack of uniform coiling

ASSOCIATED DISEASE STATES AND CONDITIONS
pathogenic spirochetes include members of the genera *Borrelia*, *Leptospira*, and *Treponema*
Borrelia: endemic and epidemic relapsing fever; Lyme disease
Leptospira: acute febrile systemic illness (leptospirosis) in humans occupationally exposed to animals or working in rat-infested surroundings, but almost never seen in peripheral blood films
Treponemes: syphilis, yaws and pinta, but also virtually never seen in peripheral blood films

Louse-born *Borrelia recurrentis* is the infectious agent of epidemic relapsing fever, while a variety of *Borrelia* species can cause the tick-borne endemic relapsing fever. *Borrelia burgdorferi* is the etiologic agent of Lyme disease, but is virtually never seen in peripheral blood, despite the successful isolation of the organism from blood culture in BSK II medium. Although both *treponemes* and *leptospires* are present in the blood of infected patients at certain phases in the illnesses caused by those organisms, they also are virtually never seen, even on dark-field examination of concentrated specimens.

Epidemic relapsing fever was an important cause of morbidity during the first half of the twentieth century, with more than 50 million people contracting the disease in Europe, Asia, Africa, and South America. Since the 1960s, it has been reported primarily in African countries and South America. Epidemics usually occur after wars, famine, or other natural disasters that result in poor living conditions and proliferation of the body louse, *Pediculus humanus*, which carries the disease. Humans serve as the only reservoir of this organism. Infection occurs from contamination of a wound with the hemolymph of infected lice rather than from the

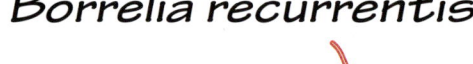

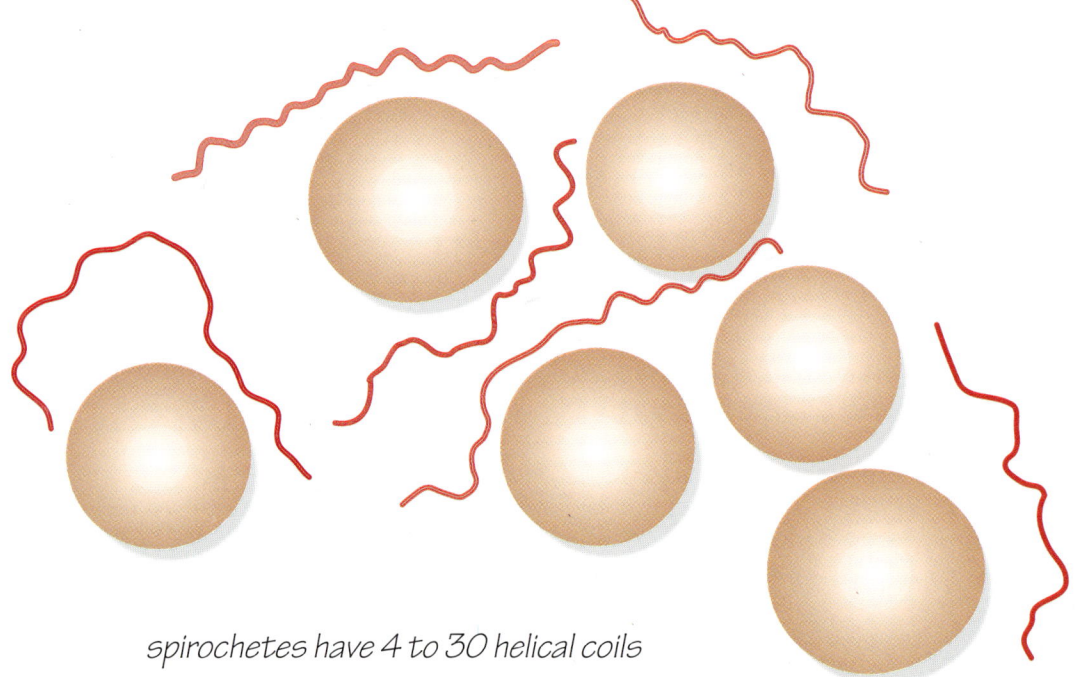

spirochetes have 4 to 30 helical coils

direct bite. The spirochetes can also directly penetrate the skin. Organisms are seen in the blood only during febrile episodes. If repeated smears are negative, examination of blood from mice inoculated with patient blood may be more sensitive in detecting the organisms.

In contrast, endemic relapsing fever is seen only sporadically during the summer in mountainous areas of the western United States and has also been reported occasionally in numerous locations around the world. The tick-borne disease is transmitted through the tick bite, unlike the louse-borne disease. Outbreaks are usually sporadic and involve only a few patients. However, the disease is probably underreported, as many patients may not be aware of the tick bite, and the disease may not be suspected during the initial febrile stage.

Symptoms of both endemic and epidemic relapsing fever include high fever, shaking chills, nausea, vomiting, abdominal pain, headache, rash, and myalgia. After three to six days, the fever suddenly breaks, coincident with the appearance of antibodies in the blood and resolution of spirochetemia. However, the organism is capable of "mutation" which leads to a new spirochetemia and relapse of symptoms, although typically milder with each reinfection.

H1-19, 1990 (Blood, Wright-Giemsa, X425)

Identification	Referee %	Participant %
Bacteria (spirochete)	100	98.8

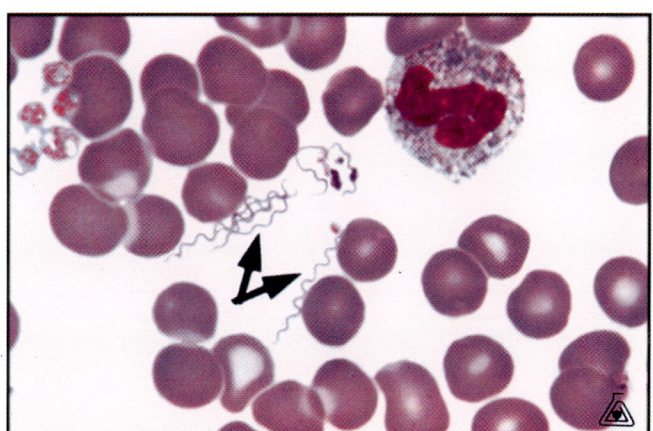

Several spiral organisms are present in the center of the field and represent *Borrelia recurrentis*. A band neutrophil is also present with toxic granules. A cluster of platelets is present in the left upper corner of the photomicrograph. The red blood cells are unremarkable, despite some overlapping and crowding. Spirochetes of *Borrelia* species have an affinity for acid dyes and can be observed in Wright-Giemsa, Leishman's, or May-Grunwald stained smears. The organisms display distinctive length, number of spirals, regularity, and tightness of the coils. When *Borrelia* is suspected in a patient, both thick and thin smears should be prepared because spirochetemia may be light, particularly after one or more febrile relapses. The organisms are not seen during afebrile intervals. If repeated direct smear examinations are negative, greater diagnostic sensitivity may be achieved by examining blood smears from mice inoculated with blood from a patient.

Fungi, Extracellular

SYNONYMS
Coccidiodes, Cryptococcus, Candida, Aspergillus, rarely others

VITAL STATISTICS
size and shape .... dependent on specific organism; *Coccidiodes* typically shows mature spherules ranging between 20-60 µm, and contain endospores ranging from 2-4 µm; *Cryptococcus* is a round to oval yeast-like fungus ranging from 3.5 to 8 µm or more in diameter, usually with a thick mucopolysaccharide capsule, and demonstrating a narrow neck when budding; *Candida* can appear in bone marrow as either yeast-like organisms with budding, or as pseudohyphae; *Aspergillus* is typically identified by its septate 4 µm-wide hyphae with characteristic 45 degree branching; *Histoplasma* is usually intracellular within macrophages, but can occasionally be seen extracellularly as 1-2 µm budding yeast forms

OTHER FINDINGS
organisms may elicit a granulomatous reaction, or may be present scattered throughout the marrow in histiocytes, neutrophils or even megakaryocytes
most organisms will stain with a PAS stain, but are accentuated by GMS staining

POTENTIAL LOOK-ALIKES
stain precipitate

ASSOCIATED DISEASE STATES AND CONDITIONS
rarely seen in bone marrow of patients with an intact immune system
immune compromise states such as:
acquired immunodeficiency syndrome
malignancy
immunosuppression

Extracellular fungi are most commonly seen in the bone marrow, but fungi such as *Candida* can rarely be identified in peripheral blood films in an extracellular location. The organisms are usually associated with intracellular organisms as well. When visualized, they indicate a serious infection which requires immediate attention.

Probably the most frequently seen fungus in the bone marrow is *Histoplasma capsulatum,* but the organisms are nearly exclusively present within macrophages. They are only rarely seen in an extracellular location, usually when the cell membranes of the macrophages have ruptured (see *Macrophage with Histoplasma, Leishmania, or Toxoplasma*, page 268, for additional information). The other organisms such as *Coccidiodes, Cryptococcus, Candida,* and *Aspergillus* occur less frequently, but are more commonly extracellular.

The presence of fungi in the bone marrow is usually indicative of a systemic infection and is therefore an ominous finding. If patients do not succumb from the fungal infection, they may suffer serious consequences from the antifungal therapy, or die as a result of the underlying disease that has led to immunosuppression. Granulomas in the bone marrow are a helpful clue to the presence of fungi, but in some patients, the organisms do not elicit a significant inflammatory response. This is particularly true in AIDS and has led some authors to advocate routine AFB and GMS stains on all bone marrow specimens from patients with that disease.

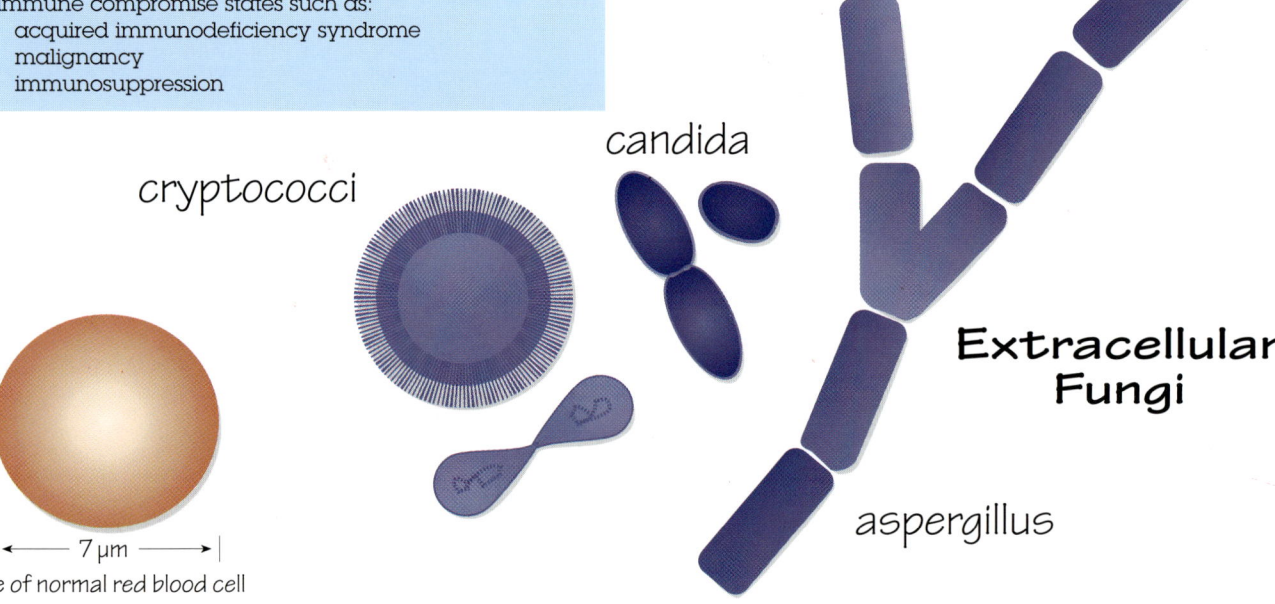

cryptococci

candida

Extracellular Fungi

aspergillus

|← 7 µm →|
size of normal red blood cell

HE-29, 1992 (Blood, Wright-Giemsa, X400)

Identification	Referee %	Participant %
Fungi, extracellular	100	86.1
Protozoan (non-malarial)	-	3.8
Macrophage with histoplasma, leishmania, or toxoplasma	-	2.5

This picture represents *Cryptococcus neoformans* in bone marrow. The slide is stained with Wright-Giemsa. Negative staining of the thick capsule is evident, as is the teardrop type of budding. Red blood cells are present in the background, but other cells in the field are distorted and difficult to identify.

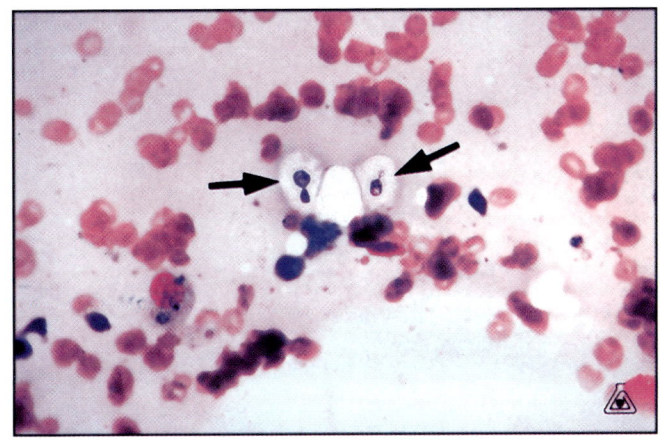

A-31, 1988 (Blood, Wright-Giemsa, X400)

Identification	Referee %	Participant %
Fungi, extracellular	100	82.8
Neutrophil necrobiosis (degenerated neutrophil)	-	9.8

This photomicrograph shows the budding yeast forms of *Torulopsis glabrata* in the peripheral blood. Small extracellular collections of coagulase-negative *Staphylococcus* are also present in the field, at 7 and 12 o'clock. The background red blood cells show mild anisocytosis.

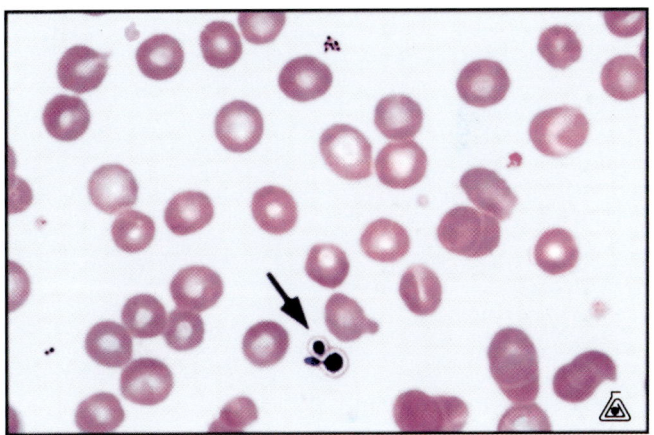

HE-28, 1992 (Tissue Biopsy, PAS-Metanil Yellow, X400)

Identification	Referee %	Participant %
Fungi, extracellular	100	97.7

This picture is from phalangeal bone in the amputated toe of a diabetic patient with *Aspergillus fumigatus* infection. The section is stained with PAS-metanil yellow and the fungal hyphae stain red. The 45 degree branching is seen to the left of the lower arrow. Background cells are difficult to identify in this field.

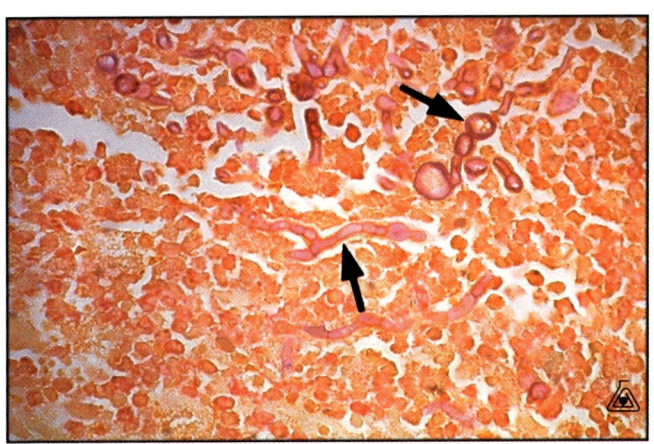

Leukocyte (Blood) with Phagocytized Bacteria

SYNONYMS
none

VITAL STATISTICS
size .... individual organisms are typically around 1 μm in size, although there is considerable variation
shape .... range from cocci to bacilli, can occur singly, as diplococci or in clusters or chains

OTHER FINDINGS
gram stain is useful in separating organisms into gram positive and negative groups

POTENTIAL LOOK-ALIKES
toxic granules in neutrophils
overlying platelets
stain precipitate

ASSOCIATED DISEASE STATES AND CONDITIONS
traumatic or surgical wounds
burns
injuries to bones and joints
brain abscess
skin infections
meningitis
pneumonia
lung abscess
empyema
mycotic aneurysm
cardiac anomalies
peritonitis
intestinal or biliary obstruction
cholangitis
carcinoma
urinary obstruction
nephropathies
post-partum endometritis
septic abortion
immunosuppressive states

As noted under the discussion of *Bacteria, Extracellular*, on page 258, it is very unusual to see bacteria on a random blood film, and this finding usually represents an overwhelming infection. When present, the organisms may be ingested by neutrophils or monocytes and can be seen within the cytoplasm of these cells. Although leukocytes with phagocytized bacteria are rare in the blood film, they are more commonly seen in infected body fluids. When present within neutrophils, bacteria can be difficult to distinguish from toxic granulation. However, toxic granulation tends to involve nearly all of the cytoplasm of the neutrophil, whereas engulfed bacteria are usually few in number and may be surrounded by a vacuole. In addition, bacteria are typically larger than toxic granules and more defined in shape. They can be accentuated on a Gram stain. Finally, only single cocci are difficult to distinguish from toxic granules; diplococci or bacilli are more easily recognized.

Intracellular Bacteria

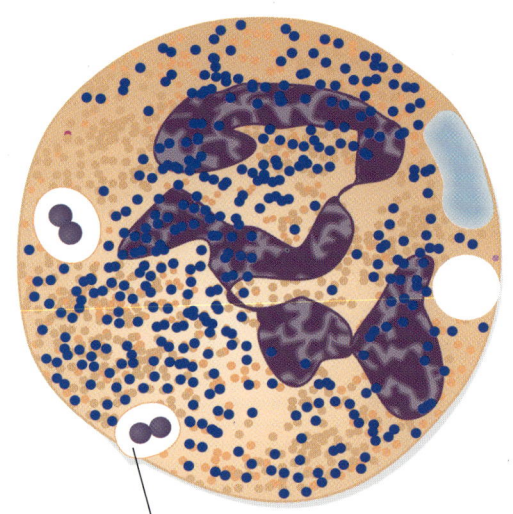

diplococci within cytoplasmic vacuole

PMN's with Toxic Changes

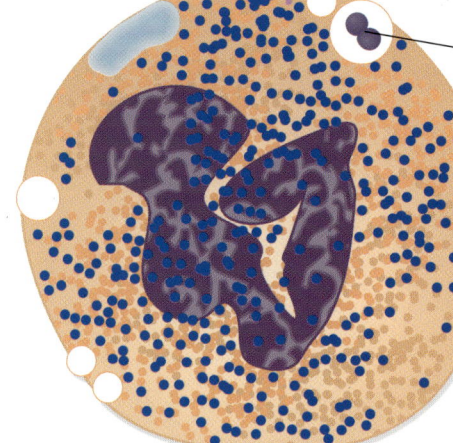

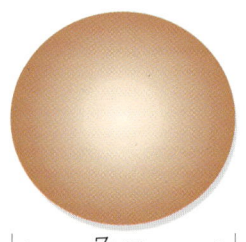

|← 7 μm →|
size of normal red blood cell

H1-41, 1985 (Blood, Wright-Giemsa, X450)

Identification	Referee %	Participant %
Leukocyte with phag. bacteria	94.4	90.8
Histiocyte, macrophage	5.6	1.7

These bacillary microorganisms are located both within the cytoplasm of the monocyte in the center of the field and extracellularly. The organisms have a uniformity of size and shape that would be unusual for stain precipitate. Adjacent red blood cells show overlapping due to this photomicrograph being taken in a thick part of the blood film.

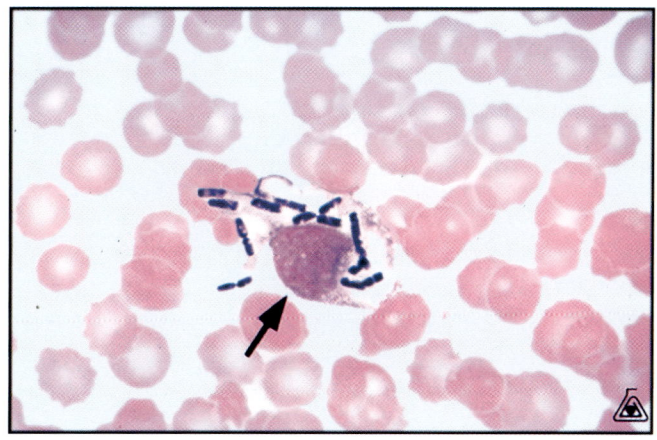

Intracellular Bacteria

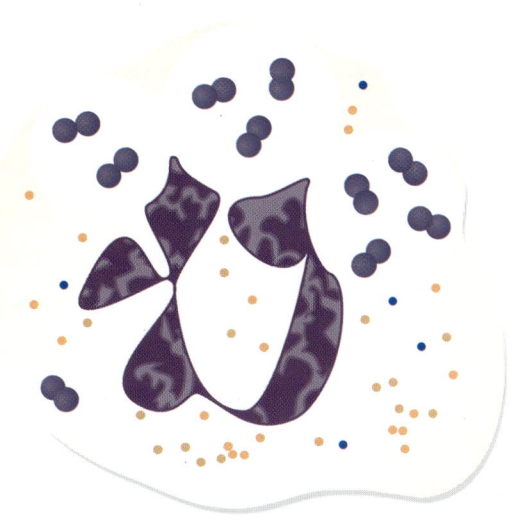 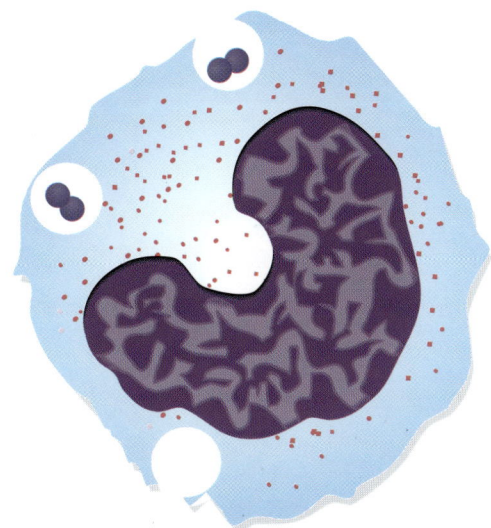

PMN with Toxic Vacuoles   Monocyte

On the left, the segmented neutrophil is distorted by toxic vacuoles containing diplococci. The cytoplasm is nearly agranular. Sometimes the cells are so degenerated and distorted that they are difficult to recognize as granulocytes. On the right, the monocyte also contains phagocytic vacuoles within which are several bacteria.

Leukocyte (Blood) with Phagocytized Fungi

SYNONYMS
none

VITAL STATISTICS
size and shape .... dependent on specific organism; *Candida* appears as a budding yeast form or as pseudohyphae; *Histoplasma capsulatum* is only rarely present in peripheral blood, but is probably the most frequently seen fungus in the bone marrow; *Histoplasma* is typically intracellular and multiple, with 1-2 µm budding yeast forms

OTHER FINDINGS
rarely visualized in peripheral blood; when seen suggest significant fungemia
blood cultures are much more sensitive in detecting the presence of fungi in the peripheral blood and should always be the method of choice for diagnosis

POTENTIAL LOOK-ALIKES
precipitated stain overlying a leukocyte
large toxic granules or Döhle bodies
large bacterial cocci

ASSOCIATED DISEASE STATES AND CONDITIONS
systemic fungal infections rarely seen in patients with an intact immune system
immune compromised states such as:
acquired immunodeficiency syndrome
malignancy
immunosuppression

Visualization of fungi in the peripheral blood is an ominous finding and should be communicated to the physician at the earliest possible moment. The phagocytized fungi may be found within neutrophils as well as monocytes. They are ensconced within a vacuole which forms a clear halo around the organism.

Usually the number of fungi present is scant, but if enough are seen, it may be possible to recognize the specific organism by morphology alone. Clinical history and blood cultures are also very important in making the appropriate identification. Blood cultures are much more sensitive in detecting the presence of fungi in the peripheral blood and should always be the method of choice for diagnosis.

Candida albicans is the fungus most commonly found circulating in the blood. *Histoplasma capsulatum* can also be seen, but is exceptionally rare. Although other fungi can be grown from blood cultures and are therefore present in the circulation, the level of fungemia is so low that they are virtually never visualized on a blood film.

Intracellular Fungi

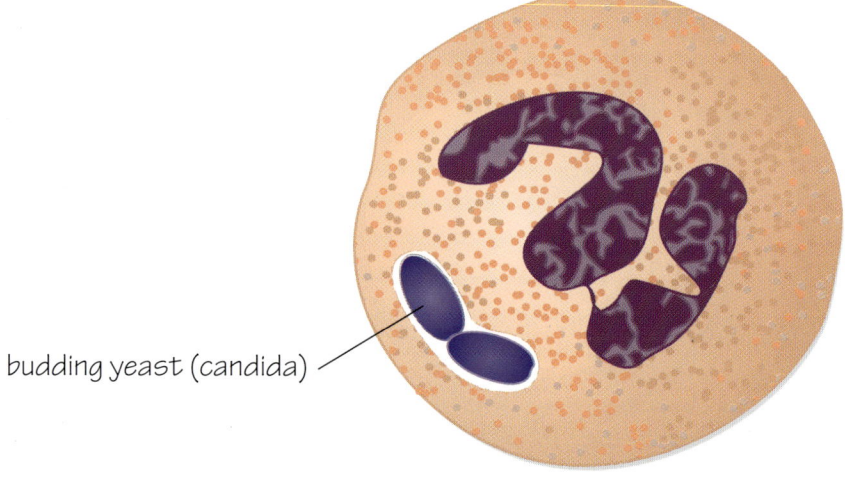

budding yeast (candida)

Segmented Neutrophil

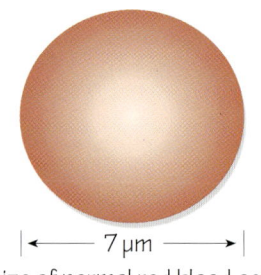

|← 7 µm →|
size of normal red blood cell

HE-13, 1996 (Blood, Wright-Giemsa, X400)

Identification	Referee %	Participant %
Leukocyte (blood) with phagocytized fungi	84.6%	56.1%
Neutrophil necrobiosis (degenerating neutrophil)	7.7%	22.1%
Segmented or band neutrophil with toxic granulation	3.8%	8.3%
Leukocyte (blood) with phagocytized bacteria	3.8%	1.8%

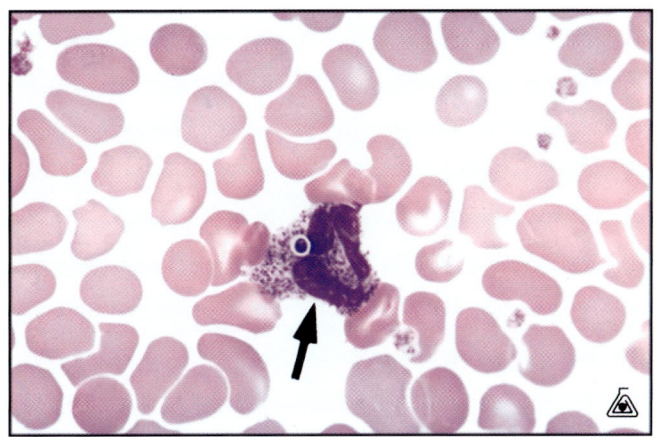

The arrowed cell exhibits a segmented nucleus with abundant pink cytoplasm containing fine azurophilic granules, consistent with a segmented neutrophil with toxic granulation. In addition, and more importantly, a round dark blue and red structure is present within the cytoplasm surrounded by a clear zone which represents a phagocytized fungal organism. Although this cell is distorted, the nuclear chromatin is still granular and the nucleus is not pyknotic.

Intracellular Fungi

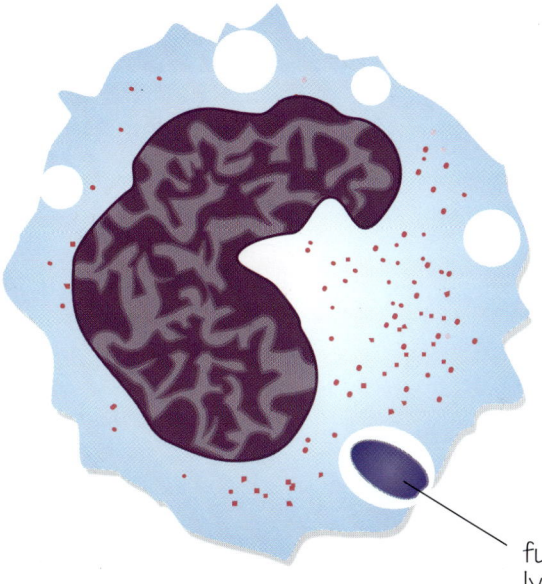

Monocyte — fungus within lysozomal vacuole

Macrophage with Histoplasma, Leishmania, or Toxoplasma

SYNONYMS
none

VITAL STATISTICS
size and shape .... *Histoplasma* is a 1-2 μm budding yeast, typically present in large numbers within the cytoplasm of macrophages in the bone marrow; have a crescent or ring-shape and also may be surrounded by a small halo, (both findings are artifacts, but helpful in diagnosis)
amastigote form of the parasite *Leishmania* has a similar size and appearance to *Histoplasma* within marrow macrophages, but is recognized by the additional presence of a dot-like kinetoplast associated with each organism
unicellular tachyzoite of *Toxoplasma gondii* also imitates *Histoplasma* morphologically, but does not stain positively with the Gomori's methanamine silver (GMS) stain

POTENTIAL LOOK-ALIKES
Histoplasma, Leishmania, and *Toxoplasma* may closely resemble each other
other look-alikes include:
  budding yeast organisms
  large bacterial cocci
  phagocytized material, particularly cells
  platelets (resemble extracellular organisms that are found when macrophage ruptures)

ASSOCIATED DISEASE STATES AND CONDITIONS
histoplasmosis
leishmaniasis
toxoplasmosis
(the presence of these organisms in the bone marrow is indicative of a systemic infection, and patients will typically manifest other symptoms or lesions associated with the specific disease)

Although all of these infections are only rarely seen in the bone marrow, *Histoplasma* is by far the most common, and in fact, is probably the most common of all fungal or parasitic infections of the bone marrow, either intracellular or extracellular. With the increasing frequency of the acquired immunodeficiency syndrome, disseminated histoplasmosis is being seen more frequently in endemic areas, including the Ohio, Mississippi and St. Lawrence river valleys, as well as other areas around the world. Dissemination typically occurs in immunosuppressed patients and normal children under the age of two. The organism can be grown from blood, urine, bone marrow, sputum, and skin.

More commonly, *Histoplasma* causes a primary pulmonary infection, which may be asymptomatic. After resolution of the initial illness, the patient may remain infection free, but there is a risk of reactivation and dissemination years later, especially involving sites such as brain, adrenal glands, and mucocutaneous surfaces.

Leishmaniasis can be divided into two main clinical groups: mucocutaneous and visceral. Mucocutaneous leishmaniasis is caused by several species and occurs primarily in Central and South America, the Mediterranean, Middle East, and Central Africa. Both the severity of disease and clinical manifestations vary with the particular species. The infection is spread by sandflies and diagnosis is best acheived by skin biopsy of affected skin, although culture is definitive. The organisms are obligate intracellular parasites and will be found in high numbers within macrophages in the dermis.

Histoplasma

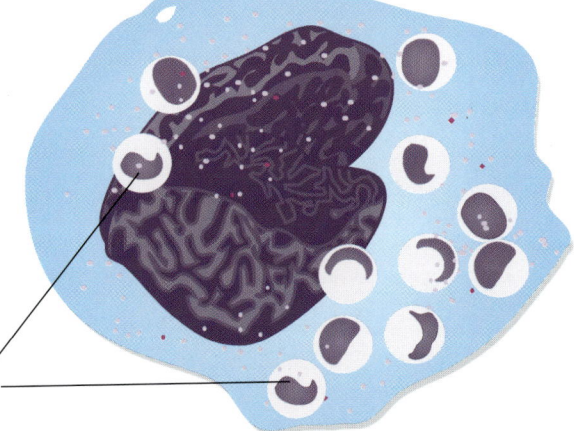

Histoplasma organisms

Bone Marrow Macrophage

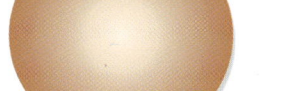

size of normal red blood cell

Visceral leishmaniasis is caused by various subspecies of *Leishmania donovani*. These organisms can tolerate higher temperatures than those causing mucocutaneous leishmaniasis, and are able to proliferate in macrophages in liver, spleen, lymph nodes, and bone marrow. Most patients have asymptomatic or mild disease, but occasional cases are severe, especially in immunodeficient patients, and can be fatal without treatment.

Toxoplasma gondii is an obligate intracellular parasite like *Leishmania* and is found in most warm-blooded animals. However, only members of the cat family serve as definitive hosts. Infection is typically asymptomatic and prevalence rates range from less than 1% in some areas to 80-90% in others. Modes of transmission include exposure to cat feces and ingestion of undercooked meat. The most serious consequences of *Toxoplasma* infection occur in the fetus (with transplacental transmission of the primary infection, especially during the first trimester), during transfusion or tissue transplantation in immunosuppressed individuals, and following reactivation, particularly in patients with AIDS. CNS toxoplasmosis is one of the leading causes of death in AIDS. In addition, the organism can cause pneumonitis and myocarditis. Reactivation, even in normal patients, can also cause a severe retinochorionitis and blindness.

HE-26, 1992 (Bone Marrow, Wright-Giemsa, X400)

Identification	Referee %	Participant %
Macrophage with histoplasma, leishmania, or toxoplasma	100	91.9

This photomicrograph shows a macrophage (arrowed cell) containing numerous organisms, most of which exhibit a dot-like kinetoplast, allowing their recognition as *Leishmania*. Immature erythroid and myeloid precursors are present in the background. A few extracellular organisms are also seen which may occur when the delicate macrophages rupture in the process of preparing the slide.

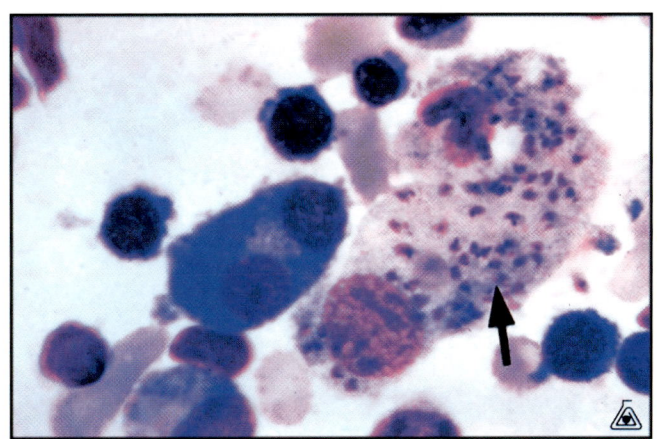

HE-30, 1992 (Bone Marrow, split screen: Left, Silver Chromate and Eosin, X170; Right, Wright-Giemsa, X400)

Identification	Referee %	Participant %
Macrophage with histoplasma, leishmania, or toxoplasma	100	93.3

This split screen photomicrograph shows a macrophage in the right panel containing numerous organisms, but no kinetoplasts are evident. The organisms, which were shown to be *Histoplasma capsulatum*, demonstrate a ring-like or crescentic appearance. The left panel is a silver chromate and eosin stain, which demonstrates the silver positive, budding yeast forms.

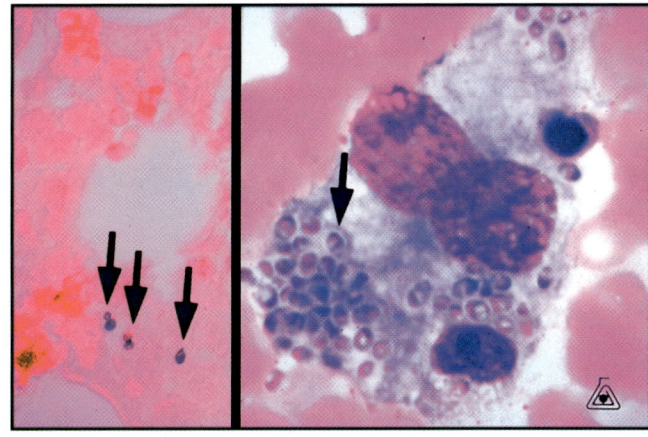

Macrophage with Phagocytized Mycobacteria

SYNONYMS
none

VITAL STATISTICS
size and shape .... straight to slightly curved bacilli varying from 0.2-0.6 μm in width and 1-10 μm in length

OTHER FINDINGS
aerobic and non-motile bacilli
acid fast stain positive (due to high lipid content in cell wall); may appear beaded
may be associated with a granulomatous inflammatory response, often with caseous necrosis (organisms are usually rare and difficult to find in such instances)
some cases (related either to the particular species or the immune status of the host) are not associated with any significant inflammatory response; organisms may be present in large numbers within the cytoplasm of histiocytes, or occasionally in an extracellular location; they appear as nonrefractile "negative images" or clear or red refractile beaded rods on Romanowsky-stained preparations

POTENTIAL LOOK-ALIKES
debris within cytoplasm
other bacterial organisms (should not be acid fast; nocardia is acid fast but is a filamentous bacteria)
in Romanovsky-stained preparations:
   intracytoplasmic immunoglobulin crystals
   scratches
   cytoplasmic cracks
   elongated areas of agranular cytoplasm
   Gaucher and pseudo-Gaucher cells

ASSOCIATED DISEASE STATES AND CONDITIONS
tuberculosis (may occur in immune competent or immune incompetent host; disseminated infections and certain species, such as Mycobacterium avium-intracellulare, are more likely to occur in the immunosuppressed patient, particularly in patients with AIDS)
tuberculous lymphadenitis (scrofula)
tuberculous spondylitis (Pott's disease)

The mycobacteria are responsible for a variety of clinical infections, with tuberculosis and leprosy probably being the best known. At least 25 species of mycobacteria are causative agents of human disease and several species can infect the bone marrow. The two species that most commonly involve the bone marrow are *Mycobacterium tuberculosis* and *Mycobacterium avium-intracellulare*. *Mycobacterium tuberculosis* elicits a granulomatous response with or without caseous necrosis, while *Mycobacterium avium-intracellulare* is usually seen in large numbers within bone marrow macrophages. The incidence of disseminated *Mycobacterium avium-intracellulare* infection has greatly increased as the population of patients with AIDS has expanded. Because this organism often does not elicit a granulomatous response, some authors have advocated routine use of the acid fast stain (and the Gomori's methenamine silver stain for fungi) on bone marrow samples from all patients with AIDS.

Mycobacterium tuberculosis is the causative agent of tuberculosis, known as consumption prior to the discovery of the tubercle bacillus as the cause of the disease by Koch in the late 1800s. The disease typically begins in childhood as a localized pulmonary infection with involvement of regional lymph nodes, known as a Ghon complex. Occasional cases become disseminated, especially in debilitated individuals. Reactivation later in life can result in a chronic progressive pulmonary disease with caseation. Clinical symptoms include

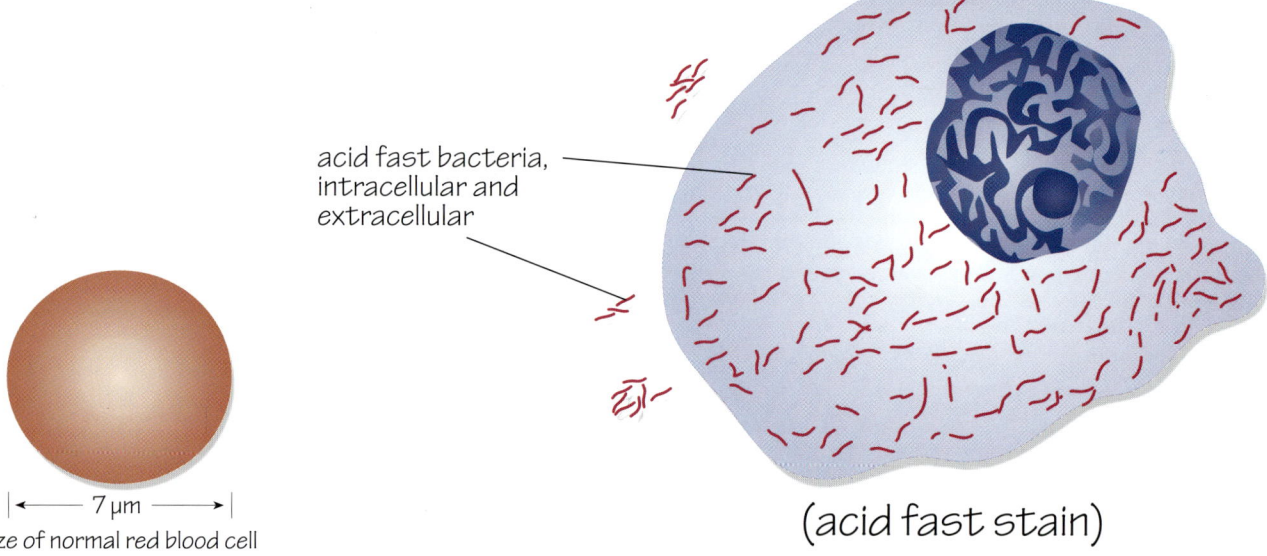

Mycobacteria in Bone Marrow Macrophage

acid fast bacteria, intracellular and extracellular

(acid fast stain)

|← 7 μm →|
size of normal red blood cell

cough, malaise, fever, chest pain, and weight loss. The incidence of tuberculosis has risen significantly in recent years. The disease has acquired a new importance in patients with AIDS; it is more aggressive and frequently disseminates, including involvement of blood and bone marrow.

The incidence of atypical mycobacterial infections has increased markedly, also in parallel to the increasing population of patients with AIDS. Of these organisms, *Mycobacterium avium-intracellulare* is the most important. This organism frequently involves the gastrointestinal tract, which probably represents the main portal of entry. The organism accumulates in large numbers within macrophages in the lamina propria. Dissemination is common, with similar accumulations of organism-laden macrophages in other organs including lung, liver, bone marrow, spleen, and lymph nodes.

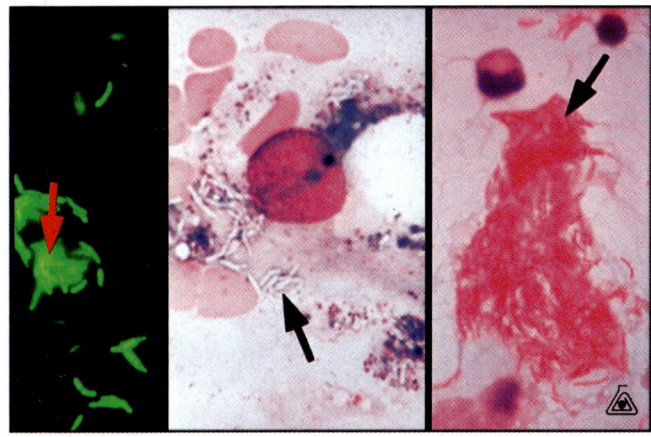

HE-27, 1992 (Bone Marrow, split screen: Left, Fluorescent Auramine-Rhodamine, X200; Middle, Wright-Giemsa, X260; Right, Kinyoun's Acid Fast, X186)

Identification	Referee %	Participant %
Macrophage with phagocytized mycobacteria	100	84.5
Bacteria (cocci/rod) extracellular	-	10.2

This picture is a tri-panel demonstrating *Mycobacterium avium-intracellulare* organisms, stained by fluorescent auramine-rhodamine, Wright-Giemsa, and Kinyoun's acid fast stains (from left to right). Numerous organisms fill the cytoplasm of the macrophage. In the Wright Giemsa stain, the organisms appear as "negative images."

Malaria (Intracellular and Extracellular)

SYNONYMS
Plasmodium falciparum, vivax, ovale, and *malariae*

VITAL STATISTICS
size .... ring forms of all four types of malaria usually less than 2 μm in diameter; trophozoites range from 3 to 8 μm depending on the species; schizonts and gametocytes range from approximately 5 to 11 μm

shape .... the different shapes and appearance of the various stages of development, and their variations between species, are distinctive, and have been reviewed in many texts (see the following *A Closer Look At...* on page 274)

OTHER FINDINGS
- infected erythrocytes enlarged in *P. ovale* and *P. vivax*
- Schüffner stippling (a golden brown to black pigment in the cytoplasm of the infected erythrocyte) is most conspicious in infections with *P. ovale* and *P. vivax*
- multiple stages of organism development are seen in the peripheral blood with all species except *P. falciparum*, where the peripheral blood usually contains only ring forms and gametocytes (unless infection is very severe)
- multiple ring forms within one erythrocyte are most common with *P. falciparum*, and are not seen with *P. malariae*
- mixed infections occur in 5 to 7% of patients

POTENTIAL LOOK-ALIKES
- platelet overlying red blood cell
- clumps of bacteria or platelets may be confused with schizonts
- masses of fused platelets may be confused with gametocyte
- precipitated stain or contaminating microorganisms (bacteria, fungi, etc.)

ASSOCIATED DISEASE STATES AND CONDITIONS
malaria

The four species of malaria are distinguished by differences in RBC and organism morphology. (See following pages for more detail.)

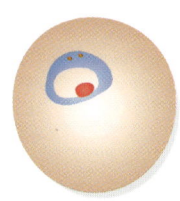
trophozoite

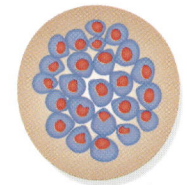
schizont

microgametocyte

There are four species of *Plasmodium* that cause the clinical disease known as malaria: *P. falciparum, P. vivax, P. ovale,* and *P. malariae. P. falciparum* typically causes the most severe disease and most fatal cases are of this type. Infection occurs through the bite of the female Anopheles mosquito, which lives in many parts of the world including the United States, but transmission of disease is most likely in areas in which the disease is endemic, particularly in tropical countries. The distribution of disease varies between species, with *P. vivax* being the most widespread (including temperate zones) and *P. falciparum* occurring primarily in the tropics. *P. ovale* infection is usually acquired on the west coast of Africa.

The organisms undergo a sexual cycle in the mosquito and only an asexual cycle in the human host. Sporozoites are injected into the human host from the saliva of the female mosquito, where they travel to the liver and inhabit hepatocytes. In the hepatocyte, organisms mature to tissue schizonts after an incubation of 8 to 25 days. These schizonts release thousands of merozoites into the bloodstream, which infect erythrocytes, forming ring trophozoites. The organisms then mature through the stages of trophozoite, schizont, and merozoite. The merozoites are again released and may either reinfect erythrocytes or mature to gametocytes. The gametocytes have no further growth in the human host, but if taken up by another mosquito, the male and female gametocytes can undergo sexual fusion, resulting in a new infectious cycle. This erythrocytic cycle takes 72 hours in *P. malariae* and 48 hours in the other three species.

Malaria is an acute infection that varies significantly in severity between different species. Both *P. vivax* and *P. ovale* can cause relapses months to years later because of reactivation of dormant phases of the organism remaining in hepatocytes. Malaria is characterized by high spiking fevers and chills that become periodic in accordance with the length of the erythrocytic phase of the organism. Patients typically have splenomegaly and varying amounts of headache, abdominal pain, diarrhea, and myalgia, with development of anemia from hemolysis, which in the most severe cases can be life-threatening or fatal (blackwater fever). High parasitemic loads can clog small capillaries in some cases, leading to severe renal and cerebral manifestations.

Diagnosis is made by identifying the organisms on either thick smears of peripheral blood stained with Giemsa, or thin smears stained with Wright-Giemsa. Speciation is most easily done on thin smears. In endemic areas, more rapid diagnosis is achieved using the upper cell layer of erythrocytes after centrifugation, staining with acridine orange, and examining the smear by fluorescent microscopy.

H1-45, 1987 (Blood, Wright-Giemsa, X380)

Identification	Referee %	Participant %
Malaria parasite	100	99.3

This picture shows several ring forms of malaria, which cannot be further speciated from this slide alone. However, other fields allowed this infection to be identified as *Plasmodium falciparum*. The background red blood cells are normochromic and normocytic.

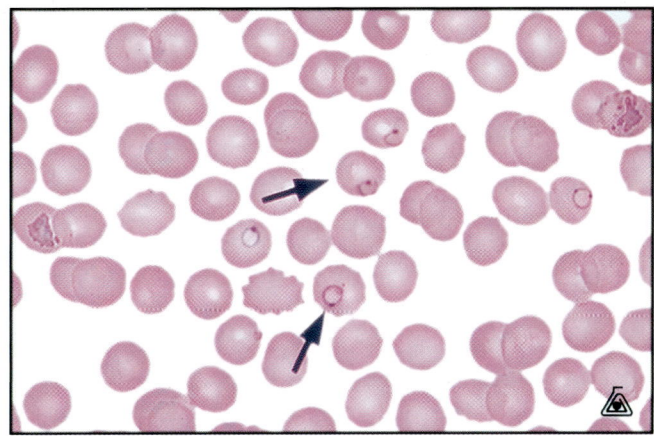

H-55, 1980 (Blood, Wright-Giemsa, X400)

Identification	Referee %	Participant %
Malaria parasite	100	98

This picture shows several trophozoites of malaria. The background red blood cells are unremarkable. The arrowed cell contains at least two microorganisms. An unarrowed red blood cell above it is also infected. The red chromatin dot is often the object first recognized and then the more indistinct blue cytoplasm is appreciated.

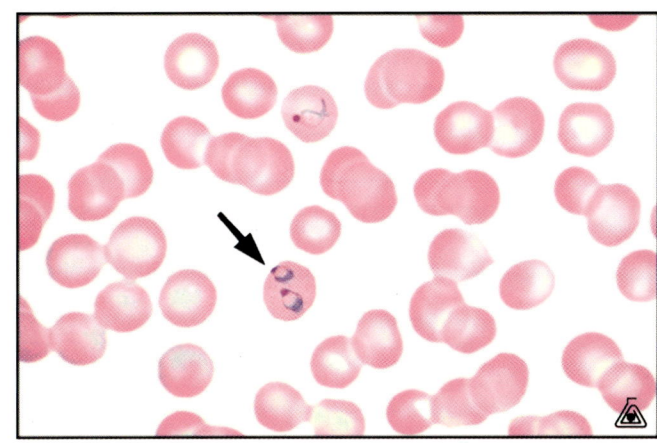

XL-28, 1988 (Blood, Wright-Giemsa, X380)

Identification	Referee %	Participant %
Malaria parasite	100	95.2

This picture shows the typical gametocyte of *Plasmodium falciparum*, which has a characteristic banana or boat shape. The background red blood cells appear normochromic, normocytic, and scattered normal-appearing platelets are also present. The organism appears to be extracellular but a thin, almost invisible veil of red blood cell cytoplasm surrounds it.

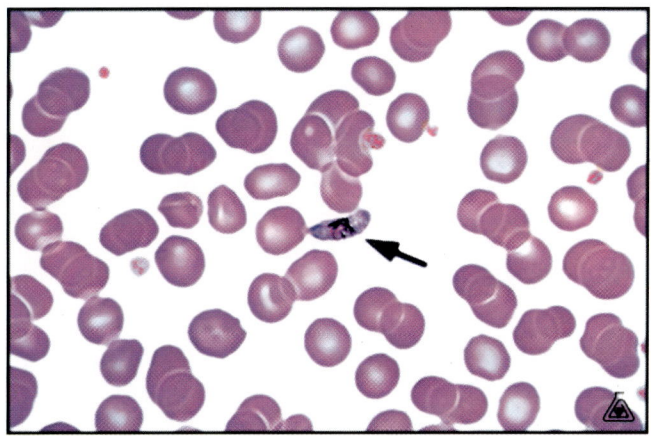

A Closer Look At...

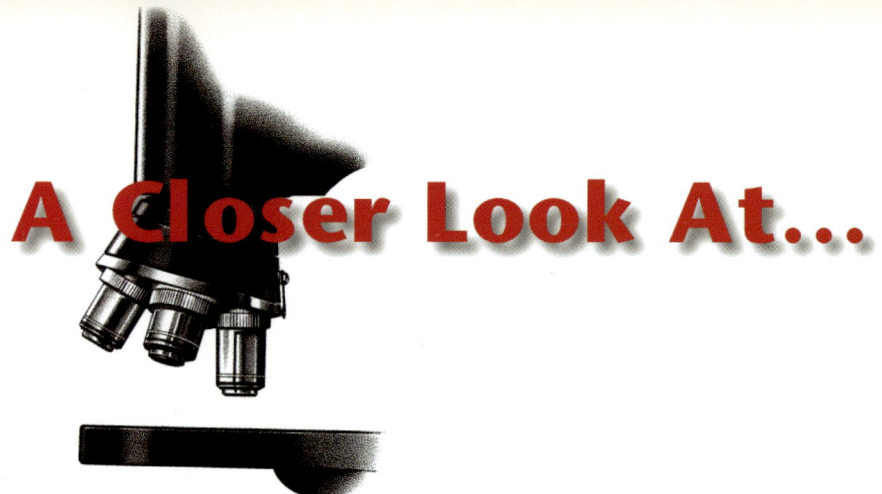

Species Differences Among Malarial Parasites

The chart below lists important morphologic differences between species of *Plasmodium*. These differences allow for accurate identification in nearly all cases, even when multiple infections are present. The most important differences include the presence or absence of various stages in the blood, the morphology of the gametocyte stage, the size of infected erythrocytes, and the presence of Schüffner's granules. *Babesia* can be easily confused with malaria, unless diagnostic tetrad forms are identified. (See *Babesia* discussion on page 254 for additional details).

SPECIES	RED CELLS	TROPHOZOITE	SCHIZONT	GAMETOCYTE	PARASITEMIA
P. vivax	larger than normal; Schüffner's dots present (coarse red granules)	>1/3 of RBC; single chromatin dot; ameboid cytoplasm	commonly present; 12-24 merozoites in random configuration; dense central yellow/black pigment	large and round; fills RBC; eccentric chromatin	1% of RBCs parasitized
P. falciparum	all sizes of RBCs infected; multiple infections of a single RBC more frequent than with other species	small rings <1/3 of RBC; delicate shape; double chromatin dots frequent	usually absent	banana-shaped; central chromatin	10% or more of RBCs parasitized (highest of all malarias)
P. malariae	normal size	>1/3 of RBC; compact cytoplasm; inverted chromatin dot; ameboid forms common (appear as band across RBC)	commonly present; 8-12 merozoites in rosette configuration; dense central yellow/black pigment	small and round; 1/2 to 1/3 size of RBC; eccentric chromatin	<0.5% of RBCs parasitized
P. ovale	oval and somewhat enlarged; fibriated edge; Schüffner's dots present (coarse red granules)	>1/3 of RBC; single chromatin dot; ameboid cytoplasm	commonly present; 8-12 merozoites in rosette configuration	small and round; 1/2 to 1/3 size of RBC; eccentric chromatin	>1% of RBCs parasitized
B. microti	no Schüffner's dots	round, ovoid, pear shaped; tetrads may be distinctive; multiple compact ring forms may occupy a single RBC; extraerythrocytic ring forms may be observed	not present	not present	5%-10% of RBCs parasitized (up to 50% in splenectomized patients)

Comparison of P. falciparum and P. vivax

The morphology of ring forms and their descendants differs among malarial species. This chart compares the morphology of the two most prevalent species, *Plasmodium vivax* and *Plasmodium falciparum*. Keep in mind that infections with two kinds of malaria are common.

P. falciparum   P. vivax

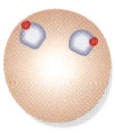

Early Trophozoite
Merozoites released from infected liver cells enter red cells and become small ring forms. *P. vivax* preferentially infects reticulocytes. At this stage, the rings are virtually indistinguishable from each other.

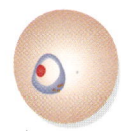

delicate ring shape; multiple parasites common, often at margins of RBC

rough shape; single chromatin dot; multiple parasites in RBC rarely seen

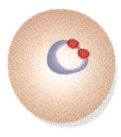

Late Trophozoite
The trophozoites feed on hemoglobin and excrete brownish hematin. In *P. vivax*, red cells enlarge as growing trophozoites become complex ameboid masses about 6–7 μm in size.

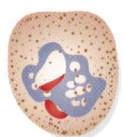 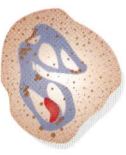

rings <1/3 of RBC; double chromatin dot frequent; no Schüffner's dots; no ameboid forms; no enlargement of RBC

ring > 1/3 of RBC; ameboid cytoplasm; single chromatin dot; Schüffner's dots

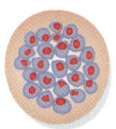

Schizont
Late trophozoites and schizonts are rarely present in *P. falciparum*. In contrast, all parasite stages coexist in *P. vivax*. The dying red cell disintegrates, releasing the merozoites which infect other red cells.

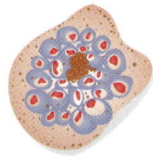

mature schizont with 24 merozoites (very rarely found)

mature schizont with 24–26 merozoites in random configuration; dense central yellow/black pigment

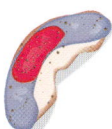 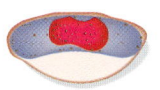

Gametocyte
A few parasites transform into large gametocytes. Crescentic or fusiform gametocytes are diagnostic of *P. falciparum*.

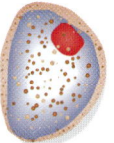 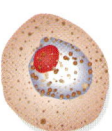

crescentic gametocytes

round gametocytes

Microfilaria

SYNONYMS
none

VITAL STATISTICS
size .... depends upon the species, but microfilariae vary from 160-315 μm in length and 3-10 μm in width (stained blood film); size is a useful criterion to distinguish various species
shape .... all microfilariae are elongate cylindrical bodies with one tapered end, one rounded end, and smooth contours; nuclei are arranged in a chain, filling most of the body; some species have a thin covering transparent sheath (see pages 278-279)

OTHER FINDINGS
size, presence or absence of a sheath, and the disposition of nuclei in the tail are most useful in speciating microfilariae found in the blood
patient's travel history is also helpful

POTENTIAL LOOK-ALIKES
fibers
chains of bacteria (especially bacilli)
contaminating fungal mycelia (such as Helicosporium)

ASSOCIATED DISEASE STATES AND CONDITIONS
elephantiasis
onchocerciasis (river blindness)

There are seven main species of filariae that infect humans and they share several characteristics in their life cycle, including an adult stage (filariae) outside the gastrointestinal tract, a blood-sucking insect as an intermediate host, and release of motile offspring (microfilariae) into the vertebrate host. The male and female worms (filaria) may reside in the lymphatic system, subcutaneous tissues, or within body cavities depending on the species. When the microfilariae are first released, they are relatively undifferentiated. They make their way to the blood stream or the skin, where they will live for one to two years. Five of the species circulate in the blood, some on a regular periodicity and others sporadically. The other two species do not circulate and are identified from small biopsies of skin.

If the microfilariae are ingested by a blood-sucking insect at this stage, they will undergo a series of additional maturation steps over 7-14 days. These organisms are now infective to a vertebrate host. If deposited on the skin, a few may enter the bite wound and undergo additional development before becoming adult worms and mating, producing new microfilariae and completing the cycle.

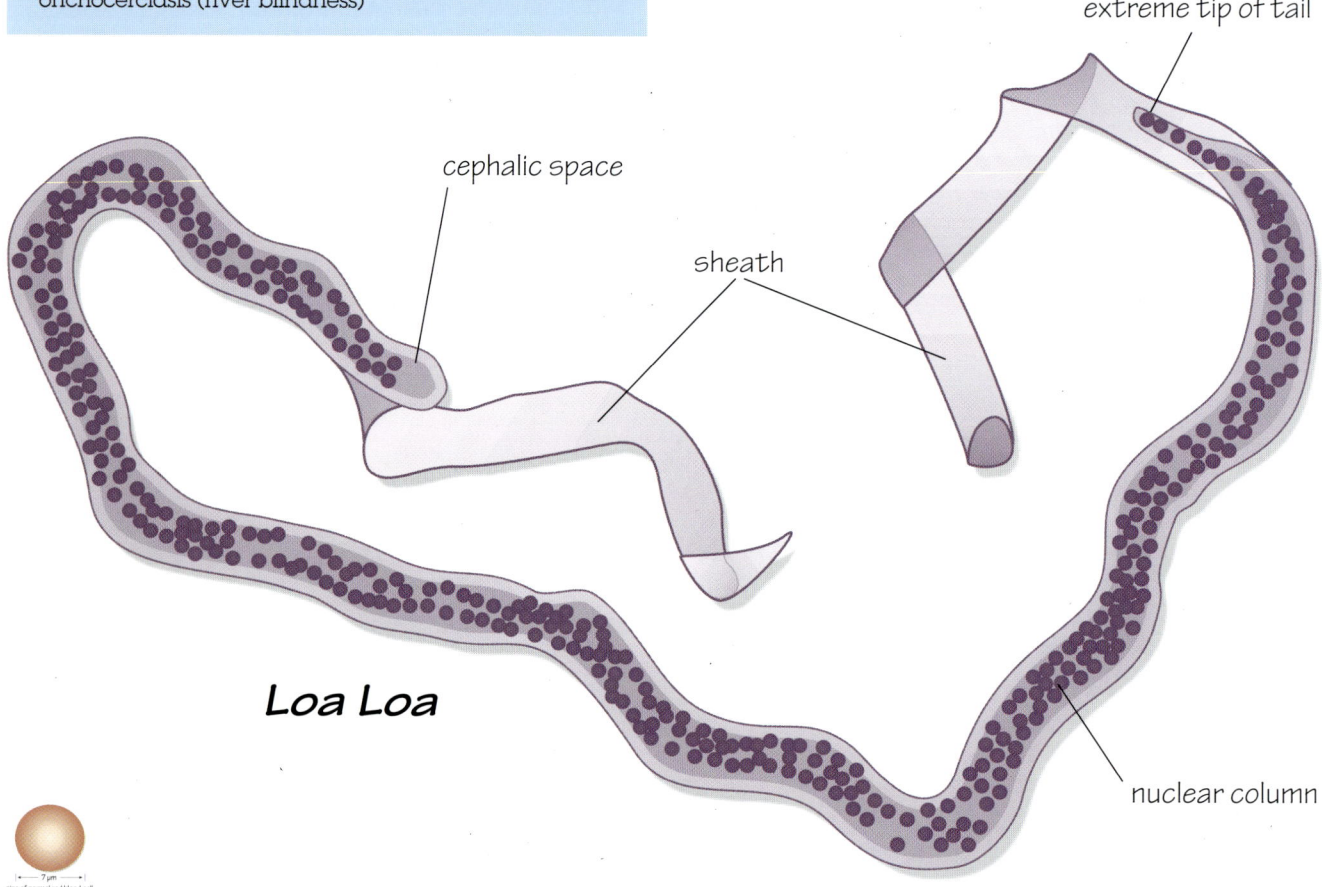

Loa Loa

The diseases associated with these parasites can be broken into three groups. The lymphatic filariae, *Wuchereria bancrofti* and *Brugia malayi*, cause obstruction of lymphatics and eventual elephantiasis. *Onchocerca volvulus* causes "river blindness" when the microfilariae invade the cornea. The adult worms reside in the skin, forming fibrous inflammatory nodules in subcutis or deeper tissues. The other microfilariae, *Loa Loa* and the *Mansonella* group, are less important causes of disease.

When microfilariae circulate in the peripheral blood, they are in low number, and as a result, they can be difficult to detect on a thin blood film stained with Wright-Giemsa. Nonetheless, this can be an effective method of diagnosis if one is lucky. In order to decrease the number of false negative results, thick smears (such as one uses in diagnosing malaria), concentration methods or membrane filtration are used. Once the organisms are identified in the blood, speciation is usually possible using the various morphologic parameters as described above and illustrated on the following pages.

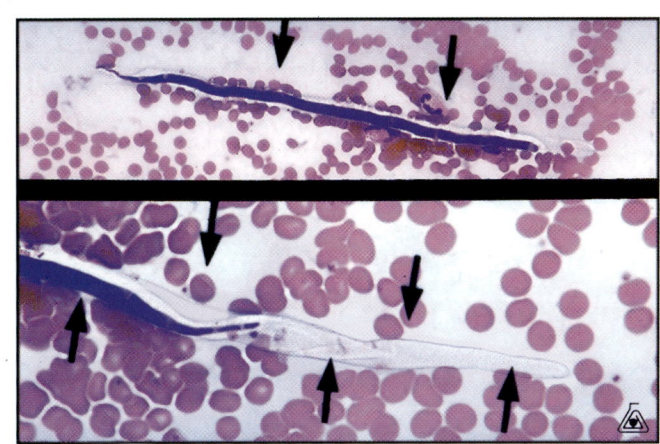

HE-21, 1996 (Blood, split screen: Upper, Wright-Giemsa, X100; Lower, Wright-Giemsa X200)

Identification	Referee %	Participant %
Microfilaria	100%	95.3%

This split screen photomicrograph shows morphologic details of *Loa Loa*, which is a sheathed microfilaria with nuclei extending to the tip and a short cephalic space. The sheath at the end of the tail is well illustrated in the lower field. Notice that the tail nuclei extend to the tip, distinguishing *Loa Loa* from *Brugia malayi* (two isolated nuclei) and *Wuchereria bancrofti* (no nuclei in tip).

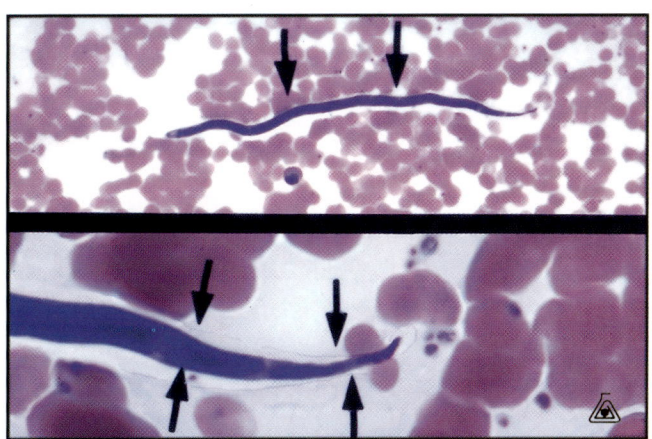

HE-22, 1996 (Blood, split screen: Upper, Wright-Giemsa, X100; Lower, Wright-Giemsa X400)

Identification	Referee %	Participant %
Microfilaria	100%	95.3%

This split screen photomicrgraph shows morphologic details of *Mansonella perstans* which is an unsheathed microfilaria. It is somewhat shorter than *Loa Loa* with a broad blunt tip containing nuclei and a longer cephalic space. The nuclei in the tail are best seen in the lower field. There is no sheath (compare to the photograph of *Loa Loa*, above). Nuclei extend to the tip of the tail, unlike *Mansonella ozzardi* and *Onchocerca volvulus*. In addition, the tail is not bent, distinguishing *Mansonella perstans* from *Mansonella streptocerca*. (See the table and illustrations on pages 278-279).

Microorganisms

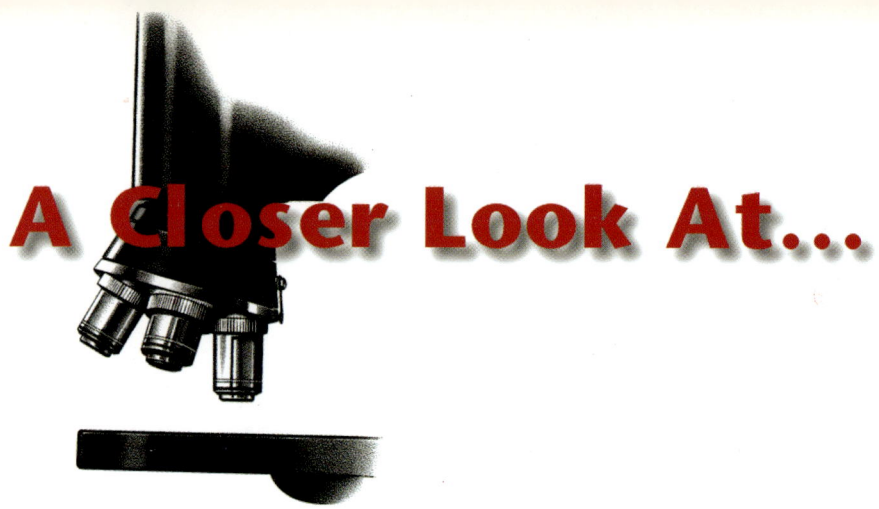

A Closer Look At...

Species Differences Among Microfilariae

Major differences among the various microfilariae are listed in the chart below and illustrated on the opposite page. The organisms can usually be separated based on the presence or absence of a sheath and the appearance of nuclei in the tail. The morphology of the head of the parasites (the cephalic space) is usually less helpful.

	Length (stained blood film)	Sheath/ Staining	Tail	Cephalic Space	Nuclear Column	Circulation	Geographic Location	Associated Disease
Wuchereria bancrofti	244-296 μm	sheath present; non-staining	pointed with no nuclei in tip	not as long as wide	distinct	yes between 22:00 and 02:00 hrs	Asia and Africa	elephantiasis
Brugia malayi	177-230 μm	sheath present; stains pink	swelling at tip with 2 nuclei	much longer than wide	may be blurred	yes nocturnal	Japan, India, SE Asia, Korea, Phillipines	elephantiasis (milder disease)
Loa Loa	231-250 μm	sheath present; non-staining	nuclei to rounded tip	short	distinct	yes diurnal	West and Central Africa	loaisis
Mansonella perstans	190-200 μm	no sheath	broad, blunt with nuclei to tip	longer than wide	distinct	yes anytime	Africa, Central and S. America	usually asymptomatic
Mansonella ozzardi	163-203 μm	no sheath	thin pointed tip without nuclei	longer than wide	distinct	yes anytime	Central and S. America, West Indies	usually asymptomatic
Mansonella streptocerca	180-240 μm	no sheath	tapered and bent hooked tip with nuclei	longer than wide	distinct	no skin only	West and Central Africa	usually asymptomatic
Onchocerca volvulus	304-315 μm	no sheath	pointed, no nuclei in tip	broad	distinct	no skin only	Africa, Central and parts of S. America	onchocerciasis (river blindness)

Tail and Sheath Morphology of Microfilariae

Sheathed Microfilariae

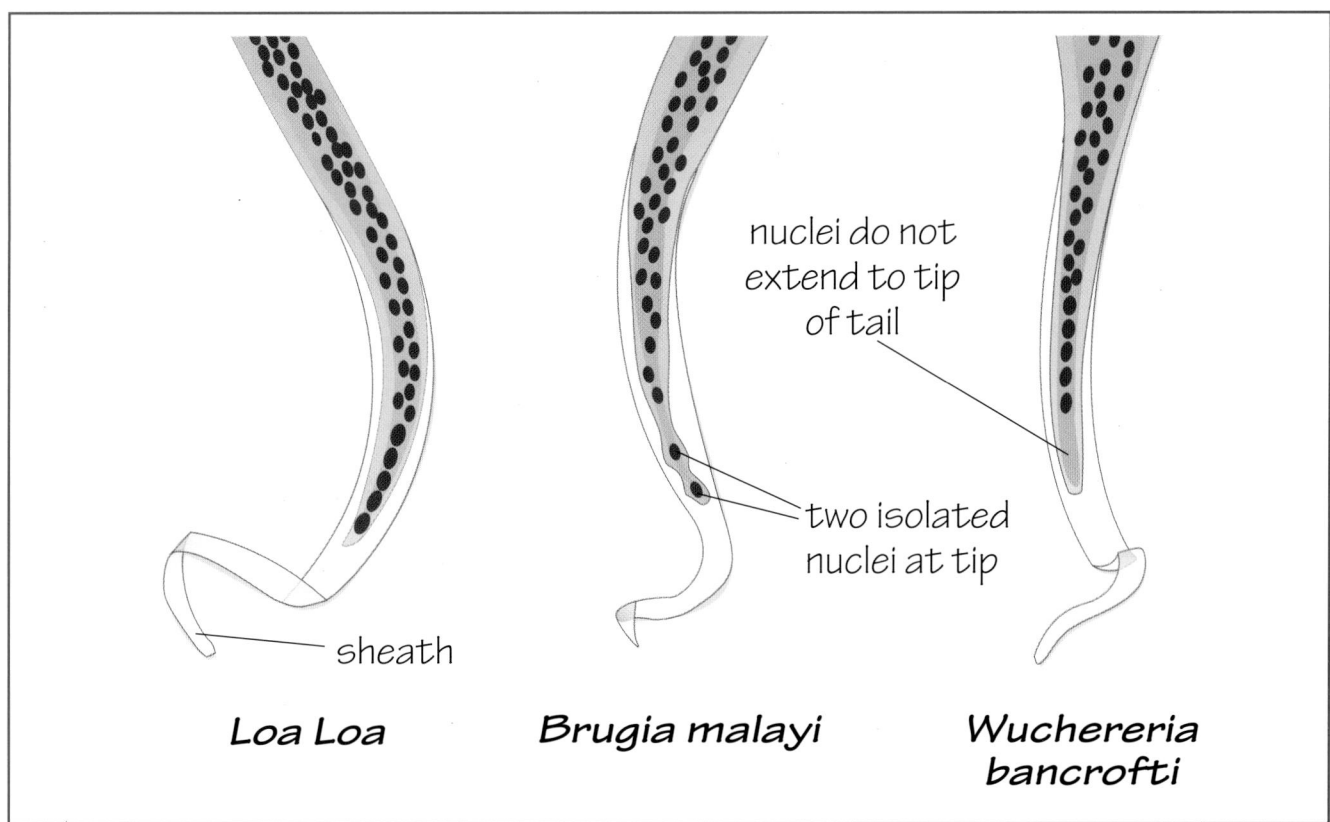

Unsheathed Microfilariae

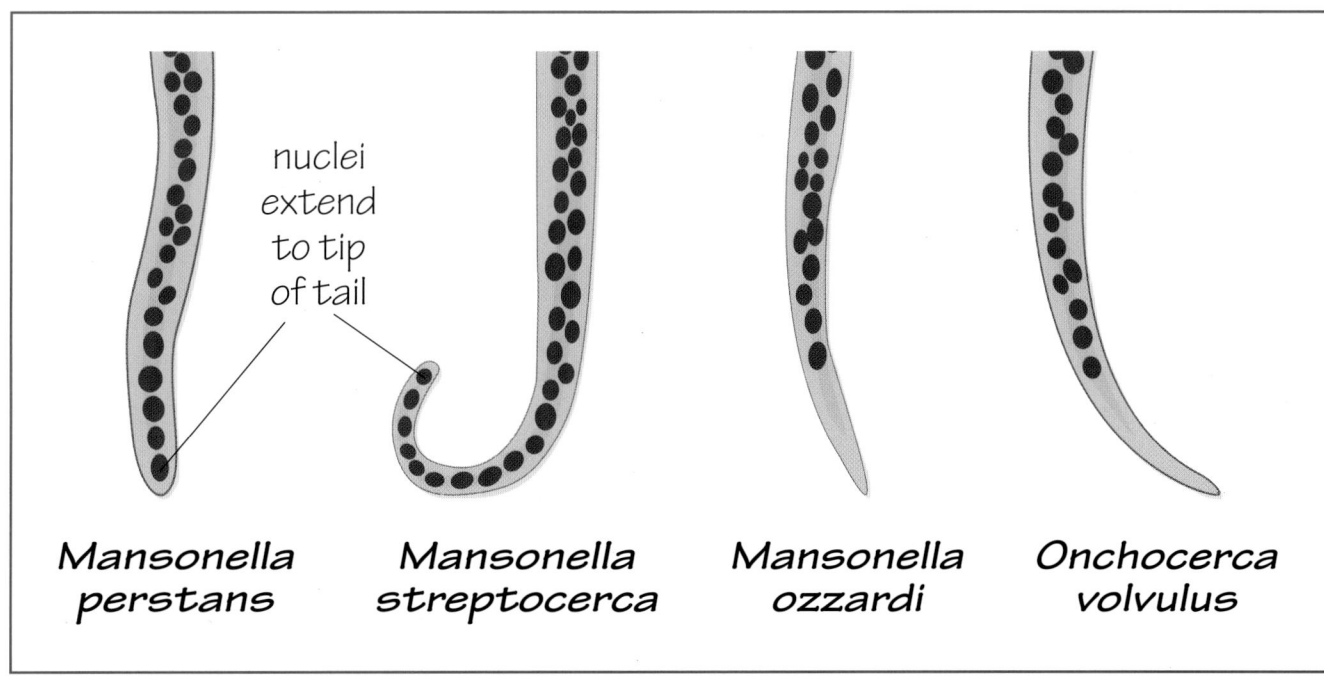

Protozoan (Non-Malarial)

SYNONYMS
none

VITAL STATISTICS
- size .... trypomastigotes of the *T. brucei* group are up to 30 µm long with graceful curves and a small kinetoplast; trypomastigotes of *T. cruzi* are shorter (20 µm) with S and C shapes and a larger kinetoplast
- shape .... trypomastigote stage is seen in the peripheral blood and shows a long slender body with a kinetoplast at the posterior end, an undulating membrane and axoneme extending the entire length, and a flagellum at the anterior end, representing an extension of the axoneme

OTHER FINDINGS
- high IgM levels in blood and CSF of patients with African trypanosomiasis
- serology is useful for diagnosis and to help distinguish American from African trypanosomiasis

POTENTIAL LOOK-ALIKES
- artefacts such as fibers, threads, etc.
- microfilaria

ASSOCIATED DISEASE STATES AND CONDITIONS
- African sleeping sickness (*T. brucei*)
- Chagas' disease (*T. cruzi*)

The trypanosomes are *hemoflagellates*, along with *Leishmania* organisms, and are characterized by the presence of a kinetoplast. The diseases caused by trypanosomes are typically divided into American trypanosomiasis (Chagas' disease) and African trypanosomiasis.

Chagas' disease occurs primarily in Central America and South America, although endogenous cases may occur in the southern, southeastern, and southwestern United States. The causative agent, *Trypanosoma cruzi*, requires both an animal reservoir (usually rodents) and an insect vector (reduviid bug). The reduviid bug defecates while biting, and if the bite site is scratched, the organisms can enter the host. They can also be introduced through intact mucosa of the mouth or conjunctiva. The organisms enter cells, where they form amastigotes and proliferate. When the cell is full, amastigotes transform to trypomastigotes and these are released into the blood to reinfect other cells.

Chagas' disease is typically acute in children and infants, with symptoms of fever, chills, hepatosplenomegaly, and myocarditis, which may be fatal. In adults, the acute infection is milder, but in both adults and children, the infection is lifelong and chronic sequelae can occur including myocardial conduction defects, myocardial scarring, megacolon, and megaesophagus.

African trypansomiasis has two forms, both of which require an insect vector (the tsetse fly) for transmission. *T. brucei rhodesiense* causes disease in East Africa, with several animal reservoirs. This disease is acute with fever, lymphadenopathy, and a rapid clinical deterioration. In contrast, *T. brucei gambiense* has a human reservoir. *T. brucei gambiense* causes the disease known as sleeping sickness with somnolence and coma as the major manifestations.

Trypanosomes in Peripheral Blood

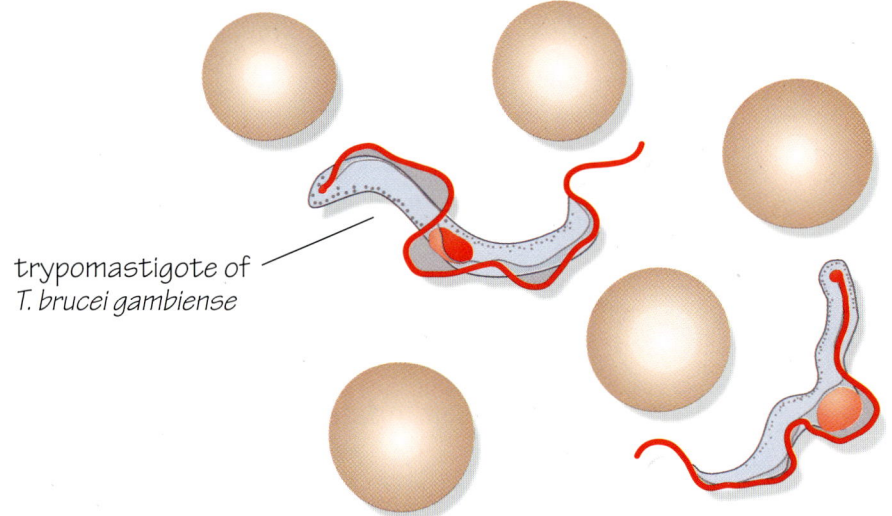

trypomastigote of *T. brucei gambiense*

HE-39, 1991 (Blood, Wright-Giemsa, X400)

Identification	Referee %	Participant %
Protozoan (non-malarial)	100	87.8

Two trypomastigotes of *T. brucei gambiense* are present in the center of the field in an extracellular location. The background red blood cells appear normochromic and normocytic. The cytoplasm of the protozoa is pale blue and contains darker granules. The nucleus is central and red-staining. A smaller kinetoplast is located at the posterior end. An undulating membrane and flagellum can also be distinguished. The morphology is distinctly different from malarial organisms and should not be confused with *P. falciparum* gametes which are smaller and more plump.

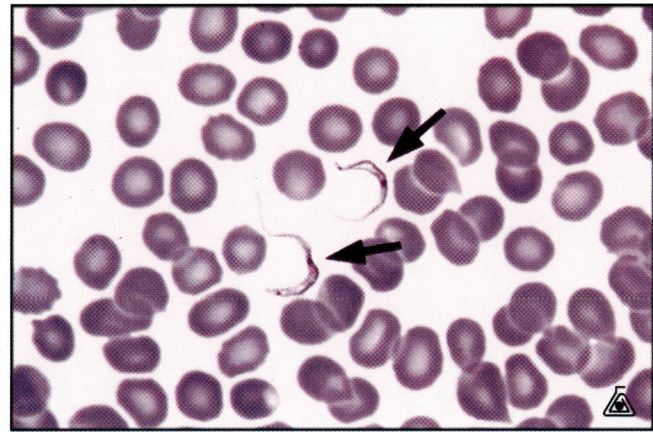

Trypomastigotes

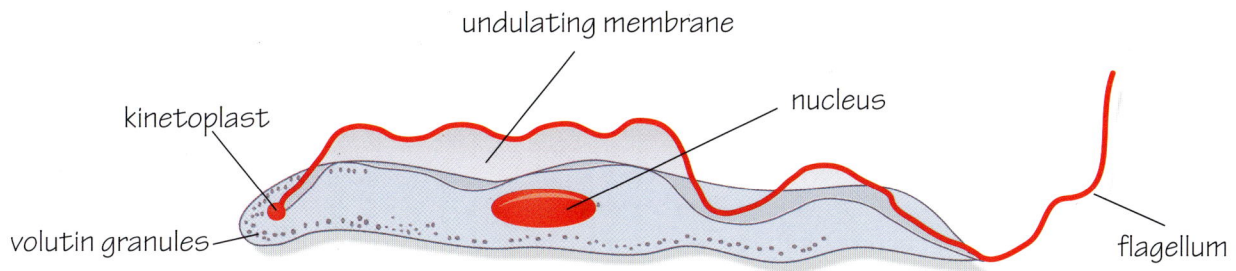

Trypanosoma brucei

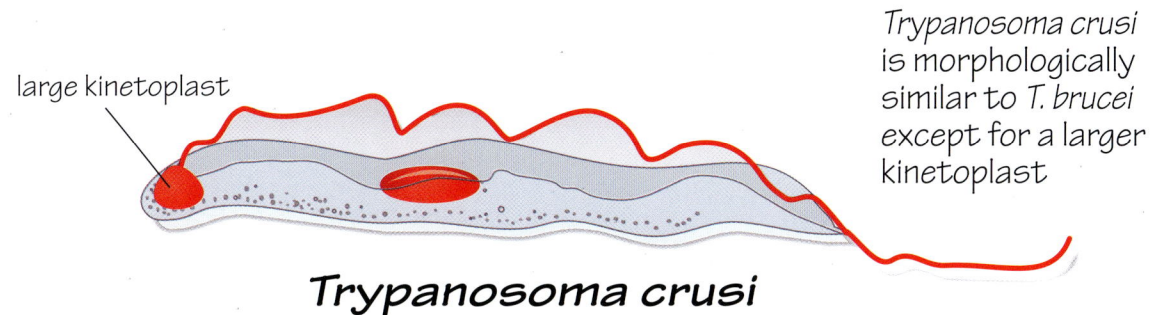

Trypanosoma crusi

Trypanosoma crusi is morphologically similar to *T. brucei* except for a larger kinetoplast

A Closer Look At...

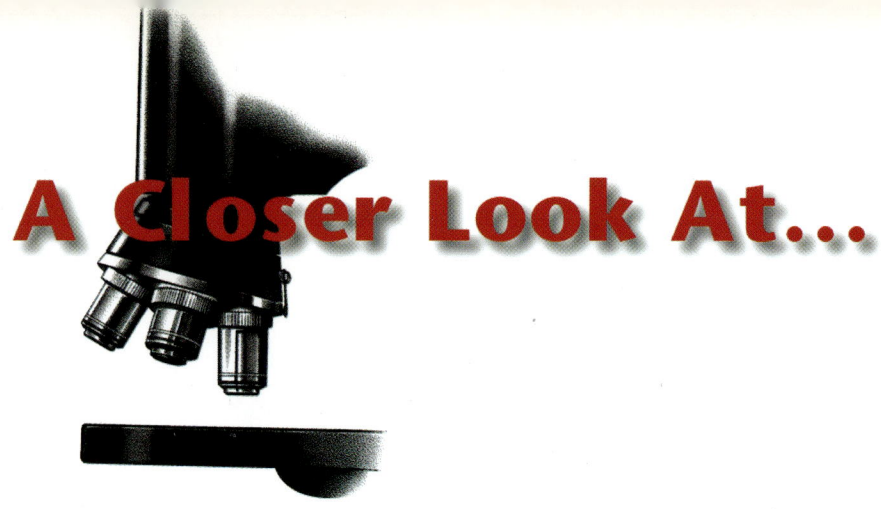

African Trypanosomiasis

The life cycle of the protozoa causing African trypanosomiasis, *Trypanosoma brucei gambiense* and *Trypanosoma brucei rhodesiense,* is depicted on the next page. Tsetse flies (*Glossina* species) are the insect vectors. Once ingested, the trypomastigotes multiply in the tsetse fly stomach and intestine for 10 to 14 days before traveling to the salivary glands. Here, the organisms transform into epimastigotes and continue to divide. After an additional week, they transform into infective metacyclic trypomastigotes. The entire cycle in the fly takes about 21 days.

When the insect feeds, the infective forms are injected with the saliva. A dose of at least 350 trypomastigotes is necessary to infect man. One to two days later the organisms leave the skin and enter the blood stream and lymphatic vessels where they continue to multiply by asexual binary division. Direct transmission may occur if feeding is interrupted and the fly quickly travels from an infected host to a susceptible one.

An inflammatory nodule or chancre often develops at the site of the tsetse fly bite. After dividing for a short time, the trypomastigotes enter the blood and lymphatics. At this point, the patient's own immune system may limit or even cure the disease. If not, replication continues and the first symptoms occur when the organisms invade lymph nodes. This triggers irregular fevers and night sweats, sometimes accompanied by headache, malaise, and anorexia. A transient skin rash is usually seen in light-skinned patients. The lymph nodes are enlarged, soft, and non-tender. Posterior cervical lymph nodes are the most common ones involved (a finding called Winterbottom's sign). The spleen and liver may become enlarged as well. Intermittent febrile episodes up to a week in duration are followed by symptom-free periods of several weeks. The trypanosomes are capable of expressing variable antigen types in order to evade the host's immune system. Each febrile episode is initiated by a new antigenic subtype of trypomastigote. Depending on the number of trypanosomes in the blood, the disease may be mild or fulminating.

As the disease progresses, the immune system is overwhelmed. This may take years. The sleeping sickness stage begins when the trypomastigote invades the brain, meninges, and spinal cord. Patients are confused, tired, show poor coordination, and often complain of a constant severe headache. Progressive apathy and drowsiness are accompanied by changes in personality such as delusions and hysteria. Eventually, the patient develops an uncontrollable desire to sleep and finally lapses into a coma. Patients die of secondary bacterial infection or malnutrition.

The Rhodesian form follows a more rapid course than the Gambian form of trypanosomiasis. Some patients develop myocarditis and die due to heart failure before the brain is involved. Tissue damage by the parasite is not responsible for the severe pathogenicity, which is more likely due to destruction of the immune system through abnormal stimulation by parasite products such as enzymes, mitogens, and hemolysins.

Definitive laboratory diagnosis is made by finding the trypanosomes in the blood, CSF, bone marrow, or material aspirated from enlarged lymph nodes. Multiple daily blood examinations may be necessary.

Drug treatment is usually effective if begun early in the disease. Once the CNS is involved, therapy is much less successful. All the drugs are toxic and require prolonged administration.

Prevention is complex and involves medical, veterinary, agricultural, entomological, and social interplay. Whole tribes of people have had to be displaced. Prophylactic medication, insect repellents, heavy clothing, nets, and screens give some protection to travelers.

Life Cycle of Trypanosoma gambiense and Trypanosoma rhodesiense

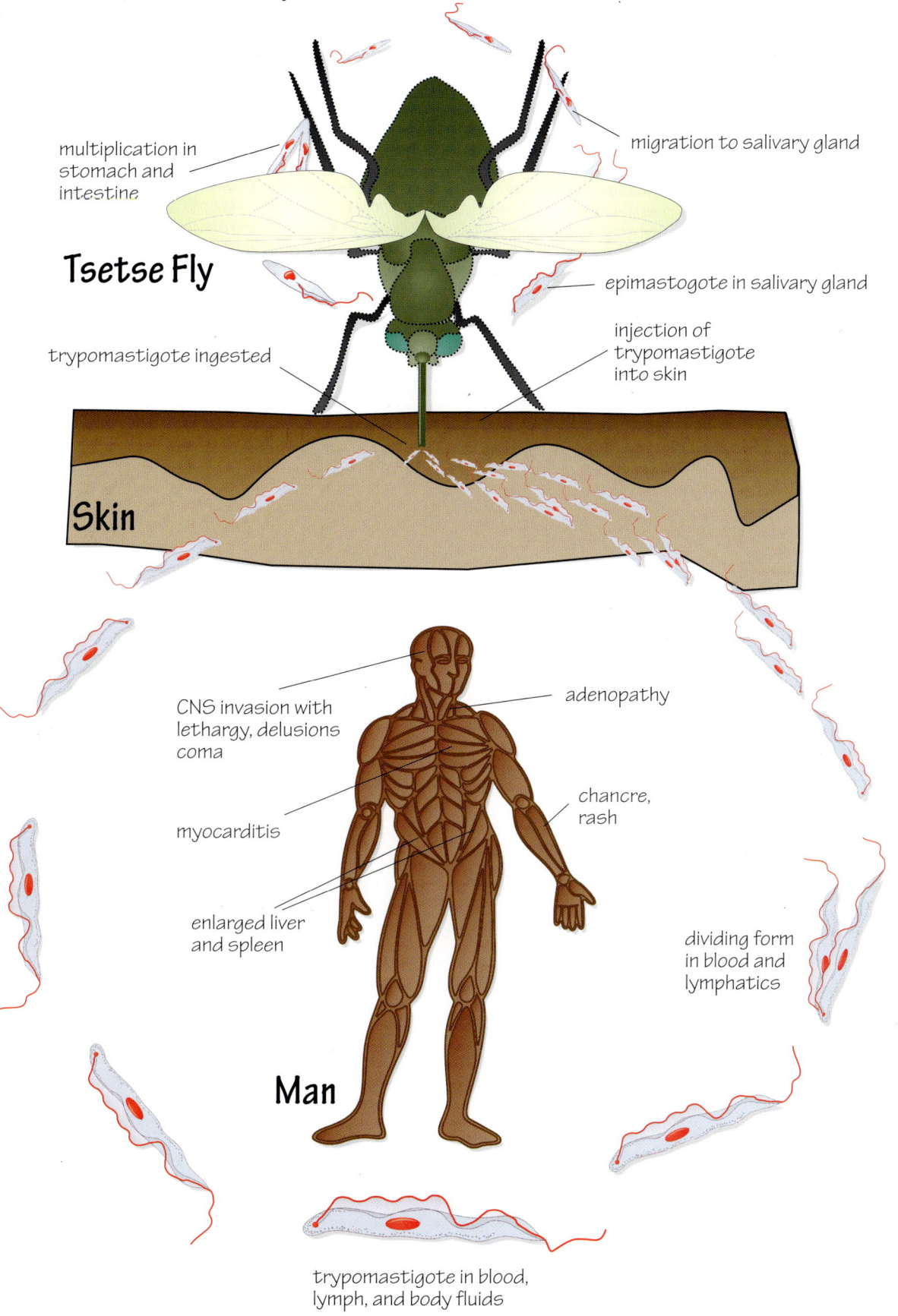

Artifacts

Introduction 285
Basket Cell or Smudge Cell 286
Neutrophil Necrobiosis 288
   A Closer Look At...Cell Death 290
Erythrocyte with Overlapping Platelet 292
Stain Precipitate 294

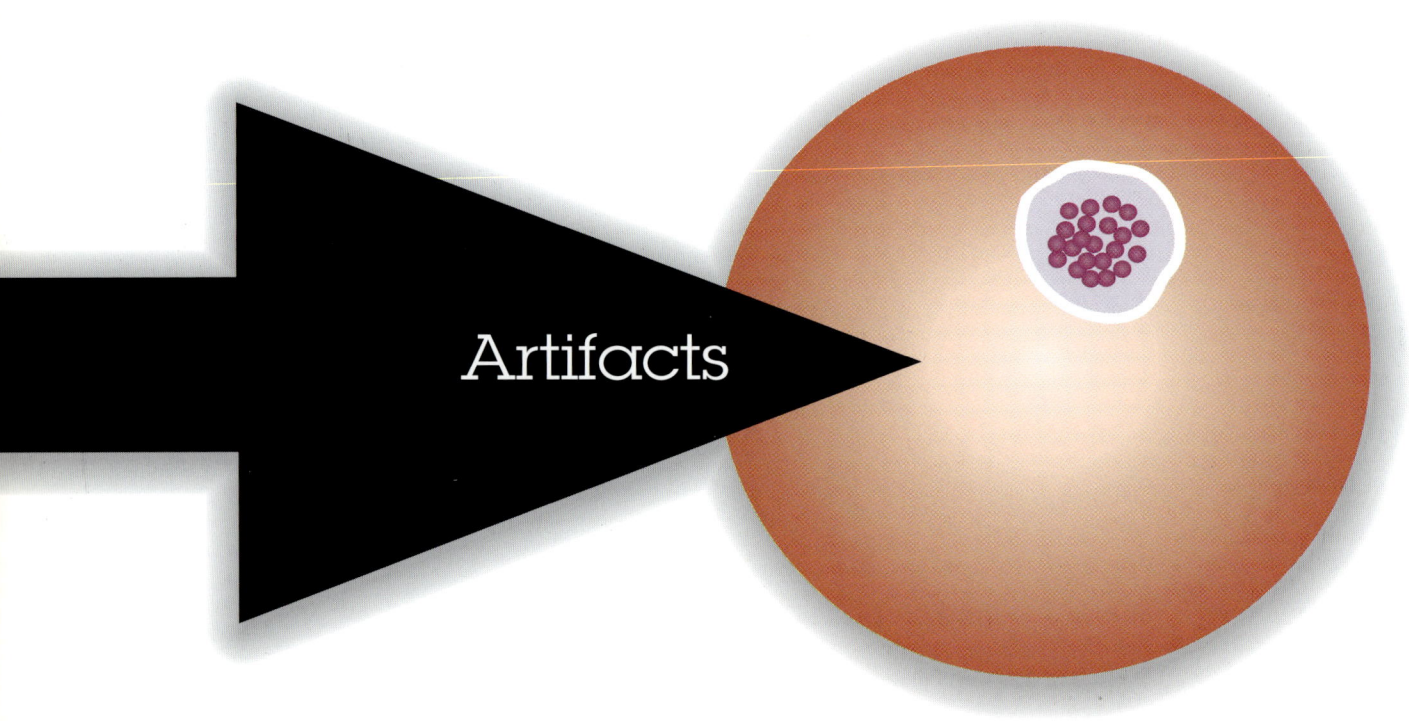

Introduction

A variety of processes, conditions, and physiologic events can mimic diagnostic elements or other cells. This short section looks at a few of these imposters. In some cases, poor technique (delay in processing) or inattention to proper staining procedures can be avoided. Other examples are physiologic and part of the natural order in hematology.

A subset of conditions are concerned with the morphology of cell death. Cellular tombstones in the form of basket and smudge cells may mimic lymphocytes and megakaryocyte nuclei. They are also helpful in their own right as an indicator of cell fragility, a common feature of chronic lymphocytic leukemia. Necrobiotic polymorphonuclear leukocytes may be mistaken for nucleated red blood cells. Other conditions suggest red cell inclusions or organisms, such as stain precipitate or platelets overying red blood cells.

Basket Cell or Smudge Cell

SYNONYMS
none

VITAL STATISTICS
- size .... variable; may be size of lymphocyte or much larger as the chromatin strands spread out over the slide
- cell/nuclear shape .... highly variable; there is often a central mass of chromatin from which wisps and strands of chromatin extend, giving the characteristic basket appearance; other cells are simply amorphous smears of chromatin
- chromatin .... homogeneous; no detail
- cytoplasm .... none or indistinct

KEY DIFFERENTIATING FEATURES
uniform purple chromatin in amorphous smear (smudge cell) or strands of chromatin arcing out from a homogenous chromatin mass (basket cell)
no cytoplasm

POTENTIAL LOOK-ALIKES
megakaryocyte nuclei and nuclear fragments
lymphocytes
stain precipitate
necrobiotic cells
metastatic circulating small cell carcinoma (neuroblastoma, oat cell carcinoma)

ASSOCIATED DISEASE STATES AND CONDITIONS
chronic lymphocytic leukemia
infectious mononucleosis
pertussis
lymphoma
rarely encountered in normal blood smears

The term basket cell or smudge cell is a form of cell death most commonly associated with cells that are fragile and easily damaged in the process of making a peripheral blood smear. The cell is usually a lymphocyte. When these cells degenerate and die or are damaged when making a wedge smear, the nucleus may either be a smudge or the chromatin strands may spread out from a condensed nuclear remnant giving the appearance of a basket. Cytoplasm is either absent or indistinct.

Basket cells are more common in some disease states characterized by lymphocyte fragility, such as infectious mononucleosis and chronic lymphocytic leukemia. They can be avoided by adding a drop of 22% bovine serum albumin to four or five drops of blood before preparing a wedge smear.

As discussed on pages 288-291, necrobiotic cells have swollen chromatin or condensed chromatin with recognizable cytoplasm; often, the cell's origin can be deciphered. Smudge cells are usually lymphocytes but there is no recognizable cytoplasm to give a clue to the origin of the cell. Basket cells should not be confused with necrobiotic neutrophils which have enough cytoplasm to determine the origin of the cell.

Basket Cells and Smudge Cells

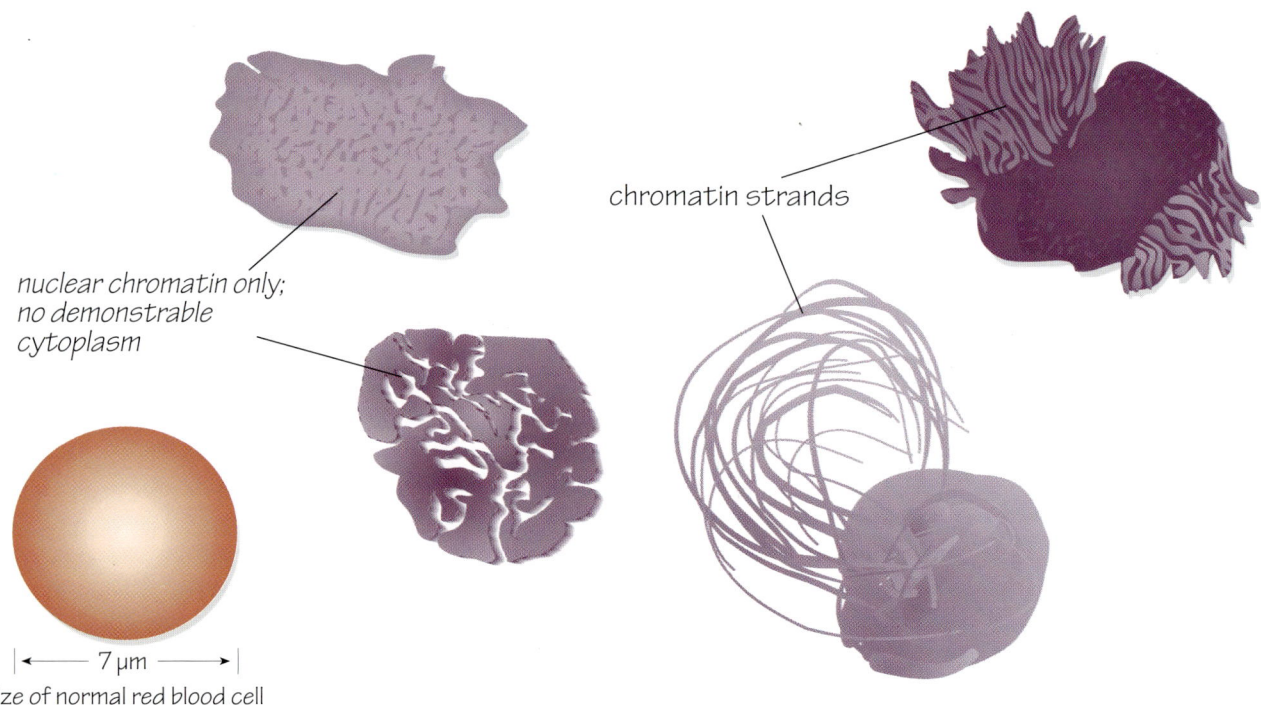

nuclear chromatin only; no demonstrable cytoplasm

chromatin strands

7 μm
size of normal red blood cell

HE-25, 1993 (Blood, Wright-Giemsa, X320)

Identification	Referee %	Participant %
Basket cell/smudge cell	96.3	87.8
Necrobiotic neutrophil	-	5.1
Stain precipitate	3.7	2.5
Megakaryocyte nucleus	-	2.0

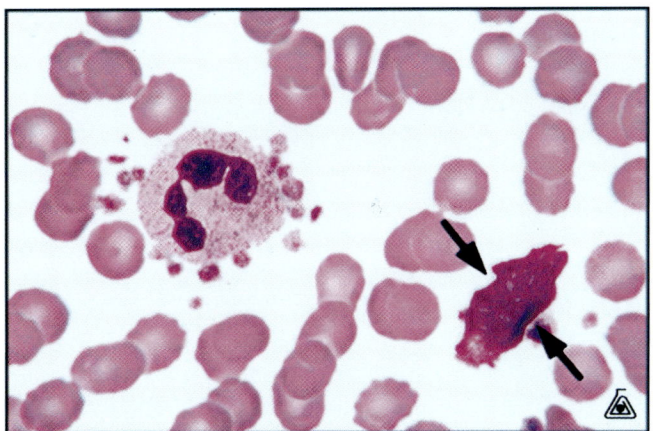

The cell illustrated here is a basket cell/smudge cell. It is most likely a degenerated lymphocyte or monocyte. There is no cytoplasm and therefore the cell cannot be identified with certainty. All that remains is condensed nuclear material. The arrowed object is not stain precipitate. Stain appears as discrete particles. It may sometimes be confused with bacterial contamination. Stain lacks any organized structure. The arrowed object does not have any specific definition but it clearly has structure and thus represents some sort of organized cellular element. The "randomness" that characterizes precipitated stain is lacking. The other leukocyte in the field is a segmented neutrophil with adherent platelets (platelet satellitism). Red cells are unremarkable.

XL-89, 1989 (Blood, Wright-Giemsa, X330)

Identification	Referee %	Participant %
Basket cell/smudge cell	100	97.5

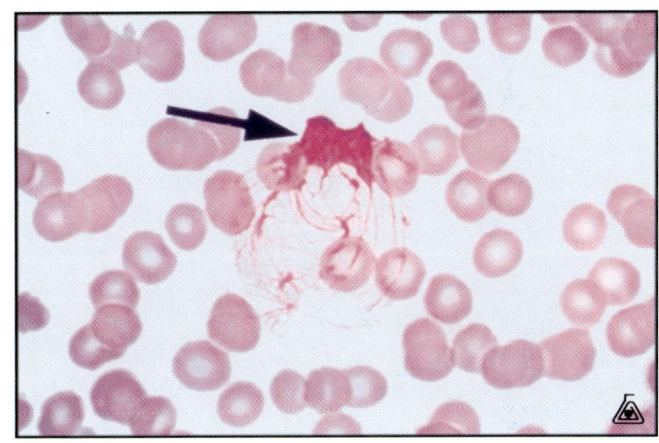

The arrowed cell is a basket cell. The cell probably originated from a lymphocyte or monocyte but because there is no cytoplasm, the exact origin cannot be determined. The nuclear remnant has burst, yielding coarse chromatin strands which extend from a condensed nuclear mass. The structure resembles a basket. Such cells are frequently seen in infectious mononucleosis and chronic lymphocytic leukemia. These artifacts are easily prevented by the addition of albumin to the blood before the peripheral blood smear is made.

H-11, 1994 (Blood, Wright-Giemsa, X330)

Identification	Referee %	Participant %
Basket cell/smudge cell	96.3%	87.8%

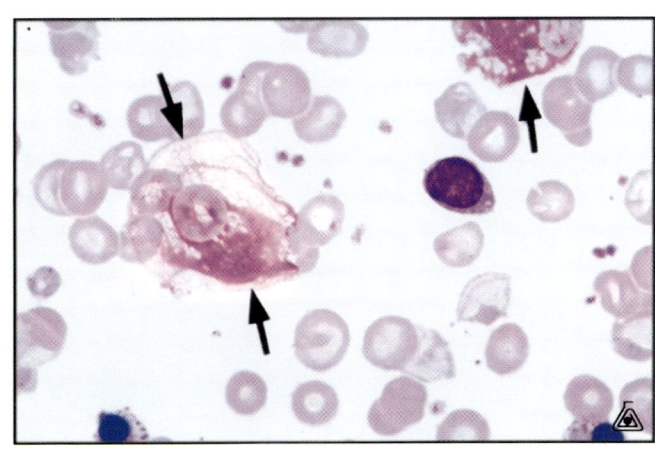

The two arrowed structures are basket cells or smudge cells. The terms are synonymous. The cells are formed in the process of smearing the blood on a glass slide. Cells that are more delicate than normal, such as the lymphocytes in chronic lymphocytic leukemia and infectious mononucleosis, are readily damaged by the mechanical process of smear preparation. Only the markedly distorted nucleus remains; the cytoplasm has been stripped free. The nuclear chromatin may take on a variety of shapes and fenestrations. The chromatin strands may extend out from a nubbin of DNA giving the cell the typical appearance of a basket. The cells are not degenerated or necrobiotic leukocytes because they lack any cytoplasm or identifiable granules.

Neutrophil Necrobiosis

SYNONYMS
degenerated leukocyte

VITAL STATISTICS
- size .... 10 to 15 μm
- N:C ratio .... 1:3 or less
- cell shape .... usually round or oval
- nuclear shape .... variable; multiple lobes which often vary in size and shape without connecting filaments; can be single; may appear fragmented and small, resembling organisms; nuclear margins may be blurred.
- chromatin .... pyknotic, dark, homogeneous and dense; parachromatin not visible
- nucleoli .... none
- cytoplasm .... abundant; generally pale pink with numerous fine, lilac granules; toxic granulation; can be hypogranular or agranular; often vacuolated; cytoplasm becomes frayed as cell degenerates; may contain ingested organisms.

KEY DIFFERENTIATING FEATURES
abundant cytoplasm containing neutrophilic granules and multiple, unconnected nuclear lobes with dark, homogeneous chromatin
based on cytoplasmic appearance and nuclear characteristics, can still be identified as neutrophils, rather than basket cells/smudge cells.

OTHER FINDINGS
signs of infection or inflammation such as neutrophilia, toxic granulation and/or vacuolation, and left-shifted myeloid maturation; may see ingested organisms (must be distinguished from small nuclear fragments)

POTENTIAL LOOK-ALIKES
nucleated red blood cells in the blood
orthochromic normoblasts in the bone marrow
neutrophils with toxic granulation and/or vacuolation
basket cell/smudge cell (degenerated leukocytes)

ASSOCIATED DISEASE STATES AND CONDITIONS
this cell type is nonspecific and can be seen in normal individuals and in a wide range of pathologic conditions including:
- infections
- inflammation
- reactive disorders

Degenerated neutrophils are generally easily identified since they resemble normal segmented neutrophils. The major distinguishing feature is karyorrhexis and/or pyknosis of the nucleus. These changes are appreciated when a cell with neutrophilic granules (pale pink cytoplasm with fine lilac granules) contains multiple, unconnected nuclear lobes (karyorrhexis) or a single, dark, round to oval nucleus (pyknosis). The chromatin is dense and homogeneous without visible parachromatin or nucleoli. The nuclear outlines may become indistinct and blurred. The nuclear lobes may also fragment into numerous small particles of varying sizes that resemble microorganisms such as bacteria or fungi. The degenerating cell may also contain real fungi or bacteria; special stains may be needed to confirm the diagnosis.

As the cellular degeneration continues, the cytoplasm will become hypogranulated and then agranular. The cytoplasmic borders may become frayed and indistinct. Sometimes, the cells will contain scattered larger azurophilic or dark blue granules (toxic granulation). Vacuolation is frequent.

Other cells that may resemble degenerated neutrophils are nucleated red cells in the blood and orthochromic normoblasts in the bone marrow. These cell types have pinkish-orange, agranular cytoplasm and have a single, often eccentric nucleus with dense chromatin and very little to no parachromatin. The nuclear to cytoplasmic ratio is about 1:2 and the nuclear and cytoplasmic borders are sharp and distinct.

If a cell is too degenerated to recognize it as a neutrophil, one should identify it as a basket/smudge cell. Basket/smudge cells have no identifiable characteristics and consist of smeared nuclear material without distinguishable cytoplasm.

Necrobiotic Neutrophils

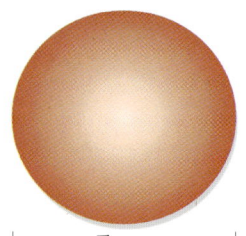
|←— 7 μm —→|
size of normal red blood cell

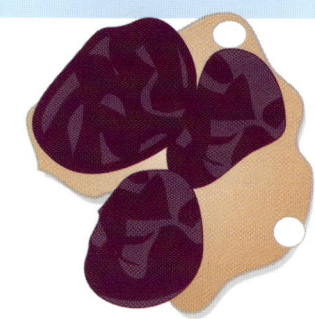

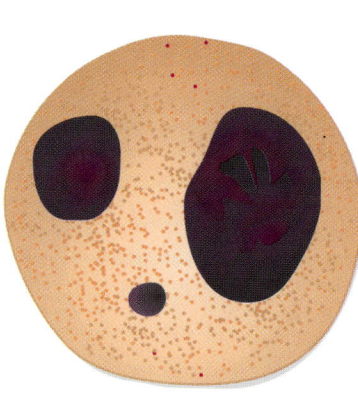

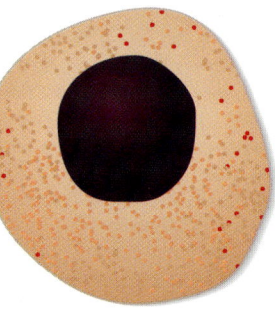
some cells may mimic nucleated red blood cells; granular cytoplasm is a helpful distinguishing feature

A-09, 1987 (Blood Wright-Giemsa, X350)

Identification	Referee %	Participant %
Neutrophil necrobiosis	100	80.1

The arrowed cell is a degenerated neutrophil. The nucleus is fragmented forming three separate remnants with dark, compact chromatin. No connecting filaments are present. The non-arrowed cell to the bottom is a mature lymphocyte. The red blood cells are normochromic and normocytic. The platelets appear abnormal and only two are present. A giant, hypogranulated platelet is noted to the right of the arrowed cell and a normal size, hypogranulated platelet is seen at the bottom of the picture, adjacent to the cell at the edge.

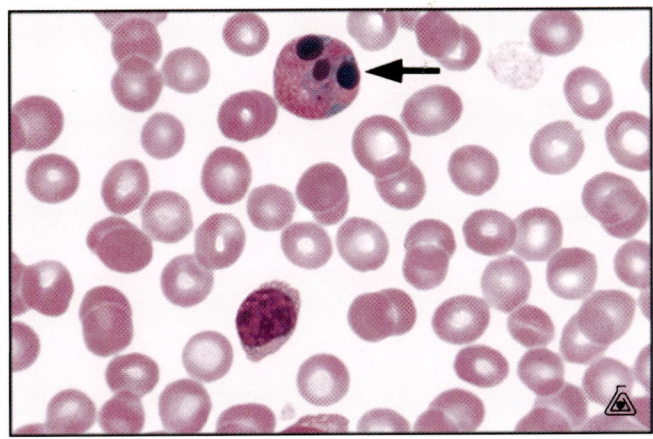

H1-18, 1984 (Blood, Wright-Giemsa, X350)

Identification	Referee %	Participant %
Neutrophil necrobiosis	100	95.7

This blood film shows crenated red blood cells in a thick area of the blood film from a case used to illustrate artifactual changes that occur in "old" blood. No platelets are present. The arrowed cell is a neutrophil which has undergone degenerative changes. The nuclear material appears as three separate remnants with dark, compact chromatin. No connecting filament is present. The cytoplasm is discolored and granular with bluish and pink/red areas. Crenated red cells are seen which exhibit rouleaux formation as commonly found in thick areas of blood films. One red cell to the right of the arrowed cell contains an apparent Howell-Jolly body which is out of the plane of focus.

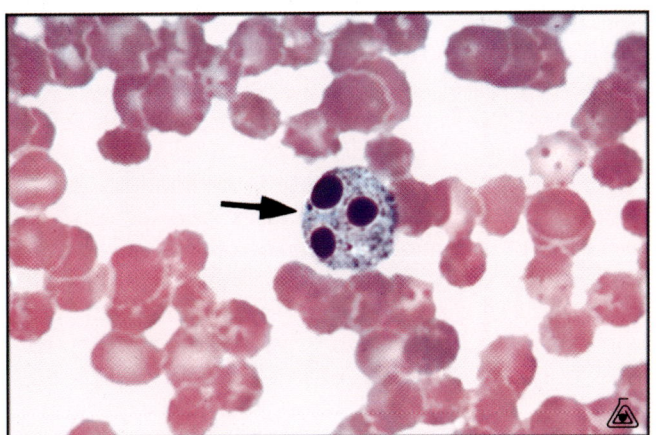

HE-45, 1994 (Blood, Wright-Giemsa, X400)

Identification	Referee %	Participant %
Neutrophil necrobiosis	75.9	83.9
Basket cell	13.8	0.5
Hypersegmented neutrophil	6.8	1.6
Neutrophil with dysplastic nucleus/agranular cytoplasm	-	4.8

The arrowed cell demonstrates neutrophil necrobiosis. The nucleus is pyknotic but still clearly segmented. The cell should not be termed hypersegmented; the numerous round nuclear remnants are artifactual and do not represent nuclear lobes. In the process of cell death, the nucleus may fragment and form multiple round aggregates. The cytoplasm contains numerous fine lilac granules, characteristic of neutrophils. The degenerated nature of the cell takes precedence over identification of cytoplasmic changes and since one can still tell that the cell is a neutrophil, the more generic term *basket cell* is incorrect.

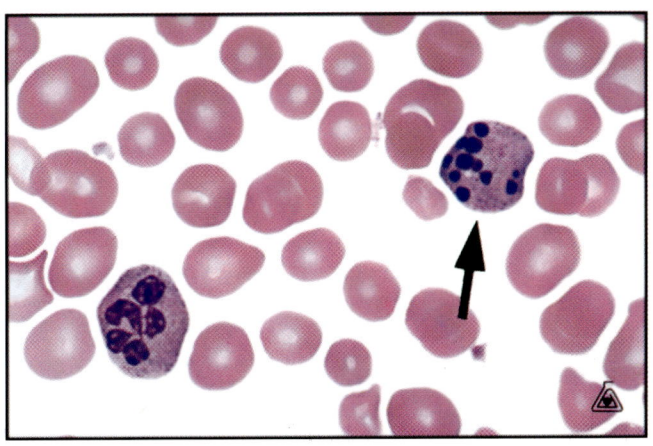

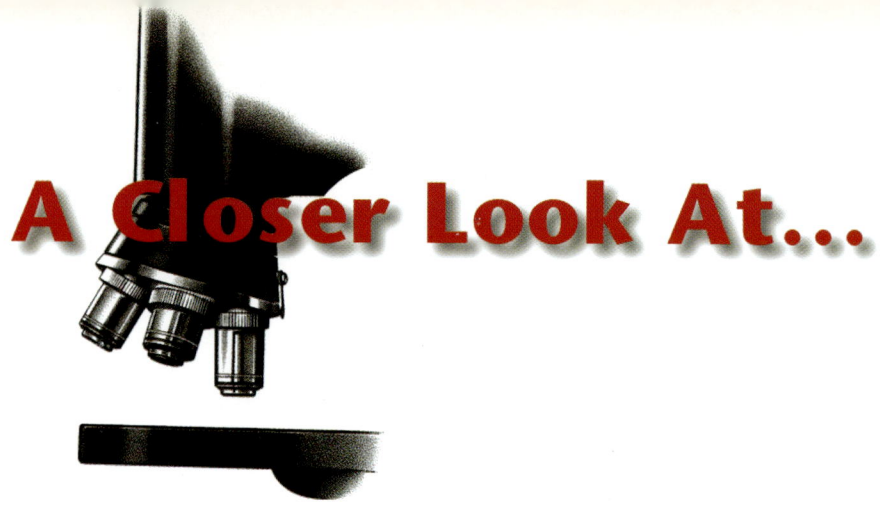

A Closer Look At...

Cell Death

Hematopoietic cell death may be either physiologic or mechanical. In the preparation of peripheral smears, mechanical distortion of fragile cells will strip away the cytoplasm leaving just nuclear strands (basket or smudge cells). Physiologic death may be due to either necrosis or apoptosis. In acute inflammation, the release of powerful enzymes causes cell necrosis. The process is indiscriminate; both the offending organism and normal cells are destroyed. Apoptosis is programmed cell death. Unlike necrosis, apoptosis does not cause an inflammatory response and therefore does not damage adjacent normal cells. It is a phenomenon that is being carefully studied because of its association with neoplastic transformation and immunologic responses.

Apoptosis is an important control mechanism for disposing of surplus or damaged cells. The process is genetically controlled. Messages are sent from the surface membrane of the cell to the mitochondria and then the cell nucleus. Neutrophils and eosinophils, for example, undergo cell death when they become senescent. External factors such as the withrawal of essential growth factors, exposure to radiation or glucocorticoids, and after cross-linking of certain surface membrane receptors such as Fas (CD95 antigen) can induce apoptosis.

Cancers develop because of an imbalance between cell generation and cell death. Defective apoptosis can promote lymphoma by allowing accumulation of lymphocytes that normally would die by apoptosis. Abnormal regulation of apoptosis may be responsible for loss of T helper lymphocytes in AIDS.

Unlike mechanical destruction, the process of cell death is a gradual one. There are three distinct endpoints, depicted on the next page: nuclear edema, pyknosis, and karyorrhexis.

The chromatin in the nucleus is composed of dense strands separated by nucleoplasm. If the nucleoplasm increases in amount due to edema, the nucleus has a fenestrated appearance. The cytoplasm breaks apart as the nucleus enlarges and is usually not visible. These cells are called basket cells or smudge cells. The cells are so distorted that they cannot be subclassified.

Nuclear pyknosis results from loss of the nucleoplasm, producing a small, dense nucleus. The cytoplasm is usually still visible and the cell lineage can often be determined.

In karyorrhexis, the nucleus becomes lobated and condensed, then breaks apart. Cytoplasm is usually visible, but reduced in amount. If the cell morphology is not too distorted, the subtype can be classified.

In apoptosis, the dying cells undergo shrinkage, chromatin compaction against the nuclear membrane, and nuclear and cytoplasmic budding to produce membrane-bound apoptotic bodies that are phagocytosed by macrophages. The morphology is similar to what happens to neutrophils when left in anticoagulant for extended periods. After 30 minutes, neutrophils swell, vacuoles develop, and granules are accentuated. The nuclear chromatin then condenses and may later break apart. Cells may resemble nucleated red blood cells. The process is accelerated if collection tubes are incompletely filled, giving a higher concentration of anticoagulant. See the atlas description of *Neutrophil Necrobiosis* on page 288 for additional information and photographic examples.

Various Forms of Cell Death

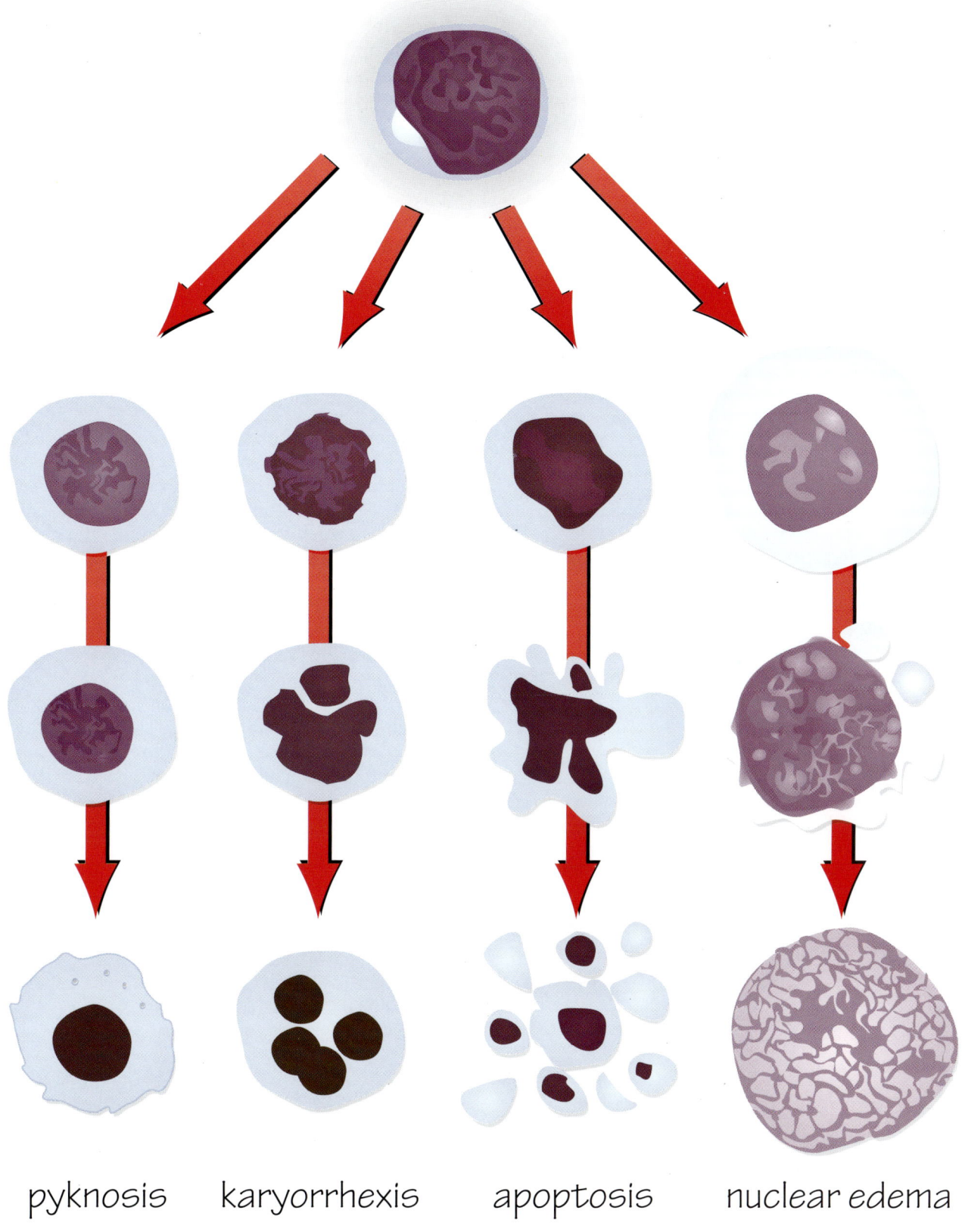

Artifacts

Erythrocyte with Overlapping Platelet

SYNONYMS
superimposition platelet artifact

VITAL STATISTICS
- size .... platelet typically 1-2 µm in diameter
- cell shape .... platelet round or oval
- nuclear shape .... no nucleus present
- cytoplasm .... platelet cytoplasm typically light blue-gray with central azurophilic granules (see platelet, normal morphology description); the overlying platelet may disperse enough hemoglobin to obliterate the pale central area of the red cell

KEY DIFFERENTIATING FEATURES
- halo around platelet
- typical granularity and morphology of platelet; compare morphology to other platelets in the background
- the platelet is not in the same plane of focus as the red cell

POTENTIAL LOOK-ALIKES
- intracellular parasites (malaria, babesia)
- extracellular organisms overlying red blood cell
- red blood cell inclusions (Howell-Jolly body, Pappenheimer body)
- vacuoles and pseudovacuoles in red blood cell

ASSOCIATED DISEASE STATES AND CONDITIONS
none; normal finding

In the preparation of a peripheral blood smear, all the formed elements are not evenly distributed over the glass surface. At the non-feather edge, red cells and leukocytes may clump together. At the feather edge, the cells form a more uniform monolayer, but some overlap may randomly occur between platelets and red cells.

Red cell morphology is usually unremarkable. In some cases the adherent platelet may press on the red cell membrane and disperse hemoglobin from the periphery to the central portion of the cell. This may obliterate any central pallor. Cells infected with malarial parasites may have variant shapes or contain pigment associated with the disease.

A platelet overlying a red cell may be mistaken for an inclusion or intra-erythrocyte infectious agents such as *Babesia* or *Plasmodia*. This is of particular concern in patients who lack functional splenic tissue because such infections tend to have a fulminent and potentially fatal course in such a host.

Differentiating a platelet from a true red cell inclusion depends on three important observations:

1) different plane of focus. The platelet lies above the red cell and careful focusing of the microscope will differentiate the two planes. Obviously, this cannot be done on a photomicrograph, so two other morphologic features are needed.

2) platelet "halo." Many times the platelet is surrounded by a thin clear zone. This halo is not a feature of any bona fide red cell inclusion.

3) morphology of the platelet. Although the overlapping platelet may look like an inclusion, compare the size, staining characteristics, and granularity with known platelets in the surrounding field. The similarity will lead to a correct identification.

Platelets Overlying Red Cells

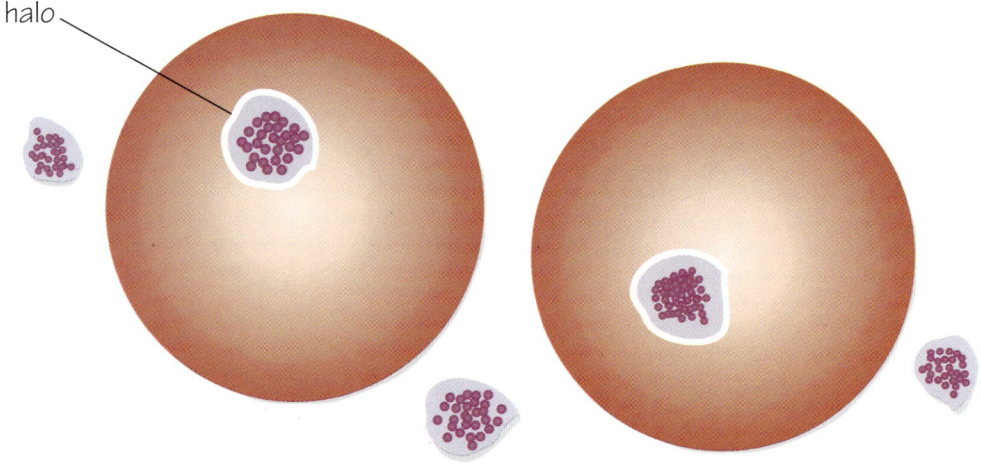

XL-59, 1989 (Blood, Wright-Giemsa, X400)

Identification	Referee %	Participant %
Erythrocyte with overlying platelet	100	90.7

The arrowed cell is an erythrocyte with overlying platelet. In the process of making blood smears, smaller elements such as platelets sometimes come to overlie larger elements such as erythrocytes. One helpful clue is difficult to demonstrate with a static photomicrograph; the overlying platelet and red cell are not in the same plane of focus so the platelet appears to be surrounded by a halo when the red cell is in focus. A second clue is the morphology of the inclusion. The platelet is a round anucleate fragment with multiple randomly distributed granules; it does not demonstrate a discrete chromocenter as would be seen in an intracellular parasite.

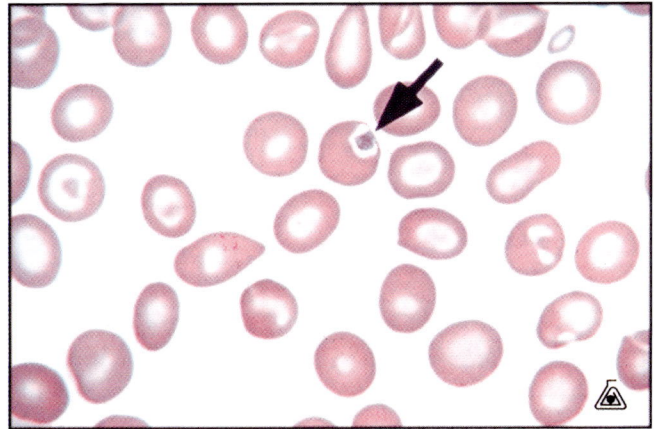

A-71, 1987 (Blood, Wright-Giemsa, X400)

Identification	Referee %	Participant %
Erythrocyte with overlying platelet	100	92.1

The photomicrograph is from a patient with hereditary ovalocytosis. The arrowed cell is an artifact of smear preparation. It is a platelet overlying a red blood cell. The platelet is well granulated and has similar morphology to other platelets in the field. Notice the well-defined halo around the pseudo-inclusion. This helps to distinguish it from a true inclusion or intracellular malarial parasite. Halos are not universally present; a few of the other platelets overlying red cells in this same field demonstrate either absent or poorly defined clear zones around them.

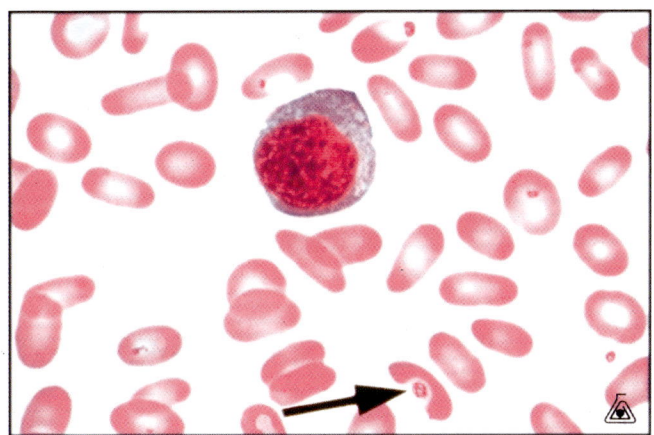

XL-29, 1988 (Blood, Wright-Giemsa, X313)

Identification	Referee %	Participant %
Erythrocyte with overlying platelet	89.5	69.2
Artifactual red cell inclusion	5.3	7.7
Malaria parasite	-	17.0
Howell-Jolly bodies	-	1.2

The arrow is pointing to an erythrocyte with overlying platelet. This is the most common erythrocyte pseudo-inclusion. Notice that the morphology of the overlying platelet is the same as the other platelets in the field. Azurophilic granules in the platelet cytoplasm are prominent and similar from cell to cell. Another clue is the halo around the overlying platelet. Some of the participants confused this artifact with a malarial parasite. The two morphologies are distinctly different. Malarial ring forms have a prominent chromatin dot and merozoites number from 8 to 24 in a single red cell. Howell-Jolly bodies are not as large as this pseudo-inclusion and stain purple-black.

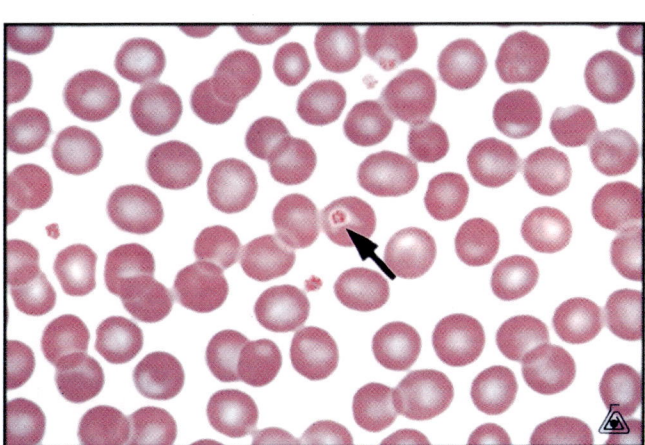

Stain Precipitate

SYNONYMS
none

VITAL STATISTICS
size .... variable; small particulates may aggregate into larger granules
shape .... granules are round but aggregates are highly variable in shape; granules dispersed in a random pattern

KEY DIFFERENTIATING FEATURES
random aggregates of metachromatic, red or purple granules
size of aggregates may be quite variable, unlike bacteria or yeast
individual red cells with single adherent stain particles may resemble inclusion (search the slide for other areas of stain precipitation that are more clumped and obviously not an inclusion; the similarity in morphology will aid in identification)

POTENTIAL LOOK-ALIKES
Howell-Jolly bodies
Pappenheimer bodies
organisms (fungi, bacteria, protozoa)
basket cells
necrobiotic cells

ASSOCIATED DISEASE STATES AND CONDITIONS
none

Stain precipitate on a Wright-Giemsa smear may be due to several different factors, depending on the staining technic used. Unclean slides, often due to dust settling on the slides, and improper drying of the stain on the smear are the two most common causes. Oxidized stain appears as metachromatic granular deposits on and between cells. The stain may adhere to red cells and be mistaken for inclusions, parasites, or infected cells. Thus the particles may mimic Howell Jolly bodies, bacteria, yeast, Pappenheimer bodies, and supravitally stained red cells containing Heinz bodies. The size of the stain droplets is variable and this can be helpful in discerning their origin. Yeast and bacteria, which are also purple, have a more uniform morphology than precipitated stain. Organisms are usually rare and dispersed throughout the slide; they do not circulate in large aggregates. Stain deposits, on the other hand, may be very focal and intense. The illustration on page 259 compares stain precipitate with extracellular bacteria.

Examples of Stain Precipitate

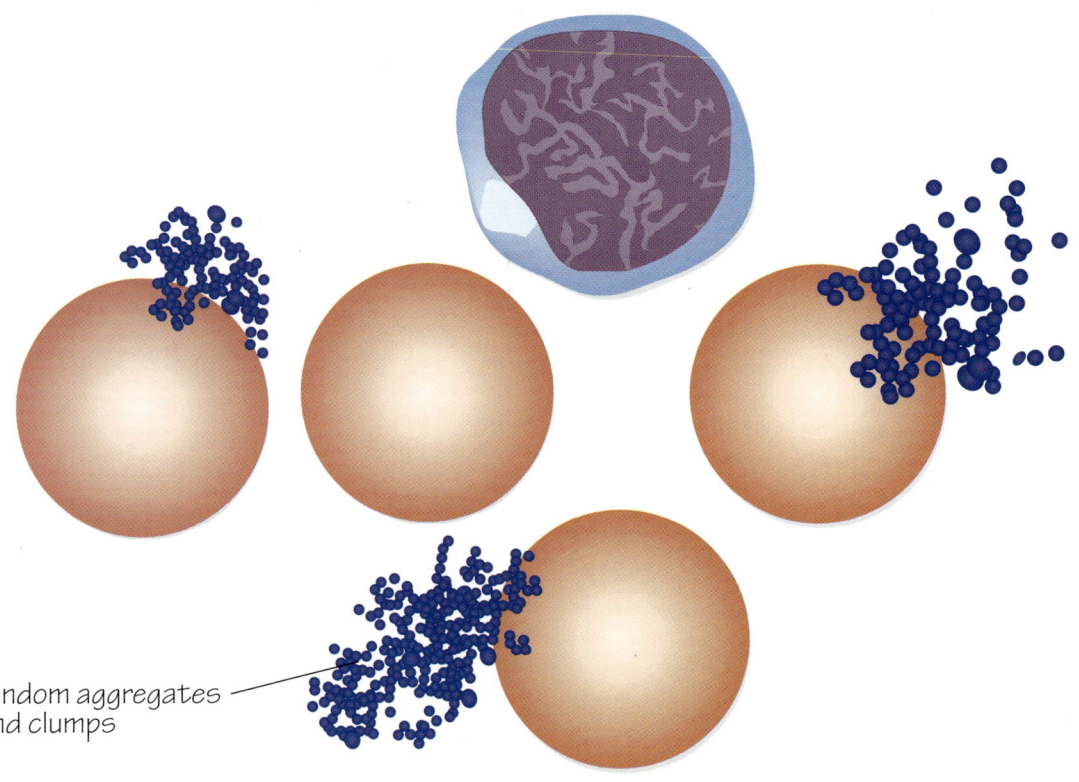

random aggregates and clumps

Artifacts

H1-18, 1990 (Blood, Wright-Giemsa, X400)

Identification	Referee %	Participant %
Stain precipitate	90	91
Spirochetes	5	5
Bacteria	-	2.3
Extracellular malarial parasite	-	1.1

This is a case of *Borellia* infection, a tick or louse-borne infection. The spirochetes are located in the center of the slide. Each organism displays a distinctive length, number of spirals, regularity, and tightness of the coils. The arrowed structures are stain precipitates. The granular, irregularly clumped purple gray material does not have any of the distinctive characteristics of spirochetes, bacteria, or malaria. The precipitate is too small to represent fungi, too finely clumped and smudged to represent bacteria, and too haphazardly arranged and without periodicity to represent spirochetes. The lone leukocyte at the top of the field is a degenerating segmented neutrophil. The cytoplasm is vaculated and exhibits toxic granulation.

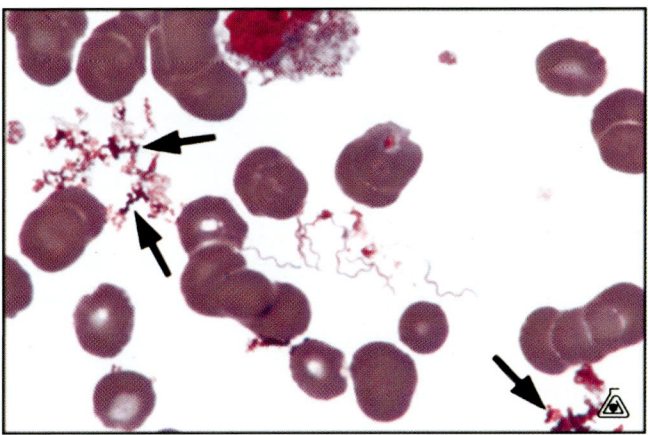

HE-40, 1991 (Blood, Wright-Giemsa, X400)

Identification	Referee %	Participant %
Stain precipitate	85	85.5
Bacteria (cocci or rod), extracellular	10	9.9
Protozoan (non-malarial)	-	1.5
Malaria, extracellular	-	1.2

The red blood cells are normochromic-normocytic without significant aniso- or poikilocytosis. The extracellular material near the arrows is precipitated stain. Cocci and fungi generally stain blue by Wright-Giemsa, unlike the material here. The material shows considerable granularity and variability in size. Portions are quite smudged and lacking in any detail. This randomness and lack of structure helps to distinguish the material from bacteria and other organisms. Although not evident on the photomicrograph, stain precipitate is also a random event on the slide, typically present in one clump. Organisms would be expected to be evenly distributed throughout the slide; they do not circulate in a large bolus.

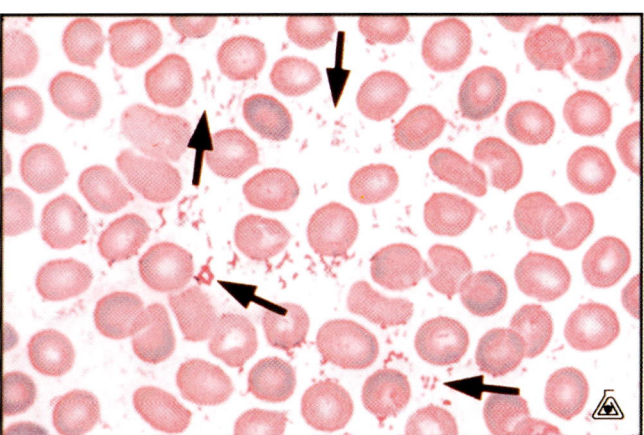

HE-25, 1996 (Blood, Wright-Giemsa, X400)

Identification	Referee %	Participant %
Stain precipitate	100	96.9
Platelet satellitism	-	1.3

The arrowed material represents a clump of precipitated stain. Like the examples cited above, the material lacks any organized morphology that would typify circulating organisms. There is a mixture of granular and smudged particles. The granular portion is too small to represent bacteria. A red cell is surrounded by the stain, which may account for the selection of platelet satellitism by a small percentage of participants. This phenomenon involves leukocytes—not red cells—which are surrounded by platelets. In addition, the stain also does not have the azurophilia and structure of platelets.

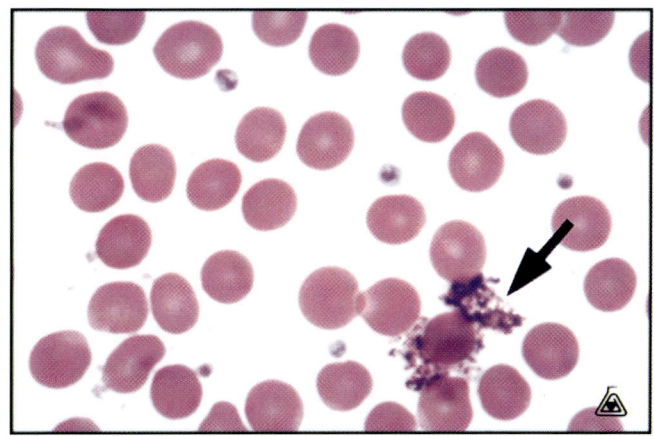

Miscellaneous Cells

Introduction 297
Blast Cell 298
   *A Closer Look At…*Antigen Markers in Blastic Cells 300
Alder's Anomaly Inclusion 302
Chédiak-Higashi Anomaly Inclusion 304
   *A Closer Look At…*Cytoplasmic Inclusions in Neutrophils 306
Endothelial Cell 308
Epithelial Cell 310
Lipocyte 312
   *A Closer Look At…*Bone Marrow Microenvironment 314
Macrophage (Histiocyte) 316
Macrophage with Phagocytized Red Cell (Erythrophagocytosis) 318
   *A Closer Look At…*Inclusions in Bone Marrow Cells 320
Gaucher Cell and Pseudo-Gaucher Cell 322
Histocyte, Sea Blue 324
Niemann-Pick Cell, Foamy Macrophage 326
Mast Cell 328
   *A Closer Look At…*Mast Cells vs. Basophils 330
Metastatic Tumor Cell 332
Mitotic Figure 334
Osteoblast 336
   *A Closer Look At…*Osteoblast vs. Plasma Cell 338
Osteoclast 340

Introduction

The *Miscellaneous* section of the CAP hematology cell identification list and glossary includes cells that do not clearly belong to the granulocytic, erythroid, megakaryocytic, or lymphoid lineages. Microorganisms and artifacts also are listed under individual headings. Most of the cells described in this section primarily are seen in the bone marrow, such as epithelial/endothelial cell, Gaucher cell/pseudo-Gaucher cell, sea blue histiocyte, lipocyte, mast cell, macrophage, macrophage with phagocytized red cells, metastatic tumor cell, mitotic figure, Niemann-Pick cell, osteoblast, and osteoclast. Others (Alder's anomaly inclusion, Chédiak-Higashi anomaly inclusion) represent hereditary abnormalities that affect multiple lineages. Finally, the blast cell is included in this section, since the lineage of origin cannot always be discerned from the morphologic appearance of this cell.

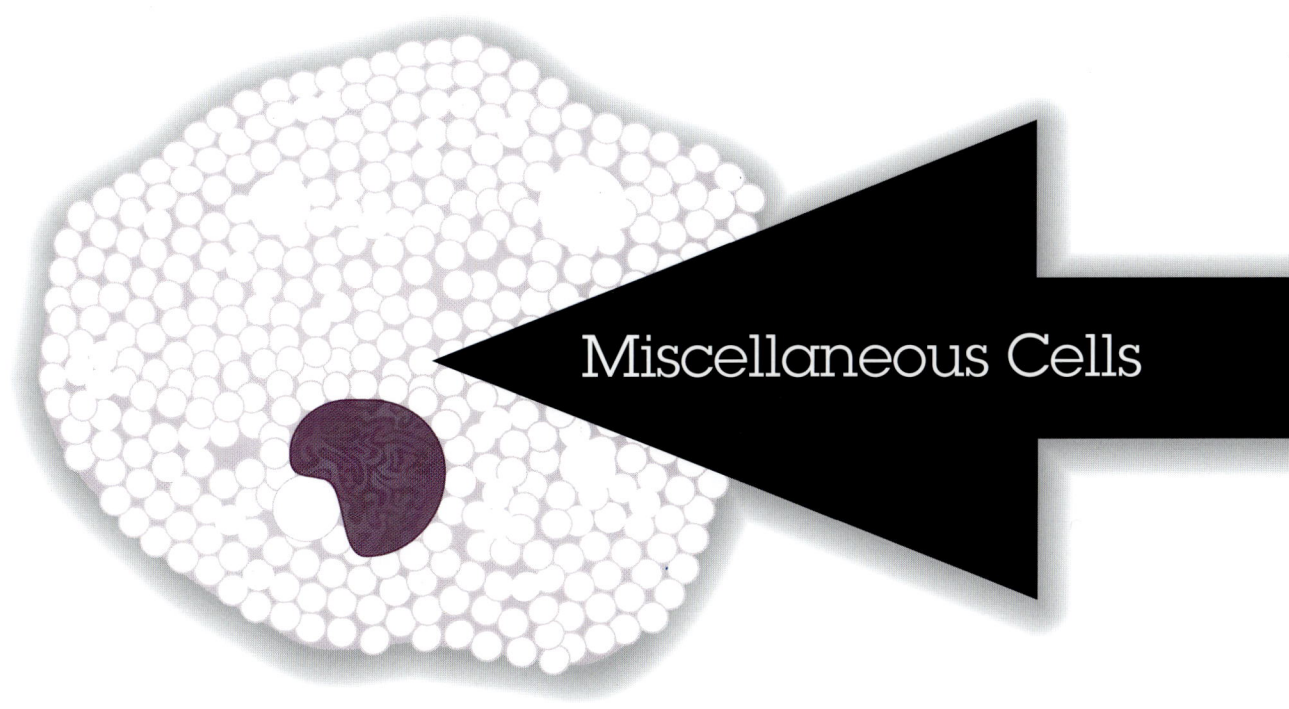

Blast Cell

SYNONYMS
none

VITAL STATISTICS
- size .... 10-20 µm
- N:C ratio .... high; approximately 7:1 to 1:1
- cell shape .... round to oval
- nuclear shape .... round, oval; may be indented or folded
- chromatin .... fine, granular
- parachromatin .... usually distinct
- nucleoli .... one or more, may be prominent
- cytoplasm .... basophilic, agranular

KEY DIFFERENTIATING FEATURES
- high N:C ratio
- finely reticulated nuclear chromatin
- prominent nucleoli

POTENTIAL LOOK-ALIKES
- reactive lymphocyte
- monocyte
- lymphoma cell

ASSOCIATED DISEASE STATES AND CONDITIONS
- acute leukemias
- myeloproliferative disorders
- myelodysplastic syndromes
- leukemic phase of lymphoma
- neonates
- regenerating marrow
- hemorrhage
- hemolysis
- severe anoxia
- severe infection
- post-splenectomy
- marrow infiltration and/or fibrosis associated with:
  - Gaucher's disease
  - lymphoma
  - Hodgkin's disease
  - non-hematopoietic malignancy

A blast is a large, round to oval cell, 10 to 20 µm in diameter. In the blood film, the cell may appear flattened or compressed by adjacent red cells. The nuclear to cytoplasmic ratio is high, varying from 7:1 to 1:1. The blast often has a round to oval nucleus, but sometimes is indented or folded, with fine, lacy to granular chromatin; one or more prominent nucleoli may be present. The cytoplasm is basophilic and agranular. In the absence of lineage associated findings, such as Auer rods, cytoplasmic granules, cytochemical data (e.g. peroxidase or sudan black B reactivity), or cell surface marker data, it is not possible to define the lineage of a given blast cell. Therefore, blastic cells without definitive cytoplasmic inclusions should be indentified as "blast, not otherwise specified" unless ancillary data is available to aid in classification as "myeloblast" or "lymphoblast."

Blasts may be found in peripheral blood in a variety of hematolymphoid malignancies, including acute leukemia, myeloproliferative disorders, myelodysplastic syndromes, and leukemic phase of lymphoma. However, the presence of an occasional blast in the blood does not always signify hematopoietic malignancy. Myeloblasts may occur in the blood in small numbers in benign states, including infancy (particularly premature neonates), regenerating marrow, hemorrhage, hemolytic anemia, severe anoxia, severe infection, and, rarely, post-splenectomy. The combination of blasts (or other immature granulocytes, such as promyelocytes or myelocytes) with nucleated red cells in the peripheral blood is termed a "leukoerythroblastic reaction." In addition, infiltration of the bone marrow with malignant lymphoma, Hodgkin's disease, non-hematopoietic tumors, or benign processes (such as Gaucher's disease) can manifest as a leukoerythroblastic reaction, often accompanied by the presence of teardrop red cells.

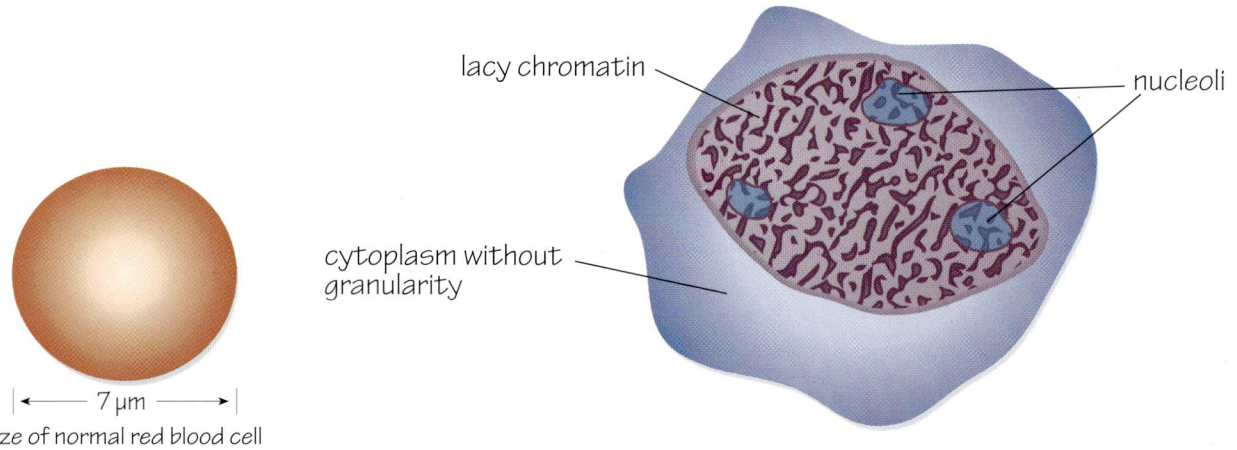

7 µm — size of normal red blood cell

H-11, 1981 (Blood, Wright-Giemsa, X400)

Identification	Referee %	Participant %
Blast cell	62.5	75.4
Lymphocyte, reactive	37.5	17.8

The nucleus of the arrowed blast has smooth, lacy chromatin with two prominent nucleoli. This nuclear appearance is common for a blast cell, but unusual for a reactive lymphocyte. The cell has a moderate amount of basophilic cytoplasm, which lacks azurophilic granules or Auer rods. Thus, it is not possible to identify cell lineage with certainty without cytochemical or immunologic data.

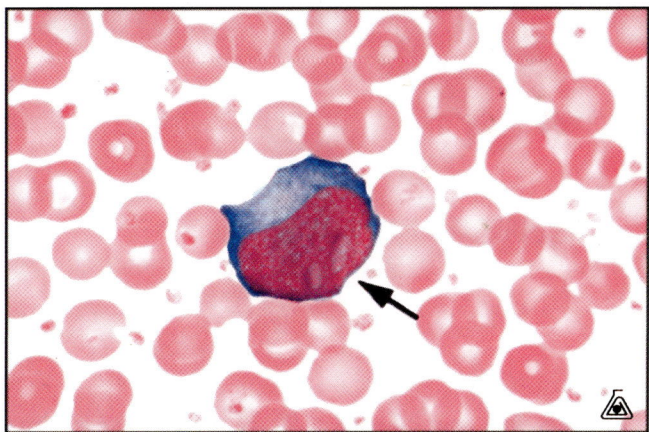

H-35, 1980 (Blood, Wright-Giemsa, X400)

Identification	Referee %	Participant %
Blast cell	100	90.5

The arrowed cell from a case of acute leukemia was identified as a blast cell of any type (i.e. myeloblast, monoblast, myelomonoblast, or lymphoblast) by 100% of referees and 90.5% of participants. The large cell has a high nuclear to cytoplasmic ratio, with granular nuclear chromatin and a single large, prominent nucleolus. The nuclear shape is irregular. The adjacent cell also is a blast, but with a very high nuclear to cytoplasmic ratio and no nucleoli. Since cytoplasmic granules cannot be identified, definitive lineage assignment cannot be made.

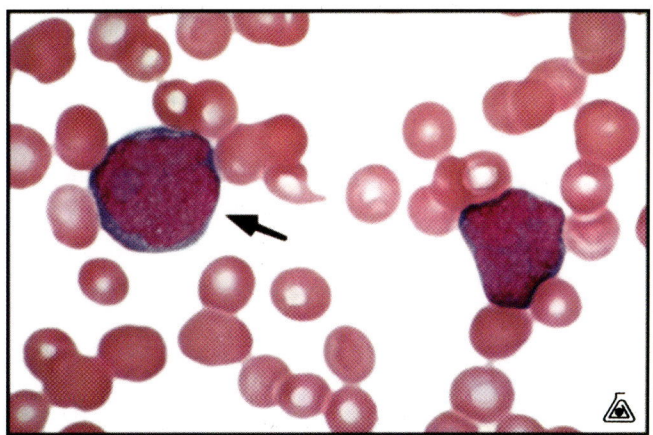

HE-13, 1994 (Blood, Wright-Giemsa, X400)

Identification	Referee %	Participant %
Blast cell	55.6	42.8
Myeloblast	25.9	26.1
Monocyte, immature	11.1	8.4
Lymphoblast	–	4.5
Lymphocyte, reactive	7.4	9.9

This cell, from a case of agnogenic myeloid metaplasia, was classified as a blast cell type (i.e., blast cell, myeloblast, lymphoblast) by most of the referees and participants. Characteristics such as a relatively high nuclear to cytoplasmic ratio, immature chromatin pattern, and multiple nucleoli all indicate a blast cell. The cytoplasm is basophilic and agranular. In the absence of cytochemistry or immunophenotyping, the more inclusive term of *blast cell* is preferred. A few participants mistakenly identified this cell as a reactive lymphocyte. Although this cell superficially resembles the immunoblastic type of reactive lymphocyte, it differs in that the nucleoli are large and well-defined, the nuclear to cytoplasmic ratio is higher, and a paranuclear Golgi region is absent.

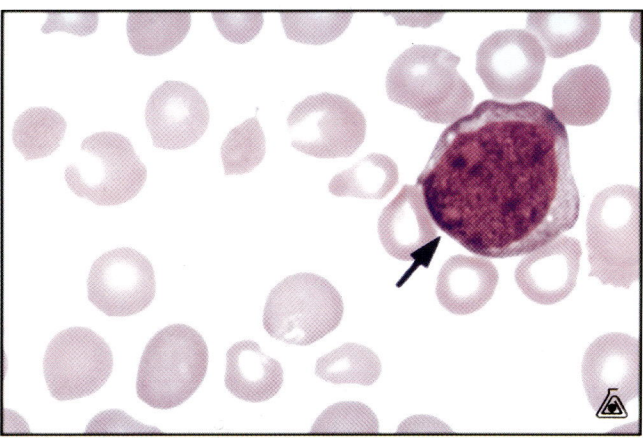

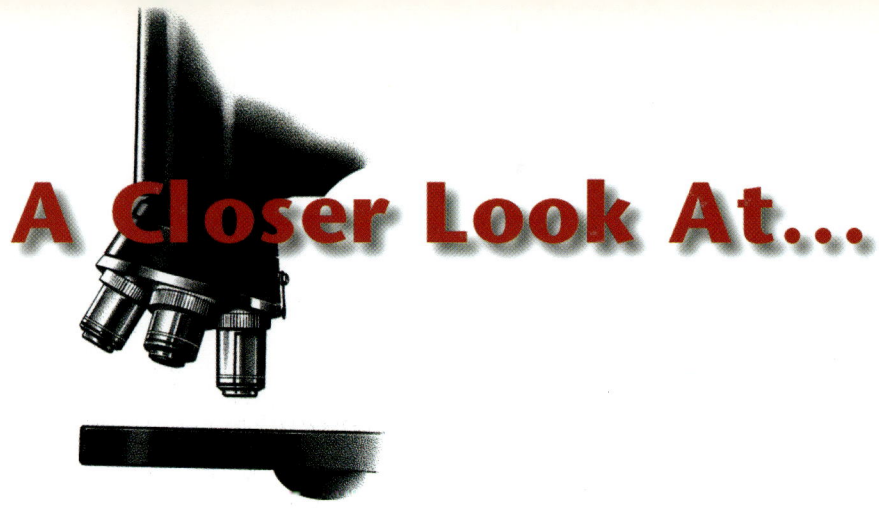

A Closer Look At...

Antigen Markers in Blastic Cells

This blast cell has lacy chromatin, multiple small nuclei, and a moderate amount of agranular cytoplasm. In the absence of cytoplasmic granules, positive cytochemistries, or antigenic markers, it is impossible to know if this is a blast of myeloid or lymphoid lineage. In addition, biphenotypic (multiple lineage markers on a single blastic cell) or biclonal (2 populations of blasts of different lineage) may occur.

The myeloblast typically has a round to oval nucleus with finely reticulated chromatin containing one or more nucleoli (see page 6). However, nuclear folding or clefting may occur in leukemic myeloblasts, particularly in monocytoid variants (sometimes referred to as monoblasts). Occasionally the myeloblast contains an Auer rod or a variable number of delicate azurophilic granules, which stain positively for myeloperoxidase or sudan black B. Normal myeloblasts as well as myeloblasts in many cases of acute myeloblastic leukemia express surface antigens CD13 and CD33. DR and progenitor antigen CD34 often are present. Myeloid leukemias with other lineage differentiation may display specific antigens such as CD14 (monocytic), CD61 (megakaryocytic), or glycophorin A (erythroid); CD34 and DR characteristically are absent in promyelocytic leukemia.

The lymphoblast (see page 216) also shows fine chromatin, although a little less so than the myeloblast. The lymphoblast may have a very high nuclear to cytoplasmic ratio with scant cytoplasm (L-1 type), or may have a small amount of cytoplasm, similar to the myeloblast (L-2 type). The nucleus often is round to oval, but may be clefted or folded. Although the cytoplasm is usually agranular, some cases of acute lymphoblastic leukemia show lymphoblasts with scant azurophilic granules (negative for myeloperoxidase or sudan black B). Antigen marker analysis is necessary for definitive identification of lymphoblasts. Examples of some of the surface, cytoplasmic, and nuclear antigens that can be seen in myeloblasts, early B-precursor lymphoblasts and T-lineage lymphoblasts are illustrated. In addition, the blasts of Burkitt's-type leukemia/lymphoma (L-3 type) are B lineage with monoclonal surface immunoglobulin expression.

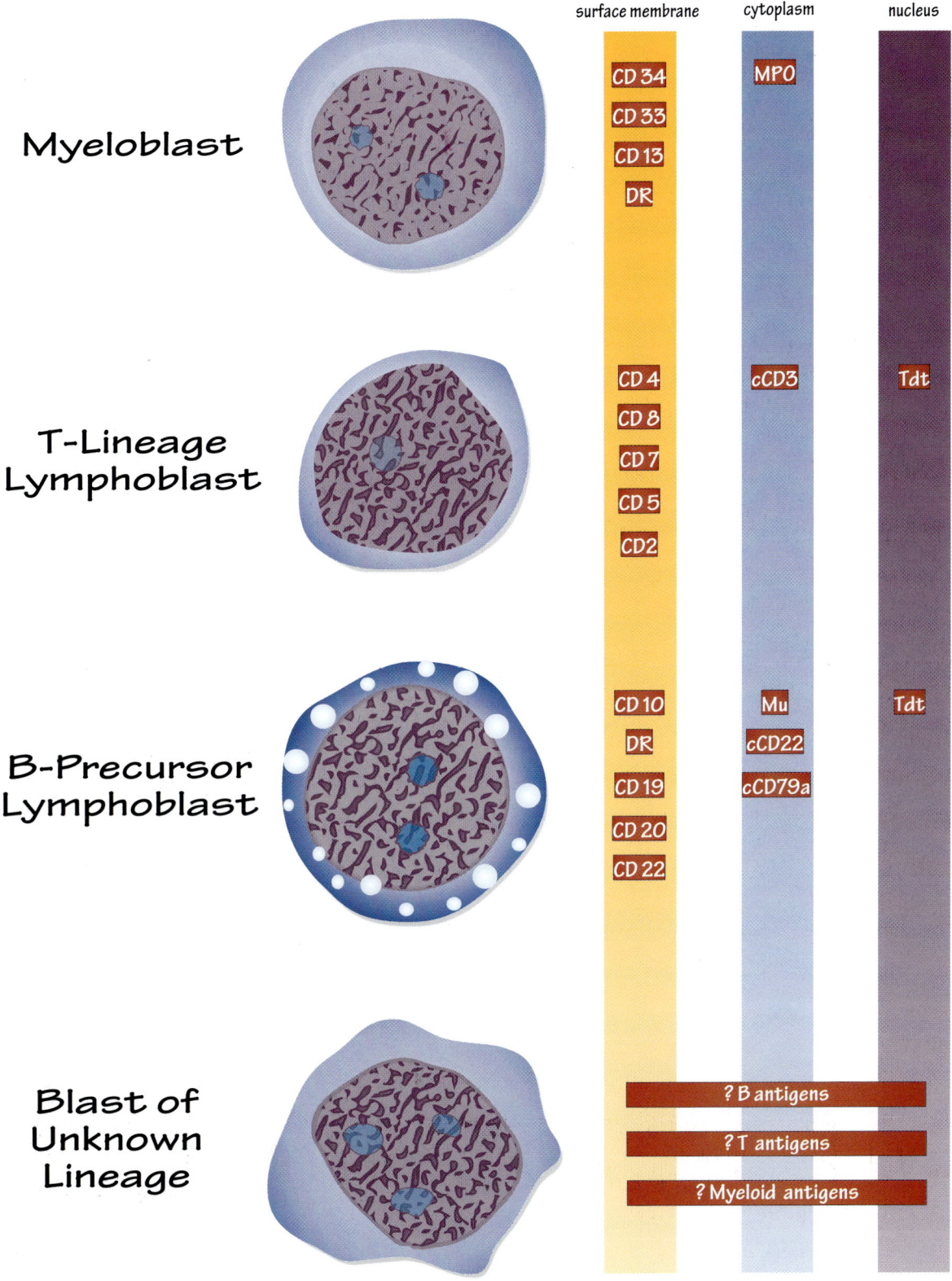

Alder's Anomaly Inclusion

SYNONYMS
Alder-Reilly granules

VITAL STATISTICS
cells .... inclusions occur in otherwise typical granulocytes, lymphocytes, and monocytes
cytoplasm .... contains large, purple or purplish-black, coarse, azurophilic granules

KEY DIFFERENTIATING FEATURES
large azurophilic granules in granulocytes, lymphocytes, and monocytes

OTHER FINDINGS
occasional granule may have a "halo" or clear zone surrounding it

POTENTIAL LOOK-ALIKES
toxic granulation
basophil
Chédiak-Higashi inclusion

ASSOCIATED DISEASE STATES AND CONDITIONS
mucopolysaccharidoses, MPS I-VII, e.g.:
   Hurler syndrome
   Scheie syndrome
   Hunter syndrome
   Sanfilippo syndrome
   Morquio syndrome
   Maroteaux-Lamy's syndrome
   Sly syndrome

Alder's anomaly inclusions are large, purple or purplish-black, coarse, azurophilic granules, resembling the primary granules of promyelocytes. They are seen in the cytoplasm of virtually all mature leukocytes and, occasionally, in their precursors. The granules in toxic granulation are nearly identical in size and staining. Toxic granulation, however, does not occur in all neutrophils and is more variable in intensity. It is also often accompanied by Döhle bodies and vacuoles, which are not found in Alder's anomaly unless there is concomitant toxic change. (See *A Closer Look At*...page 44 and *Toxic Granulation* discussion page 40).

At times, the granules may be surrounded by clear zones or "halos." The prominent granulation in lymphocytes and monocytes distinguishes these inclusions from toxic granulation, which only occurs in neutrophils.

Alder's anomaly inclusions are seen in association with the mucopolysaccharidoses (MPS), a group of inherited disorders caused by a deficiency of lysosomal enzymes needed to degrade mucopolysaccharides (or glycosaminoglycans). The inclusions represent lysosomal accumulation of undegraded or partially degraded glycosaminoglycans, such as dermatan sulfate, heparan sulfate, keratan sulfate, or chondroitin sulfate. Although variable in systemic manifestations and clinical course, the MPS share such clinical features as typical facies, skeletal dysplasia, mental deficiency, corneal opacity, and hepatosplenomegaly.

Segmented Neutrophil in Alder's Anomaly

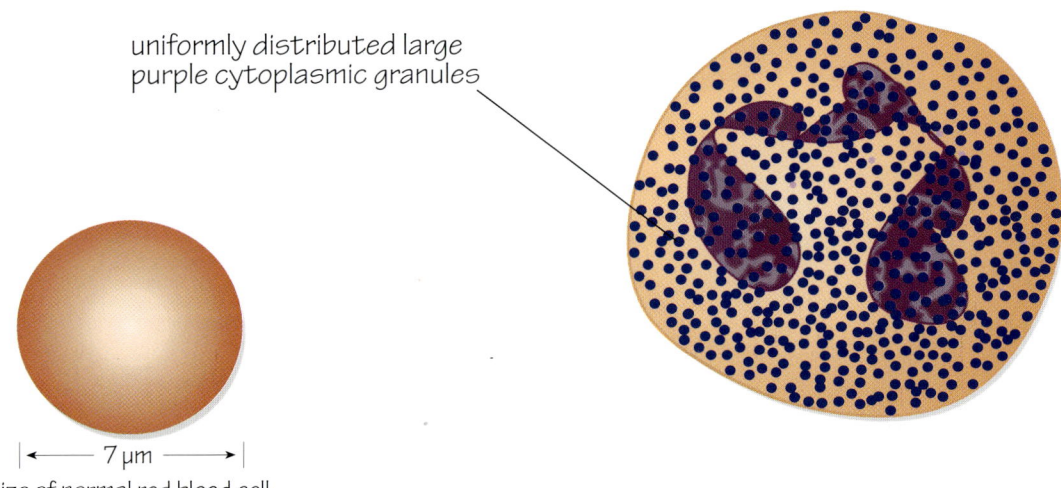

uniformly distributed large purple cytoplasmic granules

|← 7 µm →|
size of normal red blood cell

Miscellaneous Cells

HE-14, 1995 (Bone Marrow, Wright-Giemsa, X400)

Identification	Referee %	Participant %
Alder's anomaly inclusion	80.8	61.2
Segmented/band neutrophil, with toxic granulation	3.8	16.7
Eosinophil, any stage	3.8	10.6
Segmented/band neutrophil	7.7	8.0

Mucopolysaccharidosis type VII (Sly disease). All of the bone marrow precursors in this photomicrograph have large, coarse, azurophilic granules, characteristic of Alder's anomaly inclusions. In many cases, prominent granulation in lymphocytes and monocytes distinguishes these inclusions from toxic granulation, which only occurs in neutrophils. Since only neutrophils are present in this photomicrograph, the history of a mucopolysaccharidosis as well as the uniform high density of the large size granules leads one to consider Alder's anomaly rather than toxic granulation.

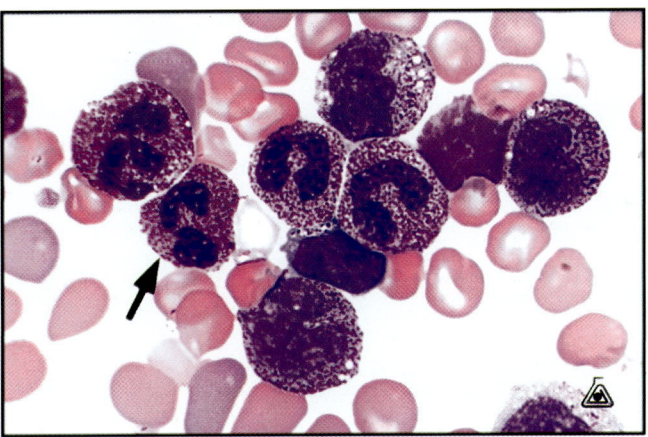

Other Cells in Alder's Anomaly

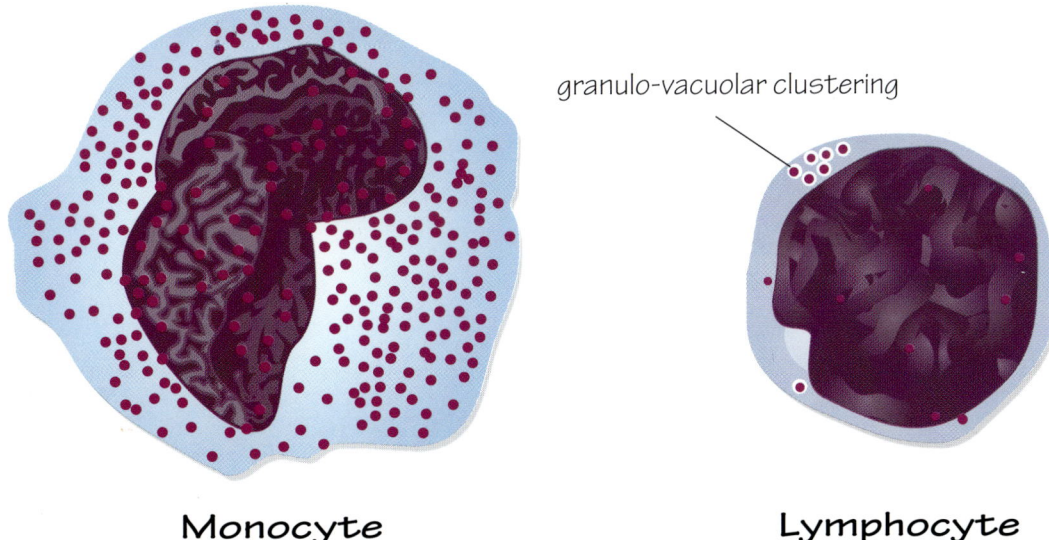

Monocyte   Lymphocyte

Miscellaneous Cells

Chédiak-Higashi Anomaly Inclusion

SYNONYMS
Chédiak-Steinbrinck-Higashi syndrome

VITAL STATISTICS
size .... inclusions occur in otherwise typical granulocytes, lymphocytes, monocytes, and rarely, in nucleated red cells
cytoplasm .... contains giant, often round, red, blue, or greenish-gray granules of variable size, often aggregated

KEY DIFFERENTIATING FEATURES
megagranules in granulocytes, lymphocytes, and monocytes

OTHER FINDINGS
accelerated lymphoma-like terminal phase

POTENTIAL LOOK-ALIKES
toxic granulation
Döhle body inclusion
Alder's anomaly inclusion

ASSOCIATED DISEASE STATES AND CONDITIONS
Chédiak-Steinbrinck-Higashi syndrome

Giant, often round, red, blue, or greenish-gray granules of variable size are seen in the cytoplasm of leukocytes (granulocytes, lymphocytes, and monocytes) and sometimes normoblasts in patients with Chédiak-Higashi syndrome. Platelets and megakaryocytes are unaffected. A poorly understood membrane abnormality results in fusion of primary (azurophilic) and to a lesser extent, secondary (specific) lysosomal granules, resulting in poor function in killing phagocytized bacteria. The Chédiak-Higashi syndrome is a rare, fatal, autosomal recessive disorder characterized by gigantic, aggregated inclusions in many of the granular body cells, including skin, hair, adrenal glands, and CNS. Clinical findings include partial oculocutaneous albinism with photophobia, nystagmus, peripheral neuropathy, pancytopenia, hepatosplenomegaly, lymphadenopathy, and recurrent severe pyogenic infections. Because the antiviral activity of the granular natural killer lymphocyte is impaired, patients are susceptible to lymphoid transformation by Epstein-Barr virus and frequently develop a lymphoma-like disorder as a terminal event.

Cells in Chédiak-Higashi

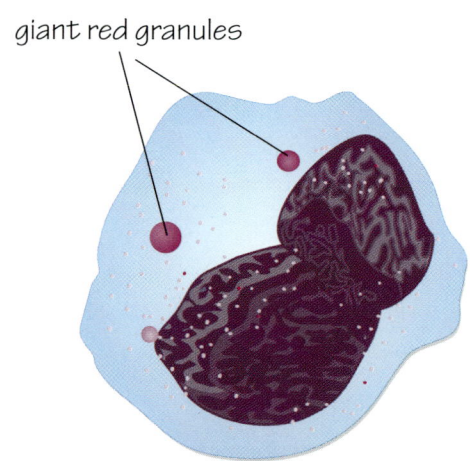

Monocyte — giant red granules

Segmented Neutrophil — slate-gray granules

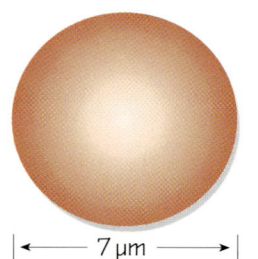

7 μm — size of normal red blood cell

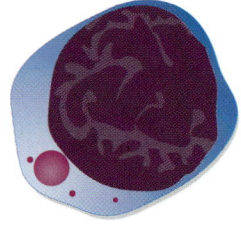

Lymphocyte

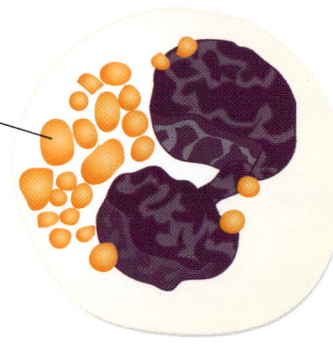

Eosinophil — giant eosinophilic granules

H-36, 1977 (Blood, Wright-Giemsa, X400)

Identification	Referee %	Participant %
Chédiak-Higashi inclusions	100	68
Döhle inclusion bodies	-	17.7
Toxic granulation	-	3.1

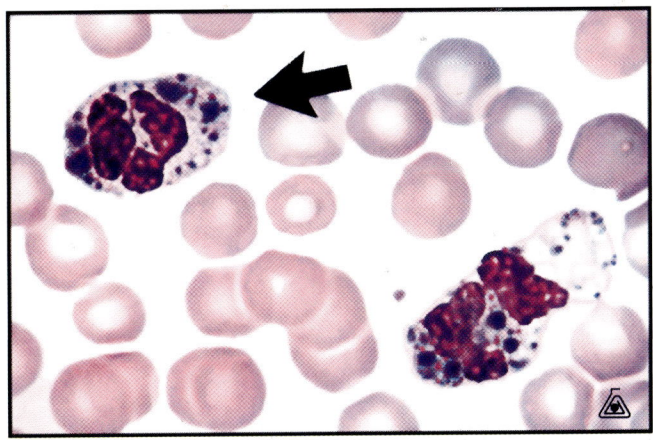

100% of referees and 68.0% of participants correctly identified the Chédiak-Higashi inclusions. Both segmented neutrophils in this photomicrograph show variably-sized and irregularly-shaped purplish-blue granules which coalesce into gigantic forms—the typical morphology of Chédiak-Higashi inclusions. In contrast, Döhle inclusion bodies are usually light blue in color and rarely this numerous. Toxic granulation appears as coarse azurophilic granules of fairly uniform size; granules would not be as large as those seen here.

H1-45, 1988 (Blood, Wright-Giemsa, X370)

Identification	Referee %	Participant %
Chédiak-Higashi inclusions	94.7	93.6
Alder's anomaly inclusion	5.3	4.2

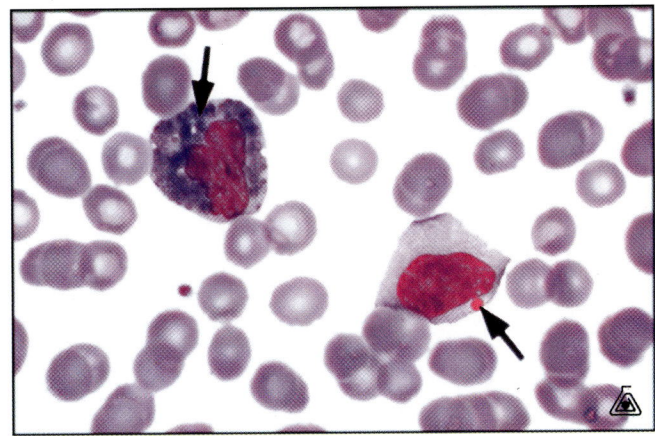

The two arrowed cells illustrate the spectrum of granules that occur as Chédiak-Higashi inclusions. The cell on the (left) is a neutrophil with numerous large slate-gray inclusions. The cell on the (right) is a large granular lymphocyte or natural killer cell with a single large azurophilic granule. Although Alder's anomaly results in abnormal granular inclusions in all leukocyte sub-classes, the granules typically are smaller and intensely magenta in color.

H1-47, 1988 (Bone Marrow, Wright-Giemsa, X370)

Identification	Referee %	Participant %
Chédiak-Higashi inclusions	84.2	77.7
Toxic granulation	5.3	15.8
Alder's anomaly inclusion	5.3	4.6

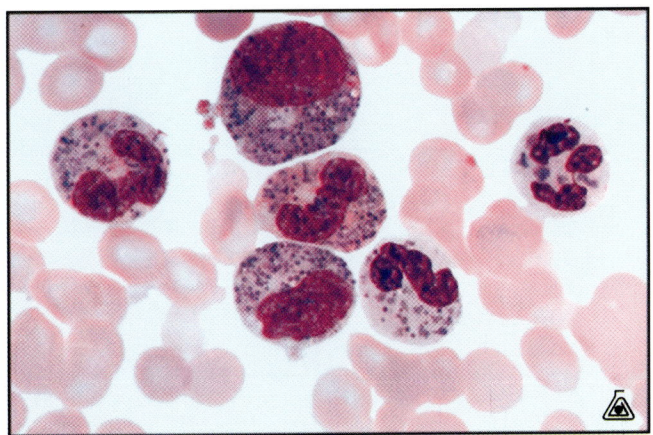

The bone marrow smear shows the diversity of granules in neutrophil precursors with Chédiak-Higashi inclusions, correctly identified by 84.2% of referees and 77.7% of participants. Although a minority of referees and participants selected "toxic granulation" or "Alder's anomaly inclusion," these inclusions would appear azurophilic rather than blue-gray in color and would not be as large as the inclusions in some of these cells. In particular, the segmented neutrophil on the (right) side of the photomicrograph shows fusion of the granules into a few very large forms.

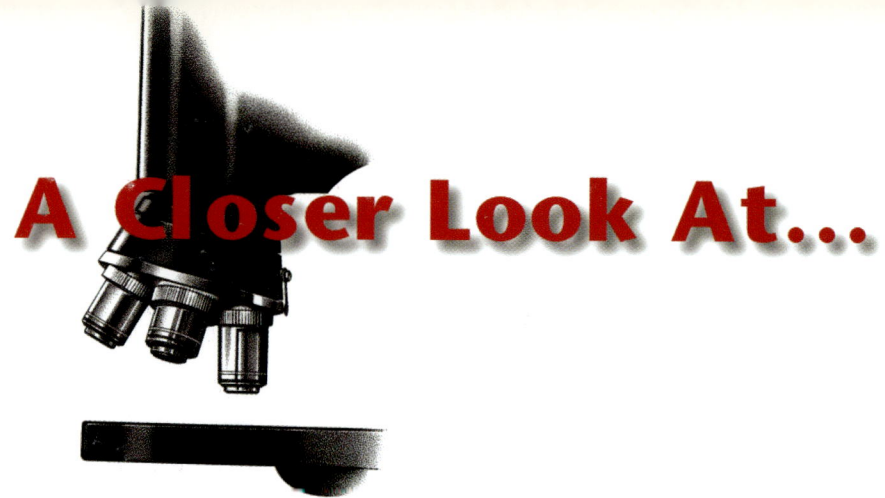

A Closer Look At...

Cytoplasmic Inclusions in Neutrophils

The table below and schematic drawing on the next page compare the various types of neutrophil inclusions. See *A Closer Look At...* page 44 and *Toxic Granulation* discussion on page 40 for additional information.

Cytoplasmic Inclusion	Inclusion Morphology	Hematopoietic Cells Involved
Döhle bodies	single to multiple gray-blue inclusions, often adjacent to the membrane; associated with toxic granulation and/or vacuolization	segmented or band neutrophils, metamyelocytes
Toxic granulation	large azurophilic (purple or dark blue) granules; may be accompanied by Döhle bodies or toxic vacuolization; number of granules vary from neutrophil to neutrophil	all neutrophil stages
Alder's anomaly	large azurophilic (purple or dark blue) granules similar to toxic granulation; granules occasionally surrounded by clear zones; all neutrophils show similar granulation (unlike toxic granulation)	neutrophils, monocytes, and lymphocytes
Chédiak-Higashi anomaly	giant fusion granules with variation in size; red, blue or greenish-gray color	neutrophils, eosinophils, monocytes, lymphocytes; rarely normoblasts
Auer bodies	agglomeration of azurophilic granules into red-pink round or rod-shaped forms; may occur in bundles (in acute promyelocytic leukemia)	blasts, promyelocytes, immature monocytes in myeloid lineage leukemias
Vacuoles	round clear zones; degenerative change due to EDTA (usually small and few in number) or drug effect (chloramphenicol, alcohol), or seen with toxic changes (Döhle bodies and toxic granulation; vacuoles are usually larger and more numerous)	all neutrophil stages
Phagocytized material	variable; bacteria, fungi, RBCs, nuclei (immunologically induced LE cells or tart cells), crystals (urate, calcium pyrophosphate, etc. in body fluids and tissue)	segmented or band neutrophils

Neutrophil Cytoplasmic Inclusions

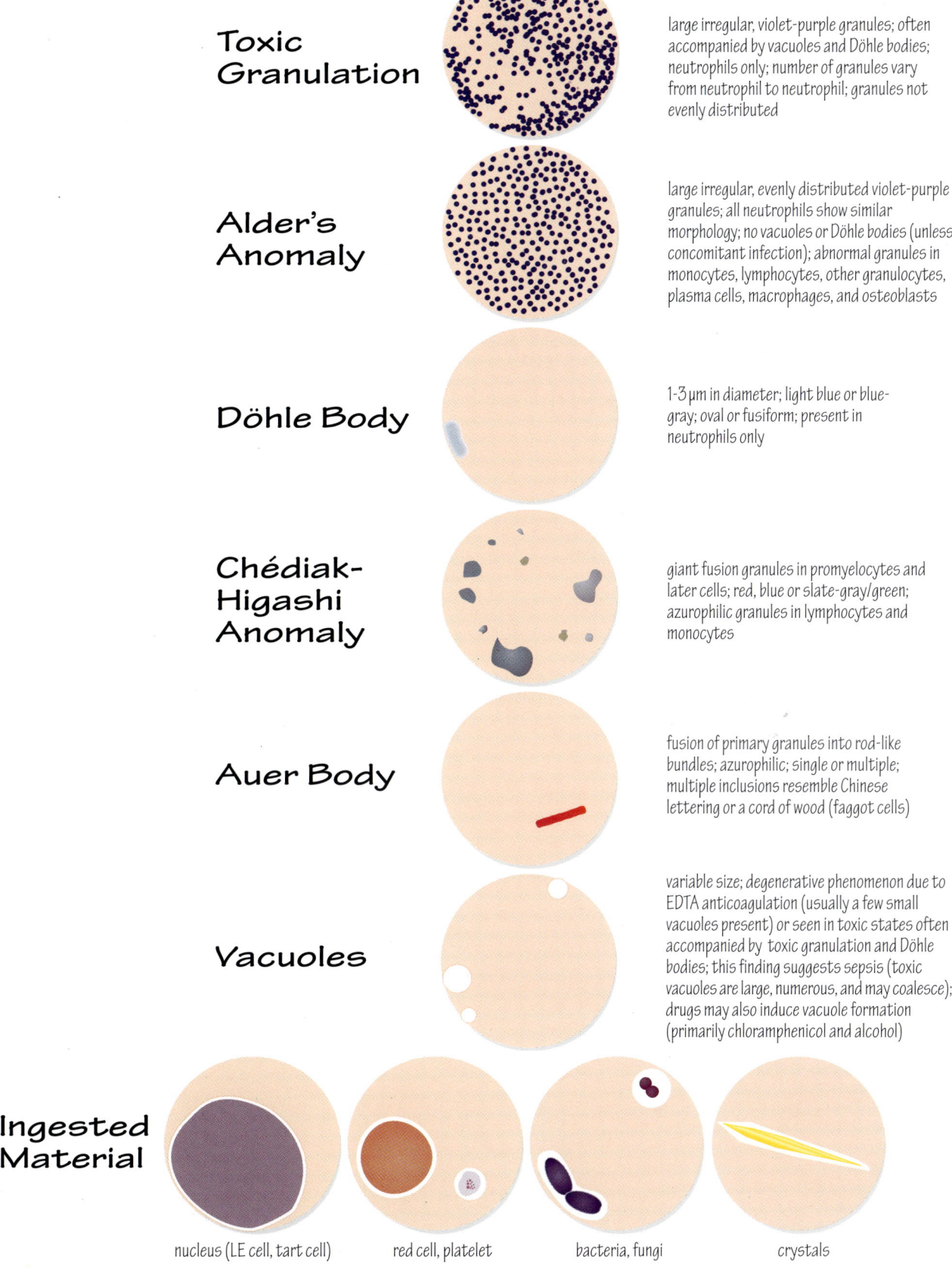

Toxic Granulation — large irregular, violet-purple granules; often accompanied by vacuoles and Döhle bodies; neutrophils only; number of granules vary from neutrophil to neutrophil; granules not evenly distributed

Alder's Anomaly — large irregular, evenly distributed violet-purple granules; all neutrophils show similar morphology; no vacuoles or Döhle bodies (unless concomitant infection); abnormal granules in monocytes, lymphocytes, other granulocytes, plasma cells, macrophages, and osteoblasts

Döhle Body — 1-3 µm in diameter; light blue or blue-gray; oval or fusiform; present in neutrophils only

Chédiak-Higashi Anomaly — giant fusion granules in promyelocytes and later cells; red, blue or slate-gray/green; azurophilic granules in lymphocytes and monocytes

Auer Body — fusion of primary granules into rod-like bundles; azurophilic; single or multiple; multiple inclusions resemble Chinese lettering or a cord of wood (faggot cells)

Vacuoles — variable size; degenerative phenomenon due to EDTA anticoagulation (usually a few small vacuoles present) or seen in toxic states often accompanied by toxic granulation and Döhle bodies; this finding suggests sepsis (toxic vacuoles are large, numerous, and may coalesce); drugs may also induce vacuole formation (primarily chloramphenicol and alcohol)

Ingested Material:
- nucleus (LE cell, tart cell)
- red cell, platelet
- bacteria, fungi
- crystals

Miscellaneous Cells

Endothelial Cell

SYNONYMS
none

VITAL STATISTICS
- size .... approximately 5 μm wide by 20-30 μm long
- N:C ratio .... 2:1 to 1:1
- cell shape .... elongated, spindle-shaped
- nuclear shape .... elliptical, may be folded
- chromatin .... dense to reticular
- parachromatin .... minimal to moderate
- nucleoli .... variable
- cytoplasm .... frayed, light blue or pink, tapering out from the ends of the nucleus; may contain a few azurophilic granules

KEY DIFFERENTIATING FEATURES
elongate cell with frayed, tapering cytoplasm at both ends

OTHER FINDINGS
frequently occur in clusters

POTENTIAL LOOK-ALIKES
metastatic tumor cell
macrophage (histiocyte)
fibroblast, fibroblast-like (reticulum cell)
lymphocyte (elongated form)

ASSOCIATED DISEASE STATES AND CONDITIONS
in vitro contamination during phlebotomy
normal bone marrow component

Endothelial cells are a normal component of the bone marrow, lining capillaries and sinuses. They have an elongated or spindle shape, approximately 5 μm wide by 20 to 30 μm long, with a moderate nuclear to cytoplasmic ratio (2:1 to 1:1). The oval or elliptical nucleus occasionally is folded and has dense to fine, reticular chromatin. One or more nucleoli may be visible. The frayed cytoplasm tapers out from both ends of the nucleus and may contain a few azurophilic granules. Endothelial cells have a similar, if not identical, appearance to fibroblast-like cells (reticulum cells) that make up the skeletal framework of the bone marrow.

Endothelial cells (lining blood vessels) rarely may contaminate peripheral blood, particularly when smears are obtained from finger or heel punctures. When accidently present in blood, endothelial cells may occur in clusters.

Endothelial Cells

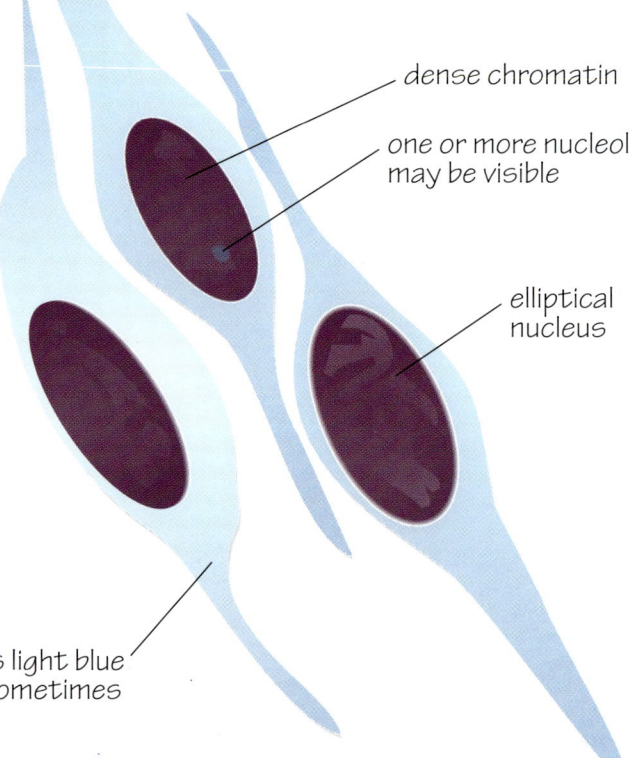

- dense chromatin
- one or more nucleoli may be visible
- elliptical nucleus
- cytoplasm is light blue or pink and sometimes tansparent

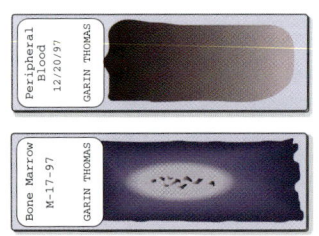

Endothelial cells are occasionally seen in bone marrow smears. They are rarely found in peripheral blood smears where they form clusters representing capillary fragments acquired during finger sticks and heal punctures.

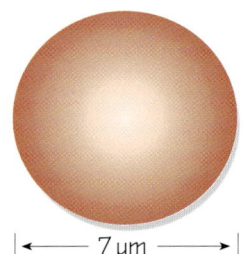

|← 7μm →|
size of normal red blood cell

HE-27, 1995 (Bone Marrow, Wright-Giemsa, X400)

Identification	Referee %	Participant %
Epithelial/endothelial cell	89.3	68.6
Osteoblast	–	8.2
Osteoclast	3.6	7.2

The arrowed structure is the nucleus of a capillary endothelial cell. There are five additional endothelial cells nuclei present that comprise a capillary, which contains a red cell within the lumen. These cells differ from osteoblasts, which have abundant blue-gray cytoplasm and a clear Golgi zone distant from the nucleus, and from osteoclasts, which are very large multinucleate cells. No other cell type other than endothelial cells would be expected to form capillary structures.

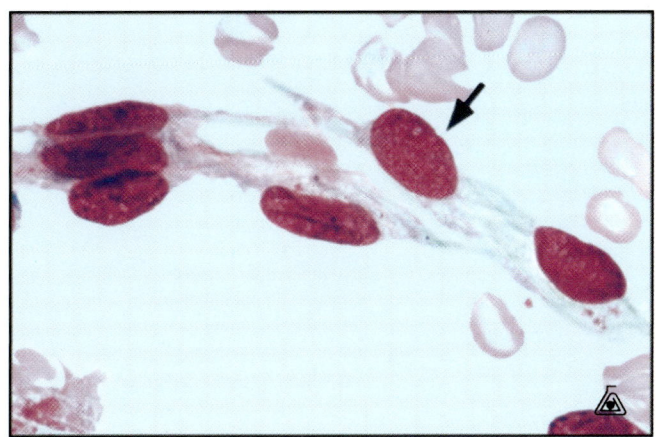

Endothelial Cells

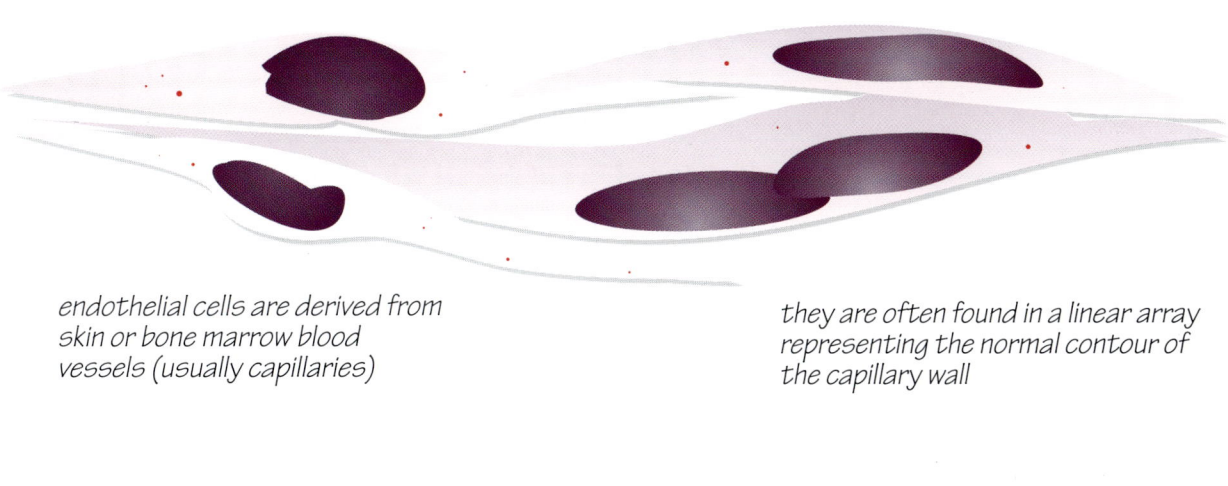

endothelial cells are derived from skin or bone marrow blood vessels (usually capillaries)

they are often found in a linear array representing the normal contour of the capillary wall

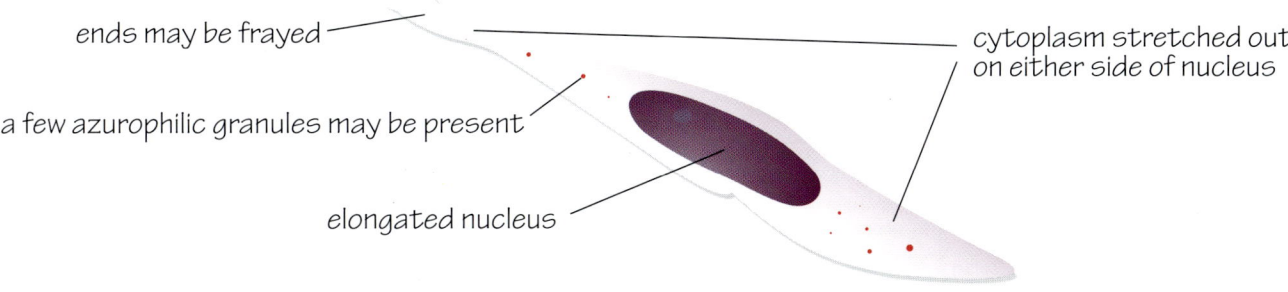

ends may be frayed

cytoplasm stretched out on either side of nucleus

a few azurophilic granules may be present

elongated nucleus

endothelial cells may also be found as single cells

Miscellaneous Cells

Epithelial Cell

SYNONYMS
skin cell

VITAL STATISTICS
- size .... 30-50 µm
- N:C ratio .... 1:1 to 1:5
- cell shape .... round to polyhedral
- nuclear shape .... round, slightly irregular
- chromatin .... dense, pyknotic
- parachromatin .... minimal
- nucleoli .... none
- cytoplasm .... abundant, lightly basophilic, may show keratinization or blue kerato-hyaline granules

KEY DIFFERENTIATING FEATURES
polyhedral-shaped cell
small, pyknotic nucleus

OTHER FINDINGS
nuclei are larger and N:C ratio is higher when derived from deeper layers of the epidermis

POTENTIAL LOOK-ALIKES
metastatic tumor cell
macrophage (histiocyte)
fibroblast

ASSOCIATED DISEASE STATES AND CONDITIONS
in vitro contamination during phlebotomy
amniotic fluid embolus

Epithelial cells are large (30-50 µm), round to polyhedral-shaped cells with a low nuclear to cytoplasmic ratio (1:1 to 1:5). The nucleus is round to slightly irregularly shaped, with dense, pyknotic chromatin and no visible nucleoli. The abundant cytoplasm is lightly basophilic and may show keratinization or a few blue kerato-hyaline granules. Epithelial cells from deeper layers of the epidermis have larger nuclei with a high nuclear to cytoplasmic ratio. In contrast to squamous carcinoma, contaminant squamous epithelial cells lack nuclear atypia. Squamous epithelial cells (derived from the skin) may rarely contaminate peripheral blood, particularly when smears are obtained from finger or heel punctures.

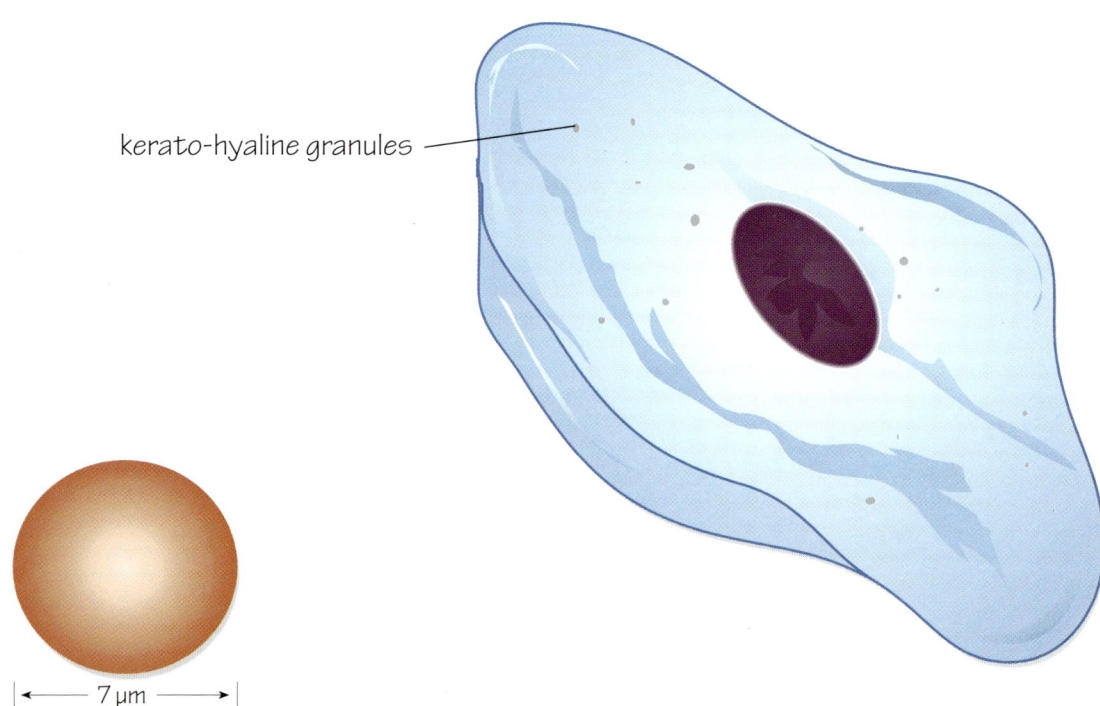

Epithelial Cell

kerato-hyaline granules

7 µm
size of normal red blood cell

HE-27, 1996 (Blood, Wright-Giemsa, X400)

Identification	Referee %	Participant %
Epithelial/endothelial cell	64	71.7
Stain precipitate	32	13.8
Lipocyte (fat cell)	4.0	1.8
Basket cell	-	4.8

This case represents skin contaminant in the preparation of a blood film from a healthy individual. The cell flanked by the two arrows is an epithelial cell. The cell is large and polyhedral. The cytoplasm is pale blue and semi-translucent. Platelets and red blood cells are seen beneath it. The cytoplasm contains blue-pink or blue-brown kerato-hyalin granules. The small dark blue-gray oval structure just above and to the right of the cell center is a pyknotic nucleus. This suggests that the cell is most likely from the superficial skin layer. Epithelial cells from deeper in the skin have larger nuclei and a higher nuclear:cytoplasmic ratio.

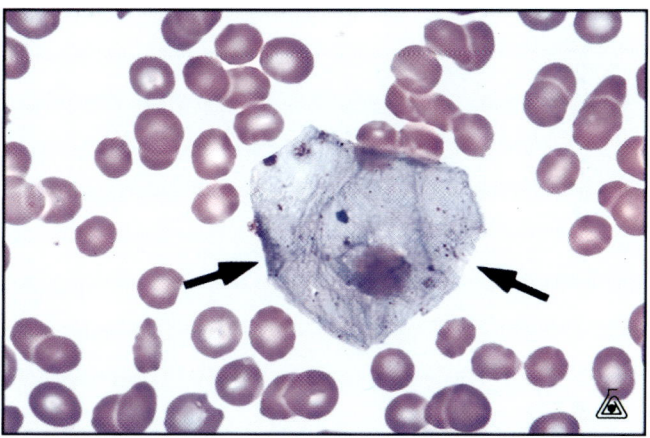

Epithelial Cell on Blood Smear

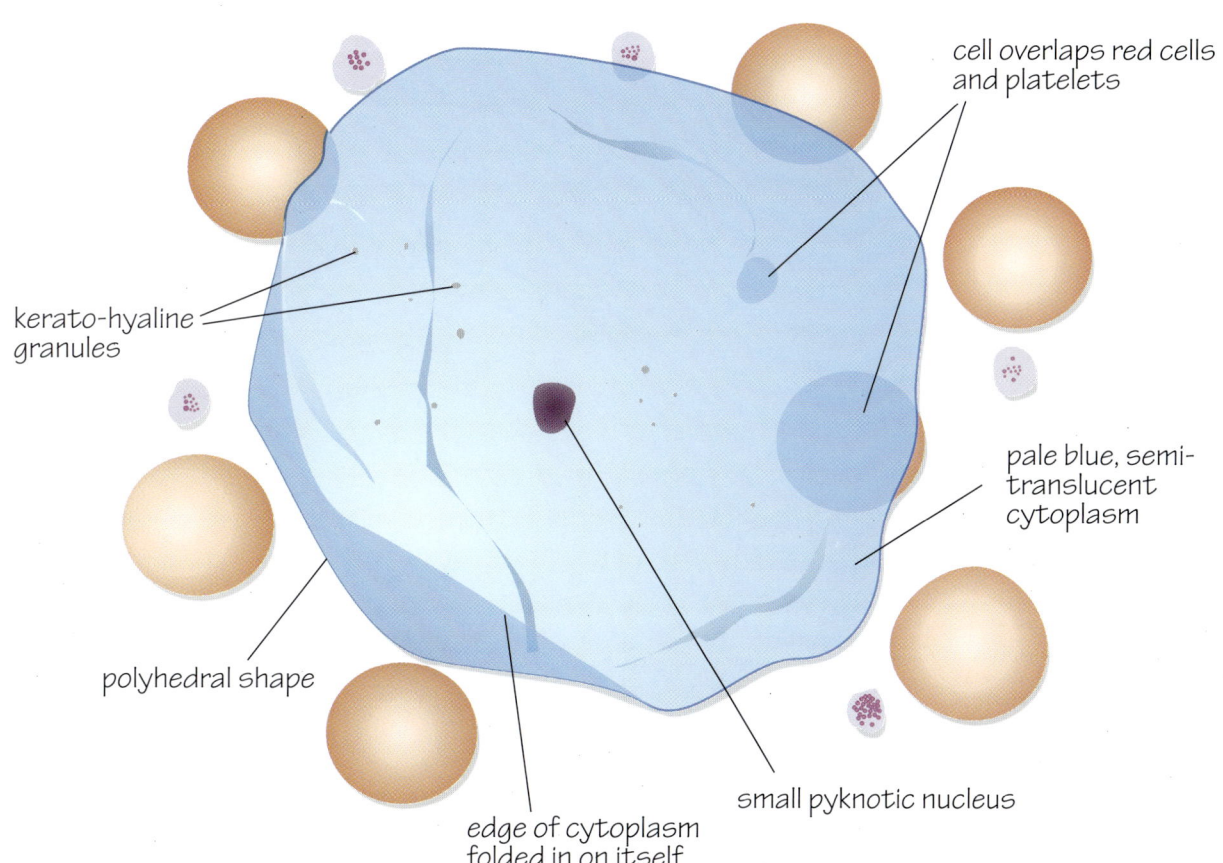

Miscellaneous Cells

Lipocyte

SYNONYMS
fat cell, adipocyte, lipid storage cell

VITAL STATISTICS
size .... 25-75 μm
N:C ratio .... very low, e.g. <1:10
cell shape .... round to oval
nuclear shape .... eccentric, flattened
chromatin .... very condensed, pyknotic
nucleoli .... none
cytoplasm .... abundant, colorless, may contain numerous large vacuoles or eosinophilic fibrils

KEY DIFFERENTIATING FEATURES
signet-ring like cell
small, condensed eccentric nucleus
colorless cytoplasm

OTHER FINDINGS
globular fat body occasionally seen within nucleus
usually occur in clusters in the bone marrow

POTENTIAL LOOK-ALIKES
macrophage (histiocyte)
plasma cell with globular inclusions
metastatic tumor cell

ASSOCIATED DISEASE STATES AND CONDITIONS
normal bone marrow constituent

The lipocyte, a normal constituent of yellow or fatty marrow, is a large (25 to 75 μm in diameter) cell with a very small, densely staining, pyknotic eccentric nucleus. Occasionally, a globular body is seen in the nucleus, thought to be fatty material. The fat-laden cytoplasm is abundant and often consists of a single, colorless fat vacuole giving the cell a signet ring appearance. Alternatively, it may appear to contain numerous large fat vacuoles, separated by delicate, light blue or pink cytoplasm. Eosinophilic fibrils may be present, both within the cytoplasm and extending outward from the cell margins. The lipocyte, a fat-producing cell, is to be distinguished from a macrophage with phagocytized fat or "lipophage." The lipid-laden macrophage contains small, uniform lipid particles, giving the cytoplasm a foamy or bubbly appearance.

Lipocyte (Fat Cell)

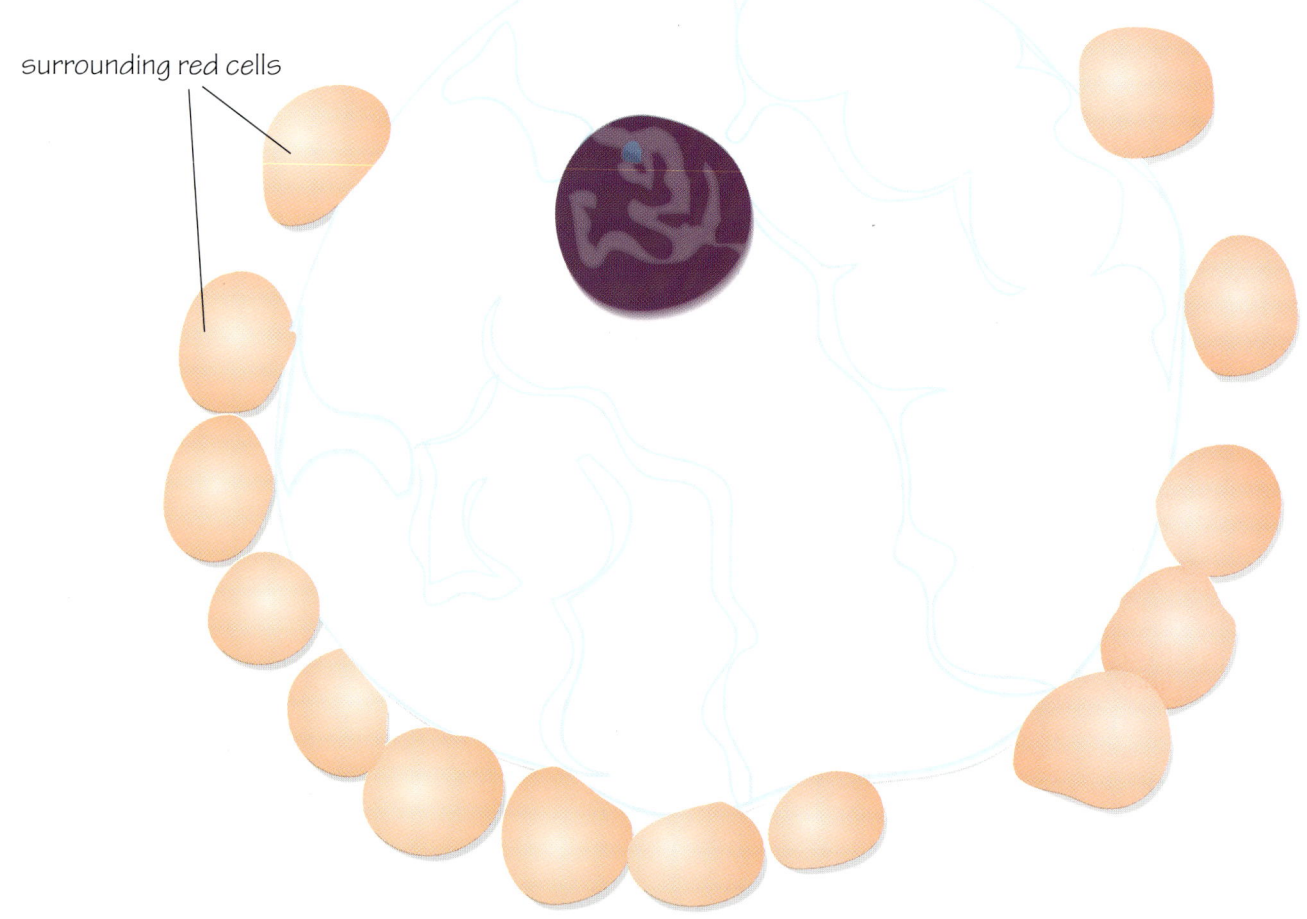

surrounding red cells

Miscellaneous Cells

HE-15, 1995 (Bone Marrow, Wright-Giemsa, X160)

Identification	Referee %	Participant %
Lipocyte (fat cell)	64.3	63.2
Macrophage with phagocytized red cells (erythrophagocytosis)	28.6	13.9
Gaucher cell, pseudo-Gaucher cell	-	12.2

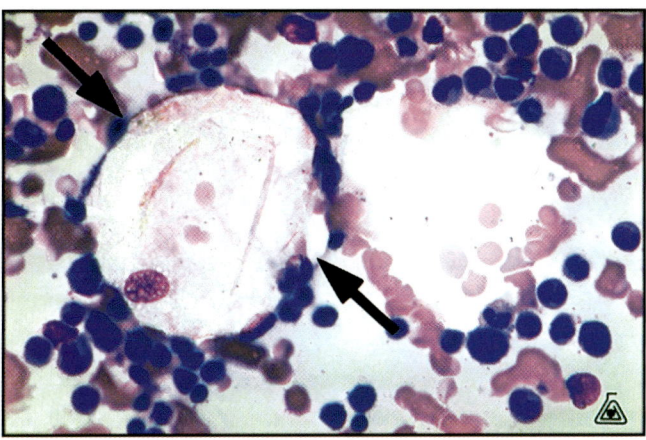

The photomicrograph shows a lipocyte or bone marrow fat cell. The cell has a small, densely staining pyknotic eccentric nucleus with numerous large fat vacuoles, separated by delicate light pink cytoplasm. Two degenerating erythrocytes overlay the cytoplasm, which may have led many participants and referees to classify this cell as a macrophage with phagocytized red cells. The Gaucher cell will have more numerous fibrillar or linear elements in the cytoplasm, rather than the occasional eosinophilic fibril seen in the cytoplasm of this lipocyte. The case is from a patient with nutritional anemia.

H-37, 1977 (Bone Marrow, Wright-Giemsa, X160)

Identification	Referee %	Participant %
Lipocyte (fat cell)	88.9	69.3
Gaucher cell, pseudo-Gaucher cell	11.1	12.1
Histiocyte	-	5.7
Niemann-Pick cell	-	6.5

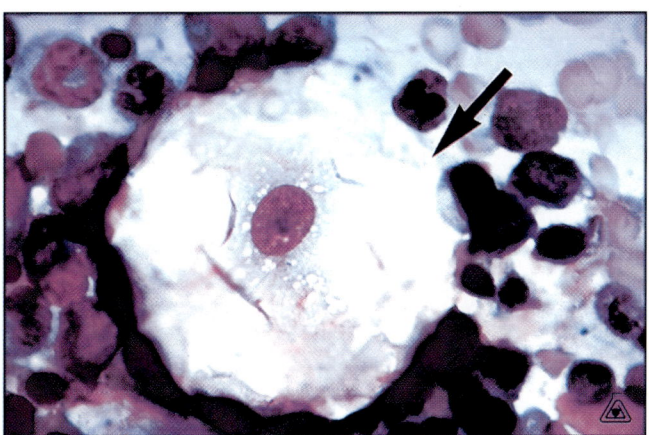

The large arrowed cell in the center of the field is a fat cell, also know as a *lipid storage cell* or *lipocyte*. The cytoplasm is slightly wrinkled and there are a few vacuoles near the centrally-located nucleus. The cell has a somewhat scalloped peripheral margin due to impingement of surrounding myeloid and erythroid cells. The nuclei of some of these cells are lighter staining where the lipocyte cytoplasm overlaps them. Lipocytes are normally found in the bone marrow, although generally only a large open space marks their presence. Gaucher cells are smaller and have a fibrillar cytoplasm. Niemann-Pick cells are also smaller and have numerous small vacuoles distributed throughout the cytoplasm. Histiocytes rarely reach this size unless they are multinucleated. The cytoplasm would also be more darkly staining. Megakaryocytes are of equivalent size but can be distinguished by their granular cytoplasm.

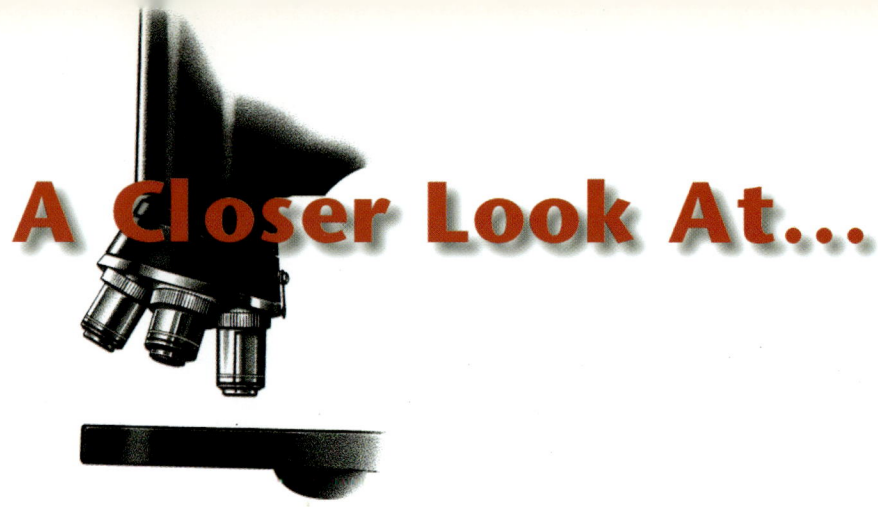

A Closer Look At...

Bone Marrow Microenvironment

Although differentiating hematopoietic cells, lipocytes, and vascular structures are apparent when examining the bone marrow, the hematopoietic stroma that mechanically supports these structures is less conspicuous. The bone marrow is surrounded by cortical bone and traversed by trabecular bone. Between the bony trabeculae is an organized framework of thin-walled venous sinuses, delicate reticulin fibers, and surrounding extracellular matrix.

The wall of a vascular sinus consists of endothelial cells, a poorly developed basement membrane, and an underlying adventitial layer. The endothelial cells control the passage of cells from the hematopoietic compartment into the venous sinus by receptor-mediated *endocytosis*, i.e. the hematopoietic cells released into the circulation must pass through the cytoplasm of endothelial cells rather than between them.

The adventitial layer supporting the sinus consists of a variety of stromal cells, sometimes collectively referred to as "reticular" or "dendritic" cells. Some of these cells have very long cytoplasmic processes and synthesize reticular fibers, both of which extend into the hematopoietic compartment. Thus, the stromal cells are ideal candidates for regulatory cells because they have a broad transportation network for targeted delivery of signaling factors and can create microenvironments within the marrow by physically separating the cells.

The stromal cells in the bone marrow are heterogeneous and consist of such cells as macrophages or histiocytes, fibroblasts, adipocytes, lymphocytes, and endothelial cells. Whether some of these cells arise from a progenitor adventitial "reticular cell" is unknown. However, it is believed that fibroblast-like cells of the adventitia can undergo lipogenesis and transform into adipocytes. As well as constituting support for the marrow vasculature, the stromal cells manufacture extracellular matrix proteins, a proteinaceous "soup" containing regulatory factors and adhesion molecules. Substances such as collagen, fibronectin, laminin, thrombospondin, vitronectin, hemonectin, and a variety of proteoglycans (e.g. heparan sulphate, chrondroitin sulphate, hyaluronic acid) provide the appropriate microenvironment for cell-to-cell contract, presentation/contact of regulatory or growth factors to cells, or recruitment of cells to specific bone marrow locations. Finally, the production of numerous growth factors and cytokines that both stimulate and inhibit hematopoietic proliferation and differentiation is largely the responsibility of the various stromal cells.

Bone Marrow Microenvironment

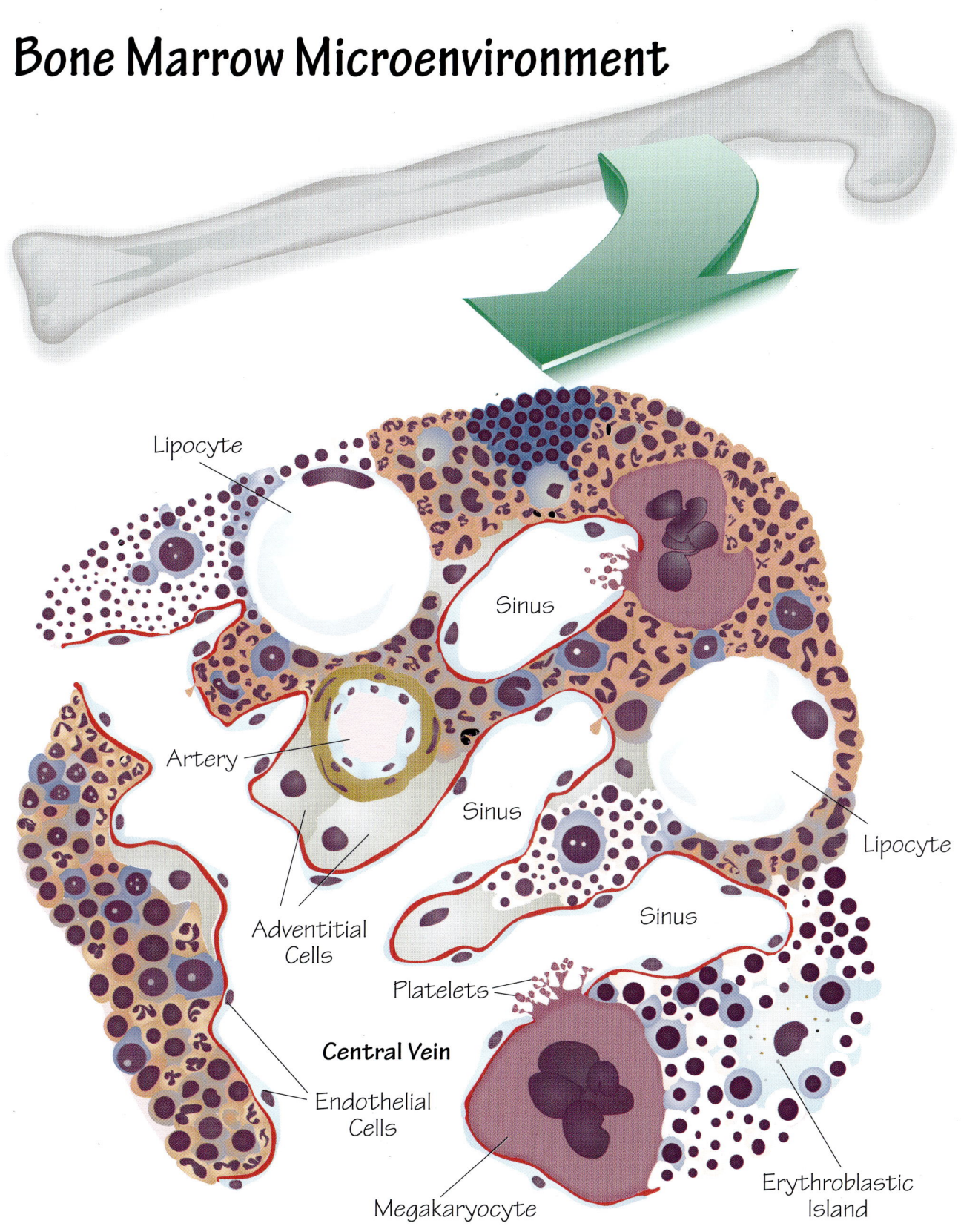

Miscellaneous Cells 315

Macrophage (Histiocyte)

SYNONYMS
reticulum cell, reticulo-endothelial cell

VITAL STATISTICS
- size .... 15-80 μm
- N:C ratio .... low, approximately 1:3; occasionally multinucleate
- cell shape .... irregular; with shaggy margins; bleb-like or filiform pseudopodia
- nuclear shape ..... round or oval, may be indented
- chromatin .... reticular pattern; distinct nuclear membrane
- parachromatin .... often visible
- nucleoli .... small; single or multiple
- cytoplasm .... frayed, abundant, pale gray-blue, often with coarse azurophilic granules and vacuoles; may have phagocytized material in native or degraded form

KEY DIFFERENTIATING FEATURES
large, bone marrow cell with abundant, streaming cytoplasm containing cytoplasmic vacuoles and/or phagocytic debris

OTHER FINDINGS
predominant component of granulomas, best appreciated in the bone marrow biopsy

POTENTIAL LOOK-ALIKES
- blast
- metastatic tumor cell
- lipocyte
- endothelial cell
- Gaucher cell
- Niemann-Pick cell
- osteoblast
- mast cell
- histiocyte, sea blue
- fibroblast

ASSOCIATED DISEASE STATES AND CONDITIONS
- inflammatory or infectious disorders
- increased intramedullary cell death, particularly following chemotherapy
- marrow neoplasias (hematopoietic and non-hematopoietic)
- histiocytic malignancies
- Langerhans cell histiocytosis

A macrophage, as the name implies, is a large (15 to 80 μm in diameter) phagocytic cell. It is irregular in shape, frequently with shaggy margins and bleb-like or filiform pseudopodia. The nucleus usually is round or oval, but occasionally may be indented. The nuclear membrane is distinct, and the nuclear chromatin is fine with a spongy, reticular pattern. One or more small nucleoli may be seen. The frayed, streaming cytoplasm is abundant, pale gray-blue, and often is granulated (coarse, azurophilic granules).

Phagocytized material (white cells, red cells, platelets, nuclei or their remnants, microorganisms) may be present in native or degraded form within the cytoplasm. Cytoplasmic vacuoles may be abundant, which contain phagocytized material or appear empty. Iron is stored in bone marrow macrophages as ferritin or hemosiderin (demonstrated with Prussian blue stain). The stored iron arises almost exclusively from phagocytosis and degranulation of senescent or defective erythrocytes.

Less phagocytic macrophages sometimes are referred to as *histiocytes*, *reticulum cells*, or *reticuloendothelial cells*. They have fewer lysosomal granules and may play a role in antigenic presentation to lymphocytes, cell-cell interactions in the immune system, and production of mediators important in inflammatory and immune responses.

Macrophage

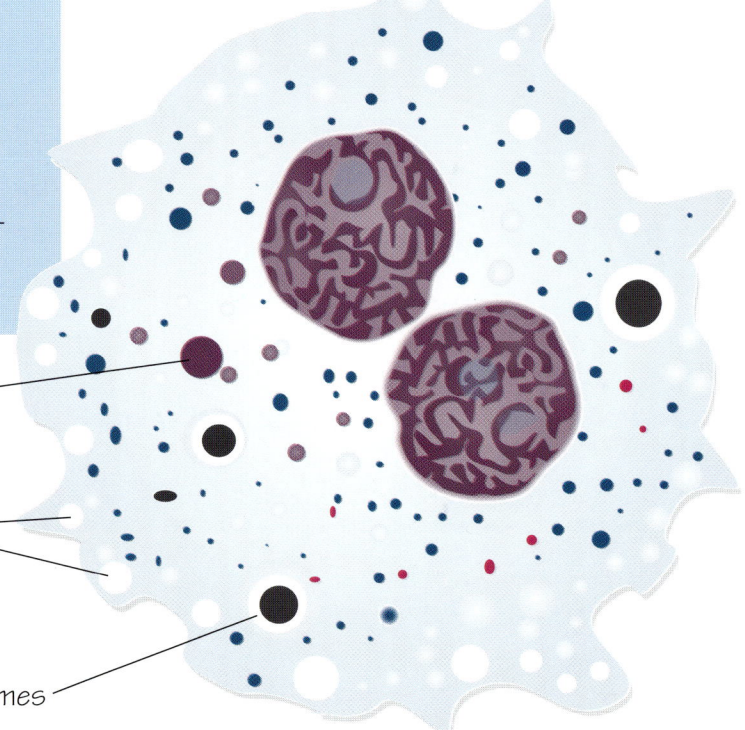

- cytoplasm containing phagocytic debris
- vacuoles
- phagolysozomes

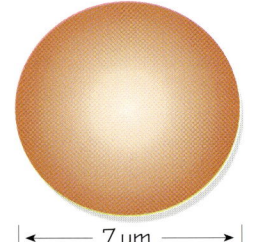

|← 7 μm →|
size of normal red blood cell

Miscellaneous Cells

Macrophages may cluster together, forming an epithelioid agglomeration, or fuse, to form multinucleated giant cells. These aggregated, epithelioid macrophages or Langhans' giant cells often are prominent components of marrow granulomas, a finding best appreciated in the bone marrow biopsy. Macrophages arise from circulating monocytes or from the marrow reticulum cells (which comprise the skeletal components of the bone marrow interstitial space, as well as bone marrow sinuses and vessels). The transformation of monocytes into macrophages is accompanied by stronger positive nonspecific esterase and acid phosphatase activity (often resistant to tartrate inhibition).

H1-20, 1988 (Bone Marrow, Wright-Giemsa, X250)

Identification	Referee %	Participant %
Macrophage (histiocyte)	100	85.7

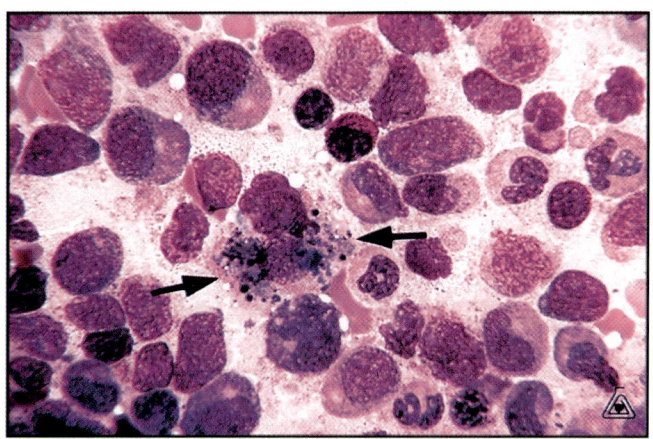

The case is from an elderly male with an unclassified myeloproliferative disorder. The bone marrow biopsy and clot demonstrated an increase in cellularity and myeloid hyperplasia. The arrowed cell is a bone marrow histiocyte. The cytoplasm contains large granular collections of cell debris and probably iron. The majority of the surround leukocytes are granulocytes. They are left-shifted with an increase in myelocytes and metamyelocytes. There is no significant dysplasia.

HE-11, 1995 (Bone Marrow, Wright-Giemsa, X250)

Identification	Referee %	Participant %
Macrophage (histiocyte)	50	33.2
Megakaryocyte or precursor, normal	17.9	30.1
Megakaryocyte or precursor, abnormal	21.4	26.7

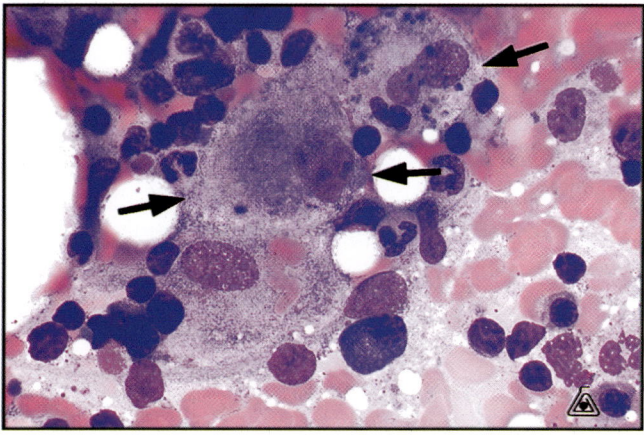

Two macrophages (histiocytes) are illustrated in this case of immune thrombocytopenia. These cells are large (approximately 65 μm in diameter), have an eccentric nucleus with finely reticulated or spongy chromatin, and show a distinct nuclear membrane. The abundant cytoplasm is pinkish-blue and contains coarse blue-black hemosiderin granules. Intact erythrocytes are seen in the third, unarrowed macrophage. Participants mistakenly identified these macrophages as megakaryocytes, probably because of the abundant azurophilic granules. However, the reticulated chromatin of the nucleus in these cells is more typical of macrophages. Furthermore, the dark hemosiderin granules in the cytoplasm of these cells would not be present in megakaryocytes.

Macrophage with Phagocytized Red Cell (Erythrophagocytosis)

SYNONYMS
erythrophage, siderophage

VITAL STATISTICS
- size .... 15-80 μm
- N:C ratio .... low, approximately 1:3; occasionally multinucleate
- cell shape .... irregular; with shaggy margins; bleb-like or filiform pseudopodia
- nuclear shape ..... round or oval, may be indented
- chromatin .... reticular pattern; distinct nuclear membrane
- parachromatin ..... often visible
- nucleoli .... one or more small
- cytoplasm .... frayed, abundant, pale gray-blue, often with coarse azurophilic granules and abundant vacuoles; contains one or more erythroid cells in native or degraded form; intact or degraded leukocytes and platelets also may be seen

KEY DIFFERENTIATING FEATURES
large macrophage containing one or more erythrocytes and/or cytoplasmic vacuoles containing erythroid phagocytic debris

OTHER FINDINGS
malignant histiocytosis (histiocytic medullary reticulosis) is characterized by a diffuse infiltration of atypical, pleomorphic histiocytes displaying multinucleation, prominent nucleoli, and vigorous erythrophagocytosis

POTENTIAL LOOK-ALIKES
other histiocytes or macrophages (Niemann-Pick cell, siderophage, Gaucher cell, sea blue histiocyte, etc.)
lipocyte

ASSOCIATED DISEASE STATES AND CONDITIONS
severe bacterial, fungal, parasitic or viral infections with immunosuppression
hemolytic anemias with immunosuppression
recent transfusion with immunosuppression
disseminated malignancy with immunosuppression
malignant histiocytosis
erythrophagocytic acute monocytic leukemia
T cell lymphoma
virus-associated hemophagocytic syndrome
familial erythrophagocytic lymphohistiocytosis
acute blood transfusion reaction
Kawasaki's disease
anticonvulsant drugs

The cytoplasm of macrophages may contain one or more intact red blood cells, as well as degraded erythroid forms within vacuoles. With further digestion, black hemosiderin granules may be evident.

Phagocytosis of erythrocytes often occurs concomitantly with macrophage ingestion of neutrophils and/or platelets (hemophagocytosis). Bone marrow histiocytic hyperplasia with hemophagocytosis results from immunologic activation of the mononuclear-phagocytic system, usually in the setting of immunosuppression. Immune stimuli can include severe bacterial, fungal, parasitic, or viral infections; recent blood transfusions, disseminated malignancy, hemolytic anemias (including those due to immune hemolysis, membrane defects, and hemoglobinopathy), and various autoimmune disorders. Striking bone marrow hemophagocytosis can be associated with some types of viral infections (virus-associated hemophagocytic syndrome), particularly Epstein-Barr virus. In addition to reactive conditions, vigorous hemophagocytosis is seen in malignant histiocytosis, T cell lymphoma, and an occasional case of acute monocytic leukemia. Malignant histiocytosis (histiocytic medullary reticulosis) is characterized by a diffuse infiltration of atypical, pleomorphic histiocytes, with prominent nuclei and multinucleation. Peripheral blood erythrophagocytosis is less commonly observed, but may be particularly striking in response to an acute transfusion reaction.

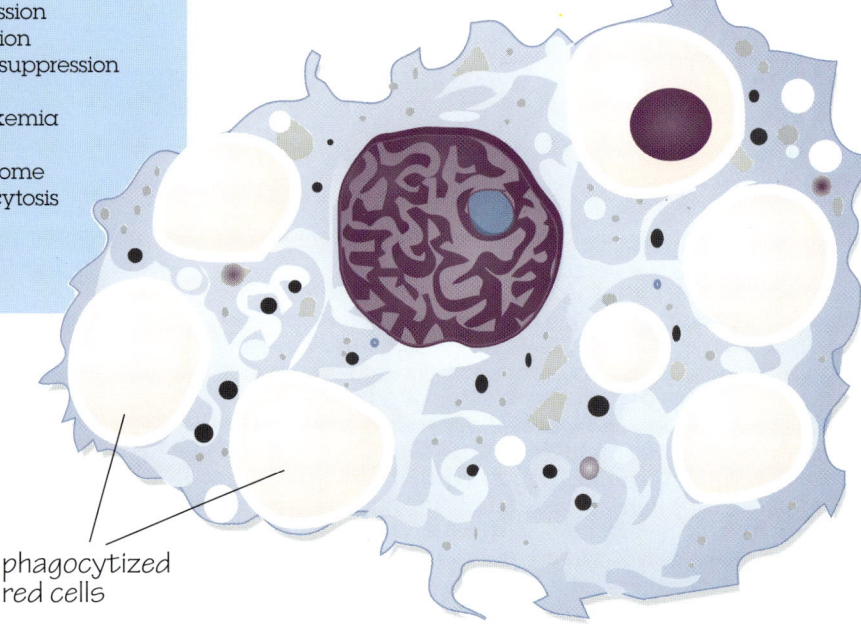

Erythrophage — phagocytized red cells

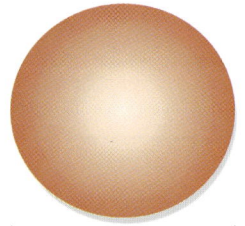

|← 7 μm →|
size of normal red blood cell

H-59, 1982 (Bone Marrow, Wright-Giemsa, X370)

Identification	Referee %	Participant %
Macrophage with phagocytized red blood cell	100	78.4
Monocyte or precursor	-	16.1

This is a case of erythrophagocytic acute monocytic leukemia. The cytoplasm of this immature monocytic precursor distinctly displays a phagocytized erythrocyte. Another immature and dysplastic monocytoid cell can be seen adjacent to the arrowed cell.

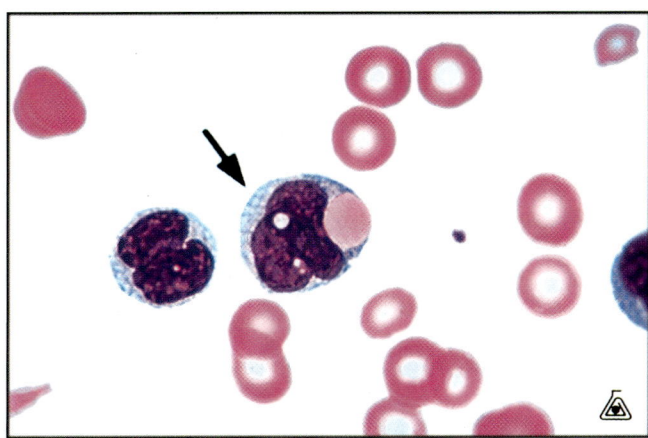

HE-15, 1994 (Blood, Wright-Giemsa, X400)

Identification	Referee %	Participant %
Macrophage with phagocytized red blood cell	100	97.1

The photomicrograph from a patient with a myeloproliferative disorder (agnogenic myeloid metaplasia) shows a rare example of erythrophagocytosis in the peripheral blood. The cytoplasm of this monocyte/macrophage is filled with readily identifable erythrocytes. Spherocytes were present in other areas of this blood smear, implying hemolysis.

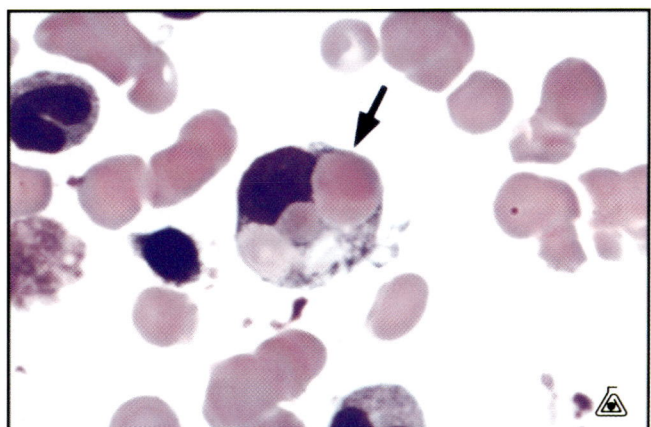

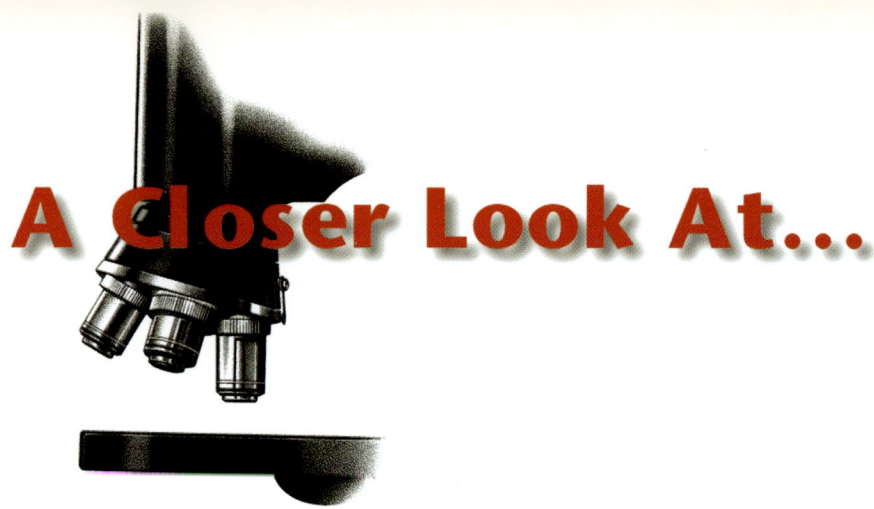

A Closer Look At...

Cytoplasmic Inclusions in Bone Marrow Cells

In contrast to the blood, cytoplasmic inclusions commonly are seen in many of the cells that reside in the bone marrow. Such inclusions may represent normal cellular breakdown products, remnants of defective digestion of cellular constituents, or synthesized material. The table on the next page lists these inclusions.

For example, *phagocytic macrophages* may contain vacuoles with partially digested cells or cellular debris, including hemosiderin granules from the degradation of senescent erythrocytes. Various inherited disorders are associated with enzyme deficiencies that result in an excess of undigested cell products in macrophages, particularly from the lipid-rich cell membrane. *Gaucher's disease* is characterized by deficiency of beta-glucocerebrosidase and an overload of glucoceramide, leading to a macrophage containing fibrillar cytoplasmic inclusions. The *sea blue histiocyte* is filled with globules of ceroid, an insoluble lipid pigment representing undigested globosides from cell membranes, seen in many lipid storage disorders. In *Niemann-Pick disease* and other gangliosidoses, deficient lysosomal enzymes lead to an accumulation of sphingomyelin or other lipid globules, giving a foamy, vacuolated appearance to the macrophage. However, excessive cell catabolism also can overload the normal capacity of macrophages to digest lipids. Thus, many of these lipid-containing cytoplasmic inclusions may accompany any disorder associated with massive cell destruction in the bone marrow.

In contrast to the lipid-laden macrophage, the *lipocyte* is a fat-producing cell. The synthesized fat appears as one or more large, colorless vacuoles, giving the cell a "signet ring" appearance. The numerous granules in the *mast cell* contain an array of substances (e.g. sulfated glycosaminoglycans, histamine, proteases, acid hydrolases, cathepsin G, and carboxypeptidase), many of which serve as mediators of inflammation and anaphylaxis. A minority of plasma cells may have globular or crystalline inclusions comprised of synthesized immunoglobulin.

Cytoplasmic Inclusions in Bone Marrow Cells

	Description
Macrophage (Histiocyte)	numerous inclusion particles including coarse azurophilic granules, blue-black hemosiderin granules, phagocytized cells or cellular debris (leukocytes, erythrocytes, platelets, microorganisms); may contain variably sized vacuoles which are empty or contain partially digested material
Macrophage with Phagocytized Red Cell	coarse azurophilic granules typical for macrophage; intact or degraded erythroid forms within vacuoles; may also contain blue-black hemosiderin granules
Histiocyte, Sea Blue	bluish-green globules or granules of variable size
Gaucher Cell, Pseudo-Gaucher Cell	fibrillar cytoplasm with wrinkled tissue paper appearance; morphologic variant may contain fibrillar inclusions and blue cytoplasmic granules
Niemann-Pick Cell (Foamy Macrophage)	numerous lipid globules which are small and relatively uniform in size
Lipocyte (Fat-Producing Cell)	single or multiple colorless vacuoles; eosinophilic fibrils may be present
Mast Cell	abundant bluish-purple or red-purple small granules, often obscuring the nucleus
Plasma Cell	may have globular or crystalline immunoglobulin inclusions within the cytoplasm

Gaucher Cell and Pseudo-Gaucher Cell

SYNONYMS
none

VITAL STATISTICS
- size .... 20-90 μm
- N:C ratio .... <1:3
- cell shape .... usually round to oval, occasional irregular
- nuclear shape .... usually round to oval, occasional irregular
- chromatin .... coarse granular, condensed
- parachromatin .... variable; none to slight amount
- nucleoli .... small or indistinct, if any
- cytoplasm .... abundant, gray, pale blue, green-blue, characteristic fibrillar appearance

KEY DIFFERENTIATING FEATURES
- large cell with abundant cytoplasm
- fibrillar cytoplasmic inclusions, resulting in distinctive linear striation of the cytoplasm

OTHER FINDINGS
- morphologic variant shows less striking linear striation of the cytoplasm and contains fine blue cytoplasmic granules, fewer in number than the sea-blue histiocyte
- pseudo-Gaucher cell may display greater amount of phagocytosis than true Gaucher's cells

POTENTIAL LOOK-ALIKES
- other histiocytes or macrophages (Niemann-Pick or Niemann-Pick-like histiocytes, siderophage, epithelioid histiocyte, sea blue histiocyte)
- lipocyte
- plasma cell with inclusions

ASSOCIATED DISEASE STATES AND CONDITIONS
- Gaucher's disease
- chronic myelogenous leukemia
- myeloma
- acute myelocytic leukemia
- idiopathic thrombocytopenic purpura
- aplastic anemia
- chronic lymphocytic leukemia
- rheumatoid arthritis
- thalassemia major
- Hodgkin's disease
- gangliosidosis

A Gaucher cell is a form of histiocyte (macrophage) that is ovoid and measures 20 to 90 μm in diameter with a low nuclear to cytoplasmic ratio (<1:3). It contains a small, round, or oval nucleus with indistinct nucleoli. The chromatin is coarse. The cytoplasm is abundant, lipid-laden (containing glucosylcerebroside), and stains gray to pale blue. Fibrillar, reticular, "crumpled cellophane," or "wrinkled tissue paper" appearance of the cytoplasm is characteristic. This distinctive linear striation results from lamellar bodies stacked within secondary phagolysosomes. A morphologic variant shows less striking linear striation and contains a small number of fine blue cytoplasmic granules. The cells stain for PAS and lysosomal enzymes such as nonspecific esterase and acid phosphatase (tartrate resistant).

Gaucher's disease is an inherited enzyme deficiency of beta-glucocerebrosidase, leading to accumulation of glucosylcerebroside in a variety of tissues, including bone, liver, lung, and brain. Page 327 illustrates the enzyme deficiency.

Pseudo-Gaucher cells, indistinguishable from true Gaucher cells on light microscopy or ultrastructurally, are phagocytic cells engaged in catabolism of glycoside from the membranes of dead cells. These macrophages have normal amounts of beta-glucocerebrosidase enzyme and are postulated to arise from excessive cell breakdown with an overload of glucoceramide. The presence of pseudo-Gaucher cells has no particular diagnostic significance.

Gaucher Cell

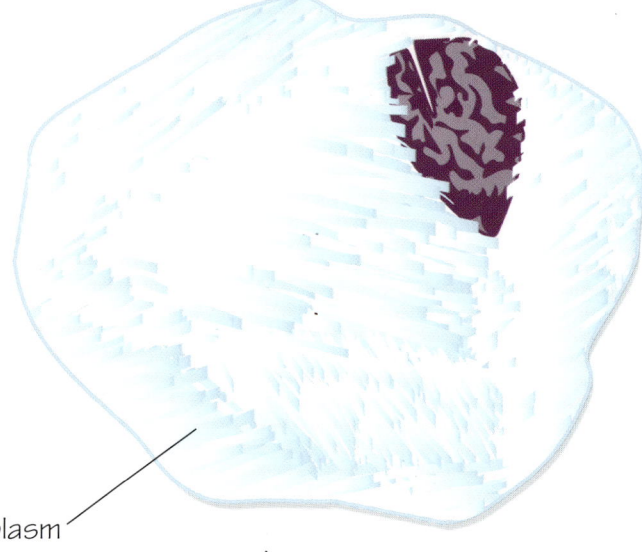

fibrillar cytoplasm (wrinkled tissue paper appearance)

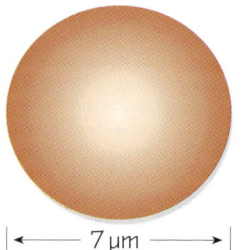

|← 7 μm →|
size of normal red blood cell

H-24, 1978 (Bone Marrow, Wright-Giemsa, X400)

Identification	Referee %	Participant %
Gaucher cell	51.9	37.5
Pseudo-Gaucher cell	9.4	50.0
Histiocyte, not otherwise specified	23.0	-

The bone marrow from a patient with Gaucher's disease shows areas of normal hematopoiesis and areas infiltrated with Gaucher cells. The prominent large cell is a Gaucher cell variant, with less striking development of the cytoplasmic lamellar structures that give rise to the characteristic fibrillar appearance. Sparse blue-green cytoplasmic granules are present.

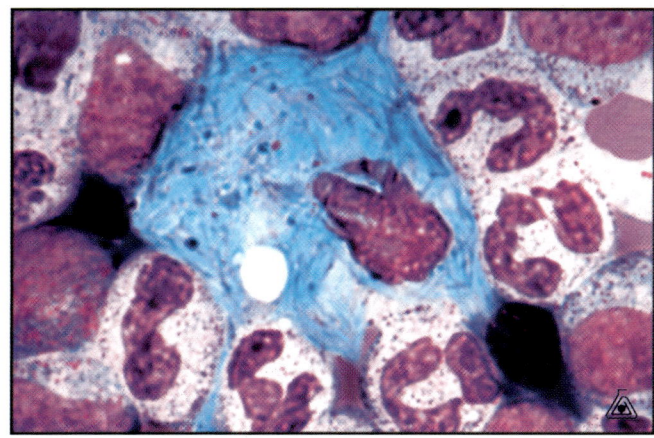

H-40, 1981 (Bone Marrow, Wright-Giemsa, X250)

Identification	Referee %	Participant %
Gaucher cell	83.3	68.7
Pseudo-Gaucher cell	16.7	11.5
Histiocyte, not otherwise specified	-	5.9
Plasma cell or precursor	-	10.1

In this case of Gaucher's disease, "Gaucher cell," "pseudo-Gaucher cell," or "histiocyte, not otherwise specified" was correctly chosen by 100% of referees and 86.1% of participants. This Gaucher cell is smaller than the one seen in photomicrograph H-24, 1978, and the striated cytoplasm is more prominent. The cell appears to have phagocytized a red cell. Approximately 10% of participants incorrectly identified this cell as a plasma cell. Although plasma cells occasionally can have needle-like immunoglobulin inclusions and eccentric nuclei similar to this cell, most are smaller in size, show more deeply basophilic cytoplasm, and a display a nuclear hof. A mature plasma cell is seen in the upper right-hand corner of this photomicrograph.

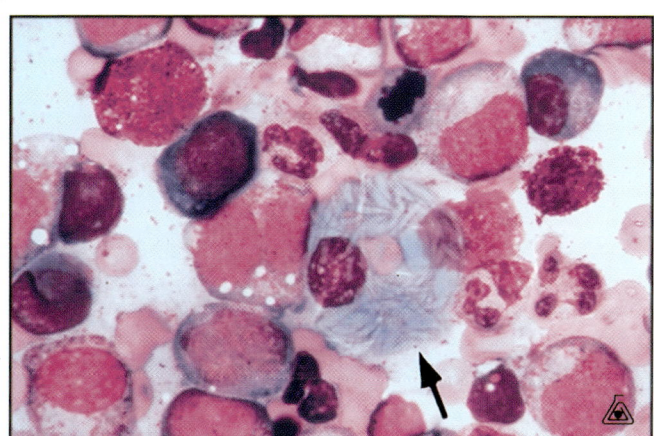

H1-46, 1987 (Bone Marrow, Wright-Giemsa, X250)

Identification	Referee %	Participant %
Gaucher cell	73.7	71.7
Pseudo-Gaucher cell	26.3	24.8

This is an example of pseudo-Gaucher cell in a patient with treated chronic myelogenous leukemia. The large arrowed cell contains very prominent cytoplasmic striations and has an identical appearance to the true Gaucher cell in H-40, 1981. 100% of referees and 95.9% of participants selected "Gaucher cell," "pseudo-Gaucher cell," or "histiocyte, not otherwise specified" as the identification.

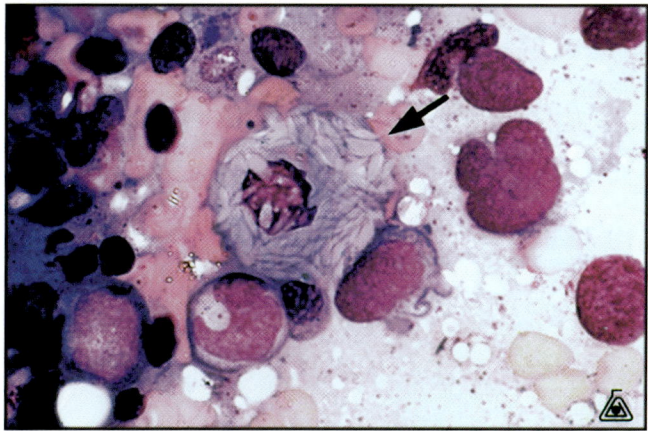

Histocyte, Sea Blue

SYNONYMS
ceroid-containing histiocytes, blue pigment macrophages

VITAL STATISTICS
- size .... 20-60 μm
- N:C ratio .... low, approximately 1:3; occasionally multinucleate
- cell shape .... irregular; with shaggy margins
- nuclear shape .... round or oval, may be indented
- chromatin .... dense
- parachromatin ... not visible
- nucleoli .... occasionally present
- cytoplasm .... frayed, abundant, filled with variably-sized globules or granules of bluish or bluish-green pigment

KEY DIFFERENTIATING FEATURES
bone marrow macrophage (histiocyte) with abundant variably-sized bluish or bluish-green cytoplasmic globules or granules

OTHER FINDINGS
in H&E-stained marrow sections, the histiocytes appear foamy or slightly eosinophilic and contain a variable number of yellow to yellow-brown granules

POTENTIAL LOOK-ALIKES
macrophage (histiocyte)
Gaucher cell, pseudo-Gaucher cell
mast cell

ASSOCIATED DISEASE STATES AND CONDITIONS
sea-blue histiocyte syndrome
Niemann-Pick disease
other lipid storage diseases, including Wolman's disease, Fabry's disease, and Tay Sachs disease
ceroid accumulation in progressive neurologic disease
hyperlipoproteinemia and hypercholesterolemia
hereditary acyltransferase deficiency
Hodgkin's disease and non-Hodkin's lymphomas
chronic myeloproliferative disorders (CML and PRV)
acute leukemias and preleukemias (myelodysplasia)
multiple myeloma
mucopolysaccharidoses
chronic granulomatous disease
immune thrombocytopenic pupura
thalassemia
sickle cell anemia
infectious mononucleosis
rheumatoid disease
sarcoidosis

These bone marrow cells are macrophages (histiocytes) that have abundant cytoplasm filled with variably-sized bluish or bluish-green globules or granules of insoluble lipid pigment, called *ceroid*. Ceroid, Latin for wax-like, is a pigment of uncertain identity, thought to represent partially digested globosides derived from cell membranes. Histiocytes containing copious amounts of the pigment have a distinctive blue-green color on Wright-Giemsa smears and give the histiocyte its colorful name. It is important to remember that ceroid pigment is not the only element that stains blue green on Wright-Giemsa; melanin, hemosiderin, and malaria pigment may also.

In H&E-stained marrow sections, the histiocytes appear foamy or slightly eosinophilic and contain a variable number of yellow to yellow-brown granules. They are distinguished from hemosiderin-laden macrophages (siderophages) by a negative Prussian blue stain.

Small numbers of sea blue histiocytes are seen in normal marrow and should not be considered a pathologic finding. Large numbers occur in marrow, spleen, and liver in an inherited disorder of unknown cause, called the *sea blue histiocyte syndrome*. The histiocytes are benign but impart morbidity due to massive sple-

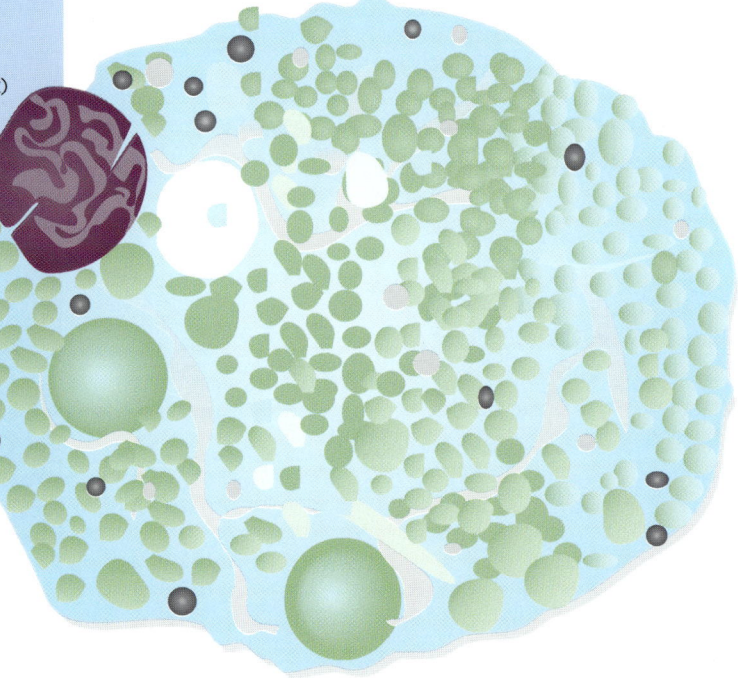

Sea Blue Histiocyte

cytoplasm contains variably-sized globules and granules of blue-green pigment

|← 7μm →|
size of normal red blood cell

Miscellaneous Cells

nomegaly and its associated risks of bleeding and rupture. The disease may be a variant of Niemann-Pick disease.

Occasional to moderate numbers of sea-blue histiocytes can be seen in other lipid storage diseases, particularly type B Niemann-Pick disease and lecithin cholesterol acyl transferase (LCAT) deficiency.

Lastly, sea-blue histiocytes are increased—sometimes markedly so—in any disorder associated with massively increased intramedullary cell destruction. Examples include chronic myelogenous leukemia, acute myelogenous leukemia, acute lymphoblastic leukemia, certain types of lymphomas, thalassemia, sickle cell anemia, and immune thrombocytopenic purpura.

HE-13, 1995 (Bone Marrow, Wright-Giemsa, X250)

Identification	Referee %	Participant %
Histiocyte, sea blue	80	86.9
Macrophage (histiocyte)	7.7	1.2

This child with sea blue histiocyte syndrome presented with hepatosplenomegaly and numerous sea blue histiocytes in the bone marrow. The cytoplasm of the macrophage in this photomicrograph is filled with globules of bluish ceroid pigment.

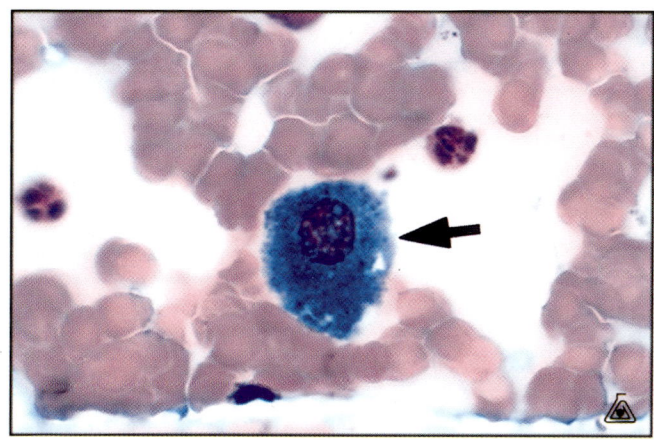

HE-30, 1995 (Bone Marrow, split screen: Left, Wright-Giemsa, X250; Right, PAS, X250)

Identification	Referee %	Participant %
Histiocyte, sea blue	51.9	59.1
Gaucher or pseudo-Gaucher cell	7.4	16.8
Niemann-Pick cell	-	7.1
Macrophage (histiocyte)	3.7	3.8

The distinctive cell in both fields is a sea blue histiocyte. The cell derives its name from the abundant blue-green or "sea-blue" globules within the cytoplasm. This is best seen in the Wright-Giemsa stained smear on the left. The major component of the material is ceroid, an insoluble lipid pigment thought to represent partially digested globosides derived from cell membranes. As shown in the PAS stain on the right, the pigment is PAS positive. Gaucher cells have gray-blue fibrillar cytoplasm. Niemann-Pick cells have vacuolated and foamy cytoplasm with a mulberry-like appearance. Some variants of Niemann-Pick disease have mixtures of foam cells and sea blue histiocytes, probably representing breakdown of the stored sphingomyelin to ceroid.

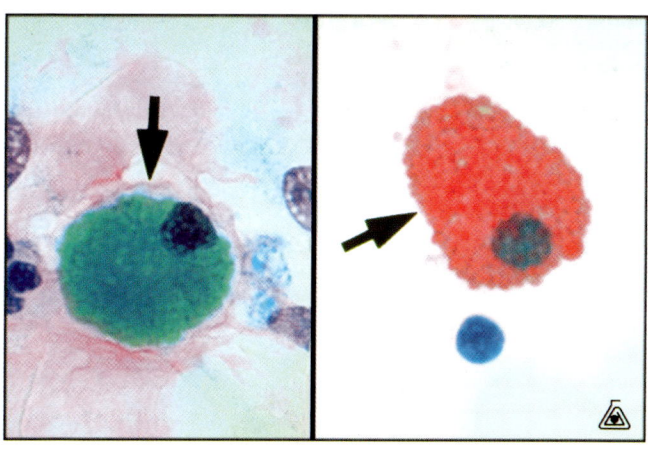

Niemann-Pick Cell, Foamy Macrophage

SYNONYMS
none

VITAL STATISTICS
size .... 20-90 µm
N:C ratio .... <1:10
cell shape .... round to oval
nuclear shape .... round, irregular margin
chromatin .... dense
parachromatin .... minimal
nucleoli .... none
cytoplasm .... foamy, vacuolated

KEY DIFFERENTIATING FEATURES
histiocyte with abundant lipid globules in cytoplasm

OTHER FINDINGS
Niemann-Pick cells show small vacuoles with uniform size
mixture of foamy macrophages and sea blue histiocytes may occur

POTENTIAL LOOK-ALIKES
macrophage (histiocyte)
Gaucher cell and pseudo-Gaucher cell
sea-blue histiocyte
lipocyte

ASSOCIATED DISEASE STATES AND CONDITIONS
Niemann-Pick disease
gangliosidoses
Fabry's disease
lactosyl ceramidosis
hyperlipidemia
thalassemias
rheumatoid arthritis
sickle cell anemia
thrombocytopenic purpura
infectious mononucleosis
chemotherapy-induced marrow aplasia
hepatitis
chronic renal failure

Niemann-Pick disease is an inherited deficiency of the lysosomal enzyme sphingomyelinase, leading to extensive accumulation of sphingomyelin in a variety of tissues, including the bone marrow. The Niemann-Pick cell is a sphingomyelin-laden histiocyte of variable size (20 to 90 µm diameter) with abundant cytoplasm (nuclear to cytoplasmic ratio <1:10). The cell has one or more small, round nuclei with coarse chromatin. The cytoplasm is vacuolated and foamy, with a mulberry-like appearance.

The enzyme deficiencies leading to Niemann-Pick disease (and Gaucher's disease) are illustrated on the next page. Macrophages digest sphingolipids released as a cell (such as a neutrophil) dies. Normally, enzymes cleave ceremide from the rest of the sphingolipid, allowing further degradation. Without sphingomyelinase, droplets of sphingomyelin accumulate in the cell.

Some variants of Niemann-Pick disease have mixtures of foamy macrophages and sea-blue histiocytes, probably representing breakdown of the stored sphingomyelin to ceroid. Blood lymphocytes and monocytes also may display cytoplasmic vacuoles containing sphingomyelin.

Foamy macrophages may be seen in other conditions, including inherited deficiencies in the metabolism of lipid materials (e.g., gangliosidoses, Fabry's disease, lactosyl ceramidosis), or excess accumulation of lipid material in bone marrow macrophages (e.g., hyperlipidemias, thalassemias, rheumatoid arthritis, sickle cell anemia, thrombocytopenic purpura, infectious mononucleosis, hepatitis). The foamy macrophages in these disorders differ slightly from Niemann-Pick cells in that their vacuoles may be larger and are more irregular in size.

Niemann-Pick Cell

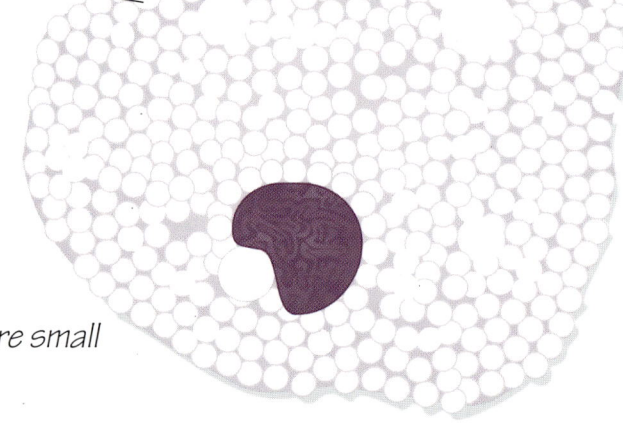

abundant lipid globules (sphyngomyelin) in cytoplasm of macrophage

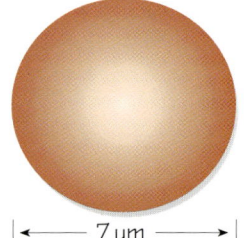

7 µm
size of normal red blood cell

the vacuoles are small and uniform

HE-12, 1995 (Bone Marrow, Wright-Giemsa, X250)

Identification	Referee %	Participant %
Niemann-Pick cell	75.0	57.3
Macrophage (histiocyte)	14.3	9.0
Macrophage with phagocytized red cells (erythrophagocytosis)	7.1	3.5
Gaucher cell, pseudo-Gaucher cell	22.2	
Lipocyte (fat cell)	3.6	4.4

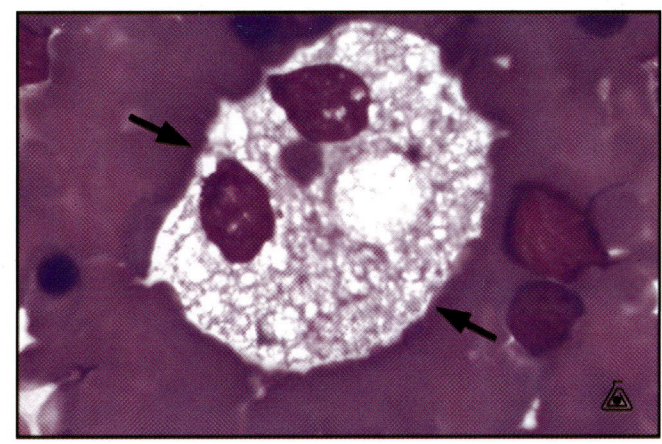

This is a case of Niemann-Pick disease. The cell is a large binucleate foamy macrophage that contains a partially digested particle, probably a phagocytized erythrocyte. Although an occasional vacuole is large, for the most part, the cytoplasmic vacuoles are small and of uniform size, giving the cytoplasm a mulberry-like appearance. Such a cell can be found in a variety of conditions in which an excess of lipid materials accumulate in macrophages (particularly in hyperlipidemias, or in diseases with excessive bone marrow cell breakdown). Given the appropriate clinical history and/or laboratory data, one can infer that this foamy macrophage most likely represents a cell diagnostic for Niemann-Pick disease. A substantial number of participants identified this cell as a *Gaucher cell*. However, the Gaucher cell is a lipid-laden histiocyte containing glucosylcerebroside, which give the cytoplasm a fibrillar or "wrinkled tissue paper" appearance.

NORMAL CELL BREAKDOWN AND DIGESTION BY MACROPHAGES

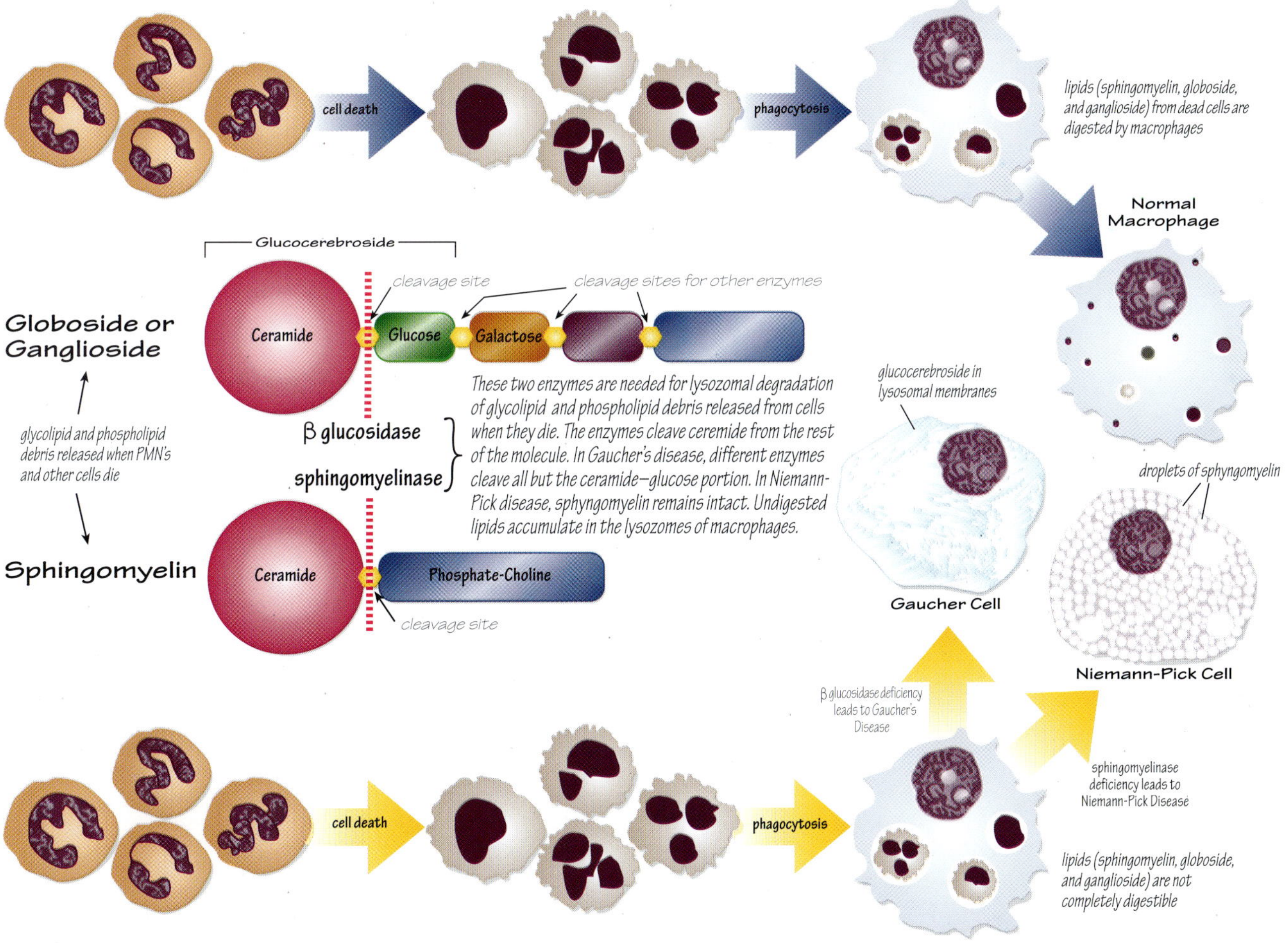

ACCUMULATION OF UNDIGESTIBLE LIPIDS DUE TO ENZYME DEFICIENCY

Miscellaneous Cells

Mast Cell

SYNONYMS
tissue basophil

VITAL STATISTICS
- size .... 15-30 μm
- N:C ratio .... approximately 1:3-1:2
- cell shape .... round or elliptical
- nuclear shape .... round
- chromatin .... condensed to fine: often obscured by granules
- parachromatin .... minimal
- nucleoli .... may have small nucleoli
- cytoplasm .... abundant black, bluish-black, or reddish-purple granules

KEY DIFFERENTIATING FEATURES
- round nuclear shape
- abundant basophilic granules that obscure the nuclear border

OTHER FINDINGS
- malignant forms may exhibit an irregular, elongated spindle shape with cytoplasmic extensions, nuclear atypia and degranulation
- systemic mast cell disease shows focal bone marrow lesions, frequently perivascular or paratrabecular
- systemic mast cell disease can be associated with a fibrotic marrow background, with osteoporosis or osteosclerosis, or with a myeloproliferative or myelodysplastic process in uninvolved marrow

POTENTIAL LOOK-ALIKES
- basophil
- promyelocyte
- hypergranular promyelocyte
- neutrophil with toxic granulation
- macrophage (histiocyte)
- sea blue histiocyte
- fibroblast

ASSOCIATED DISEASE STATES AND CONDITIONS
- systemic mastocytosis
- mastocytic leukemia
- non-Hodgkin's lymphomas
- myelodysplastic syndromes
- myeloproliferative syndromes
- aplastic anemia
- osteoporosis
- chronic liver disease
- bone marrow fibrosis
- toxic marrow damage
- marrow irradiation
- post-chemotherapy

The mast cell (tissue basophil) is a large (15-30 μm) round or elliptical connective tissue cell with a small, round nucleus and abundant cytoplasm packed with black, bluish-black, or reddish-purple metachromatic granules. Its relationship to circulating basophils or their precursors is unclear. Mast cells are distinguished from blood basophils by the fact that they are larger, (often twice the size of blood basophils), have more abundant cytoplasm, and have round rather than segmented nuclei. The cytoplasmic granules are smaller, more numerous, more variable in appearance, and less water extractable than basophil cytoplasmic granules. Although both mast cells and basophils are primarily involved in allergic and anaphylactic reactions through degranulation, the content of their granules is not identical. Both mast cell and basophil granules can be differentiated from neutrophilic granules by positive staining with toluidine blue in the former. In addition, mast cell granules stain positive for chloracetate esterase, while basophil granules contain peroxidase.

Systemic mast cell disease, best appreciated in the bone marrow biopsy, usually shows focal marrow lesions, frequently perivascular or paratrabecular. The aggregates of mast cells often are accompanied by eosinophils and can be associated with prominent lymphoid aggregates, with marrow fibrosis, or with osteoporosis or osteosclerosis. In some cases, the uninvolved marrow is hypercellular with a concomitant myeloproliferative or myelodysplastic process. Cytologically, the malignant mast cell may exhibit an irregular, elongated spindle shape with cytoplasmic extensions, nuclear atypia, and degranulation. Diffuse infiltration of the marrow by malignant mast cells is less frequently observed and may be associated with mast cell leukemia.

Mast Cell

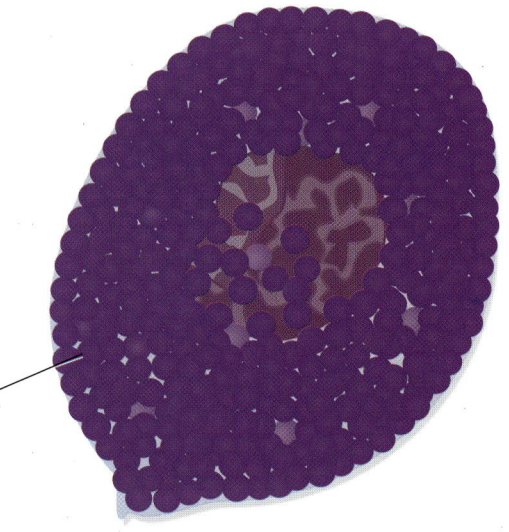

basophilic granules obscuring nuclear border

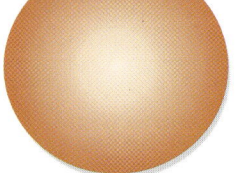

|← 7 μm →|
size of normal red blood cell

H-9, 1977 (Bone Marrow, Wright-Giemsa, X400)

Identification	Referee %	Participant %
Mast cell	100	89.3

Note the round nucleus and abundant purple-black cytoplasmic granules in this mast cell. The granules extend out to the edge of the cytoplasm obscuring the cytoplasmic border. The nuclear rim is also partially obscured and a few granules overlay the nucleus.

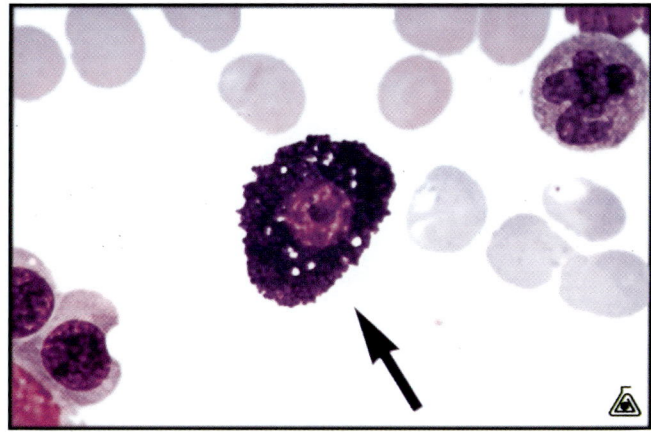

H-12, 1979 (Bone Marrow, Wright-Giemsa, X400)

Identification	Referee %	Participant %
Mast cell	88.9	78.7
Basophil or precursor	-	17.2

This is from a case of myelodysplastic syndrome. The large mast cell in the center of the field exhibits numerous purple-black granules which partially obscure the round nucleus; the cytoplasmic border is indistinct. In contrast, a basophil typically would be a smaller size cell with a segmented or "polywog-shape" rather than round nucleus, and would exhibit a lower nuclear to cytoplasmic ratio. Mast cells may occasionally be found in the peripheral blood in chronic myeloproliferative disorders.

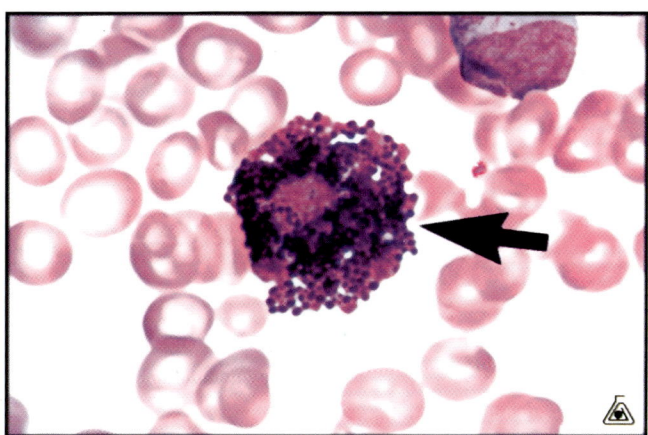

H1-43, 1987 (Bone Marrow, Wright-Giemsa, X400)

Identification	Referee %	Participant %
Mast cell	100	84.8

The large mast cell in the field has such an abundance of reddish purple granules that it is hard to discern individual granule structure. The border of the round nucleus is partially obscured by the granules. Note the excess of small, mature lymphocytes in this bone marrow aspirate, with hypercondensed nuclear chromatin. The patient has a diagnosis of small lymphocytic lymphoma.

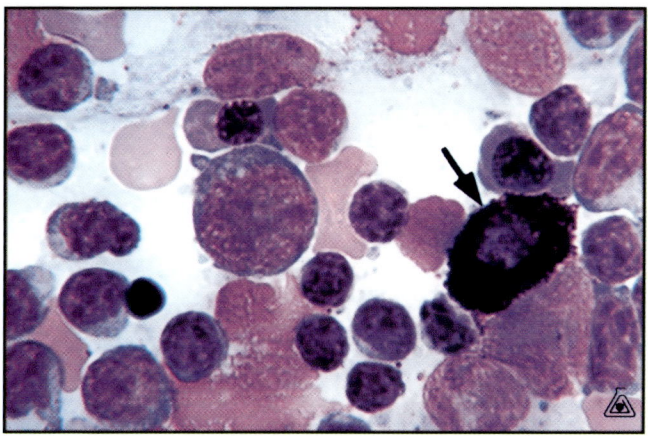

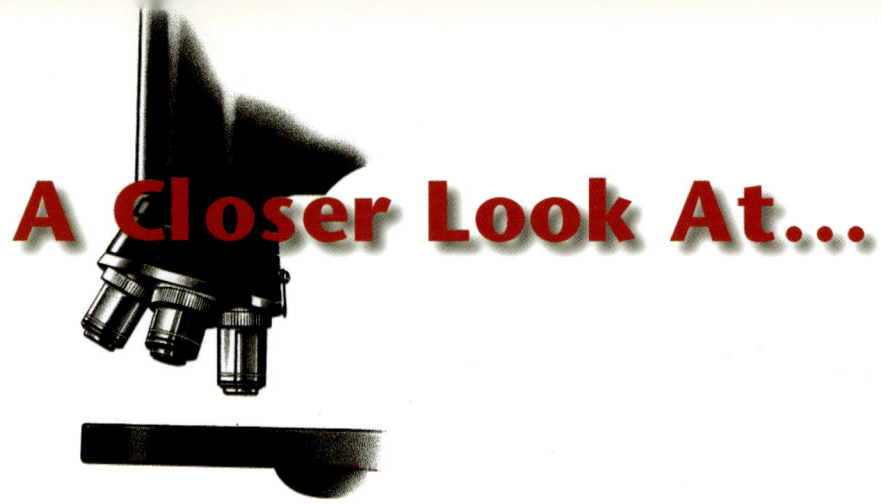

A Closer Look At...

Mast Cells vs. Basophils

The table below and the illustration on the next page highlight the important morphologic differences between mast cells and basophils. See page 28 for a more detailed discussion of basophils.

	MAST CELL	BASOPHIL
size	15-30 μm	10-15 μm
nuclear shape	round	segmented, "polywog-shaped" in mature form; round in immature forms
cytoplasm	abundant	moderate amount
metachromatic granules	numerous, evenly distributed, obscure nucleus and cytoplasmic border, insoluble	less plentiful, unevenly distributed, obscure nucleus, often extracted with staining
cytochemistry	chloracetate esterase positive	peroxidase positive
location	bone marrow; (rarely blood)	blood or bone marrow

Comparison of Mast Cells and Basophils

Mast Cell

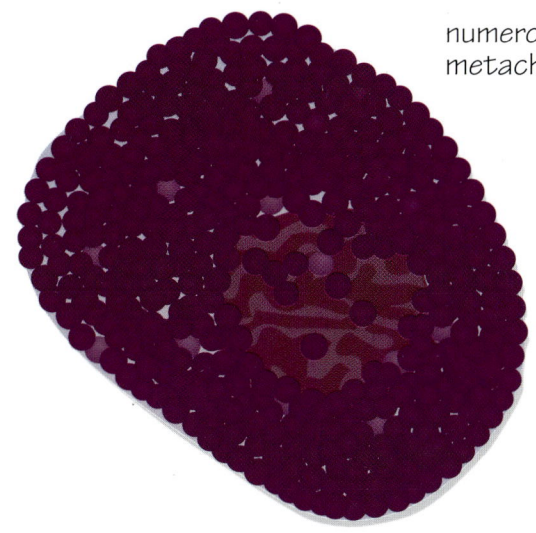

numerous, evenly distributed metachromatic granules

granules insoluble; even staining

granules obscure cytoplasmic border and nucleus

nucleus round

normally found in bone marrow and tissues; circulates in leukemic variant and rarely in chronic myeloproliferative disorders

Basophil

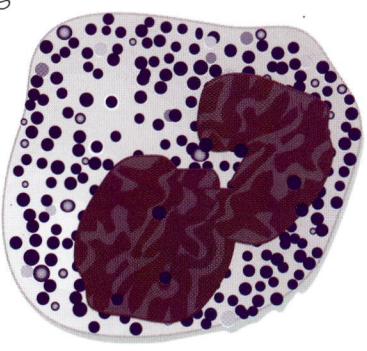

less abundant, unevenly distrubuted metachromatic granules

granules soluble with staining; some are pale

nucleus segmented in mature cells, round in earlier stages

normally found in bone marrow and blood; increased numbers in myeloproliferative conditions

Metastatic Tumor Cell

SYNONYMS
cancer cell, carcinoma

VITAL STATISTICS
- size .... large, polymorphous, varies from 15-100 μm
- N:C ratio .... variable, 7:1 to 1:5
- cell shape .... pleomorphic, round to spindle
- nuclear shape .... round or elongated to pleomorphic, may contain multiple nuclei
- chromatin .... usually finely reticulated
- parachromatin .... minimal to prominent
- nucleoli .... may be multiple, large
- cytoplasm .... variable, may be intensely basophilic, granular, finely vacuolated, frayed; may contain bluish cytoplasmic debris; large vacuoles in adenocarcinoma; keratin formation in squamous carcinoma

KEY DIFFERENTIATING FEATURES
- clusters of large pleomorphic cells (blast-like or with abundant cytoplasm)
- usually form cohesive sheets or 3-dimensional (ball-like) cell aggregates
- fine nuclear chromatin
- irregular nuclear shape
- prominent nucleoli
- multiple pleomorphic nuclei

OTHER FINDINGS
- often clump together, with lack of individual cell boundaries
- concentrated at the periphery of the bone marrow aspirate smear
- many mitotic cells
- many autolytic cells
- detected primarily in the bone marrow biopsy
- may organize into glandular or rosette structures
- associated with fibrosis or necrosis (may result in "dry tap")
- adjacent inflammatory response (macrophages, lymphocytes, plasma cells)
- leukoerythroblastic reaction in blood

POTENTIAL LOOK-ALIKES
- blasts (particularly small round tumors, e.g., oat cell carcinoma, neuroblastoma, retinoblastoma, rhabdomyosarcoma, Ewing's sarcoma)
- lymphoma cell
- mast cell (systemic mastocytosis)
- megakaryocyte or precursor, normal or abnormal
- macrophage (histiocyte)
- osteoblast
- osteoclast
- lipocyte
- epithelial/endothelial cell

ASSOCIATED DISEASE STATES AND CONDITIONS
non-hematopoietic malignancies

Metastatic tumor cells are larger than most bone marrow cells, except megakaryocytes, varying from approximately 15 μm to 100 μm in diameter with a highly variable nuclear to cytoplasmic ratio (7:1 to 1:5). They frequently adhere in tight clusters, forming syncytial sheets or mulberry-like aggregates ("morulae"), best detected in the periphery of the aspirate smear. Within a given sample, the tumor cells often are polymorphous, varying in cell size and shape. Likewise, nuclei are round, spindle-shaped, or pleomorphic; multiple nuclei of unequal size and shape may be present. The nuclear chromatin usually is finely reticulated, often with prominent parachromatin spaces; one or more large nucleoli may be seen. Rapidly proliferating tumors can show many mitotic forms and many small autolytic cells with nuclear pyknosis or karyorrhexis. The amount of cytoplasm is variable, scant in small cell tumors (e.g. oat cell carcinoma, neuroblastoma, retinoblastoma, rhabdomyosarcoma, Ewing's sarcoma) and plentiful in others, particularly adenocarcinoma. The cytoplasm may be intensely basophilic and may contain granules or fine vacuoles, bluish cytoplasmic debris, or large vacuoles (especially adenocarcinoma). The cytoplasm often appears frayed on the aspirate smear, due to pulling apart of cohesive tumor cells. Keratin formation may be apparent in squamous carcinoma. It imparts a robin's egg blue color to the cytoplasm.

Non-hematopoietic malignant cells frequently are inaspirable ("dry tap"); thus biopsy sections are preferred for the detection of metastatic tumors. In addition, the organization of tumor cells into glandular or rosette structures and tumor-associated fibrosis may not be detected in marrow smears. In the bone marrow biopsy, an inflammatory response (macrophages, lymphocytes, and plasma cells) may be seen adjacent to the metastatic site. Nests or cords of tumor cells may be trapped and compressed within dense fibrous tissue, making it difficult to discern cytological features. Cytochemistry and immunohistochemistry are useful in distinguishing metastatic neoplasia from hematopoietic malignancy and in determining tumor origin. The presence of a leukoerythroblastic reaction (i.e. immature neutrophils plus nucleated red cells) in the blood is associated with involvement of bone marrow with metastatic tumor. In very rare cases, the tumor cells may be found circulating in the peripheral blood.

H1-11, 1977 (Bone Marrow, Wright-Giemsa, X313)

Identification	Referee %	Participant %
Metastatic tumor cell	90	76.6
Blast cell	-	11.3

This patient had metastatic carcinoma to the bone marrow. The primary was unknown. The large tumor cells are heaped upon each other, forming a compact aggregate; it is impossible to discern where the cytoplasm of one cell stops and another cell begins. The nuclei have finely reticulated, blast-like chromatin and prominent parachromatin spaces; multiple nucleoli are visible in some of the nuclei. Although many participants identified these cells as "blast cells," it is unlikely that hematopoietic blasts would tightly adhere in a large cluster.

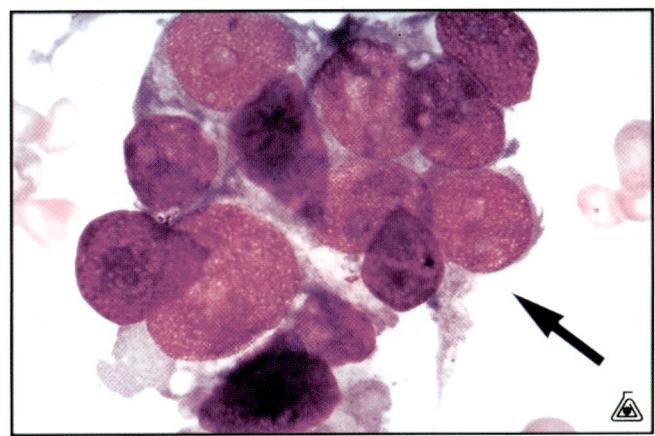

Group of Metastatic Carcinoma Cells

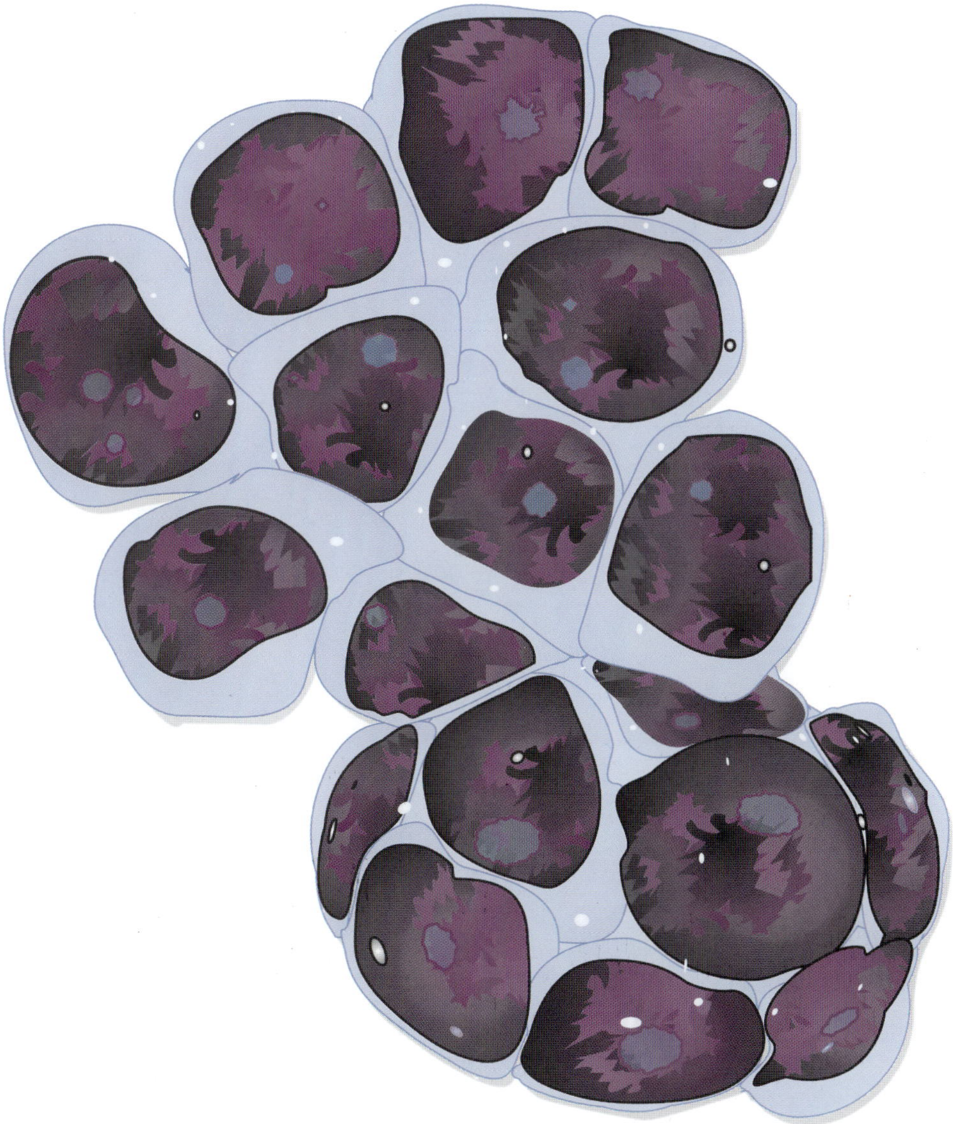

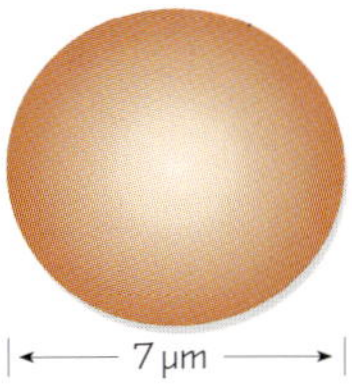

Miscellaneous Cells

Mitotic Figure

SYNONYMS
dividing cell

VITAL STATISTICS
- size .... variable
- N:C ratio .... variable
- cell shape .... variable
- nuclear shape .... irregular; separates in two in anaphase and telophase
- chromatin .... dense; individual chromosomes may be visible
- parachromatin .... not visible
- nucleoli .... none seen
- cytoplasm .... characteristic of resting cell

KEY DIFFERENTIATING FEATURES
- dense, irregularly-shaped nucleus
- nucleus often has a clear central zone
- chromosomal strands may be visible

OTHER FINDINGS
- two daughter cells are apparent in anaphase and telophase
- only a small number are seen in normal marrow aspirates

POTENTIAL LOOK-ALIKES
- neutrophil necrobiosis (degenerated neutrophil)
- basket cell/smudge cell (degenerated leukocyte)
- lymphocyte
- metastatic tumor cell

ASSOCIATED DISEASE STATES AND CONDITIONS
- acute leukemias
- myeloproliferative syndromes
- myelodysplastic syndromes
- lymphoma
- metastatic tumor
- regenerating marrow
- hemolytic anemia
- megaloblastic anemia (particularly after treatment)
- reactive lymphocytosis (marrow)

A cell containing a mitotic figure is variable in size; it may or may not be larger than the surrounding cells. The cytoplasm has color and granulation characteristic of the resting cell. When a cell undergoes mitosis, typical nuclear features no longer are present. Instead, the nucleus appears as a dark, irregular mass, often with a clear central zone. It may take various shapes, including a daisy-like form or a mass with irregular projections. In metaphase, the individual chromosomes become visible; arranged equatorially, they begin to separate and to move toward opposite poles. Rarely, the anaphase or telophase of mitosis may be seen, with two separating masses of chromosomes forming two daughter cells. A mitotic cell can be distinguished from a degenerating cell by a relatively compact nucleus (or nuclei); a degenerating cell often displays a pyknotic nucleus which has been fragmented into numerous purple, roundish inclusions. Although the bone marrow is normally a rapidly dividing tissue, only small numbers of mitotic cells are found in normal marrow aspirates. Mitotic cells are rarely seen in the blood smear, associated with hematopoietic malignancy.

Cells In Various Stages of Mitosis

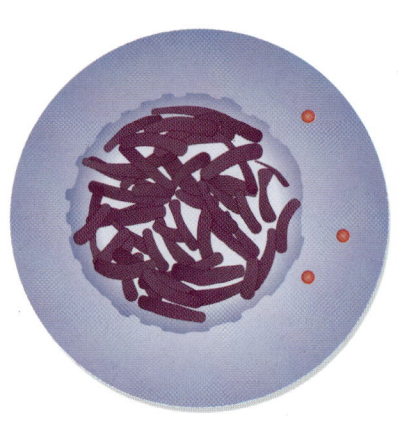
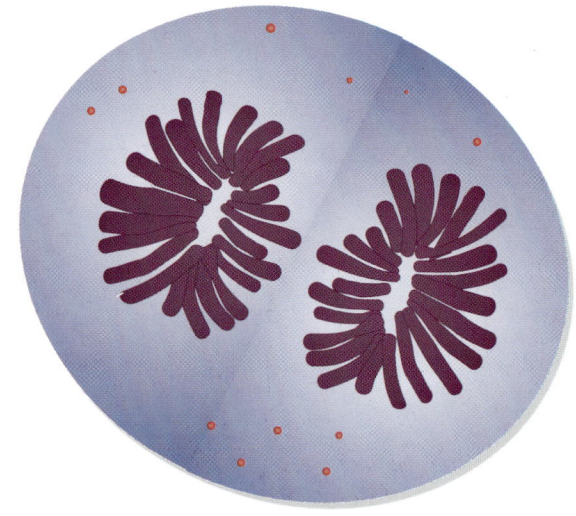

H1-19, 1987 (Bone Marrow, Wright-Giemsa, X250)

Identification	Referee %	Participant %
Mitotic figure	100	91.1

In this case of partially treated megaloblastic anemia, a mitotic cell in metaphase is arrowed. Individual chromosomes are visible, which have begun to separate to opposite sides of the cell. Note the giant band neutrophil located in the center of the photomicrograph.

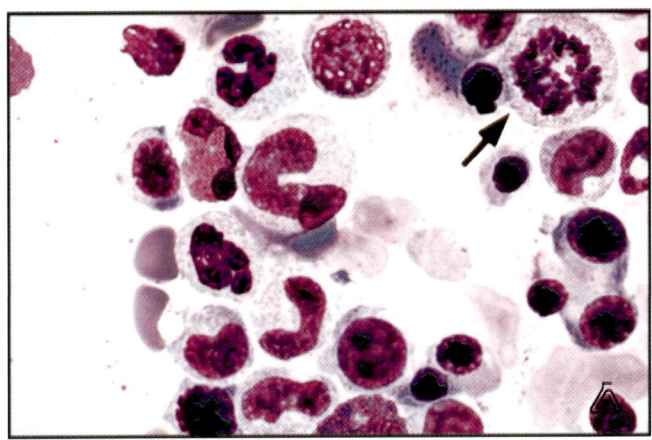

HE-13, 1991 (Bone Marrow, Wright-Giemsa, X400)

Identification	Referee %	Participant %
Mitotic figure	94.7	87.2
Myelocyte, dysplastic	5.3	3.5
Myelocyte	-	1.5
Promyelocyte	-	1.5

A mitotic cell in late telophase is arrowed. The chromosomes have coalesced into irregularly-shaped, dense masses with a clear central area and cytoplasmic partition between the two daughter cells has begun. The abundant cytoplasmic azurophilic granulation identifies this cell as a member of the neutrophil series, most likely a promyelocyte. The patient had a diagnosis of myelodysplastic syndrome (refractory anemia with excess of blasts).

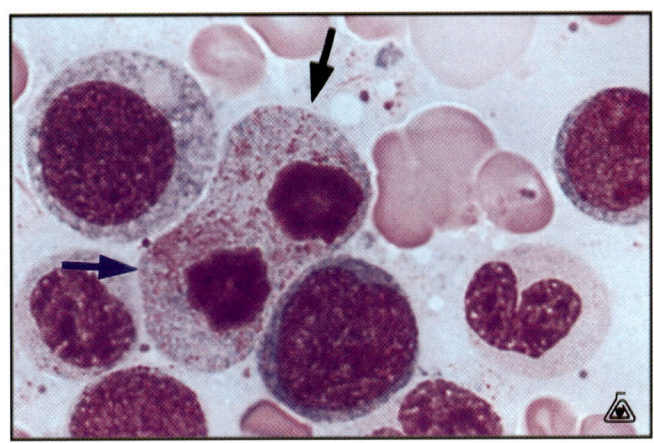

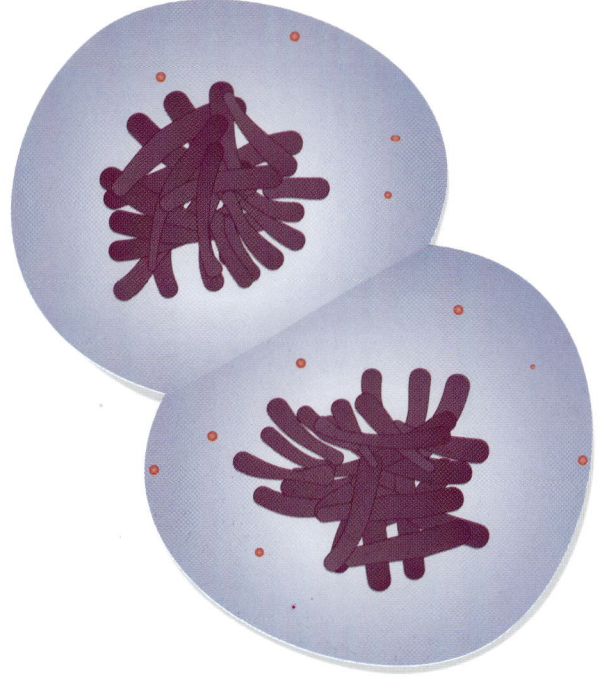

Miscellaneous Cells

Osteoblast

SYNONYMS
none

VITAL STATISTICS
- size .... 20-50 µm
- N:C ratio .... approximately 1:5
- cell shape .... ellipsoid
- nuclear shape .... round to oval
- chromatin .... reticular, fenestrated
- parachromatin .... small parachromatin spaces
- nucleoli .... one or more
- cytoplasm .... abundant, blue-gray; prominent Golgi clear zone away from nucleus (not paranuclear); border may be indistinct

KEY DIFFERENTIATING FEATURES
- ellipsoidal shape with clear Golgi zone a short distance from (rather than next to) the nucleus
- indistinct cytoplasmic border
- reticular, fenestrated nuclear chromatin with one or more nucleoli
- nucleus may be partially extruded from the cell

OTHER FINDINGS
- often occur in clusters
- located along bone trabeculae

POTENTIAL LOOK-ALIKES
- plasma cell
- metastatic tumor cell

ASSOCIATED DISEASE STATES AND CONDITIONS
- prominent in growing children
- bone marrow remodeling (prior injury)

The osteoblast is a bone-forming cell, producing bone matrix (osteoid), which becomes lamellar bone when mineralized. It is large (25 to 50 µm in diameter), often ellipsoid, and contains a round or ovoid nucleus with one or more nucleoli. The nucleus may be partially extruded from the cell. The cytoplasm is abundant, stains blue-gray, and may have an indistinct, streaming border. A prominent clear zone which represents the Golgi apparatus (called the *Hof*) is usually evident a small distance away from the nucleus. Osteoblasts often occur in clusters in the marrow of growing children; small numbers may be seen in adult specimens. In bone marrow biopsies, they often are located along the margins of the bone trabeculae.

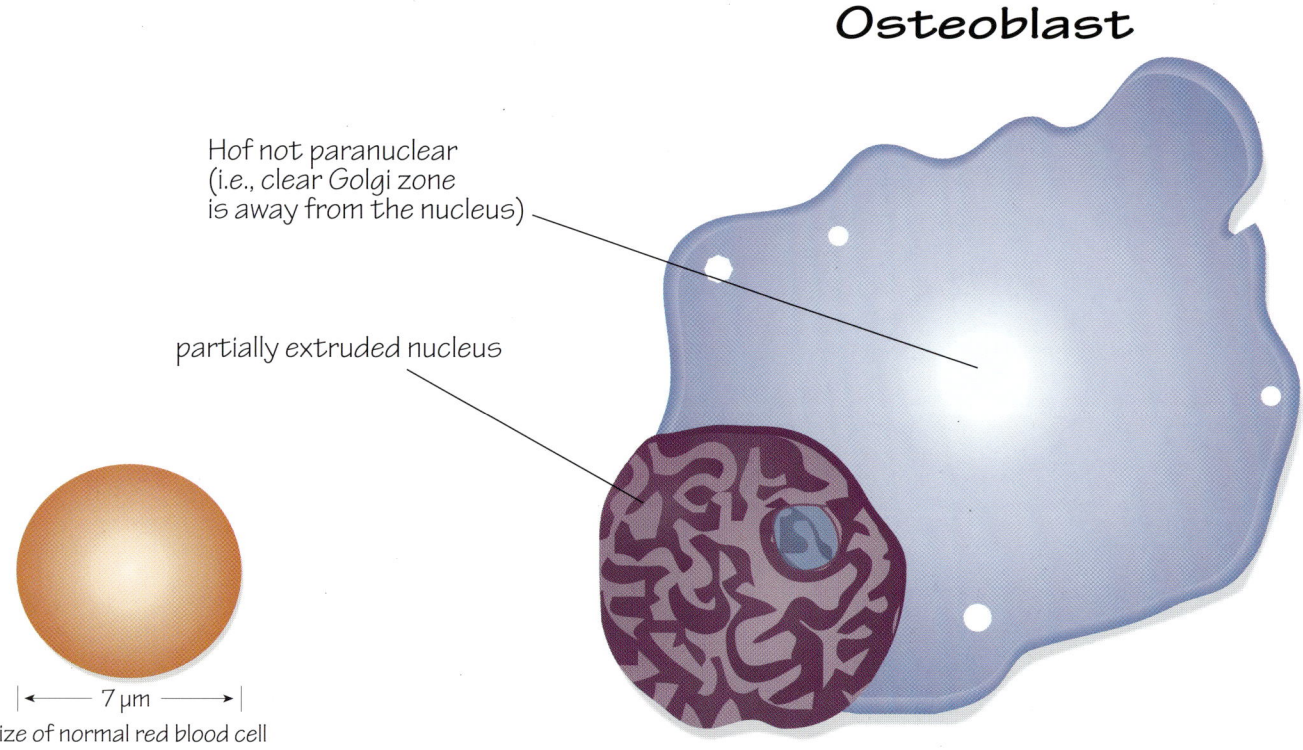

Osteoblast

- Hof not paranuclear (i.e., clear Golgi zone is away from the nucleus)
- partially extruded nucleus

7 µm
size of normal red blood cell

H-26, 1979 (Bone Marrow, Wright-Giemsa, X250)

Identification	Referee %	Participant %
Osteoblast	88.9	77.2
Plasma cell	11.1	5.5

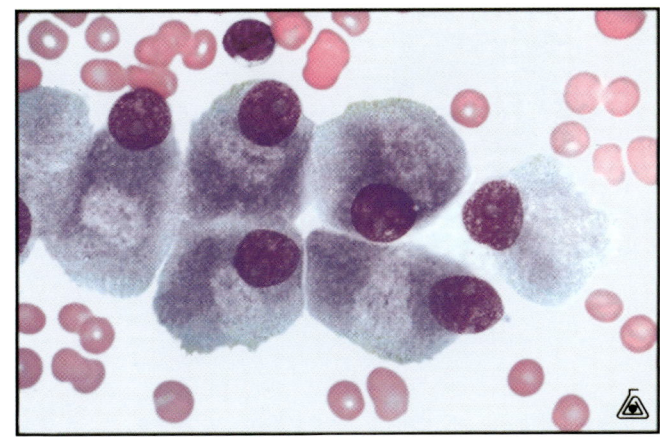

A cluster of osteoblasts is seen in this photomicrograph. The most common alternative choice was "plasma cell." However, these osteoblasts differ from plasma cells by their large size, copious cytoplasm with indistinct cytoplasmic border, and Golgi zone away from the nucleus, with cytoplasm intervening in between. Some of the nuclei appear to be extruded from the cells. In contrast, mature plasma cells show condensed, ropey nuclear chromatin and a paranuclear Golgi zone; however, immature plasma cells in myeloma may show less condensed nuclear chromatin and nucleoli similar to these osteoblasts.

H1-5, 1988 (Bone Marrow, Wright-Giemsa, X325)

Identification	Referee %	Participant %
Osteoblast	82.4	65.4
Plasma cell, normal	11.8	27.6
Metastatic tumor cell	5.9	0.7

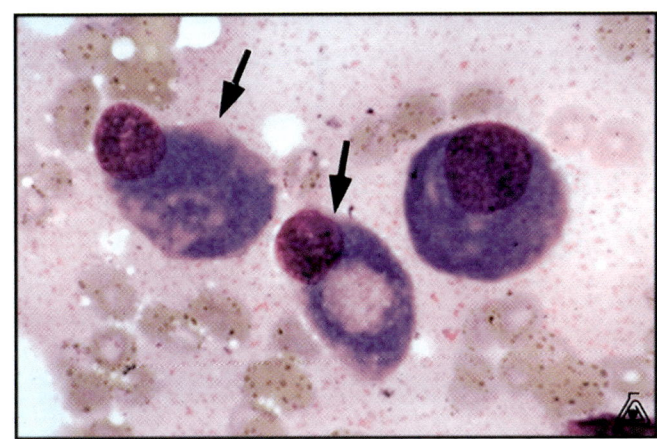

The case is from a patient with metastatic carcinoma to the bone marrow. The biopsy showed extreme fibrosis, bone destruction, and new bone formation. The two arrowed cells are osteoblasts. Their nuclei are "extruded" and appear to extend out of the boundary of the cytoplasm. The clear space representing the Golgi apparatus (hof) is at some distance from the nucleus, in contrast to plasma cells. Metastatic tumor was present in other areas of the bone marrow. The osteoclasts are indicative of new bone formation in response to the malignancy.

HE-27, 1997 (Bone Marrow, Wright-Giemsa, X250)

Identification	Referee %	Participant %
Osteoblast	82.1	80.6
Plasma cell, mature	10.7	4.8
Plasma cell, immature	7.1	8.1

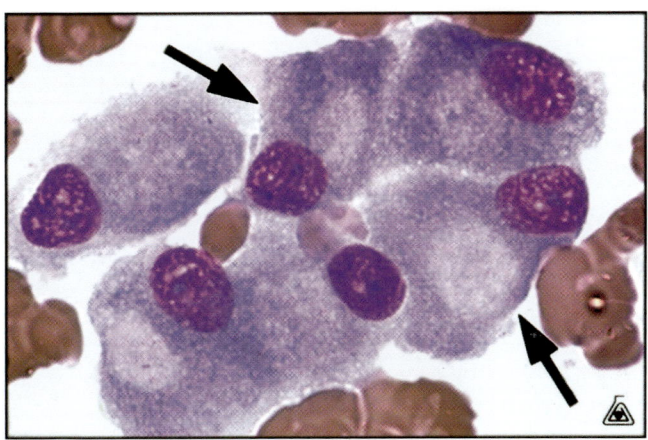

The arrowed cells are osteoblasts. Such cells are involved in bone formation. They are sometimes present in aspirates of bone marrow or touch preparations of trephine biopsies from bone marrow. They are large cells with round or oval nuclei and abundant blue-gray cytoplasm. A prominent clear area (*hof*) which represents the Golgi zone is often present in the cytoplasm away from the nucleus. The nuclei are usually eccentrically placed and may have the appearance that they are "falling off the cell." Osteoblasts may be difficult to differentiate from plasma cells, but plasma cells are usually smaller, the nuclear chromatin pattern more condensed, and the cytoplasm a deeper blue. The hof in plasma cells is located next to the nucleus.

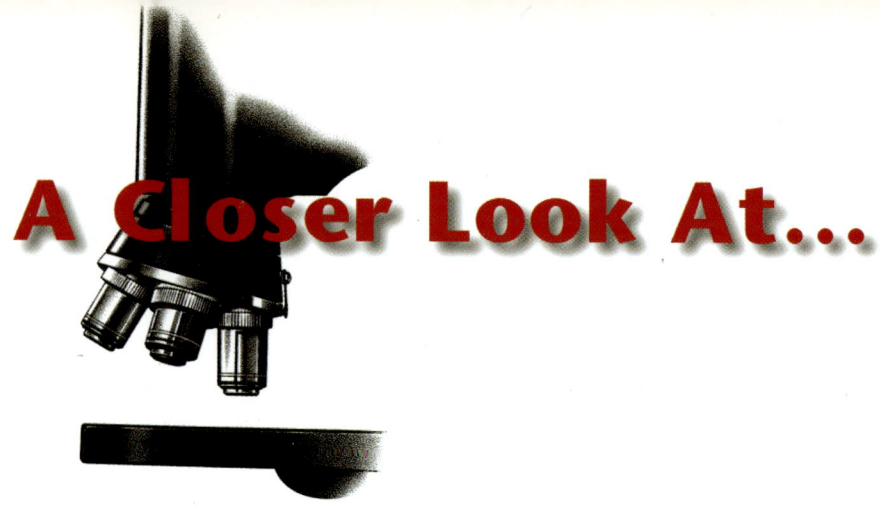

A Closer Look At...

Osteoblast vs. Plasma Cell

The table below and the illustration on the next page highlight the important morphologic differences between osteoblasts and plasma cells. See page 238 for a more detailed discussion of plasma cells.

	Osteoblast	Plasma Cell
size	20-50 μm	10-20 μm
cell shape	ellipsoid	round to oval
nucleus	round to oval; eccentrically placed; partially extruded or projecting from cytoplasm	round to oval; eccentrically placed; may be bi-nucleate; contour confined to cytoplasm
nuclear chromatin	fine, reticular	coarse and ropey; clock-face condensation (with hematoxylin/eosin stain); may be less condensed in immature forms
nucleoli	one or more	none (mature); one or more (immature)
cytoplasm	lightly basophilic	intensely basophilic; occasionally may be pink-red (flame cell)
cytoplasmic border	indistinct	distinct
Golgi clear zone	away from nucleus	paranuclear
cytoplasmic inclusions	none	may contain immunoglobulin globules or crystals
location in bone marrow	margins of trabeculae; may occur in small clusters	near blood vessels; may form large clusters if malignant (multiple myeloma)

Miscellaneous Cells

Comparison of Osteoblasts and Plasma Cells

Osteoblast

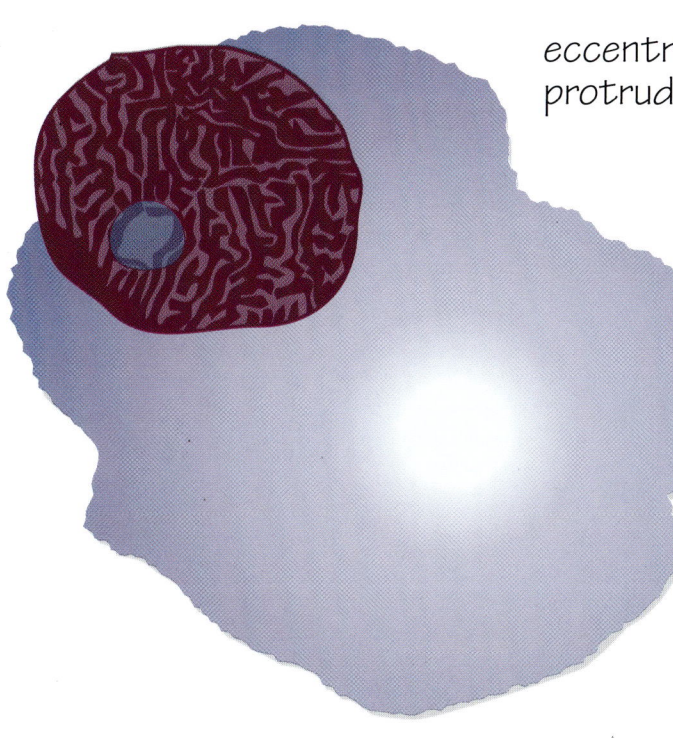

eccentric nucleus, protruding from cytoplasm

reticular fine nuclear chromatin

one or more nucleoli

Golgi clear zone away from nucleus

Plasma Cell

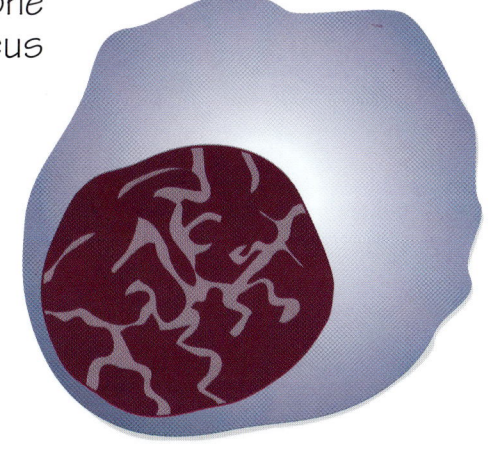

Golgi clear zone near nucleus

no nucleoli in mature cell

coarse ropey chromatin with prominent marginal condensation

eccentric nucleus that does not extend beyond cytoplasmic margin

Osteoclast

SYNONYMS
 none

VITAL STATISTICS
 size .... approximately 100 µm
 N:C ratio .... approximately 1:1
 cell shape .... oval, irregular
 nuclear shape .... round to ovoid
 chromatin .... dense or reticular
 parachromatin .... variable
 nucleoli .... one or more, small, but prominent
 cytoplasm .... blue or purple to pale pink, contains many fine reddish-purple granules

KEY DIFFERENTIATING FEATURES
 large size
 multiple, uniformly-sized, separated nuclei (even number)
 prominent nucleoli
 granular cytoplasm
 frayed cytoplasmic margins

OTHER FINDINGS
 located along bone trabeculae

POTENTIAL LOOK-ALIKES
 megakaryocyte or precursor, normal or abnormal
 metastatic tumor cell
 macrophage
 cluster of osteoblasts

ASSOCIATED DISEASE STATES AND CONDITIONS
 prominent in young children
 metastatic carcinoma
 acute leukemia
 myelofibrosis
 hyperparathyroidism
 secondary osteoporosis
 Paget's disease

Osteoclasts are involved in bone resorption, frequently located along the bone trabeculae. They are very large cells, approximately 100 µm in diameter. Though osteoclasts resemble megakaryocytes, they can be differentiated by the presence of an even number of multiple round to ovoid nuclei, relatively uniformly shaped, but widely separated. The nuclear chromatin may be dense or reticular, and each nucleus usually contains one or more small, prominent nucleoli. The cytoplasm is abundant, with frayed margins, stains blue or purple to pale pink, and contains many fine reddish-purple granules. Osteoclasts are most frequently seen in marrow samples from children or from patients with Paget's disease or hyperparathyroidism.

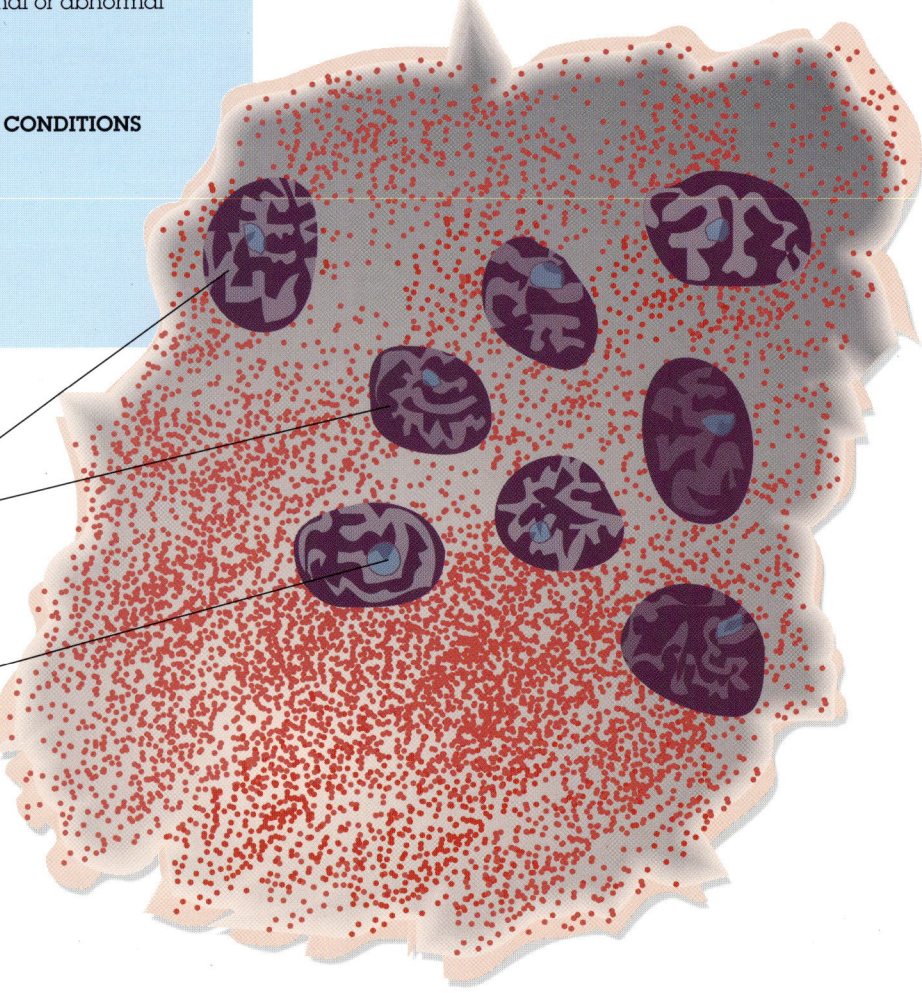

Osteoclast

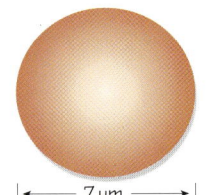

size of normal red blood cell

Miscellaneous Cells

H-41, 1979 (Bone Marrow, Wright-Giemsa, X250)

Identification	Referee %	Participant %
Osteoclast	100	91.0
Metastatic tumor cell	-	2.5
Osteoblast	-	2.4
Megakaryocyte	-	1.5

This large bone marrow osteoclast has widely separated, round to oval nuclei with reticular nuclear chromatin and prominent nucleoli. An even number of nuclei (10) are present. The pink cytoplasm has frayed margins and exhibits numerous red-purple granules.

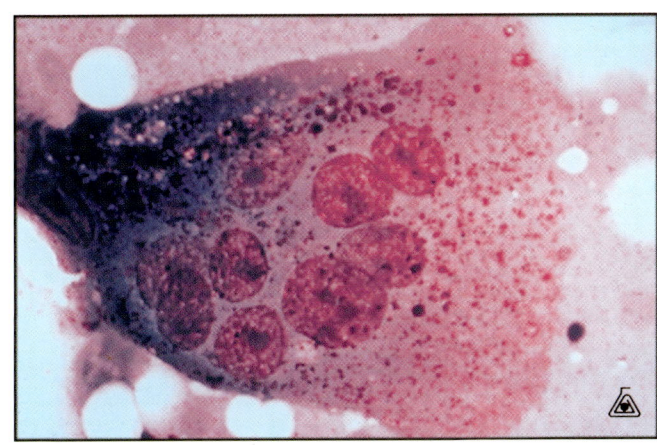

H1-4, 1988 (Bone Marrow, Wright-Giemsa, X250)

Identification	Referee %	Participant %
Osteoclast	100	91.5
Megakaryocyte	-	5.6

The biopsy of this marrow was heavily infiltrated by metastatic transitional cell carcinoma and showed fibrosis, bony destruction, and new bone formation with little normal hematopoietic tissue. The gigantic osteoclast in this photomicrograph is multinucleate, with widely-separated, uniform nuclei containing small nucleoli, and reticulated chromatin. Seventeen nuclei are visible, appearing to violate the rule that osteoclasts have an even number of nuclei (perhaps the adjacent uninucleate "cell" with granulated blue cytoplasm represents a fragment of the osteoclast). The cytoplasm is blue and shows the red-purple granulation and frayed margins characteristic of this cell. In contrast to the two osteoclasts seen in these photomicrographs, megakaryocytes have overlapping and connected nuclear lobes with dense nuclear chromatin.

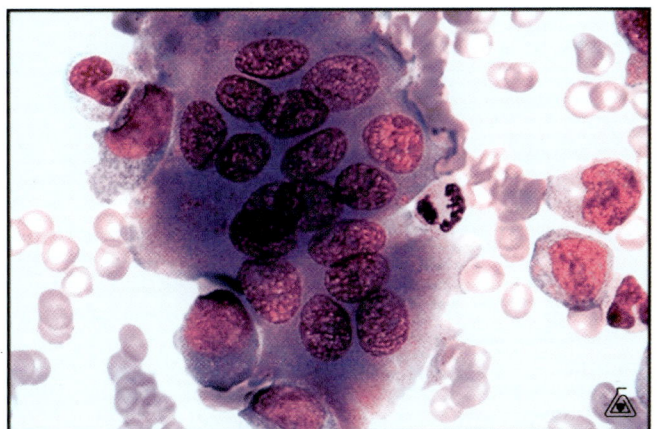

HE-28, 1997 (Bone Marrow, Wright-Giemsa, X250)

Identification	Referee %	Participant %
Osteoclast	92.0	90.8
Megakaryocyte or precursor, normal	7.1	3.7
Megakaryocyte or precursor, normal	-	1.5

The arrowed cell is an osteoclast. These cells are very large and have multiple, separate round or oval nuclei of uniform size. The nuclear chromatin is condensed. One or more nucleoli are clearly visible. The cytoplasm is abundant, blue to purple in color and contains reddish-purple granules. Osteoclasts are normal cells that are involved in bone resorption. Morphologically, they closely resemble megakaryocytes but megakaryocytes possess nuclei with multiple overlapping lobes. Nucleoli are absent except in immature cells. Megkaryocyte cytoplasm is granular but the granules are usually smaller and more uniform in appearance than in osteoclasts.

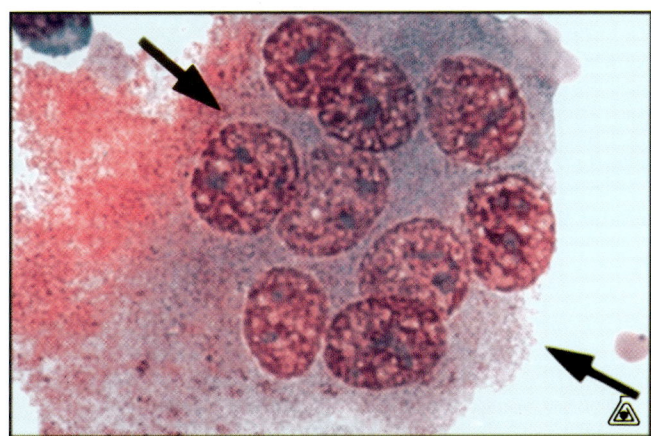

Miscellaneous Cells

Appendix A
Selected References

General Textbooks

Aycock S, Bick RL, Drennan CL, McRoyan CD. In: Powers LW, ed. *Diagnostic Hematology*. St. Louis: CV Mosby; 1989.

Babior BM, Stossel TP. *Hematology: A Pathophysiologic Approach*. 3rd ed. New York: Churchill Livingstone; 1994.

Bain BJ. *Blood Cells. A Practical Guide*. Philadelphia: JB Lippincott Company; 1989.

Begemann H, Rastetter J. *Atlas of Clinical Hematology*. 3rd ed. New York: Springer-Verlag; 1979.

Bessis M. *Blood Smears Reinterpreted*. New York: Springer-Verlag; 1976.

Bessis M. *Living Blood Cells and Their Ultrastructure*. New York: Springer-Verlag; 1973.

Beutler E, Lichtman MA, Coller BS, Kipps TJ, eds. *Williams Hematology*. 5th ed. New York: McGraw-Hill Inc; 1995.

Bick RL, Bennett JM, Brynes RK, et al, eds. *Hematology: Clinical and Laboratory Practice*. St. Louis: Mosby-Year Book, Inc; 1993.

Brücher H. *Bone Marrow Diagnosis in Clinical Practice*. Baltimore: John Hopkins University Press; 1989.

Diggs LW, Sturm D, Bell A. *The Morphology of Human Blood Cells*. 5th ed. Abbott Park, Ill: Abbott Laboratories; 1985.

Foucar K. *Bone Marrow Pathology*. Chicago: ASCP Press; 1995.

Harmening DM, ed. *Clinical Hematology and Fundamentals of Hemostasis*. 2nd ed. Philadelphia: FA Davis Company; 1992.

Hathaway WE, Goodnight SH Jr. *Disorders of Hemostasis and Thrombosis. A Clinical Guide*. New York: McGraw-Hill, Inc; 1993.

Heckner F, Lehmann HP, Kao YS. *Practical Microscopic Hematology*. 3rd ed. Baltimore: Urban & Schwarzenberg; 1988.

Henry JB, ed. *Clinical Diagnosis and Management by Laboratory Methods*. 19th ed. Philadelphia: WB Saunders Co; 1996.

Hoffman R, Benz EJ, Shatill SJ, et al. *Hematology; Basic Principles and Practice*. New York: Churchill Livingstone; 1995.

Hoffrand VA, Pettit, JE. *Color Atlas of Clinical Hematology*. 2nd ed. Boston: Mosby-Wolfe; 1994.

Hoffrand VA, Pettit JE. *Sandoz Atlas—Clinical Hematology*. London: Gower Medical Publishing; 1988.

Hyun BH, Gulati GL, Ashton JK. *Color Atlas of Clinical Hematology*. New York: Igaku-Shoin; 1986.

Jandl JH. *Blood: Textbook of Hematology*. 2nd ed. Boston: Little, Brown and Company; 1996.

Kapff CT, Jandl JH. *Blood: Atlas and Sourcebook of Hematology*. 2nd ed. Boston: Little, Brown and Company; 1991.

Kjeldsberg C, ed. *Practical Diagnosis of Hematologic Disorders*. Chicago: ASCP Press; 1989.

Koepke JA, ed. *Practical Laboratory Hematology*. New York: Churchill Livingstone; 1991.

Krause JR. *Bone Marrow Biopsy*. New York: Churchill Livingstone; 1981.

Lee GR, Bithell TC, Foerster J, et al, eds. *Wintrobe's Clinical Hematology*. 9th ed. Philadelphia: Lea & Febiger; 1993.

Li CY, Yam LT, Sun T. *Modern Modalities for the Diagnosis of Hematologic Neoplasms*. New York: Igaku-Shoin; 1996.

Lotspeich-Steininger CA, Stiene-Martin EA, Koepke JA, eds. *Clinical Hematology*. Philadelphia: JB Lippincott Company; 1992.

McDonald GA, Paul J, Cruickshank B. *Atlas of Haematology*. 5th ed. Edinburgh: Churchill Livingstone; 1988.

McKenzie, S. *Textbook of Hematology*. 2nd ed. Baltimore: William and Wilkins; 1996.

Miale, JB. *Laboratory Medicine—Hematology*. St. Louis: CV Mosby; 1982.

Mufti GJ, Flandrin G, Schaefer HE, Sandberg AA. *An Atlas of Malignant Haematology. Cytology, Histology, and Cytogenetics*. London: Lipppincott-Raven; 1996.

Naeim F. *Pathology of Bone Marrow*. New York: Igaku-Shoin Medical Publishers; 1992.

Nathan DG, Oski FA, eds. *Hematology of Infancy and Childhood*. 4th ed. Philadelphia: WB Saunders Company; 1993.

Nomura T, Furusawa S. *Essentials of Microscopic Hematology*. New York: Igaku-Shoin Medical Publishers; 1991.

O'Connor BH. *A Color Atlas and Instructional Manual of Peripheral Blood Cell Morphology*. Baltimore: Williams and Wilkins; 1984.

Rapaport SI. *Introduction to Hematology*. New York: Harper & Row; 1971.

Schumacher HR, Nand S. *Myelodysplastic Syndromes. Approach to Diagnosis and Treatment*. New York: Igaku-Shoin Medical Publishers; 1995.

Smith H. *Diagnosis in Paediatric Haematology*. New York: Churchill Livingstone; 1996.

Sun NCJ. *Hematology. An Atlas and Diagnostic Guide*. Philadelphia: WB Saunders Company; 1983.

Wiernik PH, Canellos GP, Kyle R, et al. *Neoplastic Diseases of the Blood*. 2nd ed. New York: Churchill Livingstone Inc; 1991.

Zucker-Franklin D, Greaves MF, Grossi CE, et al. *Atlas of Blood Cells. Function and Pathology*. Philadelphia: Lea and Febiger; 1981.

Granulocytic (Myeloid) Cells

Altman AJ. Cytologic diagnosis of the acute nonlymphocytic leukemias. *Am J Pediat Hemat Oncol*. 1985;7:21-44.

Bainton DF. Morphology of neutrophils and neutrophil precursors. In: Williams WJ, Beutler E, Erslev AJ, Lichtman MA, eds. *Hematology*. 4th ed. New York: McGraw-Hill; 1990:760-769.

Boggs DR, Winklestein A. *White Cell Manual*. 4th ed. Philadelphia: FA Davis; 1983.

Creutzig U, Cantu-Rajnoldi A, Ritter J, et al. Myelodysplastic syndrome in childhood. *Am J Ped Hemat Oncol*. 1989;9:324-330.

Emerson SG, Farnen JP. Hematopoiesis and the hematopoietic growth factors. In: McClatchey KD, ed. *Clinical Laboratory Medicine*. Baltimore: William and Wilkins; 1994.

Hoagland HC. Myelodysplastic (preleukemic) syndromes—the bone marrow refractory failure problem. *Mayo Clin Proc*. 1995;70:673-677.

Hyun BH, Gulati GL, Ashton JK. Hematopoiesis and blood cell morphology. In: *Laboratory Medicine. Test Selection and Interpretation*. Howanitz JH, Howanitz PJ, eds. New York: Churchill-Livingston, 1991.

Lasser A. The mononuclear phagocyte system—a review. *Hum Pathol*. 1983;14:108-126.

McKenna RW, Allison PM. Diagnosis, classification and course of myelodysplastic syndromes. *Clin Lab Med*. 1990;10:638-706.

Neame PB, Soamboonsrup P, Quigley JG, et al. The use of monoclonal antibodies and immune markers in the diagnosis, prognosis and therapy of acute leukemia. *Trans Med Rev*. 1994;8:59–75.

Peterson L, Hrisinko MA. Benign lymphocytosis and reactive neutrophilia. *Clin Lab Hemat*. 1993;13:863-877.

Erythrocytic Cells and Inclusions
Bell RE. The origin of "burr" erythrocytes. *Brit J Haemat.* 1963;9:552-555.

Borges A, Desforges JF. Studies of Heinz body formation. *Acta Haematol (Basel).* 1967;37:1-10.

Fujita T, Kashimura M, Adachi K. Scanning electron microscopy (SEM) studies of the spleen—normal and pathological. *Scanning Electron Microsc.* 1982;I:435-444.

LoBuglio AF, Cotran RS, Jandl JH. Red cells coated with immunoglobulin G: binding and sphering by mononuclear cells in man. *Science.* 1967;158:1582-1585.

Nathan DG. Thalassemia. *N Engl J Med.* 1972;286(11):586-594.

Rose WF, de Biosfleury A, Bessis M. The interaction of phagocytic cells and red cells modified by immune reactions. Comparison of antibody and complement coated red cells. *Blood Cells.* 1975;1:345-358.

Ward CJ, Schwartz BS, White JG. Heinz-body anemia: "bite cell" variant—a light and electron microscopic study. *Am J Hematol.* 1983;15:135-146.

Yoo D, Lessin LS. Drug-associated "bite cell" hemolytic anemia. *Am J Med.* 1992;92:243-248.

Nucleated Red Blood Cells
Bottomley SS. Sideroblastic anaemia. *Clin Haematol.* 1982;11:389-409.

Herbert V. Biology of disease. Megaloblastic anemias. *Lab Inves.* 1985;52:3-19.

Ross DW. The life history of individual blood cells. *Blood Cells.* 1987;12:541-542.

Megakaryocytic Cells and Thrombocytes
Bizarro N. Platelet satellitosis to polymorphonuclears: cytochemical, immunological, and ultrastructural characterization of eight cases. *Am J Hematol.* 1991;36:235-242.

Bizzaro N, Goldschmeding R, Von Dem Borne AEG. Platelet satellitism is FcgRIII (CD16) receptor-mediated. *Am J Clin Pathol.* 1995;103:740-744.

Hehlmann R, Jahn M, Baumann B, et al. Essential thrombocythemia. Clinical characteristics and course in 61 cases. *Cancer.* 1988;61:2487-2496.

Jantunen E. Inherited giant platelet disorders. *Eur J Haemotol.* 1994;53:191-196.

Kobayashi Y, Ozawa M, Maruo N, et al. Megakaryocytic ploidy in myelodysplastic syndromes. *Leuk Lymphoma.* 1993;9:55-61.

Kobayashi Y, Uoshima N, Kimura S, et al. Relationship between morphological classification of the degree of maturation and the ploidy of micromegakaryocytes in myelodysplastic syndrome patients. *Int J Hematol* (Ireland). 1995;61(3):117-122.

Ohshima K, Kikuchi M, Takeshita M. A megakaryocte analysis of the bone marrow in patients with myelodysplastic syndrome, myeloproliferative disorder and allied disorders. *J Pathol.* 1995;177:81-189.

Tefferi A, Mathew P, Noel P. The 5q-syndrome: a scientific and clinical update. *Leuk Lymphoma.* 1994;14:75-278.

Thiele J, Titius BR, Kopsidis C, et al. Atypical micromegakaryocytes, promegakaryoblasts and megakaryoblasts: a critical evaluation by immunohistochemistry, cytochemistry, and morphometry of bone marrow trephines in chronic myeloid leukemia and myelodysplastic syndromes. *Virchows Arch B Cell Pathol Incl Mol Pathol.* 1992;62:275-282.

Lymphocytic and Plasmacytic Cells
Harris NL, Jaffe ES, Stein H, et al. Revised European/American Classification of Lymphoid Neoplasms: A Proposal from the International Lymphoma Study Group. *Blood.* 1994;84/5:1361-1392.

Rebuck, JW. Hematology Check Sample No. H-80. Chicago: ASCP Press; 1976.

Schumacher HR, Cotelingam JD. *Chronic Leukemia. Approach to Diagnosis.* New York: Igaku-Shoin Medical Publishers; 1993.

Ward PCJ. The Lymphoid Leukocytoses. *Postgrad Med.* 1980; 67:2-6.

Wiernek PH, Canellos GP, Kyle R et al. *Neoplastic Diseases of the Blood.* 2nd ed. New York: Churchill Livingstone Inc; 1991:440.

Microbiology
Ash LR, Orihel TC. *Atlas of Human Parasitology.* 2nd Ed. Chicago: ASCP Press: 1984:13-17, 79-84, 91-94.

Eberhard ML, Lammie PJ. Laboratory diagnosis of filariasis. *Clinics in Lab Med.* 1991;11(4):977-1010.

Ferry JA, Pettit CK, Rosenberg AE, et al. Fungi in megakaryocytes. *Am J Clin Pathol.* 1991;96:577-581.

Godwin JH, Stopeck A, Chang VT, et al. Mycobacteremia in acquired immune deficiency syndrome. *Am J Clin Pathol.* 1991;95:369-375.

Kurtin PJ, McKinsey DS, Gupta MR, et al. Histoplasmosis in patients with acquired immunodeficiency syndrome. *Am J Clin Pathol.* 1990;93(3):367-372.

Murray PR, Baron EJ, Pfaller MA, et al, eds. *Manual of Clinical Microbiology.* 6th ed. Washington DC: American Society of Microbiology Press; 1995:Chapters 2, 31, 51-2, 61, 63-4, 104, 108.

Osborne BM, Guarda LA, Butler JJ. Bone marrow biopsies in patients with the acquired immunodeficiency syndrome. *Hum Pathol.* 1984;15;1048-1053.

Sun NCJ, Shapshak P, Lachant NA, et al. Bone marrow examination in patients with AIDS and AIDS-related complex (ARC). *Am J Clin Pathol.* 1989;92:589-594.

Sun T. *Color Atlas and Textbook of Diagnostic Parasitology.* New York: Igaku-Shoin; 1988.

Artifacts
Staunton MJ, Gaffney EF. Apoptosis. Basic concepts and potential significance in human cancer. *Arch Pathol Lab Med.* 1998;122;310-319.

Fisher, MMS, Guerra CG, Hickman JR, et al. Peripheral blood lymphocyte apoptosis. A clue to the diagnosis of acute infectious mononucleosis. *Arch Pathol Lab Med.* 1996; 120:951-955.

Miscellaneous Cells
Horny HP, Parwaresch MR, Lennert K: Bone marrow findings in systemic mastocytosis. *Hum Pathol.* 1985;15:808-814.

Hyun BH, Gulati GL, Ashton JK. Hematopoiesis and blood cell morphology. In: Howanitz J, Howanitz PJ, eds. *Laboratory Medicine. Test Selection and Interpretation.* New York: Churchill Livingstone; 1991.

Neufeld EF, Muenzer J. The Mucopolysaccharidoses. In: Scriver CR, Beaudet AL, Sly WS, et al, eds. *The Metabolic Basis of Inherited Disease.* New York: McGraw-Hill; 1989.

Savage RA. Specific and not-so-specific histiocytes in bone marrow. *Lab Medicine.* 1984; 15:467-471.

Scully RE, Mark EJ, McNeely WF, et al. Case records of the Massachusetts General Hospital. *N Engl J Med.* 1992;326:472-481.

Appendix B
Hematology Master List (1997-1998) (with Proficiency Testing Codes)

Granulocytic (Myeloid) Cells
- 011 Myeloblast
- 144 Promyelocyte
- 141 Myeloblast/Promyelocyte with Auer Rod(s)
- 013 Myelocyte, Neutrophilic
- 014 Metamyelocyte, Neutrophilic
- 187 Segmented or Band Neutrophil
- 111 Basophil
- 112 Eosinophil (any stage)
- 140 Monocytes, Immature
- 139 Monocyte
- 025 Metamyelocyte, Giant (Bone Marrow)
- 023 Band Neutrophil, Giant (Bone Marrow)
- 181 Segmented or Band Neutrophil with Toxic Granulation and/or Multiple Toxic Vacuoles
- 184 Segmented or Band Neutrophil with Döhle Body with or without Toxic Granulation
- 024 Segmented Neutrophil, Hypersegmented Nucleus
- 142 Neutrophil with Dysplastic Nucleus/Agranular Cytoplasm
- 143 Neutrophil with Pelger-Huët Nucleus

Erythrocytic Cells and Inclusions
- 037 Erythrocyte (Normocytic, Normochromic)
- 042 Acanthocyte
- 148 Bite Cell
- 189 Blister Cell (Pre-Keratocyte)
- 190 Echinocyte
- 191 Fragmented Cell (Schistocyte, Helmet Cell, Keratocyte)
- 132 Macrocyte (Oval or Round Excluding Polychromatophilic Red Cells)
- 152 Microcyte (with Central Pallor)
- 156 Nucleated Red Cell, Normal or Abnormal (Blood)
- 048 Ovalocyte
- 036 Polychromatophilic Red Cell (Non-Nucleated)
- 049 Sickle Cell (Drepanocyte)
- 050 Spherocyte
- 051 Stomatocyte
- 052 Target Cell (Codocyte)
- 053 Teardrop Cell (Dacryocyte)
- 153 Reticulocyte (Supravital Stain)
- 054 Basophilic Stippling (Coarse)
- 150 Heinz Body
- 055 Hemoglobin C Crystal
- 151 Hemoglobin H Inclusions (Supravital Stain)
- 057 Howell-Jolly Body (Wright-Giemsa stain)
- 105 Howell-Jolly Body (Iron Stain)
- 128 Pappenheimer Bodies, Presumptive (Wright-Giemsa Stain)
- 059 Pappenheimer Bodies (Iron Stain)
- 080 Red Cell Agglutinates
- 090 Rouleaux

Nucleated Red Cells
- 159 Pronormoblast (Bone Marrow)
- 154 Basophilic Normoblast (Bone Marrow)
- 157 Polychromatophilic Normoblast (Bone Marrow)
- 161 Orthochromic Normoblast (Bone Marrow)
- 203 Nucleated Red Cell, Megaloblastic (Bone Marrow)
- 156 Nucleated Red Cell, Normal or Abnormal (Blood)
- 183 Nucleated Red Cell, Dysplastic (Bone Marrow)
- 163 Sideroblast (Iron Stain)
- 164 Sideroblast, Ringed (Iron Stain)

Megakaryocytic Cells and Thrombocytes
- 072 Megakaryocyte or Precursor, Normal
- 119 Megakaryocyte or Precursor, Abnormal
- 115 Megakaryocyte Nucleus
- 073 Platelet, Normal
- 166 Platelet, Giant (Macrothrombocyte)
- 188 Platelet, Hypogranular
- 167 Platelet Satellitism

Lymphocytic and Plasmacytic Cells
083 Hairy Cell
060 Lymphoblast
168 Lymphocyte, Mature
169 Lymphocyte, Reactive (to Exclude Plasmacytoid and Immunoblastic Forms)
064 Lymphoma Cell
126 Plasma Cell, Mature
127 Plasma cell, Immature or Abnormal (Malignant Myeloma Cell)
170 Plasma cell or Precursor with Inclusion Body
133 Prolymphocyte
120 *Sézary* Cell

Microorganisms
185 Babesia
171 Bacteria (Cocci or Rod), Extracellular
172 Bacteria (Spirochete), Extracellular
173 Fungi, Extracellular
174 Leukocyte (Blood) with Phagocytized Bacteria
134 Leukocyte (Blood) with Phagocytized Fungi
175 Macrophage (Bone Marrow) with Phagocytized Histoplasma, Leishmania or Toxoplasma
135 Macrophage with Phagocytized Mycobacteria
058 Malaria (Intracellular and Extracellular)
186 Microfilaria
136 Protozoan (Non-Malarial)

Artifacts
094 Basket Cell or Smudge Cell
093 Neutrophil Necrobiosis (Degenerated Neutrophil)
182 Erythrocyte with Overlapping Platelet
123 Stain Precipitate

Miscellaneous Cells
076 Blast Cell
020 Alder's Anomaly Inclusion
021 Chédiak-Higashi Anomaly Inclusion
116 Epithelial/Endothelial Cell
138 Lipocyte (Fat Cell)
178 Macrophage (Histiocyte)
179 Macrophage with Phagocytized Red Cell (Erythrophagocytosis)
129 Gaucher Cell and Pseudo-Gaucher Cell
137 Histocyte, Sea Blue
087 Niemann-Pick Cell, Foamy Macrophage
019 Mast Cell (Tissue Basophil)
086 Metastatic Tumor Cell
107 Mitotic Figure
088 Osteoblast
089 Osteoclast

Appendix C
How to Review Proficiency Testing Photomicrographs

The College of American Pathologists Proficiency Testing Program in hematology involves a series of three challenges per year. Each challenge includes a set of photomicrographs and case histories. Participants should follow a simple strategy when selecting identifications from the Master List of possibilities.

First, read the history. Clues to the disease process are often found there. Next, match the slide with the description in the case study. Pay careful attention to the site (bone marrow or peripheral blood) and the stain used (iron, Wright-Giemsa, etc.). Many identifications are missed simply because participants chose the wrong stain for an identification. A Wright-Giemsa stained red cell inclusion is selected, for example, when the photomicrograph is labeled *iron stain*.

Next, view all the photomicrographs with appropriate lighting and magnification. It is tempting to just hold the slides up to a light source and select your answer. This is a recipe for failure. Photomicrographs are best viewed in a darkened room with a good 35 mm slide projector to maximize detail. Subtleties of color, chromatin, etc., are missed if you use a hand-held viewer or hold the slide up to the light. Such a set up also affords a more formal review of the case and creates a collaborative environment for fellow technologists, clinicians, and pathologists.

You just received the latest CAP hematology proficiency testing mailing. First, read the history and slide descriptions. Pay careful attention to the site (bone marrow, peripheral blood, etc.) and any special stains used.

Next, examine the photomicrographs, carefully matching them with the history and descriptions. The temptation is to simply hold the slides up the light and evaluate the arrowed object. *DON'T DO IT!* It may be convenient but any nuances of color and morphology will be missed.

A hand held small viewer is OK, but not ideal. Only one person can see the slide at a time and the images are small. The cheaper viewers use light bulbs that do not produce an accurate color range.

Photomicrographs are best viewed in a darkened room with a good 35mm slide projector to maximize detail. Subtleties of color, chromatin, etc., are missed if you use a hand viewer or hold the slide up to the light.

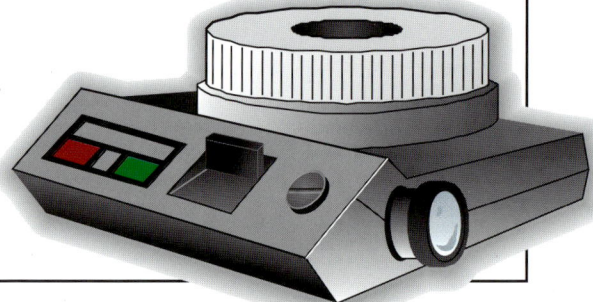

Appendix D
CAP Hematology Proficieny Testing Challenges Listed by Master List Identification

Laboratories that have participated in the CAP Comprehensive Surveys and have retained photomicrographs from these Surveys will find that Appendix D provides the identification (YR SLIDE IDENTIFICATION), referee (R%), and participant (P%) data for each photomicrograph used in the Surveys from 1978-1997. Please note that over the years, the master list of identifications has changed; some listings have been modified (e.g., segs and bands are now a single identification), while others are no longer on the current Master List.

YR	SLIDE IDENTIFICATION	R%	P%
GRANULOCYTIC (MYELOID) CELLS			
BAND NEUTROPHIL (015)			
79	H-11 Band or segmented neutrophil	100	97.1
80	H-6 Band neutrophil	55.6	57.4
80	H-9 Band neutrophil	100	81.1
82	H-40 Band neutrophil	37.5	39.0
83	H1-48 Band neutrophil	61.1	73.9
85	H1-5 Band neutrophil	100	97.3
85	XL-24 Band neutrophil	88.9	87.3
86	XL-61 Band neutrophil	89.4	86.9
87	XL-06 Band neutrophil	94.7	91.9
87	XL-72 Band neutrophil	88.9	91.1
90	H1-48 Band neutrophil	94.1	86.5
90	XH-07 Band neutrophil	78.9	23.5
91	HE-43 Band neutrophil	70	46.5
92	HE-21 Band neutrophil	95	83.4
92	HE-40 Band neutrophil	90	91.7
87	A-69 Band neutrophil	100	97
85	A-48 Band neutrophil	86.7	85.6
86	A-09 Band neutrophil	94.4	94
84	A-29 Band neutrophil	94.4	95.4
91	HE-57 Band or segmented neutrophil	100	96.6
86	XL-05 Band/segmented neutrophil	100	94.3
90	XH-30 Band/segmented neutrophil	100	96.9
94	HE-14 Band neutrophil	92.6	60.3
BAND NEUTROPHIL WITH TOXIC GRANULATION (130)			
91	HE-23 Band neutrophil with/without toxic granulation	85	89.6
85	H1-8 Band neutrophil, toxic granulation	83.3	70.3
85	H1-9 Band neutrophil, toxic granulation	100	95.4
87	H1-4 Band neutrophil, toxic granulation, pseudo Pelger-Huët	89.5	89
BAND NEUTROPHIL, GIANT (023)			
87	H1-20 Giant band, giant metamyelocyte	89.5	89.1
BASOPHIL, ANY STAGE (111)			
78	H-21 Basophil or precursor	100	94.5
81	H-08 Basophil	100	98.5
81	H-37 Basophil	83.3	87.5
89	XL-31 Basophil	100	82.6
91	HE-06 Basophil	100	97.6
91	HE-59 Basophil	84.2	66.1
92	HE-25 Basophil	100	98.3
92	XH-14 Basophil	100	98.3
84	H1-29 Basophil or precursor	100	98.4
84	A-30 Basophil or precursor	94.4	80.1
91	HE-27 Basophil, any stage	100	91.9
87	XL-50 Basophil, mature	94.1	78.6
88	H1-29 Basophil, mature or immature	90	85.5
86	XL-04 Basophil, or precursor	100	86.4
86	XL-42 Basophil, or precursor	94.4	96.6
86	A-64 Basophil	100	83.9
86	A-46 Basophil	100	95.4
94	HE-30 Basophil	65.5	44.2
97	HE-08 Basophil	100	97.8
EOSINOPHIL, ANY STAGE (112)			
77	H-21 Eosinophil or precursor	100	88.2
81	H-07 Eosinophil	100	95.4
81	H-39 Eosinophil	66.7	30.6
82	H-28 Eosinophil	77.8	41.1
83	H1-21 Eosinophil	100	98.1
85	H1-45 Eosinophil	94.4	91.1
88	XL-14 Eosinophil	100	98.9
89	H1-19 Eosinophil	100	97.3
90	H1-46 Eosinophil	94.1	98.1
91	HE-22 Eosinophil	100	99.1
92	HE-22 Eosinophil(ic) myelocyte	100	92.6
92	HE-36 Eosinophil	100	98.8
92	HE-13 Eosinophil	89.5	55.1
86	H1-20 Eosinophil or precursor	100	97.4
85	A-47 Eosinophil or precursor	100	96
84	A-10 Eosinophil or precursor	88.2	94.1
88	H1-44 Eosinophil, Chédiak-Higashi	94.7	93
88	XL-30 Eosinophil, mature	100	88.6
86	XL-45 Eosinophil, or precursor	100	94.1
87	A-49 Eosinophil	100	92.2
93	HE-41 Eosinophil	100	86.3
94	HE-29 Eosinophil	72.4	51.1
95	HE-22 Eosinophil	100	99.6
97	HE-07 Eosinophil	100	99.6
97	HE-24 Eosinophil	100	99
METAMYELOCYTE (014)			
78	H-10 Metamyelocyte, myelocyte	100	95.1
79	H-55 Metamyelocyte, myelocyte	100	86.4
81	H-09 Metamyelocyte	75.0	60.9
81	H-38 Metamyelocyte	100	73.8
90	XH-06 Metamyelocyte	100	84
85	H1-4 Metamyelocyte, band, toxic granulation	100	97.3
85	H1-6 Metamyelocyte, myelocyte	100	93.8
82	A-48 Metamyelocyte	100	73.5
83	A-10 Metamyelocyte	5.9	29.4
82	A-30 Metamyelocyte	50	61.2

YR	SLIDE IDENTIFICATION	R%	P%
82	A-I0 Metamyelocyte	57.1	68.5
94	HE-12 Metamyelocyte	92.6	90.8
96	HE-43 Metamyelocyte	78.6	71

METAMYELOCYTE, GIANT (025)

YR	SLIDE IDENTIFICATION	R%	P%
91	HE-55 Metamyelocyte/giant, band/giant	100	96

MONOCYTE (139)

YR	SLIDE IDENTIFICATION	R%	P%
77	H-34 Monocyte	88.9	92.9
79	H-22 Monocyte	100	93.6
78	H-37 Monocyte, promonocyte	75	75.2
88	XL-31 Monocyte, lymphocyte, histiocyte	100	93.2
80	H-1 0 Monocyte	77.8	52.1
80	H-40 Monocyte	100	88.1
83	H1-23 Monocyte	72.2	59.6
83	H1-33 Monocyte	66.7	66.3
86	XL-64 Monocyte	94.7	90.5
88	XL-06 Monocyte	100	77.0
90	H1-44 Monocyte	100	94.9
90	XH-05 Monocyte	100	94.4
90	XH-31 Monocyte	94.4	91.9
92	HE-24 Monocyte	85	82.7
92	HE-54 Monocyte	100	96.4
92	HE-60 Monocyte	90	72
82	H-27 Monocyte or precursor	77.8	91.6
82	H-57 Monocyte or precursor	88.9	86.5
82	H-58 Monocyte or precursor	66.7	59.7
85	H1-31 Monocyte or precursor	100	94.7
85	H1-33 Monocyte or precursor	100	92.6
87	XL-52 Monocyte or precursor	94.1	90.8
88	H1-18 Monocyte or precursor	94.1	70.9
81	A-6 Monocyte or precursor	28.6	30.1
87	A-70 Monocyte or promonocyte	94.7	80.7
87	A-50 Monocyte, macrophage, reactive lymphocyte	94.8	95.7
88	A-30 Monocyte, myelocyte, metamyelocyte	100	93.3
85	XL-43 Monocyte, or precursor	100	90.9
85	XL-63 Monocyte, or precursor	100	84.9
87	XL-05 Monocyte, or precursor	100	94.9
86	A-47 Monocyte, promonocyte	100	75.2
89	A-12 Monocyte, toxic granulation, band, giant band, seg	100	94.8
89	A-79 Monocyte	100	92.1
85	A-27 Monocyte	94.1	80.9
95	HE-24 Monocyte	96.4	91.1
95	HE-38 Monocyte	100	100
96	HE-24 Monocyte	96.4	94.3
96	HE-38 Monocyte	100	98.1
97	HE-09 Monocyte	100	98.9
97	HE-23 Monocyte	100	98.9

MONOCYTE, IMMATURE (140)

YR	SLIDE IDENTIFICATION	R%	P%
91	HE-46 Monocyte, immature	73.7	58.2
91	HE-56 Monocyte, immature monocyte	100	89.5
92	HE-09 Monocyte, immature monocyte	100	97.5
82	H-56 Dysplastic monocyte precursor	66.7	73.6

MYELOBLAST (011)

YR	SLIDE IDENTIFICATION	R%	P%
91	HE-11 Myeloblast	57.9	56.3
92	HE-53 Myeloblast, blast	100	81.7
86	H1-41 Myeloblast, blast, monoblast	100	92.9
86	H1-42 Myeloblast, blast, monoblast	100	91.3
86	H1-17 Myeloblast, blast, monoblast, lymphoblast, promyelocyte	100	90.9
87	H1-8 Myeloblast, blast, promyelocyte	89.5	74.8
80	H-36 Blast, myeloblast	100	75.6
88	H1-32 Blast, myeloblast	100	88.9
91	HE-29 Blast, myeloblast, lymphoblast	100	91.2
94	HE-26 Myeloblast	65.5	54.7

MYELOBLAST/PROMYELOCYTE WITH AUER ROD (141)

YR	SLIDE IDENTIFICATION	R%	P%
87	A-08 Auer rod, myeloblast	95	95
95	HE-06 Myeloblast/promyelocyte with Auer rod	92.9	94.4
96	HE-29 Myeloblast/promyelocyte with Auer rod	92.3	86

MYELOCYTE (013)

YR	SLIDE IDENTIFICATION	R%	P%
80	H-7 Myelocyte	66.7	67.5
81	H-06 Myelocyte	62.5	45.5
87	H1-21 Myelocyte	84.2	76.7
92	HE-06 Myelocyte	95	64.6
92	HE-45 Myelocyte	95	92.3
91	HE-58 Myelocyte, metamyelocyte, giant metamyelocyte	90	87.2
88	H1-21 Myelocyte, metamyelocyte	88.2	91.6
82	A-67 Myelocyte, metamyelocyte	100	88.4
82	A-9 Myelocyte, promyelocyte	100	89.5
82	A-47 Myelocyte	100	82.1
86	A-10 Myelocyte	22.2	17.5
82	A-29 Myelocyte	87.5	70.3
84	A-49 Myelocyte	88	66.3
91	HE-12 Myelocyte, dysplastic	52.6	18.2
94	HE-42 Myelocyte	82.8	79.9

NEUTROPHIL WITH PELGER-HUËT NUCLEUS (143)

YR	SLIDE IDENTIFICATION	R%	P%
84	H1-6 Pelger-Huët	81.3	71.6
81	H-35 Pelger-Huët anomaly	50.0	49.4
84	H1-7 Band neutrophil, Pelger-Huët	81.3	71.6

NEUTROPHIL WITH DYSPLASTIC NUCELUS AND/OR AGRANULAR CYTOPLASM (142)

YR	SLIDE IDENTIFICATION	R%	P%
86	H1-44 Pseudo Pelger-Huët, degenerated neutrophil	88.2	60.1
86	H1-45 Pseudo-Pelger-Huët	70.6	43.5

PROMYELOCYTE (144)

YR	SLIDE IDENTIFICATION	R%	P%
78	H-50 Promyelocyte	100	73.4
78	H-22 Promyelocyte, myelocyte	100	67.1
80	H-39 Promyelocyte	85.7	55.4
81	H-10 Promyelocyte	100	55.6
87	H1-9 Promyelocyte	57.9	40.2
92	HE-11 Promyelocyte	100	54.4
86	H1-43 Promyelocyte, metamyelocyte, myelocyte	100	97.4
82	A-49 Promyelocyte, myelocyte	100	87.6
95	HE-08 Promyelocyte	96.4	95

SEGMENTED NEUTROPHIL (145)

YR	SLIDE IDENTIFICATION	R%	P%
78	H-8 Segmented neutrophil	100	96.1
80	H-11 Segmented neutrophil	66.7	74.1
80	H-8 Segmented neutrophil	100	97.4
82	H-39 Segmented neutrophil	87.5	83.5

YR	SLIDE IDENTIFICATION	R%	P%
84	H1-4 Segmented neutrophil	87.5	93.4
85	XL-23 Segmented neutrophil	94.4	96.2
85	XL-45 Segmented neutrophil	84.2	93.7
86	XL-06 Segmented neutrophil	100	94.1
86	XL-44 Segmented neutrophil	88.9	93.7
87	XL-04 Segmented neutrophil	94.7	94.9
89	H1-22 Segmented neutrophil	95	97.6
89	H1-29 Segmented neutrophil	94.4	94.6
90	H1-45 Segmented neutrophil	100	94.9
90	XH-21 Segmented neutrophil	90	87.2
91	HE-47 Segmented neutrophil	78.9	35.7
92	HE-38 Segmented neutrophil	90	96.1
92	HE-56 Segmented neutrophil	85	66.2
83	A-8 Segmented neutrophil	94.1	86.7
88	A-49 Segmented/hypersegmented neutrophil	90	84.9
90	XH-15 Segmented/hypersegmented neutrophil	100	98.4
88	XL-77 Segmented/hypersegmented neutrophil	90	77.1
89	A-78 Segmented/hypersegmented neutrophil	100	98
93	HE-11-16 Segmented or band neutrophil	N/A	N/A
93	HE-27-32 Segmented or band neutrophil	N/A	N/A
96	HE-07 Segmented or band neutrophil	100	96.9
96	HE-40 Segmented or band neutrophil	96.2	96.2
97	HE-10 Segmented or band neutrophil	100	95
97	HE-15 Segmented or band neutrophil	100	91.5
97	HE-22 Segmented or band neutrophil	96	98

SEGMENTED NEUTROPHIL WITH TOXIC GRANULATION (147/181)

85	A-68 Neutrophil, toxic granulation	100	97.8
8.5	H1-46 Toxic granulation	66.7	62.0
91	HE-26 Segmented neutrophil with/without toxic granulation	100	97.9
91	HE-07 Segmented neutrophil, toxic granulation	100	96.1
87	A-31 Segmented neutrophil, toxic granulation	100	93.2
89	A-80 Segmented neutrophil, toxic granulation	89.5	93.9

SEGMENTED NEUTROPHIL WITH DÖHLE BODY, WITH OR WITHOUT TOXIC GRANULATION (146); SEGMENTED OR BAND NEUTROPHIL WITH DÖHLE BODY, WITH OR WITHOUT TOXIC GRANULATION (184)

78	H-9 Band neutrophil, Döhle body	100	84.8
90	H1-21 Toxic granulation/vacuolization, Döhle bodies	100	82.1
90	H1-31 Segmented neutrophil, toxic granulation/vacuoles, Döhle body	100	99.1
82	H-43 Döhle body inclusion	100	92.4
96	HE-51 Segmented or band neutrophil with Döhle body	91	95.3

SEGMENTED NEUTROPHIL, HYPERSEGMENTED NUCLEUS (024)

78	H-48 Hypersegmented neutrophil	100	95.5
81	H-21 Hypersegmented neutrophil	100	97.5
81	H-36 Hypersegmented neutrophil	100	97.5
82	H-9 Hypersegmented neutrophil	100	98.4
84	H1-31 Hypersegmented neutrophil	89.5	97.3
87	H1-17 Hypersegmented neutrophil	100	99.3
88	XL-78 Hypersegmented neutrophil	100	96.8
92	HE-55 Hypersegmented neutrophil	100	98.8
81	A-24 Hypersegmented neutrophil	100	94.6
82	A-8 Hypersegmented neutrophil	100	96.2
94	HE-40 Segmented neutrophil, hypersegmented	100	99.7

ERYTHROCYTIC CELLS/INCLUSIONS IN BLOOD

ACANTHOCYTE (042)

85	H1-30 Acanthocyte	64.7	53.7
85	H1-32 Acanthocyte	88.2	72.6
92	HE-51 Acanthocyte	100	98.9
81	H-51 Acanthocyte, echinocyte	100	98.9
83	H1-31 Acanthocyte, echinocyte	100	99.4
90	AH-28 Acanthocyte, schistocyte	100	94.5
90	AH-26 Acanthocyte	100	90
92	HE-51 Acanthocyte	100	98.9

BASOPHILIC STIPPLING (COARSE) (054)

77	H-47 Basophilic stippling	87.5	91.2
79	H-36 Basophilic stippling	100	98.6
81	H-54 Basophilic stippling	85.7	96.4
83	H1-44 Basophilic stippling	88.9	88.7
85	H1-7 Basophilic stippling	100	98.7
86	H1-5 Basophilic stippling	100	96
87	H1-7 Basophilic stippling	100	99.4
88	XL-80 Basophilic stippling	100	96
94	HE-08 Basophilic stippling	100	98.3
96	HE-06 Basophilic stippling	100	98.5
96	HE-37 Basophilic stippling	100	98.3

BURR CELL (ECHINOCYTE), CRENATED CELL (180/190)

84	H1-21 Crenated RBC, echinocyte	84.2	98.1
84	H1-22 Crenated RBC, echinocyte	68.4	72.6
85	H1-29 Echinocyte, crenated RBC	94.2	97.1
85	H1-34 Echinocyte, crenated RBC	94.2	96.5
91	HE-38 Echinocyte, crenated RBC	100	93.2

ERYTHROCYTE (NORMOCYTIC) (037)

84	H1-5 Erythrocyte	75.0	70.3
90	H1-04 Erythrocyte	85	72.5
90	AH-04 Erythrocyte, any hypochromic/microcytic	100	98.4
85	XL-64 Erythrocyte, normal	84.2	60.3
85	XL-05 Erythrocyte, normochromic/microcytic	100	87.3
83	A-50 Erythrocyte	88.2	69.3
89	XL-86 Erythrocyte, any microchromic/hypocytic	95	92.4
97	H-21 Erythrocyte, normal	100	97.9

HEINZ BODY (056)

79	H-53 Heinz body	85.7	71.4

HEMOGLOBIN C CRYSTAL (055)

79	H-38 Hemoglobin C crystal	100	98.8

HEMOGLOBIN H CRYSTAL (SUPRAVITAL STAIN) (151)

89	H1-7 Hemoglobin H inclusion	68.4	55

YR	SLIDE IDENTIFICATION	R%	P%
HOWELL-JOLLY BODY (107)			
77	H-49 Howell-Jolly body	100	97.9
79	H-39 Howell-Jolly body	100	99.2
90	XH-23 Howell Jolly body	100	92.3
90	AH-27 Howell Jolly body, Wright-stain	88.9	90.7
87	H1-22 Howell-Jolly bodies	84.2	68.1
86	A-65 Howell-Jolly bodies	100	96.7
85	A-09 Howell-Jolly bodies	100	96.9
81	H-23 Howell-Jolly body	100	98
82	H-11 Howell-Jolly body	100	88.8
83	H1-30 Howell-Jolly body	100	96.6
84	H1-46 Howell-Jolly body	100	98.7
85	H1-21 Howell-Jolly body	66.7	59.6
92	HE-37 Howell-Jolly body	100	97.9
84	H1-17 Howell-Jolly body	94.8	98.3
83	A-27 Howell-Jolly body	100	95.6
83	H1-22 Pseudo-Howell Jolly body	N/A	N/A
HOWELL-JOLLY BODY (IRON STAIN) (105)			
96	HE-42 Heinz body (iron stain)	84.6	80.3
HOWELL-JOLLY BODY (WRIGHT STAIN) (057)			
97	HE-40 Heinz body (Wright's stain)	100	98.1
MACROCYTE (ROUND OR OVAL) (132)			
82	H-8 Macrocyte, oval macrocyte	100	98.8
89	H1-43 Macrocytic oval/round RBC	100	98.2
81	A-23 Macrocytic RBC, ovalocyte	100	91.1
96	HE-26 Macrocyte (oval or round excluding polychromatophilic red cells)	100	99
MICROCYTE (152)			
83	H1-46 Microcyte	94.4	96.8
83	H1-47 Microcyte	88.9	78.4
86	XL-26 Microcytic erythrocyte	94.7	92.9
84	H1-32 Microcytic RBC, hypochromic/normochromic	78.9	92.2
86	A-28 Microcytic RBC, hypochromic/normochromic	100	97.3
91	HE-09 Microcytic RBC, schistocyte	100	91.6
84	A-47 RBC-normochromic/microcytic hypochromic/microcytic	94	91
85	XL-04 Erythrocyte—hypochromic	100	65.4
86	XL-63 Erythrocyte—hypochromic	100	69.9
85	XL-44 Erythrocyte—hypochromic/normal	100	94.6
89	A-55 Erythrocyte—hypochromic/microcytic RBC	95	95
86	A-29 Erythrocyte—hypochromic, normocytic or microcytic	100	88.9
NUCLEATED RED CELL IN PERIPHERAL BLOOD (156)			
85	A-30 Normoblast (any stage)	94.1	93.5
85	H1-43 Normoblastic metarubricyte	66.7	73.1
88	XL-53 NRBC, any maturation stage	95	96.3
89	XL-33 NRBC, any stage	100	96
90	XH-14 Nucleated RBC	95	93.7
91	HE-30 Nucleated RBC	100	95.9
93	HE-40 Nucleated erythrocyte in peripheral blood	96.3	98.3
94	HE-07 Nucleated erythrocyte in peripheral blood	100	93.2
94	HE-43 Nucleated erythrocyte in peripheral blood	86.2	89.3
OVALOCYTE (ELLIPTOCYTE) (048)			
85	XL-26 Ovalocyte	100	97.9
90	H1-07 Ovalocyte	100	98.3
90	XH-22 Ovalocyte	100	98
91	HE-41 Ovalocyte	100	98.3
92	HE-57 Ovalocyte	100	98.5
85	A-66 Ovalocyte	100	98.6
83	A-49 Ovalocyte	94.1	96.5
87	A-68 Elliptocyte	100	98.6
93	HE-07 Ovalocyte	100	98.7
96	HE-09 Ovalocyte	100	99.4
97	HE-06 Ovalocyte	100	99.5
PAPPENHEIMER BODIES, WRIGHT STAIN (128); IRON STAIN (059)			
78	H-36 Siderocyte	75.0	67.7
90	H1-08 Pappenheimer bodies	N/A	N/A
81	H-24 Siderotic granules, Wright stain	100	91
81	H-25 Siderotic granules, iron stain	100	95.9
96	HE-44 Pappenheimer body (iron stain)	84.6	75.2
POLYCHROMATOPHILIC RED CELL (036)			
87	XL-74 Polychromatophilic RBC, macrocytic, round or oval	94.5	94.8
85	A-11 Polychromatophilic RBC, macrocytic, oval or round	100	98.5
84	A-11 Polychromatophilic RBC, macrocytic, oval or round	100	93.4
83	H1-35 Polychromatophilic RBC	72.2	57.4
85	H1-18 Polychromatophilic RBC	94.4	91.5
86	H1-6 Polychromatophilic RBC	75.0	79.3
86	H1-9 Polychromatophilic RBC	56.2	42.0
89	H1-5 Polychromatophilic RBC	94.7	95.1
92	HE-10 Polychromatophilic RBC	100	94.7
91	HE-24 Polychromatophilic RBC, macrocyte	100	97.2
86	XL-24 Polychromatophilic RBC, macrocytic round RBC	100	97.3
90	XH-12 Polychromatophilic RBC, macrocytic round or oval	100	86.6
86	A-27 Polychromatophilic RBC	88.9	70.1
83	A-30 Polychromatophilic red cell	72.2	69.8
RED CELL AGGLUTINATES (080)			
89	A-77 RBC agglutinates	100	87.8
95	HE-26 Red cell agglutinates	100	98.8
97	HE-26 Red cell agglutinates	100	97.8
RETICULOCYTE (SUPRAVITAL STAIN) (153)			
77	H-48 Reticulocyte	100	98.2
79	H-52 Reticulocyte	57.1	47.1
85	H1-20 Reticulocyte	100	97.4
85	H1-22 Reticulocyte	94.4	96.3
89	H1-6 Reticulocyte	94.7	93.3
89	H1-8 Reticulocyte, Heinz body	94.7	86.4
84	A-9 Reticulocyte/RNA stained	100	96.4
85	A-50 Reticulocyte	73.3	67.1
95	HE-42 Reticulocyte	N/A	N/A

YR	SLIDE IDENTIFICATION	R%	P%
ROULEAUX (090)			
86	H1-30 Rouleaux	88.9	96.5
86	H1-29 Rouleaux; RBC agglutinates	100	99.8
BITE CELL (BLISTER CELL), KERATOCYTE (148)			
86	H1-7 Bite cell, helmet cell	100	99
86	H1-4 Bite cell, helmet cell	100	99.4
86	H1-8 Bite cell, helmet cell	100	97.8
SCHISTOCYTE (FRAGMENTED CELL, HELMET CELL) (047)			
90	H1-32 Schistocyte	100	95.9
92	HE-08 Schistocyte	100	97.7
92	HE-59 Schistocyte	95	93.4
80	H-54 Schistocyte, helmet cell	100	94.6
88	A-68 Schistocyte	100	95.2
90	XH-24 Fragmented RBC	100	88.2
81	H-49 Helmet cell	100	98.8
88	XL-54 Helmet cell	94.7	95.9
86	XL-25 Helmet cell, schistocyte	94.7	87.5
87	A-30 Helmet cell, schistocyte	100	92.5
87	A-29 Helmet cell, schistocyte	100	93
85	A-67 Helmet cell, schistocyte	100	97.6
83	A-47 Helmet cell, schistocyte	94.1	94.7
82	A-27 Helmet cell	100	69.2
84	A-65 Helmet cell	94.7	95.2
SICKLE CELL (049)			
79	H-37 Sickle cell	100	98.5
81	H-50 Sickle cell	57.1	84.4
85	XL-62 Sickle cell	100	99
87	XL-26 Sickle cell	100	99
87	XL-27 Sickle cell	90	58.2
82	A-68 Sickle cell	100	98.1
86	A-45 Sickle cell	100	99
85	A-28 Sickle cell	100	99.8
93	HE-42 Sickle cell	100	99.5
94	HE-23 Sickle cell	100	99.8
SPHEROCYTE (050)			
79	H-21 Spherocyte	100	96.2
80	H-51 Spherocyte	100	96.3
83	H1-34 Spherocyte	88.9	90.4
83	H1-45 Spherocyte	100	97
85	H1-17 Spherocyte	100	97.7
85	H1-19 Spherocyte	100	94.7
86	XL-07 Spherocyte	100	91.2
87	XL-73 Spherocyte	100	80.2
89	XL-32 Spherocyte	100	82.6
90	XH-32 Spherocyte	100	86.4
92	HE-07 Spherocyte	100	89.1
92	HE-23 Spherocyte	95	92.2
81	A-60 Spherocyte	100	81.2
84	A-8 Spherocyte	100	84.3
85	A-08 Spherocyte	100	90.1
89	A-10 Spherocyte	100	92.6
86	A-63 Spherocyte	100	95.1
87	A-28 Spherocyte	100	97.3
88	A-71 Spherocyte	95	96.1
93	HE-45 Spherocyte	92.5	96.3
94	HE-09 Spherocyte	100	96.5
96	HE-36 Spherocyte	100	98.2

YR	SLIDE IDENTIFICATION	R%	P%
STOMATOCYTE (051)			
80	H-52 Stomatocyte	100	97.4
86	H1-31 Stomatocyte	100	97.4
86	H1-46 Stomatocyte	100	99.2
88	A-29 Stomatocyte	100	98
95	HE-23 Stomatocyte	100	99.1
TARGET CELL (052)			
79	H-8 Target cell	100	99.5
80	H-53 Target cell	100	99.5
81	H-53 Target cell	100	99.4
83	H1-32 Target cell	100	99.5
84	H1-41 Target cell	100	99.1
85	XL-06 Target cell	100	98.6
85	XL-61 Target cell	94.7	99.4
86	XL-62 Target cell	100	99.4
87	XL-28 Target cell	100	99.3
89	XL-60 Target Cell	100	99.1
92	HE-39 Target cell	100	98.8
84	A-46 Target cell	100	92.7
80	A-58 Target cell	100	97.3
89	A-33 Target cell	100	99.3
86	A-62 Target cell	100	99.5
88	A-69 Target cell	100	99.5
85	A-29 Target cell	100	99.6
82	A-65 Target cell	88.9	90.4
93	HE-43 Target cell	100	99.5
97	HE-36 Target cell	100	99.5
TEARDROP CELL (053)			
79	H-7 Teardrop cell	100	99.3
82	A-46 Teardrop cell	100	96.3
83	A-48 Teardrop cell	100	98.7
80	H-50 Teardrop cell	100	99.4
87	XL-49 Teardrop cell	100	99.1
83	A-28 Teardrop cell	100	96.1
85	A-69 Teardrop cell	100	98.2
86	A-26 Teardrop cell	100	98.8
88	A-70 Teardrop cell	95	98.8
87	H1-6 Teardrop RBC	100	99.5
89	XL-62 Teardrop RBC	94.7	95.7
91	HE-28 Teardrop RBC	100	94.3
92	HE-52 Teardrop RBC	90	98.4
89	A-35 Teardrop RBC, hypochromic RBC, (normal/microcytic)	100	98.5
93	HE-10 Teardrop	100	98.5
94	HE-39 Teardrop	96.6	99.5

NUCLEATED RED CELLS IN BONE MARROW
NUCLEATED RED CELL, MEGALOBLASTIC (BONE MARROW) (203); NUCLEATED RED CELL, DYSPLASTIC (BONE MARROW) (183)

YR	SLIDE IDENTIFICATION	R%	P%
96	HE-14 Nucleated red cell, megaloblastic	83.3	59.4
96	HE-47 Nucleated red cell, megaloblastic	88	71.9

PRONORMOBLAST (159)

YR	SLIDE IDENTIFICATION	R%	P%
89	H1-46 Rubriblast, megaloblastic rubriblast/prorubricyte	100	96.7
96	HE-45A Pronormoblast	56	60.5

YR	SLIDE IDENTIFICATION	R%	P%
	BASOPHILIC NORMOBLAST (154)		
79	H-23 Prorubricyte, rubricyte	88.9	80.5
87	H1-41 Prorubricyte	73.7	70.5
92	HE-42 Basophilic normoblast	85	73.6
96	HE-45B Basophilic normoblast	48.8	56.1
96	HE-50 Basophilic normoblast	36	26.1
	POLYCHROMATOPHILIC NORMOBLAST (157)		
78	H-34 Rubricyte, metarubricyte	100	87.5
89	H1-32 Rubricyte, metarubricyte	94.4	87.1
80	H-38 Rubricyte, prorubricyte/ metarubricyte	100	90.7
91	HE-61 Polychromatophilic/ orthochromic NRBC	100	88.5
91	HE-44 Polychromatophilic normoblast	42.1	34.6
92	HE-41 Polychromatophilic normoblast	90	74.3
92	HE-14 Polychromatophilic NRBC	26.3	23.5
	ORTHOCHROMATOPHILIC NORMOBLAST (161)		
79	H-24 Metarubricyte, megaloblastic	100	89.6
77	H-35 Metarubricyte, rubricyte	88.9	93.6
81	H-22 Metarubricyte	100	87.2
81	H-52 Metarubricyte	85.7	94
87	H1-18 Metarubricyte, megalometa- rubricyte, rubricyte, megalorubricyte	100	98.2
87	H1-5 Metarubricyte, rubricyte	89.5	92.7
84	A-48 Metarubricyte, rubricyte	100	90.2
87	A-10 Metarubricyte, rubricyte	95	90.6
85	A-10 Metarubricyte, rubricyte	84.2	81.5
82	A-66 Metarubricyte	100	85.5
82	A-28 Metarubricyte	62.5	64.3
	PRONORMOBLAST, MEGALOBLASTIC (160)		
82	H-6 Megaloblastic rubriblast, rubriblast	100	84.6
81	A-26 Megaloblastic rubriblast	16.7	29.3
82	A-11 Megaloblastic rubriblast	85.7	40.2
	BASOPHILIC NORMOBLAST, MEGALOBLASTIC (155)		
84	H1-34 Megaloblastic prorubricyte, megaloblastic rubriblast	89.5	71.1
92	HE-12 Megaloblastic basophilic normoblast	31.6	21.3
84	H1-33 Megaloblastic prorubricyte, megaloblastic rubricyte	79.0	70.9
	POLYCHROMATOPHILIC NORMOBLAST, MEGALOBLASTIC (158)		
77	H-8 Megaloblastic RBC precursor	90	63.8
84	H1-30 Megaloblastic rubricyte	47.4	38.4
89	H1-47 Megaloblastic rubricyte/ metarubricyte /prorubricyte	100	90.9
81	A-25 Megaloblastic rubricyte	50.0	27.5
	ORTHOCHROMATOPHILIC NORMOBLAST, MEGALOBLASTIC (162)		
82	H-7 Megaloblastic metarubricyte	66.7	49.2
88	A-51 Megaloblastic metarubricyte	45.0	9.3
	SIDEROBLAST, (IRON STAIN) (163)		
79	H-51 Normal sideroblast	85.7	79.4
	SIDEROBLAST, RINGED (IRON STAIN) (164)		
79	H-50 Ringed sideroblast	85.7	93.3
81	H-26 Ringed sideroblast	83.7	81.9
87	H1-44 Ringed sideroblast, sideroblast	100	95.7
90	H1-06 Ringed sideroblast, siderotic granules, sideroblast	100	96
	MEGAKARYOCYTIC CELLS/THROMBOCYTES		
	MEGAKARYOCYTE OR PRECURSOR, NORMAL (072)		
79	H-40 Megakaryoblast	25.0	20.5
77	H-50 Megakaryocyte, any stage	100	96.3
88	H1-31 Megakaryocyte	70.0	49.0
91	HE-63 Megakaryocyte	100	86.2
92	HE-43 Megakaryocyte	100	83.5
91	HE-62 Megakaryocyte (spleen)	100	88.4
89	H1-45 Megakaryocyte, normal/ abnormal	100	94.1
92	HE-44 Megakaryocyte, immature	95	87.7
84	A-67 Megakaryocyte, megakaryoblast	94.7	75.4
	MEGAKARYOCYTE NUCLEUS (115)		
88	H1-30 Megakaryocyte nucleus, megakaryocyte or precursor	95	81.8
95	HE-44 Megakaryocyte nucleus	31.8	33.1
	MEGAKARYOCYTE OR PRECURSOR, ABNORMAL (119)		
91	HE-14 Megakaryocyte, abnormal	47.4	21.8
	PLATELET, NORMAL (073)		
90	H1-22 Platelet	80	67.8
92	HE-58 Platelet	100	96.3
82	H-10 Platelet, normal	100	96.6
82	H-41 Platelet, normal	100	92.3
91	HE-25 Platelet, normal	100	98.8
84	A-68 Platelet, normal	94.7	94.4
84	H1-8 Platelets	93.8	93.9
84	H1-19 Platelets, normal/abnormal	100	91.5
85	XL-07 Normal/giant platelet	100	85.3
94	HE-21 Platelet, normal	100	94.8
94	HE-36 Platelet, normal	100	98.3
97	HE-12 Platelet, normal	100	98.7
97	HE-37 Platelet, normal	100	99.3
97	HE-42 Platelet, normal	100	94.2
	PLATELET, GIANT (166)		
82	H-42 Giant platelet	100	96.3
87	XL-07 Giant platelet	100	92
87	XL-71 Giant platelet	94.4	85.5
91	HE-31 Giant platelet	95	80.6
91	HE-10 Giant platelet, abnormal platelet	100	92.3
91	HE-60 Giant platelet, abnormal platelet	100	96.5
90	XH-04 Giant platelet, abnormal platelet	100	92.8
84	A-66 Giant platelet	100	73.2
87	A-11 Giant platelet	100	98
83	A-69 Giant platelet	91.7	92.1
86	XL-23 Platelet, giant	94.7	85.2
93	HE-09 Platelet, giant	100	98
94	HE-06 Platelet, giant	100	98.7
96	HE-08 Platelet, giant	100	97
	PLATELET, ABNORMAL MORPHOLOGY (165)		
78	H-47 Platelet, abnormal	87.5	80.5

YR	SLIDE IDENTIFICATION	R%	P%
78	H-11 Platelet, abnormal	100	94.9
81	A-40 Platelet, abnormal	100	92.8
88	H1-33 Platelet, abnormal	85	83
87	XL-51 Platelet, abnormal, normal	94.1	96.2

PLATELET, HYPOGRANULAR (188)

YR	SLIDE IDENTIFICATION	R%	P%
95	HE-43 Platelet, hypogranular	62.5	23.3

PLATELET SATELLITISM (167)

YR	SLIDE IDENTIFICATION	R%	P%
93	HE-26 Platelet satellitism	100	96.6

LYMPHOCYTIC/PLASMACYTIC CELLS

HAIRY CELL (083)

YR	SLIDE IDENTIFICATION	R%	P%
80	H-26 Hairy cell	100	86.5
80	H-37 Hairy cell	28.6	21.2
84	H1-42 Hairy cell	100	80.7
84	H1-44 Hairy cell	100	83.6
84	H1-43 Lymphocyte, hairy cell	100	96
97	HE-11 Hairy cell	96.4	80.5

LYMPHOBLAST (060)

YR	SLIDE IDENTIFICATION	R%	P%
82	H-23 Lymphoblast, blast, myeloblast	100	81.9
82	H-24 Lymphoblast, blast, myeloblast	88.9	58
90	AH-06 Lymphoblast, blast	63.2	9.6
90	AH-05 Lymphoblast, blast	85.7	9.9
81	A-58 Lymphoblast, blast	85.7	67.0
82	H-25 Lymphoblast, blast, myeloblast/ monoblast	100	77.7

LYMPHOCYTE (168)

YR	SLIDE IDENTIFICATION	R%	P%
77	H-22 Lymphocyte	88.9	96.3
80	H-24 Lymphocyte	85.7	92
84	H1-45 Lymphocyte	100	87.3
84	H1-9 Lymphocyte	81.3	78.8
85	XL-42 Lymphocyte	100	95.7
87	H1-32 Lymphocyte	84.2	79.6
87	XL-29 Lymphocyte	100	93.6
88	H1-46 Lymphocyte	57.9	66.7
89	H1-44 Lymphocyte	95	92
90	H1-30 Lymphocyte	83.3	94.4
91	HE-45 Lymphocyte	89.5	70.6
86	A-07 Lymphocyte	100	89.3
85	A-49 Lymphocyte	100	90.4
90	AH-07 Lymphocyte	100	95.2
80	A-23 Lymphocyte	71.4	78.5
86	A-44 Lymphocyte	86.7	79.8
83	H1-19 Lymphocyte, normal	100	97.7
86	XL-43 Lymphocyte, normal	100	97.1
83	A-9 Lymphocyte, normal	88.2	74.3
83	A-66 Lymphocyte, normal	91.7	92.3
84	A-28 Lymphocyte, normal	94.4	91.9
91	HE-42 Lymphocyte, prolymphocyte, atypical lymphocyte	100	90.2
93	HE-08 Lymphocyte, normal	100	98.5
93	HE-23 Lymphocyte, normal	96.3	97.3
94	HE-22 Lymphocyte, normal	100	98.7
94	HE-38 Lymphocyte, normal	93	95.1
95	HE-21 Lymphocyte, normal	100	96.9
95	HE-25 Lymphocyte, normal	100	96.9
96	HE-39 Lymphocyte, normal	96.3	84.3
97	HE-13 Lymphocyte, normal	96.4	95.9

LYMPHOCYTE, REACTIVE (169)

YR	SLIDE IDENTIFICATION	R%	P%
78	H-23 Lymphocyte, reactive	37.5	24.5
78	H-35 Lymphocyte, reactive	87.5	93
79	H-9 Lymphocyte, reactive	88.9	82.4
80	H-22 Lymphocyte, reactive	85.7	92.9
83	H1-18 Lymphocyte, reactive	100	95.2
83	H1-20 Lymphocyte, reactive	100	96.3
87	H1-34 Lymphocyte, reactive	84.2	80.2
89	XL-61 Lymphocyte, reactive	89.5	88.4
90	XH-29 Lymphocyte, reactive	100	93.6
91	HE-54 Lymphocyte, reactive	100	98
80	H-21 Lymphocyte, reactive	85.7	95.3
84	A-27 Lymphocyte, reactive	100	87.1
83	A-67 Lymphocyte, reactive	100	91.4
86	A-08 Lymphocyte, reactive	100	95.1
81	A-43 Lymphocyte, reactive	16.7	29.5
83	A-11 Lymphocyte, reactive	82.4	54.2
89	H-14 Lymphocyte, atypical lymphocyte	100	93
89	XL-87 Lymphocyte, atypical lymphocyte	100	96.2
90	AH-14 Lymphocyte, atypical lymphocyte	90	92.1
91	HE-08 Lymphocyte, atypical lymphocyte	100	90.4
82	H-26 Atypical lymphocyte	44.4	14.4
88	XL-S6 Atypical lymphocyte	21.0	36.0
89	XL-88 Atypical lymphocyte	95	86.8
90	AH-29 Atypical lymphocyte	66.7	44.0
85	XL-25 Reactive lymphocyte	50.0	44.2
95	HE-36 Lymphocyte, reactive	100	100
97	HE-41 Lymphocyte, reactive	100	81
97	HE-44 Lymphocyte, reactive	100	74.4

LYMPHOMA CELL (064)

YR	SLIDE IDENTIFICATION	R%	P%
90	H1-47 Lymphoma cell, abnormal lymphocyte, lymphoblast, blast	88.2	82.7
87	H1-42 Abnormal lymphocyte suggestive of CLL or PDLL, lymphocyte	89.4	91.3
89	H1-30 CLL lymphocyte	27.8	18.5
89	H1-33 CLL lymphocyte	16.7	20.5
87	H1-29 Malignant lymphoma cell, lymphoblast, blast	94.7	93.9
87	H1-30 Malignant lymphoma cell, lymphoblast, blast	94.7	89.2
87	H1-31 Malignant lymphoma cell, lymphoblast, blast	94.7	91.2
87	H1-33 Malignant lymphoma cell, lymphoblast, blast	94.7	90.4
97	HE-45 Lymphoma cell, malignant	85.2	63.7

PLASMA CELL, MORPHOLOGY MATURE (126)

YR	SLIDE IDENTIFICATION	R%	P%
77	H-24 Plasma cell, any subtype	100	89.9
89	H1-31 Plasma cell	100	97.2
83	H1-3 Plasma cell or precursor	64.3	82.3
83	H1-7 Plasma cell or precursor	85.7	89.5
83	H1-8 Plasma cell or precursor	100	93
88	H1-22 Plasma cell or precursor	100	94.4
90	H1-33 Plasma cell, any level	100	95.5
90	H1-34 Plasma cell, any level, lymphoblast	94.4	96.8
92	HE-15 Plasma cell, mature	63.2	39.7
80	H-25 Plasma cell, normal/abnormal	100	89

YR	SLIDE IDENTIFICATION	R%	P%
95	HE-28 Plasma cell, morphology mature	96.4	85.4

PLASMA CELL OR PRECURSOR W/INCLUSION BODY (170)

YR	SLIDE IDENTIFICATION	R%	P%
79	H-10 Plasma cell with/without inclusions	100	87.4
86	H1-32 Plasma cell, plasmacyte/inclusions	100	98.1
86	H1-33 Plasma cell, plasmacyte/inclusions	100	98.1
91	HE-15 Plasma cell with inclusion	10.5	9.4
83	H1-6 Plasma cell with inclusions	78.6	71.7
83	A-68 Plasma cell or precursor with inclusion body	83.3	89.4
95	HE-29 Plasma cell or precursor with inclusion body	74.1	56.6

PLASMA CELL, MORPH IMMATURE (127)

YR	SLIDE IDENTIFICATION	R%	P%
83	H1-4 Plasmablast	50.0	45.9
83	H1-5 Plasmablast	21.4	15.9

PROLYMPHOCYTE (133)

YR	SLIDE IDENTIFICATION	R%	P%
77	H-23 Prolymphocyte	55.6	34.3
80	H-23 Prolymphocyte	28.6	54.2
96	HE-28 Prolymphocyte	84.6	56.6

SÉZARY CELL (120)

YR	SLIDE IDENTIFICATION	R%	P%
89	H1-18 Sézary cell, PDLL, lymphoma	95	91
89	H1-20 Sézary cell, PDLL, lymphoma	100	91.6
89	H1-21 Sézary cell, PDLL, lymphoma	100	91.3
96	HE-11 Sézary cell	80	44.8
96	HE-12 Sézary cell	78.6	45.7
97	HE-43 Sézary cell	80	66.6

MICROORGANISMS
BABESIA (185)

YR	SLIDE IDENTIFICATION	R%	P%
96	HE-15 Babesia	30.8	29.7

BACTERIA (COCCI OR ROD), EXTRACELLULAR (171)

YR	SLIDE IDENTIFICATION	R%	P%
85	H1-42 Bacteria	100	98.9

BACTERIA (SPIROCHETE), EXTRACELLULAR (172)

YR	SLIDE IDENTIFICATION	R%	P%
90	H1-19 Spirochetes	100	98.8

FUNGI, EXTRACELLULAR (173)

YR	SLIDE IDENTIFICATION	R%	P%
92	HE-29 Cryptococcus neoformans	100	86.1
92	HE-28 Aspergillus fumigatus	100	97.7
88	A-31 Fungi, bacteria	100	82.8

LEUKOCYTE WITH PHAGOCYTIZED BACTERIA (174)

YR	SLIDE IDENTIFICATION	R%	P%
88	A-28 Leukocyte with phagocytized bacteria	100	86.9
85	H1-41 Leukocyte with bacteria	94.4	90.8

LEUKOCYTE WITH PHAGOCYTIZED FUNGI (134)

YR	SLIDE IDENTIFICATION	R%	P%
96	HE-13 Leukocyte with phagocytized fungi	84.6	56.1

MACROPHAGE WITH PHAGOCYTIZED HISTOPLASMA, LEISHMANIA, OR TOXOPLASMA (175)

YR	SLIDE IDENTIFICATION	R%	P%
79	H-54 Histoplasmosis/macrophage	100	74.0
86	H1-34 Macrophage with phagocytized histoplasma	100	95.6
92	HE-30 Histoplasma capsulatum	100	93.3
92	HE-26 Leishmania donovani	100	91.9

MACROPHAGE WITH PHAGOCTIZED MYCOBACTERIA (175)

YR	SLIDE IDENTIFICATION	R%	P%
92	HE-27 Mycobacterium intracellulare	100	84.5

MALARIA, EXTRACELLULAR (176); INTRACELLULAR (177)

YR	SLIDE IDENTIFICATION	R%	P%
80	H 55 Malaria parasite	100	98
83	H1-49 Malaria parasite	100	88.2
87	H1-45 Malaria parasite	100	99.3
88	XL-28 Malaria parasite	100	95.2

MICROFILARIA (186)

YR	SLIDE IDENTIFICATION	R%	P%
96	HE-21 Microfilaria (Loa loa)	100	95.3
96	HE-22 Microfilaria (Mansonella)	100	95.3

PROTOZOAN (NON-MALARIAL), EXTRACELLULAR (136)

YR	SLIDE IDENTIFICATION	R%	P%
91	HE-39 Protozoan, non-malarial	100	87.8

ARTIFACTS
ARTIFACTUAL RED CELL INCLUSION (096); ERYTHROCYTE WITH OVERLYING PLATELET (182)

YR	SLIDE IDENTIFICATION	R%	P%
89	XL-59 Artifact, RBC inclusion, platelet	100	90.7
88	H1-43 Artifactual RBC inclusion	100	95.6
87	A-48 Platelet, artifactual RBC inclusion	100	85.1
87	A-71 Platelet, artifactual RBC inclusion	100	92.1
88	XL-29 Platelet, artifactual RBC inclusion	94.8	76.9
97	HE-38 Erythrocyte with overlying platelet	100	80.4

BASKET CELL/SMUDGE CELL (094)

YR	SLIDE IDENTIFICATION	R%	P%
84	H1-20 Basket cell	89.5	75.4
85	H1-44 Basket/smudge cell	100	99
89	A-58 Basket/smudge cell	100	98.7
93	HE-25 Basket cell	96.3	92.9

DEGENERATED NEUTROPHIL, SIMULATING NRBC (093)

YR	SLIDE IDENTIFICATION	R%	P%
84	H1-18 Degenerated neutrophil	100	95.7
87	A-09 Degenerated neutrophil, basket cell	100	80.1

STAIN PRECIPITATE (123)

YR	SLIDE IDENTIFICATION	R%	P%
91	HE-40 Stain precipitate	85	85.5
90	H1-18 Stain precipitate, smudge cell	95	91.7
96	HE-25 Stain precipitate	100	96.9

MISCELLANEOUS
ALDER'S ANOMALY INCLUSION (020)

YR	SLIDE IDENTIFICATION	R%	P%
95	HE-14 Alder's anomaly	80.8	61.2

BLAST CELL (076)

YR	SLIDE IDENTIFICATION	R%	P%
78	H-49 Blast, any type	62.5	70.2
88	H1-19 Blast cell, myeloblast	76.5	47.5
81	H-11 Blast, any type	62.5	75.4
82	H-55 Blast, any type	100	89.6
80	H-35 Blast, any type	100	90.5
86	HE-41 Blast cell, myeloblast	100	92.9
86	HE-42 Blast cell, myeloblast	100	91.3
88	HE-32 Blast cell, myeloblast	100	88.9
92	HE-53 Blast cell	100	89.8
94	HE-13 Blast cell	81.5	68.9
95	HE-07 Blast cell	92.8	90.8

YR	SLIDE IDENTIFICATION	R%	P%
CHÉDIAK-HIGASHI ANOMALY INCLUSION (021)			
77	H-36 Chédiak-Higashi anomaly	100	68.0
88	H1-45 Chédiak-Higashi anomaly	94.7	93.6
88	H1-47 Chédiak-Higashi, toxic granulation	89.5	93.5
EPITHELIAL/ENDOTHELIAL CELL (116)			
95	HE-27 Epithelial/endothelial cell	89.3	68.6
96	HE-27 Epithelial/endothelial cell	64	71.7
GAUCHER CELL (081)			
78	H-24 Gaucher, pseudo-Gaucher, histiocyte	87.5	84.3
81	H-40 Gaucher cell	83.3	68.7
87	H1-46 Pseudo-Gaucher cell, Gaucher cell	100	95.9
HISTIOCYTE, SEA BLUE (137)			
95	HE-13 Histiocyte, sea blue	88.5	88.1
97	HE-30 Histiocyte, sea blue	55.6	59.1
LIPOCYTE (ADIPOCYTE, FAT CELL) (138)			
77	H-37 Fat storage cell	88.9	69.3
95	HE-15 Lipocyte (fat cell)	64.3	63.2
MACROPHAGE WITH PHAGOCYTIZED RED CELLS (179)			
82	H-59 Erythrophagocytosis, monocyte	100	94.5
94	HE-15 Macrophage with phagocytized red cells	100	97.1
MACROPHAGE (HISTIOCYTE) (178)			
88	H1-20 Histiocyte, macrophage	100	85.7
97	HE-30 Macrophage (histiocyte)	55.6	59.1
MAST CELL (019)			
77	H-9 Mast cell (tissue basophil)	100	89.8
79	H-12 Mast cell, basophil	88.9	95.9
87	H1-43 Mast cell, mature basophil, immature basophil	100	93.9
82	H-44 May-Hegglin anomaly	100	74.5
97	HE-29 Mast cell (tissue basophil)	96.2	86.3
METASTATIC TUMOR CELL (086)			
77	H-11 Metastatic tumor cells, blasts	90	87.9
88	H1-6 Metastatic tumor cell	52.9	38.3
MITOTIC FIGURE (107)			
87	HI-19 Mitotic figure	100	91.1
91	HE-13 Mitotic figure	94.7	87.2
NIEMANN-PICK CELL (087)			
95	HE-12 Niemann-Pick cell	92.9	57.3
OSTEOBLAST (088)			
79	H-26 Osteoblast	88.9	77.2
88	H1-5 Osteoblast	82.4	65.4
88	H1-7 Osteoblast	76.5	65.1
97	HE-27 Osteoblast	82.1	80.6
OSTEOCLAST (089)			
77	H-10 Osteoclast	90	78.2
79	H-41 Osteoclast	100	91
82	H-60 Osteoclast	77.8	90.9
88	H1-4 Osteoclast	100	91.5
88	H1-8 Osteoclast	76.5	69.8
97	HE-28 Osteoclast	92.9	90.8

Appendix E
CAP Hematology Proficieny Testing Challenges Listed by Year

Laboratories that have participated in the CAP Comprehensive Surveys will find a complete listing below of the clinical histories for the challenges used in these Surveys from 1989-1997.

1989

H1-4-8, Hemoglobin H disease
These peripheral blood photomicrographs are from a 52-year-old Filipino woman, hospitalized for replacement of previous mitral and aortic prosthetic valves with porcine xenografts. Her CBC included the following: WBC = 4.9 X 10^9/L, RBC = 4.15 X 10^{12}/L, HGB = 8.9 g/dL, HCT = 30.4%, MCV = 73 fL, MCH = 21.4 pg, MCHC = 29.3%, and RDW = 20.1%. Slides H1-4 and H1-5 are stained with conventional Wright's stain; slide H1-6 is stained with brilliant cresyl blue (BCB) for 10 minutes; slides H1-7 and H1-8 are stained with BCB for 2 hours.

H1-18-22, Sézary syndrome
These peripheral blood photomicrographs are from a 56-year-old man with a four-year history of generalized exfoliative dermatitis involving large areas of his trunk. His CBC included the following: WBC = 12.5 X 10^9/L, HGB = 13.4 g/dL, HCT = 40.1% and PLT = 256 X 10^9/L.

H1-29-33, Cryoglobulinemia
Peripheral blood and bone marrow photomicrographs from this same patient are presented as part of the interpretive challenge in this Survey mailing (slides H-34, 35, 36). Please see the interpretive challenge for the patient history and other pertinent lab data.

H1-34-36, (Interpretive challenge)
There are no arrows on these slides.

H1-43-47, Vitamin B_{12} deficiency
These peripheral blood and bone marrow photomicrographs are from a 29-year-old Iranian-American woman with a two-year history of ataxia, lower extremity weakness and spasticity, and sensory abnormalities. Although no specific etiology could be identified in her previous hospitalization or outpatient visits, she was thought to have early multiple sclerosis. The current hospital admission was due to several months' worsening of leg weakness and development of personality changes, including increased emotional lability and irritability. Her CBC included the following: WBC = 3.7 X 10^9/L, RBC = 1.86 X 10^{12}/L, HGB = 8.0 g/dL, HCT = 23.3%, MCV = 125 fL, MCH = 43.0 pg, MCHC = 34.3%, PLT = 347 X 10^9/L and RDW = 21.6%.

XL-4-7, Mycosis fungoides
These peripheral blood photomicrographs are from a 56-year-old man with a four-year history of generalized exfoliative dermatitis involving large areas of his trunk. His CBC included the following: WBC = 12.5 X 10^9/L, HGB = 13.4 g/dL, HCT = 40.1% and PLT = 256 X 10^9/L.

XL-31-34 (also A-9-12), ABO hemolytic disease of newborn
These peripheral blood photomicrographs are from an 8 pound, 11 ounce term baby who was noted to be icteric. Partial CBC data included: HGB = 7.9 g/dL and MCV = 110 fL.

XL-59-62 (also A-32-35), Thalassemia trait
These peripheral blood smear photomicrographs are from a 32-year-old black female under treatment for a chronic psychiatric disorder. She was hospitalized because of increasing agitation and a 15-pound weight loss. Her CBC included the following: WBC = 5.2 X 10^9/L, RBC = 5.02 X 10^{12}/L, HGB = 10.2 g/dL, HCT = 31.9%, MCV = 63 fL, MCH = 20.3 pg, MCHC = 32.0%, and RDW = 16.4%.

XL-86-89 (also A-55-58), Infectious mononucleosis
These peripheral blood photomicrographs are from a 19-year-old white female who presented with fever (101°F), sore throat, malaise, and generalized weakness for the past nine days. On physical examination, she had mild but tender cervical lymphadenopathy. Her CBC included the following: WBC = 15.2 X 10^9/L, HGB = 14.1 g/dL, HCT = 44.0%, MCV = 87 fL, and PLT = 223 X 10^9/L.

A-77-80, Cold autoagglutinins
These peripheral blood photomicrographs are from a 64-year-old woman whose initial routine CBC yielded the following data: WBC = 16.1 X 10^9/L, RBC = 0.12 X 10^{12}/L, HGB = 8.4 g/dL, HCT = 19.7%, MCV = 164 fL, MCH = 70.0 pg, MCHC = 42.6%, and PLT = 427 X 10^9/L. Slide A-77 is a split-screen photomicrograph of unstained wet mounts with room temperature blood in the left panel and warmed blood in the right panel; slides A-78 to A-80 are Wright's stained peripheral blood smears, with A-78 being a split-screen similar to A-77 (room temperature blood on the left and warmed blood on the right).

1990

H1-04-08, Hereditary sideroblastic anemia
See interpretive challenge H1-09-11 for complete history.

H1-09-11, (Interpretive challenge)
An asymptomatic 47-year-old man was examined in September 1987 following a previous diagnosis of thalassemia with iron overloading. Peripheral blood and bone marrow photomicrographs from 1987 are shown as slides H1-04, 05, 06, and 09; histograms from a Coulter counter and Geometric Data Hematrak are printed.

In 1975, a CBC had shown slight anemia (HGB = 12.0 g/dL) with microcytosis (MCV = 65 fL). He had never been transfused. His mother was of Greek ancestry. She, her sister, and several maternal male first cousins had microcytosis, with MCVs ranging from 65-77 fL, but none was anemic. A paternal uncle and his daughter (both of whom were alcoholics) had died of complications of Laennec's cirrhosis. There was no family history of hemochromatosis. The printed genetic pedigree diagram displays the family's blood HGB concentrations and MCVs.

On examination, he was found to have moderate splenomegaly, anemia, microcytosis, and markedly elevated serum ferritin. Liver biopsy in 1987 showed the changes seen in slide H1-10 (hematoxylin and eosin) and slide H1-11 (iron stain). Laboratory data at that time included: RBC = 5.14 X 10^{12}/L, HGB = 11.0 g/dL, HCT = 34.0%, MCV = 67 fL, reticulocytes = 2.1%, ferritin = 3290 ng/mL, normal hemoglobin electrophoresis, 2.9% HGB-A2, 0.8% HGB-F.

Treatment was prescribed and a program of weekly phlebotomies was begun.

He was seen again two years later (1989). Peripheral blood photographs from 1989 are shown as slides H1-07 and 08, while histo/cytograms from a Coulter S+IV and Technicon H-1 are printed. His 1989 CBC on two different Coulters and a Technicon was as follows:

	S+IV	STKR	H-1	Units
WBC	4.9	4.7	4.28	X 10^9/L
RBC	5.40	5.46	5.49	X 10^{12}/L
HGB	13.1	13.3	13.3	g/dL
HCT	40.7	40.1	41.6	vol %
MCV	75.3	73.5	75.8	fL
MCH	24.3	24.4	24.3	pg
MCHC	32.2	33.1	32.0	g/dL
RDW	22.3	21.3	20.2	%
HDW	—	—	3.19	g/dL
PLT	165	163	138 SR	X 10^9/L
MPV	9.6	9.7	8.9	fL
LYMP	30.0	30.8	27.2	%
MONO	23.5 RM	11.6	7.5	%
GRAN	46.5 RM	57.6	—	%
NEUT	—	—	60.5	%
EOSI	—	—	2.4	%
BASO	—	—	0.7	%
LUC	—	—	1.6	%
LI	—	—	2.21	-
MPXI	—	—	-2.0	-

Using all information from the history, the photomicrographs, and the CBC particle histo/cytograms, select the best answer(s) for each of the following questions:

1. The one diagnosis that best explains the history and laboratory data is (select one only)
    A. congenital atransferrinemia.
    B. beta-thalassemia trait.
    C. alpha-thalassemia trait.
    D. hereditary sideroblastic anemia.
    E. myelodysplastic disorder (refractory anemia with ringed sideroblasts).

2. This disorder is most likely the result of (select one only)
    A. defective iron transport to erythroblasts.
    B. excess oral iron intake, as in food and alcoholic beverages.
    C. a defect in heme synthesis.
    D. accelerated hemoglobin degradation.
    E. a primary inability of the intestinal mucosa to block the absorption of iron.

3. The genetic lesion responsible for this disorder is (select one only)
    A. partial deletion of a portion of chromosome 16.
    B. a mutation in the promoter region 5' to the first intron of a globin gene.
    C. a defect involving either monosomy or partial deletion of chromosome 5.
    D. an inherited mutation of a portion of the X chromosome.
    E. a point mutation of chromosome 6 near the major histocompatibility locus.

4. The diagnosis should be confirmed by (select one only)
    A. the data provided and the response to therapy.
    B. assay of delta-aminolevulinic acid synthetase.
    C. assay of ferrochelatase (heme synthetase).
    D. assay of serum transferrin receptor.
    E. cytogenetic analysis.
    F. DNA probe (Southern blot) analysis.

5. If the condition is untreated, complications that may develop include (select one or more)
    A. bleeding due to severe thrombocytopenia.
    B. hyperglycemia.
    C. bleeding from esophageal varices.
    D. cancer of the liver.
    E. transition to acute leukemia.

H1-18-22 ; AH-12-15, Borrelia
These peripheral blood photomicrographs are from a 58-year-old female admitted with fever, chills and weakness developing over two weeks. Her counts were: WBC = 27.8 X 10^9/L and HCT = 26.5%. Three years ago, she vacationed in South Africa without malarial prophylaxis, but had no fever or history of malaria. One month ago, she visited friends in the Tehachapi mountains (elevation 6000 ft).

H1-30-34, Plasma cell leukemia
See the combined histogram/interpretive challenge for complete clinical history and related laboratory data.

H1-35-37, (Interpretive challenge)
A 78-year-old white man was admitted to hospital with disorientation, somnolence, and fever. A chest radiograph demonstrated lung infiltrates consistent with both acute bronchopneumonia and pulmonary congestion, with slight cardiomegaly. Significant hematologic data included WBC = 17.0 X 10^9/L, HGB = 8.9 g/dL, HCT = 29%, MCV = 95 fL, MCHC = 36%, PLT = 91 X 10^9/L, reticulocytes = 0.4% (uncorrected). CBC particle histograms are shown for the Technicon H-1 and the Coulter S+IV. Slide H1-35 is a high-power electron micrograph; slide H1-36 shows this patient's serum and urine protein electrophoresis and urine immunofixation electrophoresis; slide H1-37 is a bone marrow biopsy immunoperoxidase preparation reacted for immunoglobulin kappa light chains.

Using all information provided, please select the single best answer from the following questions:

1. The differential diagnoses for the findings on the Technicon H-1 patterns could include all of the following EXCEPT
    • acute lymphocytic leukemia.
    • plasma cell leukemia.
    • acute myelogenous leukemia without differentiation.
    • infectious mononucleosis.
    • acute stem cell leukemia.

2. The WBC patterns on the Coulter S+IV histogram could be explained by all of the following cells EXCEPT
   - atypical lymphocytes.
   - abundant normoblasts.
   - immature granulocytes.
   - blasts.
   - eosinophils.

3. Considering the probable diagnosis in this case, one should expect survival to be
   - relatively short (0-12 months).
   - 3-4 years before "blast crisis" occurs and leads rapidly to death.
   - 10-15 years.
   - greater than 15 years.
   - perfectly normal, as this process is completely benign with complete recovery within 2-6 weeks.

4. An expected laboratory finding in this patient would be
   - positive heterophile antibody test.
   - low leukocyte alkaline phosphatase score.
   - monoclonal cytoplasmic kappa immunoperoxidase staining.
   - cells positive for tartrate-resistant acid phosphatase.
   - coagulation test evidence for disseminated intravascular coagulation (DIC).

5. Slide H1-35 is an electron micrograph of the characteristic cell in this hematologic process. The principal cytoplasmic organelle demonstrated is
   - mitochondria.
   - lysosomes.
   - rough endoplasmic reticulum.
   - Auer rods.
   - viral particles.

6. Based on the serum/urine protein electrophoresis and immunofixation electrophoresis patterns (slide H1-36), one could conclude that
   - a monoclonal protein is not present.
   - the findings are non-diagnostic.
   - a polyclonal gammopathy is present, indicating a reactive peripheral blood process.
   - a monoclonal process is seen in the urine only.
   - monoclonal bands are seen in both the blood and urine.

7. Findings in the peripheral blood raise several possible diagnoses listed below. Which is most likely?
   - Plasma cell leukemia
   - Infectious mononucleosis
   - Rheumatoid arthritis
   - Acute prolymphocytic leukemia
   - Acute lymphocytic leukemia (FAB-L3)

H1-44-48, Peripheralized diffuse lymphoma
The patient is a 60-year-old man with a previous diagnosis of lymphoma who is now hospitalized with progressive anemia, thrombocytopenia, and renal failure. CBC data included: WBC = 11.5 X 10^9/L, RBC = 3.00 X 10^{12}/L, HGB = 9.5 g/dL, HCT = 27.9%, MCV = 93 fL, MCH = 31.7 pg, MCHC = 34.1 g/dL and PLT = 108 X 10^9/L.

XH-04-07
These peripheral blood photomicrographs are from an 83-year-old male with renal failure. His CBC data included: WBC = 25.3 X 10^9/L, RBC = 2.74 X 10^{12}/L, HGB = 8.8 g/dL, HCT = 27%, PLT = 53 X 10^9/L. Serum protein electrophoresis revealed a polyclonal increase in gamma globulin.

XH-12-15, TTP
These peripheral blood photomicrographs are from a 63-year-old man with chronic cough and a pulmonary infiltrate on chest x-ray. His CBC data included WBC – 12.3 X 10^9/L, RBC = 2.80 X 10^{12}/L, HGB = 8.1 g/dL, HCT = 26.0%, PLT = 12 X 10^9/L.

XH-21-24; AH-19-22, Hereditary elliptocytosis
These peripheral blood photomicrographs are from a 32-year-old male seen in a pre-employment physical; slides XH-21 and XH-22 are from that time. Three years later he suffered major trauma in a motorcycle accident. After extensive abdominal surgery, he recovered. Slides XH-23 and XH-24 are his most recent peripheral blood smears.

XH-29-32, Autoimmune hemolytic anemia
These peripheral blood photomicrographs are from a 37-year-old female who developed pallor, weakness, and icteric sclerae over the past two weeks. CBC data included WBC = 7.8 X 10^9/L, HGB = 7.0 g/dL, HCT = 20.0% and PLT = 350 X 10^9/L. Her reticulocytes = 8% and the direct antiglobulin (Coombs) test was positive.

AH-04-07, ALL
These peripheral blood photomicrographs are from an 84-year-old woman who presented with weakness and easy fatigue. Her CBC included WBC = 12.5 X 10^9/L, RBC = 2.60 X 10^{12}/L, HGB = 7.6 g/dL, HCT = 21.0%, PLT = 12 X 10^9/L.

AH-26-29, Liver failure
These peripheral blood photomicrographs are from a 49-year-old stable alcoholic with a moderate anemia (HGB = 10.1 g/dL). He was hospitalized with deepening jaundice, increasing splenomegaly, and a sudden drop in HGB to 7.0 g/dL.

1991

HE-06-10; XH-04-07, Sickle trait/thalassemia
These peripheral blood photomicrographs are from a 28-year-old black female with alleged iron deficiency anemia and sickle cell trait. CBC results included: WBC = 5.6 X 10^9/L, RBC = 4.59 X 10^{12}/L, HGB = 9.9 g/dL, HCT = 30.7%, MCV = 67 fL, MCH = 21.6 pg, MCHC = 32.3 g/dL, RDW = 14.2% (11.5-14.7), PLT = 371 X 10^9/L, MPV = 10 fL. Hemoglobinopathy evaluation showed the following distribution of HGB types: A = 67.5%, S = 28.4%, A2 = 4.1%.

HE-11-15, Myelodysplasia – RAEB
These bone marrow photomicrographs are from a 60-year-old white male with chronic respiratory disease. He was found to have mild anemia (HGB = 10.5 g/dL), thrombocytopenia (PLT = 95 X 10^9/L) and severe leukopenia (WBC = 2.1 X 10^9/L). The peripheral blood WBC differential consisted of 6% myeloblasts, 2% myelocytes, 8% band neutrophils, 20% segmented neutrophils, 14% lymphocytes, and 50% monocytes. The marrow photomicrographs are from this admission. A few months later, he re-presented with worsening anemia (HGB = 8.5 g/dL), thrombocytopenia (PLT = 50 X 10^9/L), and a higher WBC count (6.5 X 10^9/L) with 32% blasts in his peripheral differential.

HE-22-26 ; XH-12-15, Sickle trait
These blood photomicrographs are from a 24-year-old woman who is her first trimester of pregnancy. She has a positive sickle hemoglobin screen. CBC data include WBC = 10.4×10^9/L, RBC = 3.88×10^{12}/L, HGB = 11.7 g/dL, HCT = 34.6%, MCV = 89 fL, MCH = 30.2 pg, MCHC = 33.8 g/dL, RDW = 13.9%, and PLT = 204×10^9/L.

HE-27-31; XH-21-24, Agnogenic myeloid metaplasia
These blood photomicrographs are from a 73-year-old man with splenomegaly. He reports a 30-pound weight loss in the last 6 months. CBC data include WBC = 7.0×10^9/L, RBC = 3.01×10^{12}/L, HGB = 8.5 g/dL, HCT = 26.0%, MCV = 86 fL, MCH = 28.2 pg, MCHC = 32.6 g/dL, RDW = 16.9% and PLT = 76×10^9/L.

HE-38-42, Trypanosomiasis
One week after returning to the U.S. from an African safari, this 39-year-old man developed fevers, chills, and lymphadenopathy. CBC data included WBC = 9.0×10^9/L, HGB = 14.8 g/dL, and PLT = 87×10^9/L. Serum lysozyme was elevated.

HE-43-47, Chronic myelomonocytic leukemia
These photomicrographs are from a 62-year-old man who was admitted to the hospital with pneumonia and hepatosplenomegaly. CBC data included WBC = 9.0×10^9/L, HGB = 10.2 g/dL, and PLT = 85×10^9/L. His serum lysozyme was elevated. Slide HE-43 is of peripheral blood, while the remainder are from bone marrow. All are Wright-stained, except for HE-47, which is a combined nonspecific esterase with fluoride and chloracetate esterase.

HE-54-58; XH-29-32, Rebound leukoerythroblastosis
These peripheral blood photomicrographs are from a 24-year-old man with testicular embryonal cell carcinoma. He is presently undergoing multiple cycles of chemotherapy. CBC data include: WBC = 12.2×10^9/L, RBC = 5.32×10^{12}/L, HGB = 14.2 g/dL, HCT = 41.9%, RDW = 13.3% and PLT = 436×10^9/L.

HE-59-63, Polycythemia rubra vera
These peripheral blood and bone marrow photomicrographs are from a 69-year-old man with a history of gout and gastric ulcer. Pertinent laboratory studies included WBC = 19.0×10^9/L, HGB = 20.4 g/dL, HCT = 63%, MCV = 68 fl, PLT = 610×10^9/L, leukocyte alkaline phosphatase score = 200, and serum uric acid = 10.1 mg/dL. His liver-spleen nuclear scan showed moderate hepatosplenomegaly.

1992
HE-06-10; XH-03-06, Hemolytic uremic syndrome
These blood photomicrographs are from a 4-year-old white female taken to her pediatrician because of fever, vomiting, and left upper quadrant abdominal pain for three days. On physical examination, she appeared pale, irritable, and anxious. Her temperature was 40°C, there was tenderness at the left costovertebral angle, with guarding and tenderness at the left upper quadrant. Her CBC data included: WBC = 23.5×10^9/L, RBC = 2.05×10^{12}/L, HGB = 5.9 g/dL, HCT = 16.7%, MCV = 81 fL, and PLT = 53×10^9/L. Her absolute reticulocyte concentration was 0.075×10^{12}/L. Serum chemistry data were: BUN = 192 mg/dL, creatinine = 4.1 mg/dL, bilirubin = 0.6/0.2 mg/dL (total/direct). Urinalysis was remarkable for 3+ dipstick proteinuria and sediment microscopy showing 1-3 WBC/hpf, 100 RBC/hpf, 4-10 hyaline casts/lpf, 1-3 granular casts/lpf and 1-3 waxy casts/lpf.

HE-11-15, Myelodysplasia – RAEB
These bone marrow photomicrographs are from a 60-year-old white male with chronic respiratory disease. He was found to have mild anemia (HGB = 10.5 g/dL), thrombocytopenia (PLT = 95×10^9/L), and severe leukopenia (WBC = 2.1×10^9/L). The peripheral blood WBC differential consisted of 6% myeloblasts, 2% myelocytes, 8% band neutrophils, 20% segmented neutrophils, 14% lymphocytes, and 50% monocytes. The marrow photomicrographs are from this admission. A few months later, he re-presented with worsening anemia (HGB = 8.5 g/dL), thrombocytopenia (PLT = 50×10^9/L), and a higher WBC count (6.5×10^9/L) with 32% blasts in his peripheral differential.

HE-21-25; XH-11-14, Hereditary spherocytosis
These blood photomicrographs are from a 32-year-old white male seen for evaluation of dyspnea, cough, and fever after exposure to nitric acid fumes. He was previously asymptomatic. There is a family history of anemia, and some relatives had been splenectomized. His CBC data were: WBC = 4.2×10^9/L, RBC = 3.70×10^{12}/L, HGB = 12.6 g/dL, HCT = 35.3%, MCV = 95 fL, and PLT = 211×10^9/L. His serum bilirubin results were 1.6 mg/dL (total) and 1.2 mg/dL (direct).

HE-26-30, Deep marrow infections
Each of these bone marrow photomicrographs is from a different patient. Clinical histories and stains are as follows:

HE-26, Leishmaniasis
A 37-year-old Venezuelan male was admitted for fever of unknown origin, persistent nonproductive cough, and a few episodes of shaking, chills, and drenching night sweats. He experienced malaise, anorexia, and had lost 20 pounds in the preceding month. Members of his family noted a diffuse grayish discoloration of his skin. On physical examination, he was a tense, anxious individual with diffuse skin hyperpigmentation, but no other cutaneous abnormalities. He had a mild fever with tachycardia. He showed slight generalized lymphadenopathy and scleral icterus. There was marked hepatosplenomegaly, with the liver palpable 6 cm below the right costal margin and the spleen palpable 11 cm below the left costal margin. Significant laboratory data included: WBC = 3.2×10^9/L, HCT = 25.0%, MCV = 103 fL, PLT = 103×10^9/L, reticulocytes = 0.210×10^{12}/L, bilirubin (total/direct) = 4.2/0.8 mg/dL, ALT = 112 IU/L, AST = 85 IU/L, alkaline phosphatase = 350 IU/L, negative direct antiglobulin test. His blood WBC differential consisted of 59% segmented neutrophils, 10% band neutrophils, 21% lymphocytes, and 10% monocytes. Wright-Giemsa stain.

HE-27, AIDS with atypical mycobacteria infection
A 29-year-old man was seen for fever of unknown origin and an involuntary 25-pound weight loss in the preceding three months. On physical examination he was an apprehensive, markedly undernourished white male with a temperature of 38°C. There were a few bluish 1 cm nodules on his hard palate, and there was generalized lymphadenopa-

thy. There were crepitant rales over all lung areas. Both liver and spleen were enlarged to 2 cm below the costal margins. There were several indurated, irregular, purplish-red cutaneous nodules over both lower legs. His CBC data were: WBC = 2.8 X 10^9/L, RBC = 4.80 X 10^{12}/L, HGB = 11.9 g/dL, HCT = 37.0%, MCV = 77 fL, and PLT = 157 X 10^9/L. The blood WBC differential consisted of 84% segmented neutrophils, 8% band neutrophils, 4% lymphocytes, and 4% monocytes. Panel A = fluorescent auramine-rhodamine 200X; panel B = Wright-Giemsa, 260X; panel C = Kinyoun's acid-fast, 186X.

HE-28, Aspergillosis
The patient is a 50-year-old woman with poorly controlled diabetes and long-standing ulceration of her feet. Conservative therapy failed and she underwent amputation of several toes. This histologic section is from a phalangeal bone. Periodic acid Schiff and metanil yellow stain.

HE-29, AIDS with crytococcosis
A 58-year-old woman was admitted to hospital because of recent onset of fever, chills, and generalized headache. Three months earlier, a diagnosis had been made of cranial arteritis, subsequent to which had taken 20 mg prednisone/day. On physical examination, she was a lethargic white woman with a temperature of 39°C and a pulse of 100 bpm. There was mild nuchal rigidity, but the remainder of the physical and neurologic examinations were unremarkable. Her CBC data were: WBC = 3.0 X 10^9/L, RBC = 3.97 X 10^{12}/L, HGB = 11.0 g/dL, HCT = 33.0%, MCV = 83 fL, and PLT = 113 X 10^9/L. The blood WBC differential consisted of 84% segmented neutrophils, 5% band neutrophils, 4% lymphocytes, and 7% monocytes. Lumbar puncture revealed a slightly elevated opening pressure, protein = 68 mg/dL, 3 lymphocytes/µL and no organisms were noted in the CSF. The marrow was examined because of pancytopenia. Wright-Giemsa.

HE-30, Histoplasmosis
A 49-year-old white male farmer from Iowa was hospitalized for fever, cough and weight loss, occurring over one month and unresponsive to treatment with cephalosporins. His temperature was 39°C, and his pulse was 118 bpm. Cervical and axillary lymph nodes were enlarged. There were crepitant rales over all areas of both lung. His spleen was palpable 1 cm below the left costal margin. Chest x-ray showed diffuse patchy infiltrates. His CBC data were: WBC = 2.9 X 10^9/L, RBC = 4.40 X 10^{12}/L, HGB = 12.2 g/dL, HCT = 37.0%, MCV = 84 fL, and PLT = 129 X 10^9/L. The blood WBC differential consisted of 49% segmented neutrophils, 9% band neutrophils, 23% lymphocytes, and 19% monocytes. Panel A = silver chromate and eosin, 170X; panel B = Wright-Giemsa, 400X.

HE-36-40, ITP
These four blood and one bone marrow aspirate photomicrographs are from a 32-year-old woman with a history of scleroderma, chronic esophagitis, and Raynaud's syndrome. She is currently being treated with omeprazole. Four days prior to hospital admission, she had an upper respiratory infection with sore throat, cough, and myalgias. Her CBC data were: WBC = 6.1 X 10^9/L, RBC = 3.90 X 10^{12}/L, HGB = 11.0 g/dL, HCT = 33.7%, MCV = 86 fL, RDW = 14.1%, and PLT = 3 X 10^9/L.

HE-41-45, ITP
These bone marrow aspirate photomicrographs are from the same patient described for slides HE-36 through HE-40. Select the single best answer to the following supplementary questions:

1. Considering all of the photomicrographs, the most likely principal diagnosis is
   a. acute leukemia
   b. immune thrombocytopenic purpura
   c. viral- or drug-induced marrow hypoplasia
   d. Heinz-body hemolytic anemia
   e. myelodysplastic syndrome

2. In addition to the principal diagnosis, the morphology suggests
   a. hemoglobinopathy
   b. liver disease
   c. hereditary spherocytosis
   d. splenectomy
   e. microangiopathic hemolysis

HE-51-55; XH-27-30, Myelofibrosis
These blood photomicrographs are from a 76-year-old man who was admitted to hospital for an upper GI bleed. He experienced hematemesis and melena for one week. In addition, he has a four-year history of a chronic blood disease. He now has massive splenomegaly and is transfusion-dependent. His CBC data include: WBC = 32.5 X 10^9/L, HGB = 10.7 g/dL, HCT = 31.6%, and PLT = 61 X 10^9/L.

HE-56-60, Hb S/alpha-thalassemia
These blood photomicrographs are from a 28-year-old black female with alleged iron deficiency anemia and sickle cell trait. CBC results included: WBC = 5.6 X 10^9/L, RBC = 4.59 X 10^{12}/L, HGB = 9.9 g/dL, HCT = 30.7%, MCV = 67 fL, RDW = 14.2%, and PLT = 371 X 10^9/L. Hemoglobinopathy evaluation showed the following distribution of HGB types: A = 67.5%, S = 28.4%, A2 = 4.1%.

1993

HE-06-10; XH-06-10, Myeloproliferative disorder
These blood photomicrographs are from an 87-year-old white male who presented in 1986 with fatigue. His CBC data included: WBC = 14.0 X 10^9/L, RBC = 5.67 X 10^{12}/L, HCT = 41.0%, MCV = 73 fL, and PLT = 1,100 X 10^9/L. He was treated with intravenous P32, which resulted in normalization of the RBC concentration and reduction of the PLT concentration. Wright-Giemsa stain, 400X.

HE-22–26; XH-16–20, Platelet satellitism
These blood smear photomicrographs are from a 45-year-old woman admitted to the hospital for elective surgery. Laboratory data included: WBC = 8.8 X 10^9/L; RBC = 4.57 X 10^{12}/L; HGB = 14.0 g/dL; HCT = 40%; MCV = 87.5 fL; PLT = 163 X 10^9/L. Wright-Giemsa stain, 320X.

HE-38–42; XH 26-30, Hb SC disease
These blood photomicrographs are from a 26-year-old black, pregnant woman, known to be anemic since early childhood. She was admitted to the hospital for pain in the joints, long bones, chest, and abdomen. The patient was noted to have mild splenomegaly, but hepatomegaly and lymphadenopathy were absent. CBC data included: WBC = 12.1 X 10^9/L; RBC = 3.41 X 10^{12}/L; HGB = 11.0 g/dL; HCT =

31.1%; MCV = 91 fL; PLT = 158 X 10⁹/L. Wright-Giemsa stain. 500X.

HE-43–45, Hb SC disease
These blood smear photomicrographs are from a 25-year-old black woman in the second trimester of pregnancy. Laboratory data includes: WBC = 10.2 X 10^9/L; RBC = 4.58 X 10^{12}/L; HGB = 11.2 g/dL; HCT = 33.7%; MCV = 74 fL; RDW = 13.0 (normal: <14.5); PLT = 240 X 10^9/L. Wright-Giemsa stain, 320X.

Hemoglobin electrophoresis results on cellulose acetate (alkaline) and citrate agar (acid) were provided. The most likely diagnosis for this patient is:

A. Hemoglobin G Philadelphia trait
B. Hemoglobin S trait
C. Hemoglobin S homozygous
D. Hemoglobin S/beta-thalassemia
E. Hemoglobin S/G Philadelphia
F. Hemoglobin C trait
G. Hemoglobin C homozygous
H. Hemoglobin C/beta-thalassemia
I. Hemoglobin S/C
J. Hemoglobin E trait
K. Hemoglobin E/beta-thalassemia
L. Hemoglobin S/E

H-06–10 (AAP), Hereditary spherocytosis
The patient is a 4-year-old female, presenting to your office for the first time for a school physical examination. The mother and child voice no complaints. On examination you note an easily palpable spleen. On further questioning, the mother notes that the patient sometimes has a yellow coloring. A complete blood cell count reveals: WBC = 12.5 X 10^9/L; HGB = 10.5 g/dL; HCT = 28%; MCV = 77 fL; PLT = 450 X 10^9/L. Wright-Giemsa stain, 330X.

H-16–20 (AAP), Infectious mononucleosis
The patient is a 13-year-old boy who presents with headache, fever, and sore throat. Examinations reveals cervical lymphadenopathy and a palpable spleen. In addition, the tonsils are enlarged with a thick, white exudate, and palatal petechiae are present. A complete blood count demonstrates: WBC = 10.1 X 10^9/L; HGB = 13.6 g/dL; HCT = 42%; MCV = 81 fL; PLT = 201 X 10^9/L. Wright-Giemsa stain, 330X.

H-26–30 (AAP), Thalassemia trait
These blood smear photomicrographs are from an 18-month-old female who presented to the emergency room with fever and ear pain. Examination revealed a pale, chubby female with an acute right otitis. Because she was pale, a complete blood count was obtained, which demonstrated: WBC = 21.3 X 10^9/L; HGB = 8.9 g/dL; HCT = 28%; MCV = 63 fL; PLT = 514 X 10^9/L.

1994

HE-06–15; XH-06–11, Myeloproliferative disorder (AMM)
A 60-year-old-woman was evaluated for weakness and vague left upper quadrant pain. Physical examination revealed mild hepatomegaly, moderate splenomegaly but no lymphadenopathy. She had a WBC = 30.0 X 10^9/L; HGB = 9.5 g/dL, and PLT = 450 X 10^9/L. Wright-Giemsa stain, 400X.

H-06–11 (AAP), Homozygous beta-thalassemia
The patient is a 2-year-old white male who presents to the emergency room with a fever and sore throat. In addition to exudate on his tonsils, the physical examination reveals that he is pale and has significant hepatosplenomegaly. The mother relates that he has a chronic anemia that has required transfusions. A complete blood count reveals: WBC = 18.5 X 10^9/L; HGB = 7.1 g/dL; HCT = 21%; MCV = 63 fL, and PLT = 465 X 109/L. Wright-Giemsa stain, 330X.

HE-21–25; H-17–22, Sickle cell anemia
The patient is a 5-month-old black infant who presents to the emergency room with lethargy and irritability. On examination, there is tachycardia, thready pulses, and a large tender spleen. WBC = 8.1 X 10^9/L; HGB = 4.8 g/dL; HCT = 18%; MCV = 78 fL; and PLT = 101 X 10^9/L. Wright-Giemsa stain, 330X.

XH-17–22, Sickle cell anemia
The patient is a 20-year-old black male who presents to your office with leg pain and fatigue. On examination there is tachycardia, mild icterus, and mild hepatomegaly. WBC = 8.1 X 10^9/L; HGB = 6.5 g/dL; and PLT = 201 X 10^9/L. Wright-Giemsa stain, 330X.

HE-26–30, CML in blast crisis
The patient is a 56-year-old woman with a two-year history of chronic myelogenous leukemia (CML). She presents with worsening anemia and thrombocytopenia, as well as weight loss and increased splenomegaly. Laboratory data includes: WBC = 127.8 X 10^9/L; HGB = 8.3 g/dL, and PLT = 14 X 10^9/L. Wright-Giemsa stain, 400X.

HE-36–45, B_{12} deficiency, partially treated
The patient is an 83-year-old woman with a history of increasing dementia and confusion. She was seen by her physician after a fall and was noted to be profoundedly anemic. WBC = 3.7 X 10^9/L; HGB = 5.0 g/dL; MCV = 132 fL; and PLT = 110 X 10^9/L. She refused blood transfusion and was treated with daily injections of vitamin B_{12} for one week. The illustrated blood smear is on day six of treatment. Laboratory data at that time included: WBC = 6.7 X 10^9/L; HGB = 9.2 g/dL; MCV = 110 fL; RDW = 32.0; and PLT = 199 X 10^9/L.

Slide HE-41 is included to show a low power view of the blood smear. Wright-Giemsa, HE-41: 160X; all other slides: 400X).

XH-28–33, B_{12} deficiency, partially treated
The patient is an 83-year-old woman with a history of increasing dementia and confusion. She was seen by her primary care physician after a fall and was noted to be profoundedly anemic. WBC = 3.7 X 10^9/L; HGB = 8.2 g/dL; MCV = 132 fL; and PLT = 110 X 10^9/L. She refused blood transfusion and was treated with daily injections of vitamin B_{12} for one week. The illustrated blood smear is on day six of treatment. Laboratory data at that time included: WBC = 6.7 X 10^9/L; HGB = 9.2 g/dL; MCV = 110 fL; and PLT = 199 X 10^9/L.

Slide XH-33 is included to show a low power view of the blood smear. Wright-Giemsa, XH-33: 160X; all other slides: 400X).

H-28–33 (AAP), B$_{12}$ deficiency, partially treated

The patient is a 13-year-old male with a history of celiac disease. For the past 12 to 18 months he has not been adhering to his gluten free diet and has experienced increasing symptoms of malabsorption, including diarrhea and weight loss. He is pale and has tachycardia. WBC = 6.7 X 10^9/L; HGB = 9.2 g/dL; HCT = 28.5%; MCV = 110 fL; and PLT = 199 X 10^9/L.

Slide H-33 is included to show a low power view of the blood smear. Wright-Giemsa, H-33: 160X; all other slides: 400X).

1995

HE-06–10, Acute myelocytic leukemia

The patient is a 40-year-old woman who presents with fatigue. Laboratory data include: WBC = 22.0 X 10^9/L; RBC = 3.10 X 10^{12}/L; HGB = 11.3 g/dL; HCT = 33%; MCV = 95 fL. Wright-Giemsa Stain, 400X.

HE-A; HE-11–15, Potpourri

The following ungraded challenge is a collection of bone marrow photomicrographs from five different patients.

HE-11

The patient is a 59-year-old woman with thrombocytopenia. Laboratory data include: WBC = 9.2 X 10^9/L; HGB = 13.3 g/dL; HCT = 39 %; PLT = 115 X 10^9/L. Wright-Giemsa stain, 250X.

HE-12, Niemann-Pick disease

The patient is a 9-year-old girl with bronchitis, enlarging abdomen, and poor general nutrition. Laboratory data include: WBC = 9.2 X 10^9/L; HGB = 10.3 g/dL; HCT = 30 %; PLT = 350 X 10^9/L. Wright-Giemsa stain, 400X.

HE-13, Sea blue histiocyte syndrome

This bone marrow photomicrograph is from a child with hepatosplenomegaly. Wright-Giemsa stain, 250X.

HE-14, Mucopolysaccharidosis

This bone marrow photomicrograph is from a patient with mucopolysaccharidosis type VII (Sly disease). Wright-Giemsa stain, 400X.

HE-15, Anorexia

This bone marrow photomicrograph is from a patient with anemia and poor nutrition. Wright-Giemsa stain, 160X.

XH-06–11, Septic child
PEDIATRIC HISTORY (FOR AAP)
This blood film is from a 2 1/2-month-old child with fever, lethargy, and vomiting. Laboratory data include: WBC = 13.5 X 10^9/L; RBC = 3.27 X 10^{12}/L; HGB = 10.2 g/dL; HCT = 29%; MCV = 89 fL; and PLT = 593 X 10^9/L.

ADULT HISTORY (FOR XL/MLE/AOA/AAFP)
This blood film is from a 42-year-old woman with a history of recurrent pyelonephritis who presents with high fever and rigors. Laboratory data include: WBC = 13.5 X 10^9/L; RBC = 3.27 X 10^{12}/L; HGB = 10.2 g/dL; HCT = 29%; MCV = 89 fL; and PLT = 593 X 10^9/L. Wright-Giemsa stain, 400X.

HE-21–25; XH-17-22, Pertussis
PEDIATRIC HISTORY
This blood film is from a 3-month-old boy with paroxysms of barking cough which often lead to vomiting. Laboratory data include: WBC = 18.1 X 10^9/L; HGB = 12.4 g/dL; and PLT = 595 X 10^9/L. Wright-Giemsa, 400X.

ADULT HISTORY (FOR MLE/AOA/AAFP)
This blood film is from a 30-year-old family physician who has developed a persistent barking cough. Laboratory data include: WBC = 18.1 X 10^9/L; HGB = 12.4 g/dL; and PLT = 595 X 10^9/L. Wright-Giemsa, 400X.

HE-26–30, Potpourri
HE-26
The patient is a 57-year-old woman with a sudden and severe drop in hematocrit. Laboratory data include: WBC = 18.5 X 10^9/L; RBC = 0.15 X 10^{12}/L; HGB = 12.6 g/dL; HCT = 2.1; MCV = 136 fL; MCHC = +++. Blood, Wright-Giemsa, 400X.

HE-28
This blood photomicrograph is from a 56-year-old woman with fatigue and bone pain. CBC results include: WBC = 4.6 X 10^9/L; HGB = 4.3 g/dL; HCT = 12.8%; MCV = 95 fL; and PLT = 37 X 10^9/L. Wright-Giemsa, 375X.

HE-27, 29, 30
Identify the arrowed object(s) in this collection of bone marrow photomicrographs taken from more than one patient. Wright-Giemsa, HE-29: 250X; HE-27, 30: 400X.

HE-36–40; XH-28-33, TTP
ADULT HISTORY
This blood film is from a 48-year-old woman with bloody diarrhea and abdominal pain. Laboratory data include: WBC = 16.3 X 10^9/L; HGB = 9.2 g/dL; and PLT = 55 X 10^9/L. Wright-Giemsa, 400X.

Slide XH-33 is included to show a low power overview of the blood film and has no arrow for identification. As an ungraded educational exercise, answer the following question. The most significant morphologic features of the erythrocytes seen in this peripheral blood film include (choose the one best answer):

a. Fragmented cells (schistocytes, helmet cells), spherocytes
b. Sickle cells, target cells,
c. Oval macrocytes, teardrop cells
d. Howell-Jolly bodies, target cells, acanthocytes, spherocytes
e. Echinocytes (burr cells, crenated cells)
f. Rouleaux

PEDIATRIC HISTORY (FOR XL/AOA/AAP)
This blood film is from a 5-year-old girl with bloody diarrhea and abdominal pain. Laboratory data include: WBC = 16.3 X 10^9/L; HGB = 9.2 g/dL; and PLT = 55 X 10^9/L.

HE-41–45; HE-41, 42
This blood film is from a 45-year-old man with a history of chronic alcohol abuse who now presents with liver failure. The red cell morphology shows a number of "cookie-bite" and "blister" cells. Laboratory data include: WBC = 12.5 X 10^9/L, HGB = 9.2 g/dL, and PLT = 92 X 10^9/L. HE-41: Crystal violet; HE-42: New methylene blue, 325X.

HE-43, 44
These blood films are from two separate patients with a previous history of chronic myelocytic leukemia. Both patients are anemic and thrombocytopenic with a moderate leukocytosis. Wright-Giemsa, 313X.

HE-45
This bone marrow aspirate is from a 52-year-old woman with pancytopenia. Wright-Giemsa, 250X.

1996

HE-06–10; XH-06–11, Beta-thalassemia trait
ADULT HISTORY
The patient is a 25-year-old male evaluated in the emergency room for severe abdominal pain. Laboratory data included: WBC = 7.9 X 10^9/L; RBC = 6.89 X 10^{12}/L; HGB = 13.1 g/dL; HCT = 42%; MCV = 61 fL; and PLT = 287 X 10^9/L. Wright-Giemsa, 400X.

PEDIATRIC HISTORY
The patient is a 3-year-old female who is evaluated by you in the emergency room for an earache. Laboratory data obtained from the emergency room demonstrates: WBC = 11.9 X 10^9/L; RBC = 5.72 X 10^{12}/L; HGB = 10.5 g/dL; HCT = 35%; MCV = 61 fL; RDW = 13.5; and PLT = 287 X 10^9/L. Wright-Giemsa, 400X.

HE-11-12, Sézary leukemia
The patient is a 57-year-old woman with a skin rash and leukocytosis. Laboratory data include: WBC = 62.8 X 10^9/L; RBC = 1.82 X 10^{12}/L; HGB = 6.1 g/dL; MCV = 98.3 fL; RDW = 12.9; PLT = 156 X 10^9/L. Wright-Giemsa, 400X.

HE-13
The patient is a 48-year-old woman with a history of lymphoma. Wright-Giemsa, 400X.

HE-14
The patient is a 70-year-old man with a history of essential thrombocythemia, currently undergoing treatment with hydroxyurea. Bone marrow, Wright-Giemsa, 400X.

HE-15
The patient is a 36-year-old woman who presented with fever, drenching sweats, chills, lethargy, and myalgia. Laboratory findings include evidence of hemolytic anemia, a normal leukocyte count, and abnormal liver function tests. Wright-Giemsa, 400X.

HE-21–25, Microfilaria infection
The patient is a 34-year-old white woman seen in 1994 for a history of fever for two weeks with painless swelling of her forearm. The patient had been a Peace Corps school teacher in Zaire from 1979 to 1982, and an industrial agricultural engineering consultant in Senegal from 1984 to 1990. Laboratory data include: WBC = 8.2 X 10^9/L; RBC = 4.80 X 10^{12}/L; HGB = 13.7 g/dL; MCV = 84 fL; PLT = 331 X 10^9/L. Wright-Giemsa, HE-21: 100/200X; HE-22: 100/400X; HE-23, 24, 25: 400X.

HE-26
The patient is a 47-year-old woman admitted to the hospital for elective surgery. The CBC values were within reference ranges except for an MCV of 101 fL. Wright-Giemsa, 400X.

HE-27
The patient is a 51-year-old female business executive seen for pre-employment laboratory testing. The CBC was normal. Wright-Giemsa, 380X.

HE-28, CLL
The patient is a 68-year-old man with a history of chronic lymphocytic leukemia, with a rapidly rising leukocyte count. Laboratory data include: WBC = 80.0 X 10^9/L; HGB = 9.9 g/dL; MCV = 93 fL; PLT = 74 X 10^9/L. Wright-Giemsa, 380X.

HE-29-30, Promyelocytic leukemia
The patient is a 58-year-old man with two week history of chills, night sweats, generalized malaise, and a 5-pound weight loss. Laboratory data include: WBC = 28.0 X 10^9/L; HGB = 12.5 g/dL; PLT = 59 X 10^9/L. HE-29: Blood; HE-30: Bone marrow, Wright-Giemsa, 400X.

HE-41, Polycythemia rubra vera
The patient is a 64-year-old woman with a history of polycythemia rubra vera. The recent CBC and bone marrow examination showed evolution to acute myeloid leukemia. Bone marrow, Wright Giemsa, 400X.

HE-42-43, Folate deficiency
The patient is a 59-year-old man with a history of alcoholism and poor nutrition. Laboratory data include: HGB = 9.0 g/dL; MCV = 112 fL. The blood film is stained with Prussian Blue, while the bone marrow is stained with Wright-Giemsa. HE-42: Prussian blue, 400X; HE-43: Wright-Giemsa, 400X.

HE-44, 45A, 45B, Sideroblastic anemia
The patient is a 61-year-old man with anemia; folate and vitamin B_{12} levels are within reference ranges. Photomicrograph HE-44 is a split screen peripheral blood photomicrograph. One side is stained with Wright-Giemsa, the other with Prussian blue. HE-44: Prussian blue/Wright-Giemsa, 380X.

Photomicrograph H-45 (A, B) is a low power bone marrow smear with two identifications. (A) is the large, wide arrow and (B) is the small, thin arrow. HE-45 A, B: Wright-Giemsa, 210X.

HE-46
The patient is a 41-year-old woman with a unexplained anemia. Bone marrow, Wright-Giemsa, 380X.

XH-17–21, Iron deficiency
The patient is a 13-month-old white female who presents for a 1-year check-up. On examination, the infant is pale and has a modest tachycardia. The mother notes that the child's diet consists of 36-40 oz. of whole cow milk and 4-5 small portions of mashed fruits and vegetables per day. A complete blood count reveals: WBC = 13.6×10^9/L; HGB = 7.0 g/dL; HCT = 22%; MCV = 58 fL; and PLT = 506×10^9/L. Blood, Wright-Giemsa, 330X.

XH-22, Septic child
The patient is a 5-month-old white male who presents to his physician's office with a temperature of 101°F and a respiratory rate of 55/minute. Physical examination reveals only mild intercostal refractions and wheezing with rhonchi bilaterally. The child has had a cough and congestion for two to three days prior to the visit. A complete blood count reveals: HGB = 10.2 g/dL; HCT = 29%; MCV = 89 fL; WBC = 13.5×10^9/L; and PLT = 593×10^9/L. Blood, Wright-Giemsa, 400X.

HE-36–40, XH-28–33, Lead poisoning
ADULT HISTORY
These blood photomicrographs are from a 38-year-old Filipino woman with recurrent abdominal pain, muscle weakness, and left leg and arm paresthesia. CBC data: WBC = 6.8×10^9/L; RBC = 2.74×10^{12}/L; HGB = 7.8 g/dL; HCT = 23%; MCV = 85 fL; and PLT = 395×10^9/L. Wright-Giemsa, 400X.

PEDIATRIC HISTORY
The patient is a 24-month-old male who is evaluated for irritability and lethargy. He lives in old, poorly maintained housing in the central city. Physical examination reveals a pale irritable male with no specific findings. A complete blood count reveals: WBC = 6.8×10^9/L; RBC = 2.74×10^{12}/L; HGB = 7.8 g/dL; HCT = 23%; MCV = 75 fL; and PLT = 395×10^9/L. Wright-Giemsa, 400X.

HE-50
This bone marrow photomicrograph is from a 36-year-old female with persistent anemia of unknown etiology. Wright-Giemsa, 400X.

HE-51
The patient is a 46-year-old female previously splenectomized because of suspected idiopathic thrombocytopenic purpura. Laboratory data include: WBC = 6.5×10^9/L; RBC = 4.69×10^{12}/L; HGB = 14.5 g/dL; HCT = 43%; MCV = 91 fL; RDW = 12.1; and PLT = 54×10^9. Blood, Wright-Giemsa, 400X.

1997

HE-6-10; XH-6-10, Hereditary ovalocytosis
ADULT HISTORY (HE, XL)
The patient is a female admitted to the hospital for coronary artery bypass surgery. A slide was reviewed because of an instrument flag for the platelet count. The CBC included: WBC = 11.7×10^9/L, RBC = 4.05×10^{12}/L, HGB = 12.4 g/dL, HCT = 35.7%, MCV = 88 fL, MCH = 30.7 pg, MCHC = 34.8%, and PLT = 323×10^9/L. Blood, Wright-Giemsa, 400X.

PEDIATRIC HISTORY (AAP)
The patient is an 8-year-old female evaluated prior to elective surgery. CBC data shows: HGB = 12.4 g/dL, HCT = 35.7%, MCV = 88 fL, WBC = 11.7×10^9/L (11,700/(L), PLT = 323×10^9/L (323,000/(L). Wright-Giemsa, 400X.

XH-11, Necrotizing enterocolitis
The patient present to the emergency room with fever, chills, and generalized aching. The CBC shows: WBC = 32.4×10^9/L (32,400/L), HGB = 13.1 g/dL, and PLT = 43×10^9/L (43,000/L).

HE-11-15, Hairy cell leukemia
The patient is a 61-year-old male with splenomegaly. Laboratory data include: WBC = 3.2×10^9/L, HGB = 12.5 g/dL, and PLT = 62×10^9/L. Slide HE-15 is stained with acid phosphatase in the presence of tartrate inhibitor. HE-11–HE-14 Wright-Giemsa; HE-15 Acid phosphatase with tartrate.

HE-21-25; XH-17-22, Hb S trait
ADULT HISTORY
The patient is a 28-year-old female who is in the fourth month of pregnancy. The laboratory reports a positive sickle hemoglobin solubility test. Hemoglobin electrophoresis shows approximately 60% hemoglobin A and approximately 40% hemoglobin S. Other laboratory data include: WBC = 7.8×10^9/L, RBC = 4.21×10^{12}/L, HGB = 12.6 g/dL. HCT = 37.9%, MCV = 90 fL, RDW = 14.0, PLT = 242×10^9/L. Blood, Wright-Giemsa, 400X.

PEDIATRIC HISTORY (AAP)
The patient is a 6-year-old female who has a positive sickle cell screen. A hemoglobin electrophoresis demonstrates: HGB A = 60% and HGB S = 40%. Her CBC shows: HGB = 12.6 g/dL. HCT = 37.9%, MCV = 90 fL, WBC = 7.8×10^9/L (7,800/L), PLT = 242×10^9/L (242,000/L).

HE-26, Cold agglutinins
The patient is a 57-year-old female with severe anemia. Laboratory data include: WBC = 20.4×10^9/L, RBC = 0.25×10^{12}/L, HGB = 13.1 g/dL, HCT = 2.5%, MCV = 140 fL, MCHC = +++. Blood, Wright-Giemsa, 160X.

HE-27-30, Potpourri
These photomicrographs are a collection of bone marrows taken from different patients. HE-27 and HE-29, Wright-Giemsa, 400X; HE-28, Wright-Giemsa, 250X; HE-30, Wright-Giemsa/PAS, 250X.

HE-36-40, Splenectomy
The patient is a 10-year-old female with abdominal pain and fever. Laboratory data include: WBC = 5.4×10^9/L, HGB = 12.4 g/dL, PLT = 284×10^9/L. Blood, Wright-Giemsa, 375X.

XH-28-32, Splenectomy
The patient is a 10-year-old female who had a splenectomy for trauma at age 8 years. She is evaluated for abdominal pain and fever. The CBC shows: HGB = 12.4 g/dL, HCT = 37%, WBC = 5.4×10^9/L (5,400/L), PLT - 284×10^9/L (284,000/L). Make the most specific identity possible, e.g., if a neutrophil containing ingested bacteria is arrowed, the expected answer would be neutrophil with ingested bacteria, not simply bacteria. Wright-Giemsa, 375X.

XH-33, Burkitt-type lymphoma
The patient presents with bruising and fatigue. The CBC shows: HGB = 10.5 g/dL, HCT = 31%, MVC = 80 fL, WBC = 27.3 X 10^9/L (27,300/L), PLT - 107 X 10^9/L (107,000/L). Wright-Giemsa, 400X.

HE-41-43, Sézary leukemia
The patient is a 61-year-old male with chronic skin rash manifested as a pruritic generalized exfoliative erythroderma. Laboratory data include: WBC = 50 X 10^9/L, HGB = 9.9 g/dL, MCV = 88 fL, RDW = 12.0, PLT = 149 X 10^9/L. Blood, Wright-Giemsa, 400X.

HE-44-45, Leukemic phase of small cleaved lymphoma
These blood smear photomicrographs are from a 26-year-old female with lymphadenopathy. Laboratory data include: WBC = 14.1 X 10^9/L, RBC = 4.36 X 10^9/L, HGB = 13.5 g/dL, HCT = 39%, MCV = 89 fL, RDW = 13.0, PLT = 204 X 10 9/L. Wright-Giemsa, 400X.

Index

Acanthocytes, 64-65, 76, 79, 108
    formation of, 66-67
Acquired neutrophil abnormalities, 44-45
Acute erythroid leukemia, 154
Acute erythroleukemia, 154
Acute lymphoblastic leukemia, 216, 226, 230
Acute nonlymphocytic leukemia, 8-9
African Trypanosomiasis, 280, 282-83
Alder's anomaly, 41, 58, 306-7
Alpha chain inclusion bodies, 121, 133
Alder's anomaly inclusions, 302-3
Alpha granules, 198
Alpha storage pool disease, 205
Alpha thalassemia, 130, 133
Alpha thalassemia major, 106
Alpha thalassemia minor, 88
American trypanosomiasis, 280
Anemias
    congenital Heinz body, 126, 132, 133
    Cooley's, 132
    Coomb's positive hemolytic, 100
    fragmentation, 82
    Heinz body, 70
        diagnostic morphology in, 84-85
    hemolytic, 80
        bite cells in, 68-69
    iron deficiency, 88
    megaloblastic, 86, 138, 166
    microangiopathic, 82-83
        diagnostic morphology in, 84-85
    microangiopathic hemolytic, bite cells in, 70
    microcytic, 88
    refractory, 56-57
    sickle cell, 78, 96-97, 98-99, 108
    sideroblastic, 180, 184
    spur cell, 66
Antigen markers in blastic cells, 300-301
Anucleate biconcave disc, 153
Apoptosis, 290-1
Artifacts, 285-95
Aspergillus, 262
Auer bodies, 12-13, 14-15, 306-7
Autoagglutination, 146
Autophagosome production, 144

B cell chronic lymphocytic leukemia, 232
B cell neoplasms, 232-35
B cells, 211
B-precursor lymphoblasts, 300, 301
Babesia microti, 254-55
Babesiosis, 254-55
    versus malaria, 256-57
Bacteremia, 258
Bacteria (cocci or rod), extracellular, 258-59
Bacteria (spirochete), 260-61
Bacteria, leukocytes with phagocytized, 266-67
Band neutrophil, giant, 50-51
Band, neutrophilic, 22-23
Band vs. segmented morphology, 26-27
Bart's hemoglobin, 131
Basket cells, 286-87
Basophilic megakaryocyte, 188-89
Basophilic megaloblasts, 168
Basophilic normoblasts, 158-61
Basophilic stippling, 120, 122
    coarse, 116-17, 118, 119, 121, 137
    fine, 116, 119
    formation of, 118-19
Basophils, 28-29
    versus mast cells, 330-31
Behçet's disease, 206
Beta thalassemia, 132
Bite cells, 68-69, 124, 126
    formation and morphology, 71-73, 84-85
    types of, 71
Blast cells, 298-99
    antigen markers in, 300-301
Blister cells, 74
    pre-keratocyte, 72-73
    variants, 96
Bone marrow cells, cytoplasmic inclusions in, 320-21
Bone marrow microenvironment, 314-15
Borrelia burgdorferi, 260
Borrelia recurrentis, 260
Brugia malayi, 277

Candida, 262
Candida albicans, 266
Cells, death of, 286-87, 290-91
Ceroid, 324
CFU-MK stem cell, 188
Chagas' disease, 280
Charcot-Leyden crystals, 32
Charcot-Leyden protein, 32
Chédiak-Higashi anomaly, 14
Chédiak-Higashi anomaly inclusion, 304-5
Chédiak-Higashi syndrome, 14, 304
Chronic lymphocytic leukemia, 221, 226, 230, 246, 248-49, 286
Chronic myelogenous leukemia, 216
Chronic myelomonocytic leukemia, 56-57
Coccidiodes, 262
Codocytes. *See* Target cells
Cold agglutinins, 146, 151
Congenital Heinz body anemias, 126, 132, 133
Cooley's anemia, 132
Coombs' positive hemolytic anemia, 100
Cryptococcus, 262
Cytokine induced activation of granulocyte production, 44
Cytoplasmic inclusions
    in bone marrow cells, 320-21
    in neutrophils, 306-7

Degenerated neutrophils, 289
Delta granules, 198
Deoxyhemoglobin 5 molecules, 96
Diagnostic morphology in MAHA and Heinz body anemia, 84-85
DiGuglielmo's syndrome, 154, 174
Döhle bodies, 44
    and acquired neutrophil abnormalities, 44-45
    in May-Hegglin anomaly, 46-47
    with/without toxic granulation, 42-43
Downey cells, 220-23
Dumbbell distribution, 90
Dutcher bodies, 244
Dyserythropoiesis, 86, 172
Dysplasia, 57, 192
    differences between neoplasia and, 56
Dysplastic megakaryocytes, 187, 194-95

Dysplastic neutrophils, 54-55
Dysplastic nucleated red cells, 170-73
Dyspoiesis, 192

Echinocytes, 76-77, 79
   formation of, 76
Elephantiasis, 277
Elliptocytes, 86, 90-91
Elliptocytosis, hereditary, 92-93
Endocytosis, 314
Endomitosis, 188
Endoreduplication, 188, 190
Endosomes, 176
Endothelial cells, 308-9
Envelope forms, 101
Eosinophila-myalgia syndrome, 32
Eosinophilia, 32-33
Eosinophils, 30-31
Epithelial cells, 310-11
Erythrocytes, 70
   normocytic/normochromic, 62-63
   phagocytosis of, 319
   with overlapping platelet, 292-93
Erythrocytic cells and inclusions, 60-151
Erythroid maturation, megaloblastic versus megaloblastoid, 174-75
Erythrophagocytosis, 318-19
Extracellular fungi, 262-63

FAB classification
   non-lymphocytic leukemia, 9
   lymphocytic, 216-17
FAB M6, 154, 174
Faggot cells, 12, 14-15
Ferritin, 176, 178
Fibrin degradation products, 82
Flame cells, 245
Foamy macrophages, 326-27
Follicular center cell lymphomas, 234
Fragmentation anemias, 82
Fragmented cells, 80-81
Fungi
   extracellular, 262-63
   leukocytes with phagocytized, 266-67

G-6PD deficiency, 126, 132
Gaucher cells, 322-23
Gaucher's disease, 320-22, 326
Ghon complex, 270
Giant band neutrophil, 50-51
Giant metamyelocyte, 18-19
Giant platelets, 198
Globin chain synthesis, 182
Granular megakaryocytes, 188
Granulocytes, 5
Granulocytic (myeloid) cells, 4-59
Granulomas, 262
Grape cells, 244
Gray platelet syndrome, 205

Hairy cell leukemia, 212, 214-15, 235
Hairy cells, 212-13
H bodies, 121, 133 (see also Hemoglobin H)
Heinz bodies, 68, 70, 112, 121, 123, 124-25, 133
   formation of, 126-27

Heinz body anemia, 70
   diagnostic morphology in, 84-85
Helmet cells, 68, 79-81, 84-85
Helper T cells, 211
Hematopoietic cells, dysplastic features of, 57
Heme iron, 182
Hemoglobin C, 108, 109
Hemoglobin C crystals, 128-29
Hemoglobin formation, 182-83
Hemoglobin H, 88, 123, 130-31, 132
Hemoglobin H inclusions, supravital stain, 130-31
Hemoglobinopathy, 98
Hemoglobin S, 98
Hemolysis, immune, 103, 104
Hemolytic anemia, 80
   bite cells in, 68-69
Hemosiderin, 178
Hereditary elliptocytosis, 90, 92-93
Hereditary ovalocytosis. See Hereditary elliptocytosis
Hereditary spherocytosis, 90, 100
   and red cell membrane loss, 102-3
Hereditary stomatocytosis, 104-5
Histiocytes, 316
Histiocytes, sea blue, 320-21, 324-25
Histoplasma, 268
Histoplasma capsulatum, 262, 266
Hodgkin's disease, 32
Howell-Jolly bodies, 112, 120-21, 123
   formation of, 138-39
   iron stain, 136-37
   Wright-Giemsa stain, 134-35
Horn cell. See Keratocytes
Hyaline bodies, 204
Hypersegmentation, 52-53
Hypersegmented neutrophil, 52-53
Hypochromic microcytes, 88
Hypogranular platelets, 204-5

IgA, 211
IgD, 211
IgE, 211
IgG, 211
IgM, 211
Immature monocytes, 34-35
Immune hemolysis, 102-3
Immunoblastic lymphomas, 229
Immunoblasts, 240
Immunocytoma, 233
Immunoglobulins, 211
Infectious mononucleosis, 286
Iron deficiency, 88
Iron deficiency anemia, 88
Iron utilization, 182-83

Jaundice, obstructive, 108

Karyorrhexis, 165, 289-91
Keratocytes, 72-73, 74, 79-85

Large cell lymphomas, 229
Large granular lymphocyte leukemia, 215, 237
Lead poisoning, 118
Lecithin-cholesterol acyl transferase (LCAT) deficiency, 108, 325
Left-shift phenomenon, 18

Leishmania donovani, 269
Leishmaniasis, 268-69
    mucocutaneous, 268
    visceral, 269
Leukemia
    acute erythroid, 154
    acute lymphoblastic, 216, 226, 230
    acute nonlymphocytic, 8-9
    B cell chronic lymphocytic, 232
    chronic lymphocytic, 226, 230, 246, 248, 286
    chronic myelogenous, 216
    chronic myelomonocytic, 56-57
    hairy cell, 212, 214-15, 235
    large granular lymphocyte, 237
    precursor B lymphoblastic, 232
    prolymphocytic, 232-33, 236, 246, 248
    T cell chronic lymphocytic, 236
Leukocytes
    with phagocytized bacteria, 264-65
    with phagocytized fungi, 266-67
Lipocytes, 312-13
Liver disease, 108
Loa Loa, 277-79
Lymphoblasts, 216-17, 226
Lymphocytes
    comparison of, resembling hairy cells, 215
    mature, 218-19
    normal maturation and malignant transformation, 230-31
    normal versus reactive, 220-21
    reactive, 222-25
        versus neoplastic, 226-27
Lymphocytic and plasmacytic cells, 211-51
Lymphocytosis, 214
Lymphoglandular bodies, 204
Lymphoid cells, 211
Lymphoma cells, 226-29
Lymphomas
    follicular center cell, 234, 249
    mantle cell, 233
    small lymphocytic, 232-33
    splenic marginal zone, with or without villous lymphocytes, 234
Lymphoplasmacytoid lymphoma, 233
Lymphoproliferative disorders, 150
Lysozomes, 198

Macrocytes, oval or round, 87-88
Macrophages, 316-17
    foamy, 326-27
    phagocytic, 320
    with histoplasma, leishmania, or toxoplasma, 268-69
    with phagocytized mycobacteria, 270-71
    with phagocytized red cells, 318-19
Malaria
    extracellular, 272-73
    intracellular, 272-73
    species differences among parasites, 274-75
    versus babesiosis, 256-57
Mansonelia group, 277
Mantle cell lymphoma, 233
Marty Feldman cells, 194
Mast cells, 321, 328-29
    versus basophils, 330-31
May-Hegglin anomaly, 42, 46-47, 58

Megakaryoblasts, mononuclear, 188
Megakaryocyte nucleus, 192, 196-97
Megakaryocytes, 187, 188-89, 192-193, 200
    basophilic, 188-89
    dwarf, 192
    dysplastic, 187, 194-95
    granular, 189
    maturation of, 190-91
    polyploid, 187
    pyknotic, 197
Megakaryocytic cells and thrombocytes, 187-209
Megakaryopoiesis, 190-91
Megaloblastic anemias, 86, 138, 166
Megaloblastic erythroid maturation, 174-75
Megaloblastic morphology, 168-69
Megaloblastic myelopoiesis, 44
Megaloblastic nucleated red cells, 166-67
Megaloblastic pronormoblasts, 168
Megaloblastoid erythroid maturation, 174-75
Metamyelocyte
    giant, 18-19
    neutrophilic, 20-21
Metastatic tumor cells, 332-33
Microangiopathic anemias, 82-83
    diagnostic morphology in, 84-85
Microangiopathic hemolytic anemia, bite cells in, 70
Microangiopathic hemolytic states, 103
Microcytes
    hypochromic, 88
    with central pallor, 88-89
Microcytic anemia, 88
Microfilaria, 276-77
Microfilariae, species differences among, 278-79
Micromegakaryocytes, 192, 195, 197
Microorganisms, 253-83
Microspherocyte, 83
Mitotic cells, 334
Mitotic figure, 334-35
Monocytes, 36-37
    immature, 34-35
    life cycle of, 38-39
Mononuclear megakaryoblast, 188
Morula cells, 244
Morphologic keys to identifying early normoblasts, 158-59
Mott cells, 244
Mucocutaneous leishmaniasis, 268
Mucopolysaccharidoses, 302
Multiple myeloma, 235, 242-43
Mycobacteria, macrophages with phagocytized, 270-71
Mycobacterium avium-intracellulare, 270-71
Mycobacterium tuberculosis, 270-71
Mycosis fungoides sézary syndrome, 237
Myeloblasts, 6-7, 300, 301
    and acute nonlymphocytic leukemia, 8-9
    with auer rod(s), 12-13
Myelocytes, neutrophilic, 16-17
    post-mitotic myeloid precursors, 16-17
Myelodysplasia, 194
Myelodysplastic syndromes, 56-57
    frequency of acute leukemia transformation in, 57
Myeloma
    multiple, 235, 242-43
    plasma cell, 235
Myelopoiesis, megaloblastic, 44

Natural Killer (NK) lymphocytes, 211
Necrobiosis, 288-89
Necrobiotic neutrophils, 289
Necrosis, 290
Neoplasia, differences between dysplasia, 56
Neoplasms, B cell, 232-35
Neoplastic lymphocytes, 226-27
Neutrophilic metamyelocyte, 20-21
Neutrophil necrobiosis, 288-89
Neutrophilic band, 22-23
Neutrophilic myelocytes, 16-17
    post-mitotic myeloid precursors, 16-17
Neutrophils
    acquired abnormalities in, 44-45
    cytoplasmic inclusions in, 306-7
    hypersegmented, 52-53
    segmented, 24-25, 26-27
    toxic granulation, 40
    with dysplastic nucleus/agranular cytoplasm, 54-55
Niemann-Pick cells, 321, 326-27
Niemann-Pick disease, 320, 325, 326
Non-heme iron, 182
Non-Hodgkin's disease, 32
Non-specific poikilocytes, 80
Non-stem cell disorders, 202
Normoblasts
    basophilic, 158, 160-61
    morphologic keys to identifying early, 158-59
    orthochromic, 158, 164-65
    polychromatophilic, 158, 162-63
Normochromic erythrocytes, 62-63
Normocytic erythrocytes, 62-63
Nuclear pyknosis, 290
Nuclear shape in myeloid precursors, 18-19
Nucleated red cells, 153-85
    dysplastic, 172-73
    megaloblastic, 166-67
    normal or abnormal (peripheral blood), 170-71
Null cells, 211

Obstructive jaundice, 108
Onchocerca volvulus, 277
Orthochromic normoblasts, 158, 164-65
Osteoblasts, 336-37
    versus plasma cells, 338-39
Osteoclasts, 340-41
Oval macrocytes, 86
Ovalocytes, 86, 90-91
Ovalocytosis, hereditary, 90

Pappenheimer bodies, 120-22, 137-38, 176
    formation of, 144-45
    iron stain, 142-43
    Wright-Giemsa stain, 140-41
Paroxysmal cold hemoglobinuria, 150
PAS stain, 173
Pelger Huët cells, 54
Pelger-Huët anomaly, 58-59
Peripheral B cell neoplasms, 232-35
Peripheral T cell and NK cell neoplasms, 236-37
Phagocytic macrophages, 320
Phagocytosis of erythrocytes, 319
Phenylhydrazine, 126
Plasma cell myeloma, 235
Plasma cells, 211, 321
    immature, 240-241
    immature or abnormal, 242-43
    mature, 238-39, 240-41
    versus osteoblasts, 338-39
    with cytoplasmic inclusions, 244-45
Plasmablasts, 240, 241
Plasmacytoid reactive lymphocytes, 223
Plasmacytoma, 235
Plasmodium falciparum, 272
    comparison with Plasmodium vivax, 274-75
Plasmodium malariae, 272
Plasmodium ovale, 272
Plasmodium vivax, 272
    comparison with *Plasmodium falciparum*, 274-75
Platelet dumping, 208
Platelet granules, 198
Platelet rosettes, 206-7
Platelet satellitism, 206-7, 208-9
Platelet satellitosis, 206
Platelets
    erythrocyte with overlapping, 292-93
    formation of, 200-201
    giant, 202-3
    hypogranular, 204-5
    normal, 198-99
Pleuripotential hematopoietic stem cells, 5
Poikilocytes, 80
Polychromatophilic megaloblasts, 168
Polychromatophilic normoblasts, 158-59, 162-63
Polychromatophilic red cells, 94-95
Polyploid megakaryocytes, 187
Post-mitotic myeloid precursors, 18-19
Pre-keratocytes, 72-75, 96
Precipitated hemoglobin, 132-33
    disorders associated with, 132-33
Precursor B cell neoplasms, 232
Precursor B lymphoblastic leukemia, 232
Precursor T cell neoplasm, 236
Precursor T lymphoblastic lymphoma/leukemia, 236
Prekeratocyte, 72-73, 82-85
Proerythroblast, 153
Prolymphocytes, 226-27, 246-47, 248-49
Prolymphocytic leukemia, 215, 232-33, 236, 246, 248
Prolymphocytoid transformation, 248
Promegakaryocyte, 188-89
Promyelocytes, 10-11
    with auer rod(s), 12-13
Pronormoblasts, 154-55, 158-59
Proplasmacytes, 240, 241
Proplatelets, 200
Protozoan (non-malarial), 280-81
Pseudo-Gaucher cells, 322-23
Pseudo-vacuole, 72-3
Pseudothrombocytes, 202, 204
Pseudothrombocytopenia, 208
Pyknosis, 288, 290-91
Pyknotic megakaryocytes, 197
Pyropoikilocytosis, 92-3

5q- syndrome, 192

Reactive lymphocytes, 220-21, 222-25, 226-27
Red blood cells
    agglutinates, 146-47
    agglutination, 150-51

inclusions, 120-23
    iron staining of, 137
iron uptake, storage, and utilization in, 177
macrophages with phagocytized, 318-19
maturation and cell division, 156-57
membrane loss and spherocytosis, 102-3
polychromatophilic, 94-95
spiculated, 78-79
sticky, 150-51
vacuolated non-nucleated, 74-75
Refractory anemia, 56-57
Relapsing fever, 260-61
Reticulin fibrosis, 214
Reticulocytes, 122, 165
    supravital stain, 114-15
Reticuloendothelial cells, 316
Reticulum cells, 316
Ringed sideroblasts
    formation of, 184-85
    iron stain, 180-81
River blindness, 277
RNA degradation, 118
Rouleaux formation, 148-49, 150-51
Round macrocytes, 86
Russell bodies, 244

Satellitosis, 208
Schistocytes, 79-81, 84-85
Sea blue histiocyte syndrome, 324-25
Sea blue histiocytes, 320, 324-25
Segmented neutrophil, 24-25, 26-27
Septicemia, 40
Severe liver disease, 66
Sézary cells, 250-51
Sézary syndrome, 237, 250
Sickle cell anemia, 78, 96-97, 98-99, 108
Sickle cells, 79, 96-97
    formation of, 99
Sideroblastic anemias, 180, 184
Sideroblasts, 178-79, 182
    iron stain, 137, 176-77
    ringed
        formation of, 184-85
        iron stain, 137, 180-81
Siderocytes, 137, 142, 178-79
Siderosomes, 176-78, 182
Sleeping sickness, 280
Small lymphocytic lymphoma, 232-33
Smudge cells, 286-87
Spherocytes, 70, 76, 100-101
Spherocytosis, hereditary, 90, 92, 100
    and red cell membrane loss, 102-3
Spheroechinocyte, 76

Sphingomyelin, 66
Spiculated red cells, 78-79
Splenectomy, 104
Splenic marginal zone lymphoma with or without villous lymphocytes, 215, 234
Splenomegaly, 214
Spur cell anemia, 66
Stain precipitate, 259, 294-95
Sticky red blood cells, 150-51
Stomatocytes, 104-5
Stomatocytosis, hereditary, 92, 104-5
Stromal cells, 314
Substantia reticulofilamentosa, 114, 130
Sultan bodies, 15
Suppressor T cells, 211

T cell and putative NK cell neoplasms, 236-37
T cell chronic lymphocytic leukemia, 236
T cell lymphomas, 229
T cells, 211
T-lineage lymphoblast, 300, 301
Target cells, 106-7
    formation of, 108-9
    types of, 109
Teardrop cells, 79, 110-11, 126
    formation of, 112-13
Thalassemias, 88, 185
Thermal injury, 102-4
Thrombopoietin, 200
Toxic granulation, 44-45, 302, 306-07
    and/or multiple toxic vacuoles, 40-41
    Döhle body with/without, 42-43
Toxic vacuolization, 40, 44-45, 265
Toxoplasma gondii, 269
Transferrin-iron complex, 182
Triangulocytes, 80, 85
Trypanosoma brucei gambiense, 280, 282-83
Trypanosoma brucei rhodesiense, 280, 282-83
Trypanosoma cruzi, 280
Trypanosomes, 280

Unstable hemoglobin disease, 132, 133
Uroporphyrinogen, 182

Vacuoles
    in neutrophils, 306-7
    in red cells, 72-75
Vacuolated non-nucleated red blood cells, 74-75
Visceral leishmaniasis, 269

Waldenström's macroglobulinemia, 148
Washington monument appearance, 128
Wuchereria bancrofti, 277